# PSYCHIATRIC CARE PLANS
## Guidelines for
## Planning and
## Documenting Client Care

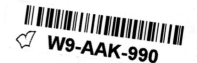

# PSYCHIATRIC CARE PLANS
## Guidelines for Planning and Documenting Client Care
### Edition 2

**Marilynn E. Doenges, MA, RN, CS**
Clinical Specialist
Adult Psychiatric/Mental Health Nursing
Private Practice
Instructor
Beth-El College of Nursing
Colorado Springs, Colorado

**Mary C. Townsend, RN, MN**
Advanced Registered Nurse Practitioner
Clinical Nurse Specialist
Psychiatric/Mental Health Nursing
Private Practice
Affiliated Psychiatric Services
Wichita, Kansas

**Mary Frances Moorhouse, RN, CCP, CCRN, CRRN**
Nurse Consultant
TNT-RN Enterprises
Colorado Springs, Colorado

 **F. A. DAVIS COMPANY** • **Philadelphia**

F. A. Davis Company
1915 Arch Street
Philadelphia, PA 19103

Printed in the United States of America

Last digit indicates print number: 10 9 8 7 6 5 4 3 2 1

*Publisher, Nursing:* Robert Martone
*Nursing Acquisitions Editor:* Joanne Patzek DaCunha
*Production Editor:* Crystal S. McNichol
*Cover Designer:* Steven R. Morrone

As new scientific information becomes available through basic and clinical research, recommended treatments and drug therapies undergo changes. The authors and publisher have done everything possible to make this book accurate, up to date, and in accord with accepted standards at the time of publication. The authors, editors, and publisher are not responsible for errors or omissions or for consequences from application of the book, and make no warranty, expressed or implied, in regard to the contents of the book. Any practice described in this book should be applied by the reader in accordance with professional standards of care used in regard to the unique circumstances that may apply in each situation. The reader is advised always to check product information (package inserts) for changes and new information regarding dose and contraindications before administering any drug. Caution is especially urged when using new or infrequently ordered drugs.

**Library of Congress Cataloging-in-Publication Data**

Doenges, Marilynn E., 1922–
    Psychiatric care plans : guidelines for planning and documenting client care / Marilynn E. Doenges, Mary C. Townsend, Mary Frances Moorhouse. —Ed. 2.
        p.  cm
    Includes bibliographical references and index.
    ISBN 0-8036-2673-8 (pbk. : alk. paper)
        1. Psychiatric nursing—Handbooks, manuals, etc.    2. Nursing care plans—Handbooks, manuals, etc.    I. Townsend, Mary C., 1941–    II.  Moorhouse, Mary Frances, 1947–  .
III. Title.
    [DNLM: 1. Nursing Assessment—handbooks.  2. Patient Care
Planning—handbooks.    3. Psychiatric Nursing—handbooks.    WY 39
D651pa 1995]
RC440.D64  1995
610.73'68—dc20
DNLM/DLC                                                                                94-30887
for Library of Congress                                        CIP

We dedicate this book to ourselves—our own intestinal fortitude, our unfailing optimism, our dogged perseverance, and our own increasing conviction in the value of Nursing Diagnosis and the future of the profession of nursing.

Special thanks to our husbands Dean, Jan, and Jim; our families who have continued to support our dreams, fantasies, and obsessions:

Nancy, Jim, Jennifer, and Jonathan Daigle; David, Monita, Matthew and Tyler Doenges; Jim Doenges, Barbara Doenges, and Bob Lanza; John, Holly, Nicole, and Kelsey Doenges; Paul Moorhouse; Jason, Ellaina, and Alexa Moorhouse; Kerry and Tina Townsend;

Alice Geissler, for being available when we need help; the staff at Memorial Hospital library, for cheerfully filling in all the blanks and patiently helping us find those elusive references; and

our colleagues, who continue to provide a sounding board and feedback for our professional beliefs and expectations.

Kudos to the F.A. Davis staff, Robert Martone and Ruth DeGeorge, who have shown great patience and helped maintain our sanity (or contributed to our insanity); and Joanne DaCunha, Crystal McNichol, and Herb Powell, who facilitated the revision process to get this project completed in a timely fashion.

Lastly, to the nurses who have patiently awaited this revision, we hope it will help in applying theory to practice and enhance the delivery and effectiveness of your care.

# CONTRIBUTORS FOR THE FIRST EDITION

**ALICE Y. ANDERSON, CAPTAIN (P), AN, BSN, MSN**
Head Nurse, Inpatient Psychiatry
Tripler Army Medical Center, Hawaii

**IDA MARLENE BEAM, BSN**
Retired, Army Nurse Corps
Private Home Respite Care
Colorado Springs, Colorado

**PAULETTE BOTKIN, RN**
Institute of Forensic Psychiatry
Colorado State Hospital
Pueblo, Colorado

**MARTI DAVIS BUFFUM, RN, MS**
Nursing Faculty/Lecturer, San Francisco State
    University
Staff Nurse III, Inpatient Psychiatry, Marin General
    Hospital
Greenbrae, California
Private Practice, Clinical Specialist
San Anselmo, California

**WM G. CANTIN, Lt, NC, USN**
Consultant/Liaison Nurse
Alcohol Rehabilitation Facility
Tripler Army Medical Center, Hawaii

**VERNA CARSON, RN, MS, DOCTORAL CANDIDATE**
Assistant Professor in Psychiatric/Community Health
    Nursing
University of Maryland School of Nursing
Baltimore, Maryland

**KATHLEEN K. DUNCANSON, BSN, CRRN, CRC**
Senior Rehabilitation Specialist
Intracorp
Woodland Park, Colorado

**ROSEMARIE GEISER, RN, MSN, CS**
Clinical Nurse Specialist, Adult Psychiatry
Palo Alto Veterans Administration Medical Center
Menlo Park Division
Palo Alto, California

**MARYANNIE LEWIS HUGHES, MSN, BSN, RN, CS**
Captain, US Army Nurse Corps
Clinical Head Nurse
Clinical Specialist at Tri-Services Alcoholism Recovery
    Facility (TRI-SARF)
Tripler Army Medical Center, Hawaii
Nurse Recruiter-Counselor
Ft. Sheridan, Illinois

**NOLA LANGE, BSN, MA**
Contract Practitioner
Colorado Springs, Colorado

**NAOMI K. LEDERACH, RN, BSN, MN**
Director of Education
Philhaven Hospital
Mount Gretna, Pennsylvania

**MARGARET D. McCOMB, RN, MN, CS**
Clinical Specialist for Nursing Process
Nursing Quality Assurance Coordinator
Veterans Administration Medical Center
Portland, Oregon

**JILL G. MEIDER, MS, RN, CS**
Clinical Specialist Child/Adolescent Psychiatric Nurse
N.E.E.D. Foundation Day Treatment Program and
    Mental Health Clinic
Colorado Springs, Colorado

**JOANNE BARNES MULLANEY, RN, PhD**
Associate Professor
Salve Regina College
Newport, Rhode Island

**EARLENE PETERSON, RNC, BSN**
Ob/Gyn Nurse Practitioner
Academy Women's Clinic
Colorado Springs, Colorado

**LEANN G. RYNIER, RN, BSN Ed, MEd**
Patient Care Education Specialist
Philhaven Hospital
Mount Gretna, Pennsylvania

# CONTRIBUTORS FOR THE SECOND EDITION

**CHRISTIE A. HINDS, RN, NP**
Director
HIV Patient Care,
FHL Health Care, Inc.
Colorado Springs, Colorado

**NOLA LANGE, RN, MA, CS**
Psychiatric Nurse Liaison
Penrose-St. Francis Healthcare System
Colorado Springs, Colorado

**LESLIE MURTAGH, RN, MS, CS**
Clinical Liaison, First Choice/Private Practice
Colorado Springs, Colorado

**BARBARA THOMAS, RN, BSN, C**
CEO, Cheyenne Mesa Residential Treatment Center
Colorado Springs, Colorado

**SANDRA F. YANEY, RN, NM, NPH, CS**
Retired, Army Nurse Corps
Family Nurse Practitioner
Collaborative Practice Consultant
Cedar Springs Psychiatric Hospital
Colorado Springs, Colorado

# REVIEWERS FOR THE FIRST EDITION

**PAM BRICKER, RNC**
Unit Coordinator
Cedar Springs Psychiatric Hospital
Colorado Springs, Colorado

**NANCY LEA CARTER, RN, BSN, MA**
Hospital Nursing & Management
Counseling of Children
Child Care Provider
Albuquerque, New Mexico

**KAREN DANNEWITZ, RN, MS, CS**
Private Practice, Consultant
Colorado Springs, Colorado

**SUZANNE SAYLE JIMERSON, RN, MS, CS**
Clinical Specialist in Adult/Family Psychiatric Nursing
Dover, Massachusetts

**NOLA LANGE, RN, MA, CS**
Psychiatric Nurse Liaison
Penrose-St. Francis Healthcare System
Colorado Springs, Colorado

**BARBARA E. THOMAS, RN, BSN, C**
Coordinator of Partial Hospitalization and Specialty
  Groups
Cedar Springs Psychiatric Hospital
Colorado Springs, Colorado

Special thanks to **DAVID U. CASTER, MD, FAPA**, Psychiatrist, Colorado Springs, Colorado.

# CONTENTS IN BRIEF

# DETAILED CONTENTS

# INTRODUCTION

One of the most significant achievements in the health-care field during the last 20 years has been the emergence of the nurse as an active coordinator and initiator of client care. While the transition from helpmate to health-care professional has been painfully slow and is not yet complete, the importance of the nurse within the system can no longer be denied or ignored. Today's nurse designs nursing care interventions that will move the total client toward a positive outcome and optimal health. This is especially true in the area of mental health nursing, where health-care reform and managed care are attempting to bring more available and affordable care to all clients.

The current state of the theory of nursing process, diagnosis, intervention, and evaluation has been brought to the clinical setting to be implemented by the nurse. This book gives definition and direction to the development and use of individualized nursing care for nurses in the psychiatric setting (hospital, clinic, private practice) who are using the nursing process to identify client needs. A holistic/humanistic focus is presented in which the nurse serves as advocate for the client. Plans of care are formulated using nursing diagnoses with interventions and rationale based on current scientific premises. They encompass psychosocial/psychodynamic concepts and have been organized according to psychiatric diagnoses as listed in the fourth edition of *Diagnostic and Statistical Manual of Mental Disorders*. DSM III-R information is included to assist in the transition to the fourth edition. ANA standards are used as a basis for the nursing process and development of plans of care, which serve as guides to the therapeutic nurse/client relationship. Therefore, the book is not an end in itself but a beginning for the future growth and development of the profession.

Professional care standards, physicians, and clients will continue to increase expectations for nurses' performance as each day brings advances in the struggle to understand the mysteries of normal body/mind function and human response to actual and potential health problems. With this increased knowledge comes greater responsibility for the nurse. To meet these challenges competently, the nurse must have up-to-date physical and psychiatric assessment skills and a working knowledge of pathophysiologic concepts concerning the changes occurring in the health-care field. This book is a tool, a means of attaining that competency.

In the past, plans of care were viewed principally as learning tools for students and seemed to have little relevance after graduation. However, the need for a written format to communicate and document individualized client care has been recognized in all care settings. In addition, governmental regulations and third-party payor requirements have created the need to validate the appropriateness of the care provided, as well as the need to justify client care charges and staffing patterns. Thus, although the student's "case studies" were too cumbersome to be practical in the clinical setting, the client plan of care meets the above identified needs. The practicing nurse, as well as the nursing student, will welcome this text as a ready reference in clinical practice.

The primary focus is early intervention to enable the client to maintain quality of life and independent living within individual capabilities. This book is designed for use in the psychiatric setting, serving as a guide for nurses who plan and promote health care for the psychiatric client and his or her family. Sample plans of care addressing specific psychiatric illnesses are organized by categories and identified by the DSM classification for easy reference. Rationales (which not only state why an intervention is important but also provide related pathophysiology, when applicable) enhance the reader's understanding of the intervention. This information also serves as a catalyst for thought in planning and evaluating the care being rendered.

Chapter 1 examines current issues/trends and their implications for the nurse caring for the client and family who are experiencing emotional difficulties. Trends in health care such as cost containment, shortened hospital stays, outpatient care, and increased use of alternative treatments are examined in light of possible effects on the delivery of care. There has been a dramatic growth of scientific knowledge into the biologic side of mental illness. Many psychiatric disorders are being reappraised as "diseases of the brain" rather than "disorders of the mind." A growing body of evidence suggests that biochemical dysfunction of the brain and central nervous system is etiologic in the development of some disorders, particularly schizophrenia, bipolar disorder, and some anxiety disorders. Research into the genetic factors involved will also provide new insights into mental illness and its treatment.

An overview of cultural, community, sociologic, and ethical concepts impacting on the psychiatric nurse in a variety of health-care settings is included. The importance of the nurse's role in cooperation and coordination with other health-care professionals is integrated throughout the plans of care.

Chapter 2 reviews the historic use of the nursing process in formulating plans of care and the nurse's role in the delivery of that care. Nursing diagnosis is discussed to assist the nurse in understanding its role in the nursing process.

In Chapter 3, a nursing-based assessment tool is provided to aid the nurse in identifying nursing diagnoses for use with the psychiatric client. A sample client situation with individual database and corresponding plan of care is included to demonstrate how to adapt the nursing process theory to practice. Finally, evaluation and documentation are addressed to complete the nursing process cycle.

Chapters 4 through 15 provide plans of care that include information from multiple disciplines to assist the nurse in providing holistic care for the client/family within the community or acute care setting. Each plan includes a client assessment database (presented in a nursing format) and associated diagnostic studies. After the database is collected, nursing priorities are sifted from the information to help focus and structure the care provided. Discharge goals are listed to identify

which general goals should be accomplished in situations in which care is expected to be terminated and not simply progress to another stage. The nursing diagnoses contain "related to" and "evidenced by" statements that provide an explanation of client problems/needs. Desired client outcomes are stated in behavioral terms that can be measured to evaluate the client's progress and the effectiveness of care provided. The interventions are designed to promote problem resolution.

A decision-making model is used to organize and prioritize nursing interventions based on the nurse acting independently/collaboratively within the health team. No attempt is made to indicate whether independent or collaborative actions come first, as this must be dictated by the individual situation. Inclusion of rationale for the nursing actions will assist the nurse to decide whether the interventions are appropriate for an individual client. A bibliography follows the text to allow for further reference/research as desired.

In summary, each plan of care in this text is an informational guide, designed to provide generalized information on the associated psychiatric/medical condition; therefore, this book is a ready reference for the practicing nurse as well as a catalyst for thought in planning and evaluating care.

Additionally, students will find the plans of care helpful as they learn and develop skills in applying the nursing process using nursing diagnoses in the psychiatric setting. The plan-of-care guides can be modified either by using portions of the information provided or by adding additional client care information to the existing guides. We appreciate that not all diagnoses presented in these plans of care may be appropriate for a particular client or locale, in which case alternatives should be chosen to meet individual client needs. We support the belief that practicing nurses and researchers need to study, use, and evaluate the diagnoses as presented. As new nursing diagnoses are developed, the information they encompass must be reflected in the database. The nurse is encouraged to share insights and ideas with the Diagnosis Review Committee of the North American Nursing Diagnosis Association (NANDA), 1211 Locust St., Philadelphia, PA 19107; 1-800-647-9002.

As a final note, this book is not intended to be a procedure manual, and efforts have been made to avoid detailed descriptions of techniques/protocols that might be viewed as individual/regional in nature. Instead, the reader is referred to a procedure manual/standards of care book for in-depth direction regarding these concerns.

## CHAPTER 1

# ISSUES AND TRENDS IN PSYCHIATRIC NURSING

Within the past century, psychiatry began to emerge from behind the veil of mystery and superstition. Two significant factors in bringing psychiatric care to the arena of scientific study and therapeutic modalities are the work of Sigmund Freud and the advent of psychotropic drugs. Although there now are many theories and techniques of communication therapies, Freud was most responsible for establishing communication as therapy and for studying mental and emotional dysfunction in a scientific manner. Research into the biologic and genetic causes of mental illness has produced a dramatic increase in the scientific knowledge available. Many psychiatric disorders are being reappraised as "diseases of the brain" rather than "disorders of the mind." A growing body of evidence suggests that biochemical dysfunction of the brain and central nervous system is the etiology of some disorders, particularly schizophrenia, bipolar disorder, and some anxiety disorders. Increasing information supports a relationship between stress and immunosuppression, providing insights about the link between stressful life events and the development of physical and emotional illness. Knowledge about substances that can poison the brain and nervous system (neurotoxicology) has enhanced our awareness of environmental pollutants and provoked us to look at what kinds of preventive measures can be taken. Efforts to treat brain diseases by the use of neural transplants and nerve regeneration have led to controversy and ethical discussions about how to accomplish these procedures.

Coupled with these ideas of brain disease is a growth in technology that allows sophisticated examination of the structure and function of the brain. Technologies such as computerized tomography (CT) scans, nuclear magnetic resonance imagery (MRI), and positron emission tomography (PET) have provided information about brain functioning that has served to guide diagnosis and intervention with some clients. Computer-assisted enhancements of the information provided by EEGs (e.g., brain electrical activity map [BEAM]) show distinctive brain patterns associated with dyslexia and other learning problems. Studies of the workplace regarding individual biologic rhythms and shift work and the potential for behavioral and neurologic harm are ongoing.

Psychotropic drugs, many of which have been available only since the 1950s, have made it possible to control symptoms of psychiatric illnesses. The major psychotropic medications may be used as therapy by themselves, but more often they are used as an adjunct to individual or group psychotherapy. They do not cure the underlying condition or emotional problem, but they do enable the client to benefit from other therapies and live as normal a life as possible.

Within the last 20 to 30 years, there has emerged a movement to release chronically ill clients from state hospitals and other mental health institutions. The reason for this was partially economic. It is expensive to keep people institutionalized and unproductive in large hospital settings. Another reason was the growing awareness of the civil rights of the individual and a belief that the rights of the chronic psychiatric client were being violated. Changes in treatment made it possible to begin to look at what could be done to help this population become more self-sufficient, contributing members of society. Clinics, day treatment programs, and other alternate facilities were proposed, and to some extent established, in an attempt to meet these goals.

However, the move in the 1960s to community

mental health care did not fulfill the promises anticipated at that time. Professional education and payment structures did not fully support the concept of community-based care, and many caregivers did not understand the mission of this movement. Although much has been learned in the past 20 years about how to treat severe mental illnesses effectively in both acute care and community-based programs, present community facilities still are not sufficient to meet the increasing need for mental health treatment and care.

Because mental illness can now be defined in the same way as physical illness, effective treatments are usually available. However, access to care remains a problem. Studies indicate that targeting at-risk groups for early intervention, the availability of appropriate treatment, and the use of employee assistance plans have proved cost-effective. Intensive community services for children that prevent separation from the family and its resultant problems also provide the opportunity for promoting family interaction and problem-solving. In addition, it has been reliably demonstrated that mental health care can reduce costs for physical illnesses (e.g., chronic pain conditions).

## ISSUES AFFECTING MENTAL HEALTH CARE

### Current Treatment

In spite of these advances, the stigma of mental illness persists as the "mysteries" surrounding psychiatry are slow to resolve. True scientific study of the relationship between therapy and change in human behavior is difficult at best, and the etiology of many disorders is still unknown or only partly understood or accepted. Biomedical research has greatly increased in recent years, providing information about the biologic, genetic, and psychologic bases for mental illness. However, intervention is still based on theory and on the personality and style of the therapist. Although theoretic approaches are many and varied, e.g., psychoanalytic, family systems, and behavioral, there are three basic forms of treatment in use today. These are (1) the use of drugs (neuropsychopharmacology), (2) conditioning or behavior modification, and (3) communication therapies.

Today there are many economic and social factors that influence the care given to psychiatric clients. Psychiatric nursing has also been changing in many ways. Nurses no longer give only long-term custodial care. Psychiatric nurses are qualified

and expected to participate in therapy, including group therapy. The role of the nurse administering medications has expanded to include discussions of side effects and expected therapeutic results to assist clients in making informed choices about their care. Psychiatric rehabilitation and the use of case management provide the nurse with the opportunity to help those who are disabled by major mental illnesses to relearn skills—how to care for their daily needs, how to become productive/ return to school or the workforce, and how to get along with colleagues and family—thus increasing the individual's ability to live independently.

## Financial Considerations

The need to provide an economic base for long-term, treatment-oriented psychiatric care remains a challenge for the health-care system. Medical costs are escalating, and there is a strong push to economize in all areas. A major step in cost cutting was the passage by Congress of prospective payment by diagnostic related groups (DRGs), in which Medicare reimburses a predetermined amount for hospitalization for each admission diagnosis. Although DRGs are not applicable for psychiatry at this time, they do influence reimbursement because third-party payors use this method for establishing payment for all health care. Health-care reform is being debated, with many different options offered to reduce costs while increasing the access to care. It is clear that community settings, e.g., community mental health centers, schools, homes, halfway houses, and even shopping malls, will increasingly be used to deliver mental health care.

This trend indicates to health-care providers that psychiatric nurses need to develop new methods of providing effective client care. Primary health care is an important concept of health-care reform. Psychiatric/mental health nurses need to begin to apply these ideas in the care of psychiatric clients. Addressing the needs of the whole person includes promoting optimal mental and physical health, preventing illness, maintaining health, and using referrals and rehabilitation. Goal-oriented, time-limited interventions are necessary if we are to continue to provide quality mental health care to our clients. The nursing process as a model for problem-solving can be used to achieve this goal, providing a framework for systematic nursing care based on scientific knowledge. Additionally, the development of nursing diagnoses has provided the impetus to more effective planning, delivery, and documentation of client care.

## Cultural Factors

The study of mental illness in relation to culture has been limited and often localized. However, available research suggests that both mental illnesses and therapeutic approaches differ among the world's cultures. Thus, there is a growing awareness that cultural factors do affect mental health and that clients from different cultural backgrounds require culturally appropriate diagnosis and care combining different care methods.

"Normal behavior" is relative to a specific culture, and different psychologic characteristics are promoted by each culture. Other variables influencing mental health include family relationships, child-rearing practices, attitudes toward illness, and social/economic status. Misdiagnosis may occur because of many factors, including differences in language, mannerisms, personality traits, religious dogma, and acceptability of the presence of and communication with ancestors or supernatural powers. For example, an individual from a gentle, mild, passive culture may create the impression of being guarded or reticent or may even be misdiagnosed as passive-aggressive. Furthermore, when a problem does exist, the culture may dictate that seeking help from outsiders is inappropriate, and the family may choose to tolerate "unusual" behavior rather than seek treatment or attempt to manage the individual on its own, thus delaying therapy. Diagnosis may be further impacted by racial and ethnic differences in the clinical presentation as variations of biologic markers for various psychiatric disorders are identified, e.g., serum creatinine phosphokinase, platelet serotonin, and HLA-A$_2$ determinations.

Once therapy is begun, the practice of self-medication, use of folk remedies, and cultural dietary preferences impact drug use/choice as well as individual cooperation with the therapeutic regimen. Additionally, racial and ethnic differences in response to psychotropic medications affect dosage requirements and potential side effects. For example, research reveals that as a rule, Asians require lower dosages and closer monitoring of several psychotropic drugs (e.g., lithium, antidepressants, and neuroleptics).

Separate from, but in conjunction with, cultural issues, religious beliefs can greatly impact the client's view of the existence and etiology of mental illness and acceptance of therapy needs and options. It is therefore imperative that psychiatric nurses be sensitive to the potential for racial and ethnic differences or needs and promote awareness by other team members.

## Community Impact

The movement from institutional to community-based care has resulted in a dramatic reduction in the number of long-term clients in institutions. However, new problems have been created, and the system has failed to care adequately for the clients who have been returned to their community. The decrease in cost of care is dubious since many nonfunctional or borderline individuals have been released only to become dependent on other community agencies and/or to wander the streets.

Care providers find themselves working with persons who have difficulty adapting to, or cannot adapt to, society as self-sufficient members because of chronic illness and/or long-term institutionalization. Nurses are challenged to assist these clients to reach realistic goals with a minimum of dependency on community resources.

Concern for civil rights has also had an impact on involuntary commitment. It must be demonstrated that a person poses a danger to self or others and/or the community before legal commitment to an institution can be accomplished. While this protects the individual from unjust confinement, there seems to be little recourse for families of disturbed persons who will not voluntarily seek treatment. Inevitably, some people who would greatly benefit receive no treatment and, without adequate care, join the chronically psychotic or nonfunctional clients in board-and-care facilities or other community agencies. Others fade into the anonymity of street or bag people subsisting by whatever means possible. Occasionally much publicity is given to the infrequent client who commits violent acts after having been discharged from the psychiatric system, creating fear and anger among the general populace with an accompanying demand for tighter controls.

## Age-Related Factors

Ours is an aging society. More and more people are reaching middle and late years. An increasing awareness of midlife crisis and the emotional impact that it has on the individual has encouraged more people to seek help with the problems that may be created at this time. Additionally, more individuals are willing to disrupt their lives (e.g., change relationships or careers) to seek happiness and "find themselves," which also impacts those around them.

As a person ages, many losses occur, e.g., jobs, loved ones, health, and ability to function (sexually and otherwise), and often the individual's self-image suffers. Chronic depression and substance abuse are increasing problems in the older population. There is also an increase of suicide in this neglected segment of our society, as depression may go unnoticed simply because no one pays attention. Nurses are in an excellent position to detect these problems and initiate goal-setting and treatment referrals with the elderly. In the past, because of limited life expectancy, goals for the elderly were not given much consideration. Obviously, this view is quite short-sighted and clearly discriminating. With this awareness comes a need for more programs to meet the needs of this group.

On the other end of the spectrum, children's and adolescents' psychiatric needs are growing and requiring the expansion of facilities and programs. More recognition is being given to the reality that delinquent youngsters are often troubled and may in fact be mentally ill. Issues of physical and sexual abuse, incest, neglect, changes in family configuration, and gender identity problems create the additional need for both inpatient and community treatment. While facilities and programs specifically designed for children and/or adolescents and their families are becoming more available, there is still a reluctance to acknowledge the reality of mental illness, substance abuse, and suicide in young people, resulting in insufficient resources to meet the need.

## Substance Abuse

Substance abuse has come full force to national and worldwide attention. Society's awareness of this problem has brought both legal and therapeutic means of solving it to the forefront. Specific modalities have been developed to work with the addicted client. Increased knowledge of the frequency of issues of dual diagnosis (presence of psychiatric illness in combination with substance abuse) has led to more effective treatment for these individuals. Additionally, recognition of the effect on the family, as well as issues of codependence, has led to a "broader" approach to what was once believed to be an "individual problem." With the substance abuser, psychiatric nurses need to be aware of such specific concerns as chemical imbalances, as well as the unique problems and needs of the individual/family unit, because many of the therapy needs for addicted individuals remain unfulfilled.

## Suicide

As noted, suicide is on the increase. The statistical rise may be due in part to the identification of some deaths as suicide that formerly may have been labeled accidental. However, pressures of life in a world where television brings the reality of global concerns into the home daily, fears about debilitating and/or terminal illnesses, and adolescent developmental issues of independence and gender identity present individuals with problems of coping that may lead to suicide. With an alarming rise in the incidence of suicide among children, adolescents (suicide is currently the second cause of death in this group), and the elderly, specific interventions are necessary in determining what kinds of preventive actions can be helpful. The nurse is often in a position to recognize the potential for suicide in the client and to take effective action.

## Stress

An increased awareness of the effects of stress on our lives is emerging. Of special interest is the influence of stress in the development of many psychologic problems. Manifestations of stress, e.g., ulcers, asthma, and perhaps any or all of the physical illnesses humans experience, have also been acknowledged. While many psychiatric treatment modalities, e.g., biofeedback, relaxation skills, and guided imagery, are directed at stress reduction/management, it is often a neglected area for the client with physical illness.

As life stressors have increased, the numbers of people who are victims of physical, sexual, and emotional abuse continue to rise in epidemic proportions. In psychiatry, the phenomenon of delayed stress reactions (the belated response of victims to violence or chronic deprivation) is being given more attention. This is now recognized as a significant cause of many disorders, which may appear years after the occurrence of the stressor. Identification of victims of, or those at risk for, abuse and intervention to prevent further victimization are also within the scope of nursing practice. Family intervention, crisis intervention, and group support can help to interrupt the pattern of violence, as well as provide assistance for victim recovery.

Societal changes, such as the increase in the number of divorces and remarriages, which result in single-parent homes and stepfamilies, create problems that demand new and creative approaches to treatment. Role changes include fathers taking on more child-rearing responsibilities and mothers combining careers with homemaking. Increased mobility of individuals often results in the lack of extended family available for role-modeling and assistance, leaving nuclear families vulnerable to added stress. Unrealistic television models of the "perfect family" and the "quick" solution of the 30-minute situation comedy lead people to believe that there is something wrong with them when problems persist. In addition, with the wide use of television, rapid travel, and the opening of third-world countries to the west, our world is shrinking, and happenings in one area affect and influence all other areas. Changes in manufacturing including the decline in jobs and downsizing in major companies, which also affect the health-care industry, have the work force in a constant state of turmoil. As a result, workers fear layoffs, look for other positions, and/or decide to return to school to train for new jobs, often at lower salary levels. Finally, advances in science and technology fuel changes in all areas of life.

## TRENDS AFFECTING DELIVERY OF CARE

### The Role of the Nurse

New developments and changes in the nursing profession are impacting the psychiatric nursing field. One of these changes is the development and implementation of nursing diagnoses, which is making written plans of care more useful for the provision and documentation of care. Identification of specific problems and determination of individual interventions necessary for reaching timely goals have enhanced the care-planning process. Additionally, more recognition is being given to the need for the client to be an active participant in the therapeutic process. Nurses enter into therapeutic relationships with clients, which become the cornerstone of quality care. Assessments are made, nursing diagnoses are identified, and nursing care is implemented and evaluated with the active involvement of the client.

Psychiatric nursing is a specialized area of nursing that uses theories of human behavior as its science and the purposeful use of self as its art. The development of Standards of Psychiatric and Mental Health Nursing Practice (ANA, 1991) provides a beginning framework for the nurse to use to guide professional practice. In conjunction with the growth of specialty professional groups and the expansion of the psychiatric nursing practice arena, nursing involvement in the interdisciplinary team approach to psychiatric care is now more frequently acknowledged and valued. In addition, nursing organizations, such as the American Nurses' Association (ANA), have established programs to credential nurses, e.g., Clinical Specialist in Psychiatric/Mental Health Nursing. These specialty certification programs share common goals: to provide consumer protection, to enhance nursing knowledge and competency, to increase nursing au-

tonomy, and to strengthen collaboration. Specialty certification will take on more importance in this cost-conscious era as managers seek to hire competent professionals.

Furthermore, independent roles for the nurse, such as private practice and liaison/consultant positions in institutions/community settings, are beginning to affect how health (psychiatric) care is delivered. The nurse requires greater clinical expertise, maturity, critical thinking ability, assertiveness, and client-management skills to meet these challenges.

### Managed Mental Health Care

This is the "Golden Age" for managed mental health care. There are over 40 million lives covered by managed care companies nationwide. Virtually all corporations have entered into HMO, PPO, and carve-out plans to provide employees and their dependents with psychiatric and substance abuse treatment benefits.

Managed care is purposefully designed to control the balance between cost and quality of care. However, many view it as a two-edged sword. On the one hand, it is a method of providing attention to goal-oriented brief therapy, strengthening accountability, and focusing on treatment and outcomes. On the other hand, health-care provider autonomy and client choices are restricted. Additionally, many in the multidisciplinary settings have high and perhaps unrealistic expectations and may become discouraged or sabotage the efforts when problems arise. Problems of conflicts between disciplines may also become more apparent, creating further conflict and interfering with establishment of the system.

Managed care exists in many settings, such as insurance-based programs, employer-based medical providerships, social service programs, the public health sector, and virtually any setting in which medical providership services exist, that is, in any setting in which an organization is responsible for *payment* of health-care services for a group of people.

Managed care includes a wide range of organized delivery systems that attempt to balance access, quality, and cost. Strategies to bring expenditures under control by managed mental health care include preauthorization, concurrent review, and external case management. With the advent of managed care, opportunities for nurses to practice in different settings have been in abundance. Many nurses have assumed the role of case manager, while others have established private case management practices. In these endeavors, they consider the client's health status and diagnosis, treatment plans, payment resources, and health-care options. Physicians are making referrals to these nurses for their clients who require assistance with their recovery/rehabilitation and health maintenance. This type of managed care has been especially beneficial to clients with *chronic* physical or mental disorders.

## Case Management

Case management is the method used to achieve managed mental health care. It is the actual coordination of services required to meet the needs of the client. In the acute care setting, case management is viewed as ". . . a methodology for organizing client care through an episode of illness so that specific clinical and financial outcomes are achieved within an allotted time frame" (Zander, 1988).

Case management and utilization review have been met with much resistance in the hospital industry. However, a survey by the National Association of Private Hospitals (*Report on Utilization Management Firms Conducting Psychiatric Reviews,* 1992) indicates that the tension between managed care firms has lessened. This is attributed to the ways in which managed mental health has positively affected the delivery of care. Quality measures are more explicit, and the criteria designated by the case managers and utilization reviewers have been more defined.

The goals of case management include:

1. To determine what the expected clinical outcomes would be in an individual with a specific illness at a specific point in time
2. To ensure that use of resources is appropriate to contain health-care costs
3. To promote collaborative practice among multidisciplinary team members and provide continuity of care for the patient
4. To discharge the client within a designated length of time (often determined by DRGs or insurance company designations)

Given the commonly shorter length of stays and the higher acuity of clients at discharge, these services have come to be known as "high-speed" care.

The case manager assumes the authority and accountability to negotiate with multiple health-care providers to obtain a variety of services required by the client. Generally, nurses or social workers are identified as case managers in the acute care setting. In the ideal situation, the nursing case manager initiates the relationship with the client prior to admission, coordinates all inpatient activities, actively engages in discharge planning, and follows the client for a designated period of time after discharge. During this process, the nursing case manager must identify those elements of the client's care that are *critical.* For example, if the

client can be in the hospital for only 5 days, what are the critical components of care that must be addressed? These critical components of care become the established guidelines for the provision of care by the health-care team. These guidelines form the basis for the clinical (or critical) pathway of care (CPC). The CPC becomes the "blueprint" for care during the time the client is in the hospital. Clinical pathways of care are best used for acute problems for which there are predictable outcomes. Most chronic psychiatric clients could benefit from managed care on a long-term basis, but clinical pathways define care that is determined by outcomes that must and can be achieved within a specific time frame.

In a clinical pathway of care, client, family, and staff behaviors are charted along a time line for which a specific outcome has been predicted. CPCs may be standardized, or they may be used as guidelines from which a more individualized CPC may be developed for a specific client. Reports from hospitals that have used these tools have suggested that there has been a definite improvement in quality of client care and significant containment of costs during the shortened hospital stays.

## Computer Applications

Many nurses believe that their limited time can be better spent with the client, giving care, rather than generating written plans of care. Computerization can decrease time spent in generating and maintaining plans of care and improve the quality of record keeping. Computerized plans of care provide psychiatric nurses with a more efficient means to develop comprehensive, continuous, individualized, and legible plans of care for each client. Nurses may quickly enter, display, evaluate, update, and print a revised plan of care.

Standardized plans of care establish priorities of care and define minimum standards of safe practice. They provide an outline for documentation of the care that has been given and the way the client responded to that care. They also serve to jog the nurse's memory when caring for clients not usually seen in that nurse's area of clinical practice. Easy access to computerized plans of care provides information and promotes safe, effective care. Standardized plans of care are not intended to be all-inclusive. Nursing judgment is required to individualize the plan of care for each specific client.

Many computerized systems providing standardized client plans of care use the nursing diagnoses accepted for testing by the North American Nursing Diagnosis Association (NANDA). These basic plans of care reflect standards of care for particular client problems and are designed to meet specific needs. Since the plans reflect a wealth of varied nursing experience, they allow even novice practitioners to formulate effective care strategies and individualize care.

## Conclusion

Up to this time, the major focus of psychiatric care has been largely on inpatient care. As we travel into the 21st century, psychiatric services are moving out of the inpatient arena and into the ambulatory care setting. Today the community mental health-care system is the fastest growing subgroup of health care. As previously noted, the factors affecting mental health and the health-care system are many and varied. In this era of rapid change with the public expectation of instant cures and the demand to contain health-care costs, increasing pressure is placed on health-care providers. New and inventive approaches are being developed in an attempt to find effective solutions and improve the delivery of mental health care.

There is no doubt that psychiatric/mental health nursing will change as a result of these developments in the health-care arena. Nursing is in a position to assist with the planning and to contribute to the provision of care in a cost-effective manner. Psychiatric nurses can work in the community to provide preventive therapy as well as supportive, transitional, or continued therapy for clients discharged from inpatient settings. To meet these challenges, nurses must continue their professional growth and accept accountability for their practice.

## CHAPTER 2

# THE NURSING PROCESS: PLANNING CARE WITH NURSING DIAGNOSIS

There is a growing awareness that nursing care is a key factor in client recovery and in the maintenance, rehabilitation, and prevention aspects of mental health care. Publication of the American Nurses' Association (ANA) Social Policy Statement (1980), which defined nursing as the diagnosis and treatment of human responses to actual and potential health problems, in combination with the ANA Standards of Clinical Nursing Practice (1991), has provided the impetus and support for the use of nursing diagnosis in the practice setting. Prospective payment plans, movement from acute care (in a hospital) to community settings (mental health centers, group homes/foster care), and other changes in the health-care system are highlighting the need for a common framework of communication and documentation. Such a framework promotes continuity of care for the client who moves from one area of the health-care system to another while maintaining the confidentiality of the client. Evaluation and documentation of care are an important part of this process.

Nurses have visionary ideas for delivery of quality care to all clients. Often, turning those ideas into action seems to be a frustrating exercise in futility, as what appears easy to do in theory seems difficult in practice. With their hectic schedules, many nurses believe that time spent in writing plans of care is time taken away from client care. In reality, the delivery of quality care involves planning and coordination. It is our belief that as the nurse works with nursing diagnosis, learning the etiology and defining characteristics, goals become apparent and interventions for attaining these goals become clear, facilitating the planning process. Properly written and used, plans of care provide tools for client care assessment, guidelines for documentation, and direction for continuity of care among nurses and other caregivers. This is particularly true in the routinely multidisciplinary approach of psychiatric care.

## NURSING PROCESS

The term *nursing process* was introduced in the 1950s, but it has taken many years to develop national acceptance of the process as an integral part of nursing care. It is adapted from the scientific approach to problem-solving and requires the skills of: (1) assessment (systematic collection of data relating to clients and their problems), (2) problem identification (analysis/interpretation of data), (3) planning (choice of solutions), (4) implementation (putting the plan into action), and (5) evaluation (assessing the effectiveness of the plan and changing the plan as indicated by the current needs). While nurses use these terms separately, in reality they are interrelated and form a continuous circle of thought and action, providing an efficient method of organizing thought processes for clinical decision-making. Nursing process is now included in the conceptual framework of most nursing curricula and accepted in the legal definition of nursing in most nurse practice acts. It is also the basis of the Standards of Psychiatric and Mental Health Nursing Practice (Table 2–1).

To use this process, the nurse must demonstrate fundamental abilities of knowledge, intelligence, and creativity, as well as expertise in interpersonal

## TABLE 2–1. Psychiatric Standards of Care (ANA, 1991)

**STANDARD I: THEORY**

The nurse applies appropriate theory that is scientifically sound as a basis for decisions regarding nursing practice.

**STANDARD II: DATA COLLECTION**

The nurse continuously collects data that are comprehensive, accurate, and systematic.

**STANDARD III: DIAGNOSIS**

The nurse uses nursing diagnoses or standard classification of mental disorders to express conclusions supported by recorded assessment data and current scientific premises.

**STANDARD IV: PLANNING**

The nurse develops a nursing care plan with specific goals and interventions delineating nursing actions unique to each client's need.

**STANDARD V: INTERVENTION**

The nurse intervenes as guided by the nursing care plan to implement nursing actions that promote, maintain, or restore physical and mental health; prevent illness; and effect rehabilitation.

**STANDARD V-A: INTERVENTIONS: PSYCHOTHERAPEUTIC INTERVENTIONS**

The nurse uses psychotherapeutic interventions to assist clients in regaining or improving their previous coping abilities and to prevent further disability.

**STANDARD V-B: INTERVENTION: HEALTH TEACHING**

The nurse assists clients, families, and groups to achieve satisfying and productive patterns of living through health teaching.

**STANDARD V-C: INTERVENTION: ACTIVITIES OF DAILY LIVING**

The nurse uses the activities of daily living in a goal-directed way to foster adequate self-care and physical and mental well-being of clients.

**STANDARD V-D: INTERVENTION: SOMATIC THERAPIES**

The nurse uses knowledge of somatic therapies and applies related clinical skills in working with clients.

**STANDARD V-E: INTERVENTION: THERAPEUTIC ENVIRONMENT**

The nurse provides, structures, and maintains a therapeutic environment in collaboration with the client and other health-care providers.

**STANDARD V-F: INTERVENTIONS: PSYCHOTHERAPY**

The nurse uses advanced clinical expertise in individual, group, and family psychotherapy; uses child psychotherapy and other treatment modalities to function as a psychotherapist; and recognizes professional accountability for nursing practice.

**STANDARD VI: EVALUATION**

The nurse evaluates client responses to nursing actions in order to revise the database, nursing diagnoses, and nursing care plans.

**STANDARD VII: PEER REVIEW**

The nurse participates in peer review and other means of evaluation to ensure quality of nursing care provided for clients.

Continued

TABLE 2–1. **Psychiatric Standards of Care (ANA, 1991)** (Continued)

**STANDARD VIII: CONTINUING EDUCATION**

The nurse assumes responsibility for continuing education and professional development and contributes to the professional growth of others.

**STANDARD IX: INTERDISCIPLINARY COLLABORATION**

The nurse collaborates with other health-care providers in assessing, planning, implementing, and evaluating programs and other mental health activities.

**STANDARD X: UTILIZATION OF COMMUNITY HEALTH SYSTEMS**

The nurse participates with other members of the community in assessing, planning, implementing, and evaluating mental health services and community systems that include the promotion of the broad continuum of primary, secondary, and tertiary prevention of mental illness.

**STANDARD XI: RESEARCH**

The nurse contributes to nursing and the mental health field through innovations in theory and practice and participation in research.

and technical skills. Some *critical assumptions* for the nurse to consider in the decision-making process are that:

- The client is a human being with worth and dignity.
- There are basic human needs that must be met. When they are not, problems arise requiring intervention by another person until the individual can resume responsibility for self.
- The client has a right to quality health and nursing care delivered with concern, compassion, and competence, and focusing on wellness, prevention, and restoration.
- The therapeutic nurse-client relationship is a critical element in this process.

## NURSING DIAGNOSIS

Nurses have struggled for years to define nursing by identifying its parameters with a goal of attaining/verifying professional status. To this end, nurses have been meeting and conducting research to develop nursing diagnoses. The North American Nursing Diagnosis Association (NANDA) has accepted the following working definition:

Nursing diagnosis is a clinical judgment about individual, family, or community responses to actual and potential health problems/life processes. Nursing diagnoses provide the basis for selection of nursing interventions to achieve outcomes for which the nurse is accountable.

Nursing diagnosis provides a framework for using the nursing process and is the crux of the nursing plan of care, focusing attention on client needs/responses (identifying problems, nursing interventions, and evaluation tools) and serving as the prime determinant of the style of nursing care to be delivered. Historically, nursing actions have often been based on variables such as signs and symptoms, tests, and medical diagnosis. Accurate diagnosis of a client problem can become a standard for nursing practice, understood by all who are using the plan of care, and thus can lead to improved delivery of care. The nursing diagnosis is as precise as the data will allow. It communicates the client's situation at the present time and reflects changes as they occur. It is necessary to seek, incorporate, and synthesize all the relevant data and make the statement meaningful so as to provide appropriate direction for nursing care.

The affective tone of the nursing diagnosis can shape expectations of the client's response and influence the nurse's behavior toward the client. For instance, if the nurse sees the client as noncompliant, the nurse's attitudes and behavior may reflect anger and mistrust, and judgmental decisions may be made that do not accurately treat the client's problem. However, accurate identification of a client's problem (e.g., Altered Compliance related to medication side effects) can become a standard for nursing practice, understood by all who are using the plan of care, and thus can lead to improved delivery of care. In addition, the nurse needs to be aware of biases that may interfere with reaching an accurate diagnosis. Keeping a mind open to numerous possibilities and not getting stuck on a single symptom/thought will facilitate this process. For example, as cues are identified, e.g., restlessness, an inference may be made by the nurse that the client is anxious. If the nurse assumes that this is only psychologic, the possibility that it may be physiologically based may be overlooked.

As previously noted, nursing diagnosis provides a common language for identifying client problems, nursing interventions, and evaluation and documentation tools. This common language is important as it facilitates communication between nurses, shifts, units, alternate care settings, and other health-care professionals. It also provides a base for clinicians, educators, and researchers to document, validate, and/or alter the nursing process.

## PLANNING CARE

Medicine, psychiatry, and nursing, as well as other health disciplines, are interrelated with implications for each other. This interrelationship should include exchanging data, sharing ideas or thoughts, and developing plans of care that include all data pertinent to the individual client/family.

The written plan of care communicates the past and present status and needs of the client to all members of the health-care team. It identifies problems solved and those yet to be solved, approaches that have been successful, and patterns of client responses. It provides a mechanism to help ensure continuity of care. It can document client care in areas of accountability, quality improvement, and liability.

The written plan of care should contain more than actions initiated by medical/psychosocial orders. It needs to contain the written coordination of care given by all disciplines. The use of plans of care reflecting only functional divisions of tasks/duties perpetuates the notion that plans of care are busywork, unrelated to caregiving. Restructuring plans of care using nursing models can increase usage and provide succinct documentation/relevance, demonstrating the relationship between planning and documentation.

The nurse becomes the person responsible for coordinating these different activities into a functional plan necessary to provide holistic care for the client. Independent nursing actions are an integral part of this process. Interdependent/collaborative actions are based on the therapeutic regimen, including suggestions and orders from all disciplines involved with the care of the client. The nurse should plan care with the client/significant other as appropriate because all are accountable for that care and for achieving the desired goals.

## COMPONENTS OF THE PLAN OF CARE

For each plan of care presented, the *Client Assessment Database* is constructed from information obtained from the *History, Physical Examination,* and *Diagnostic Studies. Nursing Priorities* are then determined and serve as a general ranking system for the nursing diagnoses in the plan of care. In this book each psychiatric condition has established *Discharge Goals,* which are broadly stated and reflect the desired general status of the client on discharge or transfer. An example of discharge goals for a client with panic disorder would include:

1. When discomfort is experienced stays in feared situation gradually increasing level of tolerance
2. Techniques to lower/keep fear at manageable level are being used
3. Phobia confronted and desensitized to the stimulus
4. Greater independence with an increasingly freer lifestyle demonstrated

Nursing priorities, along with the discharge goals, may be reworded and reorganized with time lines according to the individual client/situation to create short-/long-term goals.

The *Client Diagnostic Statement* is validated by the *Related to/Evidenced by* statements, which reflect the etiology and defining characteristics (signs and symptoms) most consistent with a specific psychiatric situation. *Desired Outcomes/Evaluation Criteria* for each problem/need area are followed by appropriate independent and collaborative interventions (with accompanying rationales) in this text.

## Assessment

As noted, construction of the plan of care begins with the collection of data (assessment). The *Assessment Database* consists of subjective and objective information encompassing the various nursing concerns reflected in the current list of nursing diagnoses developed by NANDA. Subjective data are those that are reported by the client and significant other(s). This information includes the individual's perceptions that he or she wants to share. It is important to accept what is reported, because the client/significant other is the "expert" in this regard. However, the nurse needs to note incongru-

## TABLE 2-2. Nursing Diagnoses (through 11th NANDA Conference) 1994*

Activity intolerance
Activity intolerance, high risk for
Adjustment, impaired
Airway Clearance, ineffective
Anxiety [specify level]†
Aspiration, high risk for
Body Image disturbance
Body Temperature, altered, high risk for
Bowel Incontinence
Breastfeeding, effective
Breastfeeding, ineffective
Breastfeeding, interrupted
Breathing Pattern, ineffective
Cardiac Output, decreased
Caregiver Role Strain
Caregiver Role Strain, high risk for
Communication, impaired, verbal
Constipation
Constipation, colonic
Constipation, perceived
Coping, defensive
Coping, Individual, ineffective
Decisional Conflict (specify)
Denial, ineffective
Diarrhea
Disuse Syndrome, high risk for
Diversional Activity deficit
Dysreflexia

Family Coping, compromised
Family Coping, disabling
Family Coping, potential for growth
Family Processes, altered
Fatigue
Fear
Fluid Volume deficit [Active Loss]†
Fluid Volume deficit [Regulatory Failure]†
Fluid Volume deficit, high risk for
Fluid Volume excess
Gas Exchange, impaired
Grieving, anticipatory
Grieving, dysfunctional
Growth and Development, altered
Health Maintenance, altered
Health-Seeking Behaviors (specify)
Home Maintenance Management, impaired
Hopelessness
Hyperthermia
Hypothermia
Incontinence, functional
Incontinence, reflex
Incontinence, stress
Incontinence, total
Incontinence, urge
Infant Feeding Pattern, ineffective
Infection, high risk for
Injury, high risk for

encies/dissonances that may indicate the presence of other factors, such as lack of knowledge, myths, misconceptions, or fear.

Objective data are those that are observed (quantitatively or qualitatively) and may be verified by others. They include findings from the *physical examination* and *diagnostic testing.* Evaluation of both subjective and objective data leads to the identification of problems or areas of concern or need. These problems or needs are expressed as nursing diagnoses (Table 2-2).

## Problem Identification/ Analysis

Analysis involves examining assessment findings, grouping related findings, and comparing the findings against the established normal parameters. The key, then, to accurate nursing diagnosis is problem identification, which focuses attention on a current or high-risk physical, psychologic, or be-

havioral response that interferes with the quality of life the client desires or to which he or she is accustomed. It addresses the concerns of the client, significant other(s), and/or nurse that require nursing intervention and management. In this text, the choice of individual nursing diagnosis is validated by the *Related to/Risk factors and Evidenced by* statements most consistently associated with a specific psychiatric situation/medical condition.

Nurses may feel at risk in committing themselves to documenting a nursing diagnosis; however, many references are currently available to aid in identifying and formulating the diagnostic statement. In addition, unlike medical diagnoses, nursing diagnoses change as the client progresses through various stages of illness or maladaptation to problem resolution. From the specific information obtained in the client assessment database, the related factors, signs, and symptoms can be identified, and an individualized statement of the client's problem/need and diagnosis can be formulated. For example, a client may report fear of becoming

## TABLE 2–2. Nursing Diagnoses (through 11th NANDA Conference) 1994* (Continued)

Knowledge Deficit [Learning Need]† (specify)
Noncompliance, [Compliance, altered]† specify
Nutrition, altered, less than body requirements
Nutrition, altered, more than body requirements
Nutrition, altered, high risk for more than body requirements
Oral Mucous Membrane, altered
Pain [acute]†
Pain, chronic
Parental Role Conflict
Parenting, altered
Parenting, altered, high risk for
Peripheral Neurovascular Dysfunction, high risk for
Personal Identity disturbance
Physical Mobility, impaired
Poisoning, high risk for
Post-Trauma Response
Powerlessness
Protection, altered
Rape-Trauma Syndrome
Rape-Trauma Syndrome: compound reaction
Rape-Trauma Syndrome: silent reaction
Relocation Stress Syndrome
Role Performance, altered
Self-Care deficit: feeding, bathing/hygiene, dressing/grooming, toileting
Self-Esteem, chronic low
Self-Esteem disturbance

Self-Esteem, situational low
Self-Mutilation, high risk for
Sensory/Perceptual alterations (specify): visual, auditory, kinesthetic, gustatory, tactile, olfactory
Sexual Dysfunction
Sexuality Patterns, altered
Skin Integrity, impaired
Skin Integrity, impaired, high risk for
Sleep Pattern disturbance
Social Interaction, impaired
Social Isolation
Spiritual Distress (distress of the human spirit)
Spontaneous Ventilation, inability to sustain
Suffocation, high risk for
Swallowing, impaired
Therapeutic Regimen, ineffective management of
Thermoregulation, ineffective
Thought Processes, altered
Tissue Integrity, impaired
Tissue Perfusion, altered (specify): cerebral, cardiopulmonary, renal, gastrointestinal, peripheral
Trauma, high risk for
Unilateral Neglect
Urinary Elimination, altered
Urinary Retention [acute/chronic]†
Ventilatory Weaning Response, dysfunctional (DVWR)
Violence, high risk for, directed at self/others

* Pending official publication, expected in December, 1994.
† [Author recommendations].

obese and recurrent familial focus on eating habits/changes in weight, leading to a choice of the nursing diagnosis: Body Image, disturbance related to morbid fear of obesity as evidenced by negative feelings about body/view of self as fat in presence of normal body weight.

## Planning

Goals are established and outcome statements are formulated to give direction to nursing care. *Desired Outcomes* emerge from the diagnostic statement and are defined as the results of nursing interventions and patient responses that are achievable, desired by the client and/or nurse, and attainable within a defined time, given the present situation and resources. They have been stated in general terms in this book to permit the practitioner to modify/individualize them by adding time lines, considerations of client circumstances and needs, and other specifics as appropriate. The terminology needs to be concise, realistic, measurable, and stated in words that the client can understand. Beginning the outcome statement with an action verb provides direction that is measurable (e.g., Client will: *verbalize* an increased sense of self-worth). Psychiatric nurses often work in settings in which they are members of a multidisciplinary team, requiring highly coordinated and frequently interdependent planning based on the separate and distinct roles of each team member. In this setting, it is important that the goals of each discipline do not conflict.

*Interventions* communicate actions to be taken to achieve desired client outcomes. Again, using an action verb (e.g., "instruct," "demonstrate") provides direction for the nurse. The rationale for interventions needs to be sound and feasible with the intention of providing individualized care. Actions may be inde-

15

pendent or collaborative and encompass orders from nursing, medicine/psychiatry, and other disciplines. In this book, collaborative actions in conjunction with other disciplines are identified to assist the nurse in choosing appropriate interventions for the individual/setting. The educational background/expertise of the nurse, standing protocols, and areas of practice (rural/urban, acute/inpatient, or community care settings) can influence whether an individual intervention is actually an independent nursing function or requires collaboration. Finally, the written interventions need to be dated and signed to identify the person who is initiating and coordinating the care.

## Implementation

Once the goals, outcomes, and interventions have been identified, the nurse is ready to perform the activities recorded in the client's plan of care. In putting the plan of care into action and providing cost-effective and timely care, the nurse first identifies the priorities for providing that care. To determine the current priorities, the nurse reviews resources (such as diagnostic studies and progress reports from other health-care providers), while consulting with and considering the desires of the client.

Next, there are many activities, ranging from simple tasks to complex procedures, which can be involved in carrying out interventions to provide the planned care. The nurse needs to consider which interventions can be combined to facilitate accomplishing the activities within the time constraints. Then as care is provided, data on the client's response to each of the interventions is noted. The nurse also monitors the patient and related resources for changes in status/development of complications.

## Evaluation

Evaluation of the client's response to the care delivered and achievement of the desired outcomes (which were developed in the planning phase and documented in the plan of care) are the final step of the nursing process. The evaluation phase is necessary for the determination of how well the plan of care is working and is an ongoing process. The revision of the plan of care is an essential component of the evaluation phase.

Reassessment is an ongoing evaluation process that occurs not just when a desired client outcome is due to be reviewed or when a determination is needed as to whether or not the client is ready for discharge; instead, it is a constant "monitoring" of the client's status.

## Rationale

Although rationales do not appear on agency plans of care, they are included in this book to assist the student and practicing nurse in associating the psychologic and/or pathophysiologic principles with the selected nursing intervention.

## DOCUMENTING THE NURSING PROCESS

In general, the goals of the documentation system are to:

- Facilitate the quality of client care.
- Ensure documentation of progress with regard to client-focused outcomes.
- Facilitate interdisciplinary consistency and the communication of treatment goals and progress.

Two recent publications provide the nurse with guidelines for documenting the nursing process and support the need for a written (or computer-generated) plan of care. The *Standards of Clinical Nursing Practice* (ANA, 1991) ". . . delineate care that is provided to all clients of nursing services," and each standard includes a measurement criterion addressing documentation. In addition, the Nursing Care Standards (Joint Commission on Accreditation of Healthcare Organizations [JCAHO], 1992) also focus our attention on documentation as presented in Table 2–3. These revised standards delineate the professional responsibilities of all registered nurses and provide criteria to assist in measuring achievement of identified standards.

From a nursing focus, documentation provides a record of the use of the nursing process for the delivery of individualized client care. The initial *assessment* is recorded in the *client history* or *database*. The *identification* of client problems/needs and the *planning* of client care are recorded in the plan of care. The *implementation* of the plan is recorded in progress notes and/or flow sheets. Finally, the evaluation of care is documented in progress notes and/or the plan of care.

The maintenance of a medical record is one of the most essential requirements for accreditation of health-care facilities by JCAHO and/or other credentialing and licensing agencies. JCAHO standards state that the medical record should be documented accurately and in a timely manner. Therefore, the importance of completing notes on schedule and in a manner that facilitates retrieval of data should be emphasized.

Documentation is not only a requirement for ac-

**TABLE 2–3. A Sample Portion of One Nursing Care Standard from the Joint Commission on Accreditation of Healthcare Organizations**

NC.1. Patients receive nursing care based on a documented assessment of their needs.

NC.1.3.4. The patient's medical record includes documentation of:

NC.1.3.4.1   The initial assessments and reassessments

NC.1.3.4.2   The nursing diagnosis and/or patient care needs

NC.1.3.4.3   The interventions identified to meet the patient's nursing care needs

NC.1.3.4.4   The nursing care provided

NC.1.3.4.5   The patient's response to, and the outcomes of, the care provided

NC.1.3.4.6   The abilities of the patient and/or, as appropriate, his/her significant other(s) to manage continuing care needs after discharge

creditation but also a permanent record of what happens with each client and is a legal requirement, in any health-care setting. In our society, with its many lawsuits and aggressive malpractice emphasis, all aspects of the medical record may be important for legal documentation. The plan of care that has been developed for a particular client serves as a framework or outline for charting administered care. Progress notes and flow sheets therefore reflect implementation of the treatment plan by documenting that appropriate actions have been carried out, precautions taken, etc. Both the implementation of interventions and progress toward the measurable outcomes need to be documented in the progress notes. They should be written in a clear, objective fashion and in a manner that reflects progress toward desired measurable outcomes with the use of planned staff interventions. These notations also need to be date- and time-specific and to be signed by the person making the entry. Any errors in the document must be crossed out with one line so that it is still legible, identified by the author as "error," and then initialed. White-outs or cross-outs that make the information unreadable are not acceptable, because they could be construed to mean that the individual or facility is trying to alter facts.

The medical record is also the primary source of providing proof of services, which is necessary for maintaining revenues. Third-party reimbursers are insistent that the *why, when, where, how, what,* and *who* of services be clearly documented. Absence of such documentation may result in loss of funding for individual clients and termination of funded treatment. Therefore, progress notes must document what is happening to the client during all phases of treatment—acute/inpatient, outpatient, and rehabilitation. It is important to record information and observations that will assist both the oncoming nurse and other health-care providers in maintaining the continuity of planned care. Table 2–4 provides examples of information to be documented in the client's record.

There are several charting formats that are currently used for documentation (e.g., problem-oriented medical record [POMR] and Focus® Charting). Regardless of the form you use, entries should be concise and consistent in style and format to avoid confusion and to comply with existing agency policies and procedures. Examples of documentation formats are included in Chapter 3.

## SUMMARY

The nurse's therapeutic relationship with the client creates a milieu in which the art of nursing can be practiced. As the primary coordinator of overall client care, the nurse strives to ensure that the client receives quality and cost-effective care through the use of the nursing process. Creation of, and effective use of, the client plan of care helps ensure that the psychiatric client receives individualized quality care in the midst of cost containment. The plan of care further serves as the vehicle for, and documentation of, ongoing communication among nurses and those in other disciplines and provides documentation of the impact of nursing on client care. Although nursing diagnosis is an essential component of nursing practice in the acute care setting, the use of nursing diagnosis within the nursing case management delivery system has yet to realize its full potential. Its value will come to be appreciated as the concept of case management evolves and is continually refined. Additionally, other disciplines will come to realize what nursing

## TABLE 2–4. Contents of a Progress Note

- Unsettled or unclear problems or "issues" that need to be dealt with, including attempts to contact other client care providers.
- Noteworthy incidents or interviews involving the client that would benefit from a more detailed recording.
- Other pertinent data such as notes on phone calls, home visits, and family interactions.
- Additional critical incident data such as seemingly significant or revealing statements made by the client, an insight you have into a client's patterns of behavior, client injuries, the use of any special treatment procedure, or other major events such as episodes of pain, respiratory distress, panic attacks, medication reactions, or suicidal comments.
- Administered care, activities, or observations if not recorded elsewhere on flow sheets (e.g., physician visits, completion of ordered tests, PRN medications.)

has discovered: that nursing diagnosis is the key to executing and preserving the independent practice component of nursing.

Given the rapid changes affecting the health-care system, nurses need resources to help them stay current and provide quality care for their clients. This book is designed as a resource to assist the psychiatric nurse in planning and delivering care to the client in the hospital and/or community setting, with consideration of family/significant other(s). The plans of care provided are intended to facilitate the use of the nursing process and identify nursing diagnoses for many of the most common psychiatric conditions the nurse/student deals with in daily practice. Chapter 3 will assist you in applying and adapting theory to practice.

# CHAPTER 3

# APPLYING THEORY TO PRACTICE

Client assessment is the foundation on which identification of individual needs, responses, and problems is based. To facilitate the steps of assessment and diagnosis in the nursing process, a psychiatric assessment tool has been constructed using a nursing focus instead of the familiar medical approach of "review of systems."

To achieve this nursing focus, we have grouped the current NANDA nursing diagnoses into related categories titled Diagnostic Divisions (Table 3–1), which reflect a blending of theories, primarily Maslow's hierarchy of needs and a self-care philosophy. These divisions serve as the framework or outline for collecting data (Table 3–2). The nurse is directed to the appropriate corresponding nursing diagnosis as the client information is recorded.

Since these divisions are based on human responses and needs and not specific "systems," the information gathered may occasionally be recorded in more than one area. For this reason, the nurse is encouraged to keep an open mind, pursue leads, and collect as many of the data as are available before choosing the nursing diagnosis label that best reflects the client's situation. For example, when the nurse identifies the cue of restlessness in a client, the nurse may infer that the client is anxious. The nurse may believe that the restlessness is psychologically based, overlooking the possibility that it is physiologically based. Once the appropriate nursing diagnosis is identified, appropriate goals and interventions can be established.

Recognizing and reflecting on current changes in the delivery and utilization of health care, and realizing that many people may not be seen in the health-care system except when their illness has become exacerbated, this assessment tool is not restricted to "psychiatric" data but includes general health information. Physiologic well-being may affect or be affected by the individual's psychologic state, and baseline information is necessary to assist in recognizing changes that may occur in relation to subsequent therapies or state of wellness.

From the specific data recorded in the database, the related/risk factors (etiology) and signs and symptoms can be identified, and an individualized client diagnostic statement can be formulated using the problem, etiology, signs/symptoms (PES) format to represent the client's situation accurately. The plan-of-care guidelines in this text were developed using the nursing diagnosis labels recommended by NANDA except in a few examples where the authors felt that more clarification and enhancement were required. The ongoing controversy on the validity of the NANDA-approved nursing diagnosis, Knowledge Deficit, is one example where further clarification was added. The term *Learning Need* has been added to the nursing diagnosis Knowledge Deficit. For example, the diagnostic statement may read: "Knowledge Deficit [Learning Need] regarding condition, prognosis, and treatment, related to learned maladaptive coping skills, lack of exposure to/unfamiliarity with information evidenced by questions and expressions of concern." Additionally, some diagnoses have been combined for convenience, indicating that two or more factors may be involved, e.g., Body Image disturbance/Self-Esteem, chronic low. We anticipate that the nurse will choose what is applicable in the individual situation or leave them combined if both diagnoses are indicated because the interventions address both problems.

Desired client outcomes are identified to facilitate choosing appropriate interventions and to serve as evaluators of both nursing care and client response. These outcomes also form the framework for documentation.

## TABLE 3–1. Diagnostic Divisions: Nursing Diagnoses Organized According to Diagnostic Divisions

After data are collected and areas of concern/need identified, the nurse is directed to the Diagnostic Divisions to review the list of nursing diagnoses that fall within the individual categories. This will assist the nurse in choosing the specific diagnostic label to describe the data accurately. Then with the addition of etiology or related/risk factors (when known) and signs and symptoms (defining characteristics), the client diagnostic statement emerges.

**ACTIVITY/REST**—Ability to engage in necessary/desired activities of life (work and leisure) and to obtain sleep/rest

Activity intolerance
Activity intolerance, high risk for
Disuse Syndrome, high risk for
Diversional Activity deficit
Fatigue
Sleep Pattern disturbance

**CIRCULATION**—Ability to transport oxygen and nutrients necessary to meet cellular needs

Cardiac Output, decreased
Dysreflexia
Tissue Perfusion, altered (specify): cerebral, cardiopulmonary, renal, gastrointestinal, peripheral

**EGO INTEGRITY**—Ability to develop and use skills and behaviors to integrate and manage life experiences

Adjustment, impaired
Anxiety [specify level]
Body Image disturbance
Coping, Defensive
Coping Individual, ineffective
Decisional Conflict (specify)
Denial, ineffective
Fear
Grieving, anticipatory
Grieving, dysfunctional
Hopelessness
Personal Identity disturbance
Post-Trauma Response
Powerlessness
Rape-Trauma Syndrome
Rape-Trauma Syndrome: compound reaction
Rape-Trauma Syndrome: silent reaction
Relocation Stress Syndrome
Self-Esteem, chronic low
Self-Esteem disturbance
Self-Esteem, situational low
Spiritual Distress (distress of the human spirit)

**ELIMINATION**—Ability to excrete waste products

Bowel Incontinence
Constipation
Constipation, colonic
Constipation, perceived
Diarrhea
Incontinence, functional
Incontinence, reflex
Incontinence, stress
Incontinence, total
Incontinence, urge
Urinary Elimination, altered
Urinary Retention [acute/chronic]

**FOOD/FLUID**—Ability to maintain intake of and utilize nutrients and liquids to meet physiologic needs

Breastfeeding, effective
Breastfeeding, ineffective
Breastfeeding, interrupted
Fluid Volume deficit [Active loss]
Fluid Volume deficit [Regulatory Failure]
Fluid Volume deficit, high risk for
Fluid Volume excess
Infant Feeding Pattern, ineffective
Nutrition, altered, less than body requirements
Nutrition, altered, more than body requirements
Nutrition, altered, high risk for more than body requirements
Oral Mucous Membrane, altered
Swallowing, impaired

**HYGIENE**—Ability to perform activities of daily living

Self-Care deficit: feeding, bathing/hygiene, dressing/grooming, toileting

**NEUROSENSORY**—Ability to perceive, integrate, and respond to internal and external cues

Peripheral Neurovascular Dysfunction, high risk for
Sensory/Perceptual alterations (specify): visual, auditory, kinesthetic, gustatory, tactile, olfactory
Thought Processes, altered
Unilateral Neglect

**PAIN/DISCOMFORT**—Ability to control internal/external environment to maintain comfort

  Pain [acute]
  Pain, chronic

**RESPIRATION**—Ability to provide and use oxygen to meet physiologic needs

  Airway Clearance, ineffective
  Aspiration, high risk for
  Breathing Pattern, ineffective
  Gas Exchange, impaired
  Spontaneous Ventilation, inability to sustain
  Ventilatory Weaning Response, dysfunctional (DVWR)

**SAFETY**—Ability to provide safe, growth-promoting environment

  Body Temperature, altered, high risk for
  Health Maintenance, altered
  Home Maintenance Management, impaired
  Hyperthermia
  Hypothermia
  Infection, high risk for
  Injury, high risk for
  Physical Mobility, impaired
  Poisoning, high risk for
  Protection, altered
  Self-Mutilation, high risk for
  Skin Integrity, impaired
  Skin Integrity, impaired, high risk for
  Suffocation, high risk for
  Thermoregulation, ineffective
  Tissue Integrity, impaired

Trauma, high risk for
Violence, high risk for, directed at self/others

**SEXUALITY** [Component of Ego Integrity and Social Interaction]—Ability to meet requirements/characteristics of male/female role

  Sexual Dysfunction
  Sexuality Patterns, altered

**SOCIAL INTERACTION**—Ability to establish and maintain relationships

  Caregiver Role Strain
  Caregiver Role Strain, high risk for
  Communication, impaired verbal
  Family Coping, ineffective, compromised
  Family Coping, ineffective, disabling
  Family Coping, potential for growth
  Family Processes, altered
  Parental Role Conflict
  Parenting, altered
  Parenting, altered, high risk for
  Role Performance, altered
  Social Interaction, impaired
  Social Isolation

**TEACHING/LEARNING**—Ability to incorporate and use information to achieve healthy lifestyle/optimal wellness

  Growth and Development, altered
  Health-Seeking Behaviors (specify)
  Knowledge Deficit [Learning Need] (specify)
  Noncompliance [Compliance, altered] (specify)
  Therapeutic Regimen (Individual), ineffective management

# TABLE 3–2. Psychiatric Nursing Assessment Tool

This is a suggested tool for development by an individual or institution to create a database reflecting diagnostic divisions of nursing diagnoses. Although the divisions are alphabetized for ease of presentation, they can be prioritized or rearranged to meet individual needs.

## GENERAL INFORMATION

Name: _____
Age: _____ DOB: _____ Sex: _____ Race: _____
Admission Date: _____ Time: _____ From: _____
Source of Information: _____ Reliability (1–4 with 4 = very reliable): _____

## ACTIVITY/REST:

### Reports (Subjective)

Energy level/pattern: _____
  Fatigue: _____
Occupation: _____
Usual activities/hobbies: _____
Leisure time activities: _____
Exercise program: _____
Feelings of boredom/dissatisfaction: _____
Limitations imposed by condition(s): _____
Sleep: Hours: _____ Naps: _____
Aids: _____ Insomnia: _____
Related to: _____
Nightmares: _____ Orthopnea: _____
Rested upon awakening: _____
Excessive grogginess: _____
Other: _____

### Exhibits (Objective)

Observed response to activity:
  Cardiovascular: _____
  Respiratory: _____
Mental status (e.g., withdrawn/lethargic): _____
Neuro/muscular assessment: _____
  Muscle mass/tone: _____
  Posture: _____ Tremors: _____
  ROM: _____ Strength: _____
  Deformity: _____

## CIRCULATION:

### Reports (Subjective)

History of: Hypertension: _____
  Heart trouble: _____
  Rheumatic fever: _____ Ankle/leg edema: _____
    Phlebitis: _____ Slow healing: _____
    Claudication: _____
  Bleeding tendencies/episodes: _____
Palpitations: _____ Syncope: _____
Extremities: Numbness: _____
Tingling: _____
Cough/hemoptysis: _____
Change in frequency/amount of urine: _____

### Exhibits (Objective)

B/P: R and L: lying/sitting/standing: _____
Pulse pressure: _____ Auscultatory gap: _____
Pulse (palpation): Carotid: _____
  Temporal: _____ Jugular: _____
  Radial: _____ Femoral: _____
  Popliteal: _____ Posttibial: _____
  Dorsalis pedis: _____
Cardiac (palpation): _____
  Thrill: _____ Heaves: _____
Heart sounds: _____ Rate: _____
  Rhythm: _____ Quality: _____
  Friction rub: _____ Murmur: _____
Breath sounds: Vascular bruit: _____
  Jugular vein distention: _____
Extremities: Temperature: _____
  Color: _____ Capillary refill: _____
  Homan's sign: _____ Varicosities: _____
  Nail abnormalities: _____
  Distribution/quality of hair: _____
  Trophic skin changes: _____
  Edema: _____

| Reports (Subjective) | Exhibits (Objective) |
|---|---|
| | Color: Mucous membranes: _____ |
| | Lips: _____ Nail beds: |
| | Conjunctiva: _____ Sclera: |
| | Diaphoresis: _____ |

## EGO INTEGRITY:

| Reports (Subjective) | Exhibits (Objective) |
|---|---|
| What kind of person are you (positive/negative, etc.)? _____ | Emotional status (check those that apply): |
| What do you think of your body? _____ | Calm: _____ Friendly: _____ |
| How would you rate your self-esteem (1–10)? _____ | Cooperative: _____ Evasive: _____ |
| What are your moods? | Anxious: _____ Angry/hostile: _____ |
| Depressed: _____ Guilty: _____ | Withdrawn: _____ Fearful: _____ |
| Unreal: _____ Ups/downs: _____ | Irritable: _____ Restive: _____ |
| Apathetic: _____ Separated from the world: _____ | Passive: _____ Dependent: _____ |
| Detached: _____ | Euphoric: _____ Other (specify): _____ |
| Are you a nervous person? _____ | Observed physiologic response(s): _____ |
| Are your feelings easily hurt? _____ | Defense mechanisms: Projection: _____ |
| Report of stress factors: _____ | Denial: _____ Undoing: _____ |
| Previous patterns of handling stress: _____ | Rationalization: _____ Passive-aggressive: _____ |
| Financial concerns: _____ | Repression: _____ Intellectualization: _____ |
| Relationship status: _____ | Somatization: _____ Regression: _____ |
| Work history/military service: _____ | Identification: _____ Introjection: _____ |
| Cultural factors: _____ | Reaction formation: _____ Isolation: _____ |
| Religion: _____ Practicing: _____ | Displacement: _____ Substitution: _____ |
| Lifestyle: _____ Recent changes: _____ | Consistency of behavior: _____ |
| Feelings of: Helplessness: _____ | Verbal: _____ Nonverbal: _____ |
| Hopelessness: _____ | Characteristics of speech: _____ |
| Powerlessness: _____ | Motor behaviors: _____ Posturing: _____ |
| | Under/overactive: _____ Stereotypic: _____ |

## ELIMINATION:

| Reports (Subjective) | Exhibits (Objective) |
|---|---|
| Usual bowel pattern: _____ | Abdomen: Tender: _____ Soft/firm: _____ |
| Laxative use: _____ Character of stool: _____ | Palpable mass: _____ Size/girth: _____ |
| Last BM: _____ | Bowel sounds: _____ |
| History of bleeding (urine/stool): _____ | Rectal exam: _____ Hemorrhoids: _____ |
| Hemorrhoids: _____ | Bladder palpable: _____ |
| Constipation: _____ Diarrhea: _____ | Overflow voiding: _____ |
| Usual voiding pattern: _____ | CVA tenderness: _____ |
| Incontinence/when: _____ | Stool guaiac: _____ |
| Urgency: _____ Frequency: _____ | |
| Retention: _____ | |
| Character of urine: _____ | |
| Pain/burning/difficulty voiding: _____ | |
| History of kidney/bladder disease: _____ | |
| Diuretic use: _____ | |

*Continued*

# TABLE 3–2. **Psychiatric Nursing Assessment Tool** *(Continued)*

## FOOD/FLUID:

### Reports (Subjective)

Usual diet (type): _____
   Number of meals daily: _____
Last meal/intake: _____
   Dietary pattern/content: _____ Fat intake: _____
Loss of appetite: _____ Nausea/vomiting: _____
Heartburn/indigestion: _____
   Related to: _____ Relieved by: _____

Allergy/food intolerance: _____
Mastication/swallowing problems: _____
   Dentures: _____
Usual weight: _____ Changes in weight: _____
Diuretic use: _____

### Exhibits (Objective)

Current weight: _____ Height: _____
   Body build: _____
Skin turgor: _____
   Mucous membranes moist/dry: _____
Edema: General: _____ Dependent: _____
   Periorbital: _____ Ascites: _____
Halitosis: _____ Condition of teeth/gums: _____
   Appearance of tongue: _____
   Mucous membranes: _____
Jugular vein distention: _____
Thyroid enlarged: _____
Hernia/masses: _____
Bowel sounds: _____
Breath sounds: _____
Urine S/A or Chemstix: _____
Blood glucose level: _____

## HYGIENE:

### Reports (Subjective)

Activities of daily living: _____
   Independent/dependent: _____
   Mobility: _____ Feeding:
   Hygiene: _____ Dressing:
   Toileting: _____
Preferred time of bath: _____
Equipment/prosthetic devices required: _____
   Assistance provided by: _____

### Exhibits (Objective)

General appearance: _____
Manner of dress: _____ Personal habits: _____
   Body odor: _____ Condition of scalp: _____
Presence of vermin: _____

## NEUROSENSORY:

### Reports (Subjective)

Dreamlike states: _____ Walking in sleep: _____
   Automatic writing: _____
Believe/feel you are another person: _____
Reports perception different than others: _____
Fainting spells/dizziness: _____
   Blackouts: _____
Headaches: Pain location: _____
   Frequency: _____
Tingling/numbness/weakness (location): _____
Stroke (residual effects): _____
Ability to follow directions: _____
Perform calculations: _____
Accomplish ADLs: _____
Seizures: _____ Type: _____ Aura: _____
   Frequency: _____
   Postictal state: _____ How controlled: _____
Eyes: Vision loss: _____ Last examination: _____
   Glaucoma: _____ Cataract: _____
Ears: Hearing loss: _____ Last examination: _____

### Exhibits (Objective)

Mental status: _____
   Oriented/disoriented: Time: _____
   Place: _____ Person: _____
Check all that apply:
   Alert: _____ Drowsy: _____
   Lethargic: _____ Stuporous: _____
   Comatose: _____ Cooperative: _____
   Combative: _____ Delusions: _____
   Hallucinations: _____ Affect (describe): _____
Memory: Immediate: _____ Recent: _____
   Remote: _____
Comprehension: _____
Thought processes (assessed through speech):
   Patterns of speech (spontaneous/sudden
      silences): _____ Change in topic: _____
   Content: _____ Delusions: _____
   Hallucinations: _____ Illusions: _____
   Rate or flow: _____ Clear, logical
      progression: _____ Expression: _____

**Reports (Subjective)**

Epistaxis: _____ Sense of smell:

**Exhibits (Objective)**

Mood: _____ Affect: _____
  Appropriateness: _____ Intensity: _____
  Range: _____
Insight: _____
Attention/calculation skills: _____ Judgment:
  Ability to follow directions: _____
  Problem-solving: _____
Glasses: _____ Contacts: _____ Hearing aids: _____
Pupil size/reaction: R/L: _____ Shape: _____
Facial droop: _____ Swallowing: _____
Hand grasp/release, R/L: _____
Posturing: _____ Deep tendon reflexes: _____
  Paralysis: _____

## PAIN/DISCOMFORT:

**Reports (Subjective)**

Location: _____ Intensity (0–10
  with 10 most severe): _____
  Frequency: _____ Quality: _____
  Duration: _____ Radiation: _____
  Precipitating factors: _____
How relieved: _____
Associated symptoms: _____

**Exhibits (Objective)**

Facial grimacing: _____
  Guarding affected area: _____
Emotional response: _____
  Narrowed focus: _____

## RESPIRATION:

**Reports (Subjective)**

Dyspnea: _____ Related to: _____
Cough/sputum: _____
History of Bronchitis: _____
  Asthma: _____ Tuberculosis: _____
  Emphysema: _____ Recurrent pneumonia: _____
  Exposure to noxious fumes: _____
Smoker: _____ Pack/day: _____
  Number of years: _____
Use of respiratory aids: _____
Oxygen: _____

**Exhibits (Objective)**

Respiratory: Rate: _____ Depth: _____
  Symmetry: _____
Use of accessory muscles: _____
  Nasal flaring: _____
Fremitus: _____
Breath sounds: _____
Egophony: _____
Cyanosis: _____
Clubbing of fingers: _____
Sputum characteristics: _____
Mentation/restlessness: _____

## SAFETY:

**Reports (Subjective)**

Allergies/sensitivity: _____
  Reaction: _____
Exposure to infectious diseases: _____
History of sexually transmitted disease
  (date/type): _____
Previous alteration of immune system: _____
  Cause: _____
Blood transfusion/number: _____
  When: _____ Reaction: _____ Describe: _____
High-risk behaviors (work/hobby/sexual): _____
Seat belt/helmet use: _____ _____

**Exhibits (Objective)**

Temperature: _____ Diaphoresis: _____
Skin integrity: _____ Scars: _____ Rashes: _____
  Lesions (describe): _____ Lacerations: _____
  Ulcerations: _____ Ecchymosis: _____
  Blisters: _____ Burns: (degree/percent): _____
  Drainage: _____
General strength: _____ Muscle tone: _____
  Gait: _____ ROM: _____
  Paresthesia/paralysis: _____
Results of cultures: _____
Immune system testing: _____

*Continued*

## TABLE 3–2. Psychiatric Nursing Assessment Tool (Continued)

**SAFETY:**

| Reports (Subjective) | Exhibits (Objective) |
|---|---|
| History of accidental injuries: _____ <br>    Fractures/dislocations: _____ <br>    Arthritis/unstable joints: _____ <br>    Back problems: _____ <br> Changes in moles: _____ Enlarged nodes: _____ <br> Delayed healing: _____ <br> Impaired vision: _____ Hearing: _____ <br> Prosthesis: _____ Ambulatory devices: _____ <br> Expressions of ideation of violence <br>    (self/others): _____ <br> Suicidal plan: _____ Means available: _____ | TB testing: _____ |

**SEXUALITY: [Component of Social Interaction]**

| Reports (Subjective) | Exhibits (Objective) |
|---|---|
| Sexually active: _____ Age: _____ <br>    Use of condoms: _____ <br>    Sexual concerns/difficulties: _____ <br>    Recent change in frequency/interest: _____ <br> Sexual orientation/variant preferences: _____ | Comfort level with subject matter: _____ |

**Female:**

| Reports (Subjective) | Exhibits (Objective) |
|---|---|
| Age at menarche: _____ Length of cycle: _____ <br>    Duration: _____ No. of pads used/day: _____ <br>    Last menstrual period: _____ Menopause: _____ <br>    Vaginal discharge: _____ <br>    Bleeding between periods: _____ <br> Practices breast self-exam: _____ <br> Frequency/last mammogram: _____ <br> Frequency/last PAP smear: _____ | Breast exam: _____ Genital warts/lesions: _____ <br>    Discharge: _____ |

**Male:**

| Reports (Subjective) | Exhibits (Objective) |
|---|---|
| Penile discharge: _____ Prostate disorder: _____ <br>    Circumcised: _____ Vasectomy: _____ <br> Practice self-exam, breast/testicles: _____ <br> Last proctoscopic/prostate exam: _____ | Examination: Breast/penis/testicles: _____ <br>    Genital warts/lesions: _____ Discharge: _____ |

**SOCIAL INTERACTIONS:**

| Reports (Subjective) | Exhibits (Objective) |
|---|---|
| Marital status: _____ Years in relationship: _____ <br>    Living with: _____ Concerns/stresses: _____ <br> Extended family: _____ <br>    Other support person(s): _____ <br>    Role within family structure: _____ <br> Memory of early years: _____ <br> Genogram: _____ <br> Family dynamics: _____ <br> Geographic areas lived in: _____ <br> Performance/interactions: <br>    Work: _____ School: _____ <br> Problems related to illness/condition: _____ | Verbal/nonverbal communication with <br>    family/SO(s): _____ Family interaction <br>    (behavioral) pattern: _____ <br> Speech: Clear: _____ Slurred: _____ <br>    Unintelligible: _____ Aphasic: _____ <br>    Unusual speech pattern/impairment: _____ <br>    Use of speech aids: _____ |

| Reports (Subjective) | Exhibits (Objective) |
|---|---|

Change in speech: _____
    Use of communication aids: _____
    Laryngectomy present: _____

**TEACHING/LEARNING:**

| Reports (Subjective) | Discharge Plan Considerations |
|---|---|

Dominant language (specify): _____
    Literate: _____ Education level: _____
    Learning disabilities (specify): _____
    Cognitive limitations: _____

Employment/education goals: _____
Health beliefs/practices: _____
    Special health-care concerns, e.g., impact of
    religious, cultural practices: _____
Familial risk factors (indicate relationship):
    Diabetes: _____ Thyroid (specify): _____
    Tuberculosis: _____ Heart disease: _____
    Strokes: _____ High B/P: _____
    Neuromuscular conditions:
    Epilepsy: _____ Kidney disease: _____
    Cancer: _____ Mental illness: _____ Other: _____
Prescribed medications: Drug: _____ Dose: _____
    Times: _____ Take regularly: _____
    Purpose: _____
Nonprescription drugs:
    OTC _____ Street _____
    Tobacco: _____ Smokeless tobacco: _____
    Use of alcohol (amount/frequency): _____
Admitting diagnosis per psychiatrist/
    primary therapist: _____
Reason for hospitalization per client: _____
History of current complaint: _____
    Client expectations of this hospitalization: _____
Previous illnesses and/or hospitalizations/
    surgeries: _____
Evidence of failure to improve: _____
Last complete physical exam: _____

**Discharge Plan Considerations**

Date information obtained: _____
Anticipated date of discharge: _____
    Resources available: Persons (specify): _____
    Financial: _____

Anticipated changes in living situation after
    discharge: _____
Areas that may require alteration/assistance:
    Food preparation: _____ Shopping: _____
    Transportation: _____ Ambulation: _____
    Medication: _____ Self-care assistance
    (specify): Wound care: _____
Homemaker/maintenance assistance: _____
Living facility other than home (specify): _____
Vocational rehabilitation: _____
    Interest/abilities: _____ Resources: _____
Community supports: _____ Groups: _____
    Socialization: _____
Referrals: Home care: _____
    Therapy: _____ Social services: _____
Needs: Equipment: _____
    Supplies: _____ Oxygen: _____

---

Interventions are designed to specify the action of the nurse, the client, and/or significant other(s). Interventions need to promote movement toward independence in addition to achieving psychologic/physiologic stability. This requires involvement of the client in his or her own care, including participation in decisions about the care and projected outcomes. In addition, while the individual is the primary client, significant other(s)/family members will also need consideration and inclusion in care. Nurses can be creative as they work with the standardized format presented here, redefining and sharing interventions as they are used with individual clients.

To assist in visualizing this process, a client situation and sample plan of care (Anorexia Nervosa/Bulimia) provides an example of data collection and construction of the plan of care. As the *Client Assessment Database* is reviewed, the nurse can identify the related or risk factors and defining characteristics (signs/symptoms) that were used to formulate the client diagnostic statements. Adding time lines to specific client outcomes reflects anticipated length of stay and individual client and nurse expectations. Interventions have been chosen based on concerns/needs identified by the client and nurse during data collection, as well as the interdisciplinary team. Although not normally in cluded in a plan of care, rationales are included in this sample for the purpose of explaining or clarifying the choice of interventions and enhancing the nurse's learning. Additionally, because the diagnosis of anorexia is an acute problem with predictable outcomes to be achieved within a predetermined time frame (e.g., 28 days), a sample clinical pathway is also provided. Finally, to complete the learning experience, samples of documentation based on the client situation are presented.

# Sample Client Situation: Anorexia Nervosa/ Bulimia Nervosa

MJB, a 33 year-old female, presented at the doctor's office with reports of lightheadedness, fatigue, weakness, and history of eating disorders. She was admitted to the Eating Disorders Program on referral by her family physician for controlled environment and monitoring of physiologic well-being.

## ADMITTING PHYSICIAN'S ORDERS

CBC, electrolytes, blood sugar on admission.
ECG in AM.
Endocrine studies, dexamethasone suppression test (DST) in AM.
Urinalysis in AM.
Regular diet with selective menu; schedule dietary consult.
Weigh on admission and according to protocol.
Trilafon 8 mg/tid.

## CLIENT ASSESSMENT DATA BASE

Name: Mary Jane B.   Age: 33   DOB: Feb. 13, 1959   Sex: F   Race: W   Admission date: 6/23/93   Time: 3:30 PM   From: Home   Source of information: Self-Reliability: 2–3   Family member/Significant other(s): Family not in area, no contact   Friend: Mrs. CP

### Activity/Rest

**Subjective**

Energy level: Low; tires easily but works hard
Fatigue: Always.
Occupation: Receptionist, city
  government office.
Usual activities/Hobbies:
  Volunteers for church, says has lots of
  projects, but can't get them completed,
  would like to learn new vocation.
Leisure time activities: "Not much. I don't
  like to get out with people, and I just
  don't seem to have the energy."
Exercise program: Aerobics sometimes,
  twice a day, 5 days/wk.
Limitations imposed by condition: "Afraid
  people will know about my problem."
Sleep: Not enough, maybe 4–5 hours/night
Insomnia: "I have some problem, usually
  because I don't get to bed." Says this is
  her binge time, finds things to do to
  avoid going to bed.
Not rested on awakening, tired all the time.

**Objective**

Observed response to activity:
  Respiratory: Tachypnea/28.
  Cardiovascular: Elevated pulse/120.
  Mental status: Withdrawn.
  Posture: Sits hunched over, not looking
  up.

### Circulation

**Subjective**

History of: Occasional ankle/leg edema.
Palpitations: Occasional.

**Objective**

B/P: 106/68 lying; 90/63 sitting.
Pulse: 104 at rest.

### Subjective

Syncope: "Fainting spells" several times a week, feels lightheaded/weak.

## Ego Integrity

### Subjective

What kind of person are you? "I'm a nothing, a zero."

What do you think of your body? "I don't like my body, it's too fat." Doesn't do anything where she has to expose her body. Would like to learn massage but doesn't want to have a man touch her body (a requirement of the class is that students practice on one another).

How would you rate your self-esteem (1–10)? "Zero."

What are your moods? Depressed, lonely, feels tense and anxious, empty.

Are you a nervous person? "Yes."

Are your feelings easily hurt? "Yes. I'm afraid I'm a bother to other people. They think I'm not doing a good job."

Report of stress factors: Worries about everything, binge eating, having to deal with people in her job, limited income, no savings/health insurance.

Previous patterns of coping with stress: Previously anorectic, avoided eating, distance running (frequently 10 miles a day); withdrawal (ran away from the hospital last time she was hospitalized).

Financial concerns: Is in a low-paying job, no resources.

Relationship status: Single, has never been married or had a relationship. Says "I don't like men, can't trust them."

Cultural factors: White, middle class.

Lifestyle: Has no home of her own, house-sits for people who are gone, stays with church friends between house-sitting jobs ("helps with the money"). Is alone a lot in this situation.

Significant losses/changes (Date): Left home and moved to another state 10 years ago. Does not have contact with family. Father died 4 years ago; did not see him or return for funeral.

Stage of grief/manifestations of loss: Stated matter-of-factly, "I don't want to have any contact with family. I was glad to get away from them and really don't want to have any contact with them now."

Religion: Catholic. Practicing: Yes.

### Objective

Heart/Breath sounds: Deferred.
Color: Skin, pale.
Conjunctiva/mucous membranes/lips: Pale.

### Objective

Emotional status: Calm, cooperative, fearful, anxious, dependent.

Behavior: Consistent. Verbal responses are congruent. Speech is modulated, congruent; voice low.

Defense mechanisms: Uses rationalization, "I ate lunch, some lettuce and sunflower seeds"; denial, "I'm not a worthwhile person"; and projection, "I don't like the way people act. They lie, cheat, and steal."

Body language: Sitting quietly with head down; looks up occasionally and maintains eye contact when she does; playing with a tissue.

## Elimination

### Subjective

Usual bowel pattern: Irregular, constipation an ongoing problem. Uses an herbal laxative once or twice a week.

Last BM: 2 days ago.

Character: Dry, light-colored.

Usual voiding pattern: No problem, but voiding less frequently (once/twice a day).

Character of urine: Dark yellow.

### Objective

Examinations: Deferred.

## Food/Fluid

### Subjective

Usual diet: Vegetarian, does not eat eggs or chicken. Eats 1 meal a day; no breakfast; snacks on lettuce, nuts, may have tuna for lunch. Afraid to eat for fear she cannot stop. Binges on whatever is available, usually carbohydrates (candy bars, cookies). Drinks occasional glass of water, diet colas (2–3/day)

Usual weight: 130 pounds, no recent weight changes. Weighed 85 pounds when she was hospitalized for anorexia the first time 12 years ago.

Vomiting: Usually once a day, sometimes only 2 or 3 times/wk.

Swallowing problem: Sore mouth and throat frequently.

### Objective

Current weight: 128 pounds   Height: 5 feet 4 inches   Body build: Slight.

Skin turgor: Tight.

Mucous membranes/lips: Dry.

Edema: None.

Halitosis: Sour breath.

Condition of teeth/gums: Tooth decay/ erosion evident, gums inflamed, salivary glands slightly swollen.

Bowel/breath sounds: Deferred.

## Hygiene

### Subjective

Independent in self-care.

### Objective

General appearance: Neatly dressed in boxy-style blue suit; oxford-type shoes, in good condition; dark, short hair curled around face; eye makeup lightly applied; nails well kept, no nail polish; no jewelry noted.

## Neurosensory

### Subjective

Perception different from others: Reports sees self as fat, even though others do not.

Fainting spells/dizziness: Several times a week.

Headaches: Occasionally all over head, 2–3 times/wk last 3 months. Says did not have headaches until recently when vomiting became more frequent.

Ability to follow directions: Concerned because she is not remembering things, being forgetful.

### Objective

Mental status: Alert and oriented to time, place, and person.

Memory: Intact

Intellectual functioning: Testing deferred.

Thought processes: Speech pattern is normal. Thinking seems fairly rational and logical with organized, coherent flow of ideas. Occasional evidence of distorted thinking, e.g., "I'm afraid my electrolytes are out of balance, but I take vitamins every day." Speaks in a quiet voice. Defensive thinking is

| **Subjective** | **Objective** |
|---|---|
| States has a problem concentrating, difficulty making decisions.<br><br>Eyes: No reports of eye strain or change in acuity. Does not wear glasses. | apparent with occasional ideas of reference; "people will say I'm weird if they find out about me."<br>Mood: Depressed, fearful, consistent, verbalizes feelings appropriate to the situation.<br>Affect: Behavior is consistent with expression of feelings.<br>Insight: Demonstrates some awareness of extent of condition, "I think my electrolytes are out of balance." Verbalizes awareness of not being sure she wants to give up behavior: "What will I have if I don't binge/purge anymore?" States it makes her feel, knows she is alive, in control. |

## Pain

| **Subjective** | **Objective** |
|---|---|
| No reports of pain at present, has headaches occasionally. | None noted. |

## Respiratory

| **Subjective** | **Objective** |
|---|---|
| Respiratory rate: 28 with activity/22 at rest.<br>Dyspnea related to: Exertion.<br>Does not smoke. No cough except with colds. | Breath sounds: deferred. |

## Safety

| **Subjective** | **Objective** |
|---|---|
| No history of accidents/injuries.<br>No known allergies.<br>States has frequent colds every few months.<br>Notes accidental injuries (e.g.,cut finger chopping celery), slow to heal.<br>Expressions of ideation of violence (self/others): Has suicidal thoughts occasionally, recognizes behavior as suicidal. No specific plan. | Temperature: 99.4 PO.<br>Hands dry/flaky.<br>Exam of skin: deferred.<br>No physical evidence of self-harm. |

## Sexuality

| **Subjective** | **Objective** |
|---|---|
| Is not sexually involved with anyone, states she is a virgin and does not use birth control.<br>Age at menarche: 12 years.<br>Length of cycle: Irregular.<br>Duration: 2 days.<br>Last menstrual period: 2 months ago.<br>Breast self-exam: No.<br>Routine PAP smear: No, refuses gynecologic exams. | Deferred. |

## Social Interactions

### Subjective

Memory of early years: Father alcoholic, mother rejecting person who often told the children she wished she had not gotten married or had children. Physical abuse common in the family. Reports father occasionally "belted" mother (struck her with open hand), children were frequently beaten when they had displeased parents/done something wrong.

Marital status: Single. Living with church friends, house-sitting.

Genogram: Deferred.

Family dynamics: Mother was angry with father most of the time. Sister and brother are 2 and 5 years younger, says felt responsible for them when they were little, grew apart as she became older. Has not had contact with them in past 10 years.

Extended family: None.

Other support persons: Employer; church friends, including Mr. and Mrs. S, an older couple she describes as surrogate parents.

Role within family structure: Oldest child with younger sister and brother.

Performance/interaction—work: Excellent job ratings, states she is a perfectionist.

Talks with coworkers but not about self/personal issues. Rarely socializes with coworkers.

Report of problems: Says feels lonely, does not have friends, knows she has to stop the binging/vomiting cycle. Does not trust people. Does have limited relationship with church friends, does not want them to know about her problem.

Coping behaviors: Preoccupation with food and compulsive need to binge/purge, withdrawal from interaction with others.

Frequency of social contacts (others than work): None other than church, attends mass once or twice a week.

### Objective

Not observed with family/significant other(s).

## Teaching/Learning

### Subjective

Dominant language: English.

Education Level: HS, graduated from business program, secretarial.

### Discharge Considerations

Date data obtained: 6/23.

Anticipated date of discharge: 7/21 (28 days).

Resources available: Persons: Employer

## Subjective

Learning disabilities/Cognitive limitations: Not aware of any.

Employment/Education goals: Wants a job with less public contact, no specific plan.

Health beliefs/practices: Vegetarian. Believes if she eats something, cannot stop. Believes if she eats sugar, her body craves it and she will just keep on eating.

Familial risk factors: Father died of stroke, age 67; maternal grandmother had a bad heart. Not aware of any other significant family history, although mother was not well.

Prescribed medications: None.

Nonprescription drugs: Does not take any OTC or illicit drugs. Takes an herbal laxative once or twice a week. Takes vitamins because "I know I don't eat right."

Use of alcohol: None.

Admitting diagnosis (psychiatrist): Anorexia/bulimia.

Reason for hospitalization (client): "To get my electrolytes under control."

History of current complaint: Long-standing eating problems (20 years), anorectic as an adolescent, binging and purging for last 10 years.

Client expectations of this hospitalization: "I want to begin to feel good about myself and my work, spiritually, mentally, and physically."

Previous hospitalization: Hospitalized twice 10 and 12 years ago. Ran away from the hospital the last time and moved to another state.

Evidence of failure to improve: Physical: Having blackouts, fainting spells, says electrolytes are out of balance.

Mental: States has difficulty thinking, relaxing, complains of inferiority feelings.

Date of last physical exam: 1987.

## Discharge Considerations

and church friends. Financial: Has job (not doing what she was trained to do), which employer will hold for her.

Anticipated changes in living after discharge: None, at the moment. Would like to get own place as soon as feasible.

Living facility other than home: Would like to continue to house-sit, helps financially.

Community supports: Church.

Socialization: No social activities.

# Sample Plan of Care: Anorexia Nervosa/ Bulimia Nervosa

## NURSING PRIORITIES

1. Reestablish adequate/appropriate nutritional intake.
2. Correct fluid and electrolyte imbalance.
3. Assist MJB to develop realistic body image/improve self-esteem.
4. Encourage identification and expression of feelings, especially anger.
5. Coordinate total treatment program with other disciplines.
6. Provide information about disease, prognosis, and treatment to MJB/significant other(s).

## DISCHARGE GOALS (ANTICIPATED LENGTH OF STAY: 28 DAYS)

1. Adequate nutrition and fluid intake maintained.
2. Maladaptive coping behaviors and stressors that precipitate anxiety recognized.
3. Adaptive coping strategies and techniques for anxiety reduction and self-control implemented.
4. Self-esteem increased.

| CLIENT DIAGNOSTIC STATEMENT: | NUTRITION, ALTERED, LESS THAN BODY REQUIREMENTS |
| --- | --- |
| **Related To:** | Inadequate food intake and self-induced vomiting. |
| **Evidenced By:** | Pale conjunctiva and mucous membranes, poor skin turgor, inflamed gums, tooth decay/erosion, slightly swollen salivary glands, reports of sore mouth/throat. |
| **Desired Outcomes/Evaluation Criteria— MJB Will:** | Establish a dietary pattern with caloric intake adequate to maintain appropriate weight within 72 hours (6/26 4 PM). |
| | Verbalize/demonstrate understanding of nutritional needs within 2 weeks (7/7 9 PM). |
| | Select and consume appropriate foods for healthy diet 80% of the time within 3 weeks (7/14 9 AM). |
| | Maintain weight between 125 and 135 pounds throughout program (ongoing). |

| ACTIONS/INTERVENTIONS | RATIONALE |
| --- | --- |
| Establish a minimum weight goal to be maintained. (6/24 Client conference: minimum goal 125 pounds.) | When this is agreed on, psychologic work can begin. Malnutrition is a mood-altering condition leading to depression and agitation so that adequate nutrition is important for psychologic well-being. |
| Maintain a regular weighing schedule, M-W-F immediately on arising and following first voiding in same attire, and graph results. | Provides accurate ongoing record of weight loss and/or gain. Also diminishes obsession about gains and/or losses. |

| ACTIONS/INTERVENTIONS | RATIONALE |
|---|---|
| Provide selective menu and review MJB's choices. | Client needs to gain confidence in self and feel in control of environment. More likely to eat preferred foods but may require guidance to make healthy choices. |
| Be alert to choices of low-calorie foods; hoarding food; disposing of food in various places such as pockets or wastebaskets. | Client may try to avoid taking in what she views as excessive calories. |
| Provide dietary information per teaching plan. | Understanding nutritional needs, clarifying misconceptions may enhance client's willingness to choose a more balanced diet. |
| Use a consistent approach. Present and remove food without persuasion and/or comment. Sit with MJB while eating (30 minutes maximum), also without comment. | Client detects urgency and reacts to pressure. When staff responds in a consistent manner, client can begin to trust her responses. Avoids manipulative games. Any comment that might be seen as coercion provides focus on food. Client may experience guilt if forced to eat. The one area in which she has exercised power and control is food/eating. Structuring meals and decreasing discussions about food will decrease power struggles with client. |
| Provide 1:1 supervision. Have MJB remain in the room with no bathroom privileges for 1 hour following eating or involve in group program as scheduled. | Prevents vomiting during/after eating. Note: Sometimes clients desire food and use a binge-purge syndrome to maintain weight. Purging may occur for the first time in a client as a response to establishment of weight program. |
| Avoid room checks and control devices. | Reinforces feelings of powerlessness and are usually not helpful. |
| Establish controlled exercise program with MJB, discussing likes and dislikes, e.g., walking, aerobics, swimming. | A gradually increasing exercise program can help client begin to improve muscle tone and control weight in a more satisfactory manner. MJB's excessive exercising has been counterproductive to her overall well-being. |
| Monitor exercise program and set limits on physical activities. Chart activity/level of work (pacing, etc.). | Client may exercise excessively to burn calories. |
| Provide regular diet and snacks with substitutes and preferred foods available. | Having a variety of foods available will enable client to have a choice of potentially enjoyable foods/may enhance intake. |
| Carry out program of behavior modification. Involve MJB in setting up program. Provide reward for maintaining weight, ignore gain/loss. | Provides structured eating situation while allowing client some control in choices. Note: Behavior modification may be effective only in mild cases or for short-term weight maintenance. |
| Avoid giving laxatives. Encourage use of bran or provide Metamucil as indicated. | Use of laxatives is counterproductive as they may be used by client to rid body of food/calories. May require short-term use of Metamucil initially to assist with the management of constipation. |
| Schedule dietary consultation. | Helpful in establishing individual dietary needs/program and provides educational opportunity. |

## ACTIONS/INTERVENTIONS

Administer perphenazine (Trilafon) 8 mg tid
(8 AM, 2 and 10 PM).

Review laboratory studies, e.g., blood sugar, CBC,
endocrine studies.

## RATIONALE

Antipsychotic drug that blocks postsynaptic
dopamine receptors in the brain. Given to manage
underlying pathology, e.g., depression/anxiety.

Provides information about dietary status/needs/
effectiveness of therapy.

---

| CLIENT DIAGNOSTIC STATEMENT: | FLUID VOLUME DEFICIT, active loss |
|---|---|
| Related To: | Inadequate intake of food and liquids, consistent self-induced vomiting |
| Evidenced By: | Dry skin/mucous membranes, decreased skin turgor, increased pulse rate (104), body temperature (99.4°F), orthostatic hypotension (90/63), concentrated urine/decreased urine output, change in mental state (states she is flaky, forgets things she ought to remember). |
| Desired Outcomes/Evaluation Criteria— MJB Will: | Report fluid intake of 2000 ml/day with increased urine output within 36 hours (6/25 8 AM). |
| | Demonstrate improvement in vital signs, skin turgor, and moisture of mucous membranes within 72 hours (6/26 4 PM). |
| | Verbalize understanding of causative factors and behaviors necessary to correct fluid deficit within 1 week (6/30 9 AM). |

---

## ACTIONS/INTERVENTIONS

Discuss strategies to stop vomiting, e.g., saying
positive affirmation of "I can stop vomiting,"
talking to friend/therapist, use of imagery/relaxation.

Have MJB measure urine output accurately each day.

Monitor amount and types of fluid intake. Be
aware of use of caffeinated beverages and diet
soft drink intake.

Monitor vital signs per protocol, capillary refill,
and dizziness. Recommend rising slowly, sitting,
then standing.

Note reports of muscle pain/cramps, generalized
weakness, paresthesia, nausea.

Discuss actions necessary to regain optimal fluid
balance, e.g., drinking a glass of fluid every 2 hours.
Encourage use of calorie-containing beverages
as well as water.

## RATIONALE

Helping the client to deal with anxiety feelings that
lead to vomiting and supporting decision to stop will
prevent continued fluid loss.

Reduced urinary output may be a direct result of
reduced food/fluid intake and continued vomiting.

Increased intake of diet pop results in adequate
output, even though there is no protein/calorie
intake. Caffeine can promote output, negatively
affecting fluid balance.

Orthostatic hypotension can occur with fluid deficit.

Signs of potassium deficit and may reflect inadequate
intake, starvation state, deficit from self-induced
vomiting.

Involving client in plan to correct fluid imbalances
may enhance success and provide sense of control
over what is happening to her.

37

| ACTIONS/INTERVENTIONS | RATIONALE |
| --- | --- |
| Review laboratory studies, e.g., electrolytes, CBC, urinalysis. | Syndrome may result in electrolyte imbalances, hemoconcentration. |

| **CLIENT DIAGNOSTIC STATEMENT:** | **THOUGHT PROCESSES, ALTERED** |
| --- | --- |
| **Related To:** | Malnutrition/electrolyte imbalance, psychologic conflicts, e.g., sense of low self-worth, perceived lack of control |
| **Evidenced By:** | Impaired ability to make decisions, problem-solve, non–reality based verbalizations ("I need to lose 30 pounds"; "I ate a lot of food today, sesame seeds and lettuce"); ideas of reference (says people think she is not doing a good job); altered attention span, distractibility, delay in seeking health care, does not perceive personal relevance of symptoms/danger of behavior. |
| **Desired Outcomes/Evaluation Criteria— MJB Will:** | Verbalize awareness and understanding of relationship of lack of food intake to problems of concentration and decision-making within 48 hours (6/25 4 PM). |
| | Demonstrate improved ability to make decisions, problem-solve, and memory of daily/recent events within 3 weeks (7/14 9 AM). |
| | Acknowledge reality of situation that eating behaviors are maladaptive within 3 weeks (7/14 9 AM). |
| | Verbalize ways to gain control in life situation within 4 weeks (7/21 9 AM). |
| | Decrease use of manipulative behaviors in interactions with others within 4 weeks (7/21 9 AM). |

| ACTIONS/INTERVENTIONS | RATIONALE |
| --- | --- |
| Establish a therapeutic nurse/MJB relationship. | Within a helping relationship, the client can begin to trust and try out new thinking and behaviors. |
| Be aware of MJB's distorted thinking ability. | Allows the caregiver to lower expectations and provide information and support appropriate to MJB's needs/abilities. |
| Listen to and do not challenge irrational, illogical thinking. Present reality concisely and briefly. | It is not possible to respond logically when thinking ability is physiologically impaired. The client needs to hear reality, but challenging leads to distrust and frustration. |
| Encourage strict adherence to nutrition regimen. | Improved nutrition is essential to improved brain functioning. |
| State limits matter-of-factly. Avoid arguing/bargaining. | Client who denies reality of the situation often uses manipulation to achieve control. Consistency and firmness of staff help decrease use of these behaviors. |

| CLIENT DIAGNOSTIC STATEMENT: | BODY IMAGE DISTURBANCE/SELF-ESTEEM, CHRONIC LOW |
|---|---|
| **Related To:** | Morbid fear of obesity; perceived loss of control in some aspect of life (e.g., ability to interact satisfactorily with others, eating); unmet dependency needs; dysfunctional family system |
| **Evidenced By:** | Distorted body image, view of self as fat, even in the presence of normal body weight (states needs to lose 30 pounds); expresses concern, uses denial as a defense mechanism, and feels powerless to prevent binge/purging and make changes in her life; perceptual disturbances with failure to recognize hunger; reports of fatigue, anxiety, and depression. |
| **Desired Outcomes/Evaluation Criteria— MJB Will:** | Identify/be involved in other life interests within 1 week (6/30 9 AM). |
| | Identify individual assets/strengths, accept compliments within 2 weeks (7/7 9 AM). |
| | Verbalize a more realistic body image within 3 weeks (7/14 9 AM). |
| | Acknowledge self as an individual who has responsibility for own actions and voluntarily stops binging and purging by the end of the 4-week program (7/21 9 AM). |
| | Recognize reality of areas of life where she has control within 4 weeks (7/21 9 AM). |

| ACTIONS/INTERVENTIONS | RATIONALE |
|---|---|
| Identify individual strengths and reflect positives noted without moral judgment. Encourage MJB to recognize positive characteristics related to self. | Promotes self-concept. Individual often sees self as weak-willed, even though a part of the person may feel a sense of power and control. Discussion of positive aspects of the self-system, such as social skills, work abilities, education, talents, and appearance, can reinforce client's feelings of being a worthwhile/competent person. |
| Explore MJB's expectation of self regarding need to "be perfect." | Recognizing unrealistic expectations may enhance ability to accept self as fallible. |
| State rules regarding weighing schedule, remain in sight during medication and eating times, and make known the consequences of not following the rules. Be consistent in carrying out rules, without undue comment. | Client is obsessed with fear of weight gain. Regular monitoring of client's weight is important to nutritional status. Consistency is important in establishing trust. As part of the behavior modification program, the client knows the risks involved in not following established rules (e.g., decrease in privileges). Failure to do so is viewed as the client's choice and accepted by the staff in matter-of-fact manner so as not to provide reinforcement for the undesirable behavior. |

| ACTIONS/INTERVENTIONS | RATIONALE |
|---|---|
| Respond (confront) with reality when MJB makes unrealistic statements, such as, "I've stopped vomiting so there's nothing really wrong with me." | Provides constructive feedback about how improving nutrition will give her energy to look at other aspects of her life so that food will not be so all-consuming. Individual needs to be confronted because she denies the psychologic aspects of her situation and often expresses a sense of inadequacy and depression. |
| Be aware of own reaction to MJB's behavior. Avoid arguing. | Feelings of disgust, hostility, and fury are not uncommon when caring for these clients. Prognosis remains poor even with stabilization of weight, as other problems may remain. Many continue to see themselves as fat, and there is also a high incidence of affective disorders, social phobias, obsessive-compulsive symptoms, substance abuse, and psychosexual dysfunction. The nurse needs to deal with own response/feelings so they do not interfere with care of the client. |
| Assist MJB to assume control in areas other than dieting/weight loss, e.g., management of own daily activities, work/leisure choices. | Feelings of personal ineffectiveness, low self-esteem, and perfectionism are often part of the problem. Client feels helpless to change and requires assistance to problem-solve methods of control in life situations. |
| Help MJB formulate goals for self not related to eating, e.g., choice of a satisfying vocation/avocation, and formulate a manageable plan to reach those goals, 1 at a time, on a short-/long-term basis. | Client needs to recognize ability to control other areas in life and may need to learn problem-solving skills in order to achieve this control. Client may not know how to set realistic goals, and choices may be influenced by altered thought processes. |
| Assist MJB to confront sexual fears. Provide sex education as necessary. | Major physical/psychologic changes in adolescence can contribute to development of this problem. Feelings of powerlessness and loss of control of feelings, particularly sexual feelings, sensations, and physical development lead to an unconscious desire to desexualize self. Client often believes that these fears can be overcome by taking control of bodily appearance/development/function. |
| Encourage MJB to take charge of own life in a more healthful way by making own decisions and accepting self as is. Encourage acceptance of inadequacies as well as strengths. Let MJB know that it is acceptable to be different from family, particularly mother. | Client often does not know what she may want for self. Parents (mother) made decisions for her. Client also believes she has to be the best in everything and holds self responsible for being perfect. She needs to develop a sense of control in other ways, besides dieting and weight loss. |
| Involve in personal development program. | Learning about proper application of makeup and methods of enhancing personal appearance may be helpful to long-range sense of self-esteem. |
| Use interpersonal psychotherapy rather than interpretive therapy. | More helpful for the client to discover feelings/impulses/needs from within own self. Client has not learned this internal control as a child. |
| Encourage MJB to express anger and acknowledge when it is verbalized. | Important to know that anger is part of self and as such is acceptable. Expressing anger may need to |

| ACTIONS/INTERVENTIONS | RATIONALE |
|---|---|
| | be taught to client, as anger is generally considered unacceptable in the family and therefore client does not express it. |
| Assist MJB to learn strategies other than eating for dealing with feelings. Have MJB keep a diary of feelings, particularly when thinking about food. | Feelings are the underlying issue, and clients often use food instead of dealing with feelings appropriately. May need to learn to recognize feelings and how to express them. |
| Assess feelings of helplessness/hopelessness. | 54% of clients with anorexia have a history of major affective disorder; 33% have a history of minor affective disorder. |
| Be alert to suicidal ideation/behavior. | Intensity of anxiety/panic about weight gain, depression, hopeless feelings may lead to suicidal attempts, particularly if client is impulsive. |
| Involve in group therapy daily to include Goals group and creative, occupational, and recreational sessions per protocol. | Provides an opportunity to talk about feelings and try out new behaviors. |

| CLIENT DIAGNOSTIC STATEMENT: | KNOWLEDGE DEFICIT [LEARNING NEED] regarding condition, prognosis, therapy needs |
|---|---|
| Related To: | Learned maladaptive coping skills; lack of exposure to/unfamiliarity with new information |
| Evidenced By: | Verbalization of misconception of relationship of behaviors (preoccupation with extreme fear of obesity and distortion of own body image; refusal to eat, binging, and purging; and current hospitalization), request for new information, and expressions of desire to learn more adaptive ways of coping with stressors. |
| Desired Outcomes/Evaluation Criteria— MJB Will: | Identify relationship of signs/symptoms (e.g., weight loss, tooth decay, skin problems) to behaviors of not eating or binge-purging within 3 days (6/26 4 PM). |
| | Verbalize awareness of and plans for lifestyle changes to maintain normal weight without aberrant eating pattern within 2 weeks (7/7 9 AM). |
| | Assume responsibility for own learning within 2 weeks (7/7 9 AM). |
| | Verbalize intention to attend community support group within 4 weeks (7/21 9 AM). |

| ACTIONS/INTERVENTIONS | RATIONALE |
|---|---|
| Orient to unit. Discuss rules/behavior modification program, involving MJB in establishing parameters. | Helps allay anxiety. Client involvement in establishing treatment program increases likelihood of success. |

| ACTIONS/INTERVENTIONS | RATIONALE |
|---|---|
| Determine level of knowledge and readiness to learn. | Learning is easier when it begins where the learner is. |
| Note blocks to learning, e.g., physical/intellectual/ emotional. | Malnutrition, family problems, affective disorders, and obsessive-compulsive symptoms can interfere with learning. |
| Review dietary needs, answering questions as indicated. | May need assistance with planning for new way of eating. |
| Encourage MJB to keep a diary of feelings, especially when thinking about food. | Provides avenue for client to identify feelings associated with maladaptive behaviors. Promotes discussion of more appropriate coping methods. |
| Provide information about and encourage the use of relaxation and other stress-management techniques. | New ways of coping with feelings of anxiety and fear will help client to manage these feelings in more effective ways, assisting in giving up maladaptive behaviors of not eating/binging-purging. |
| Assist with establishing a sensible exercise program. Caution regarding overexercise. | Exercise can assist with developing a positive body image and combat depression. |
| Review appropriate skin care needs. Encourage bathing every other day. Use skin cream twice a day and after bathing; massage skin, especially over bony prominences. Observe for reddened/ blanched areas. | Frequent baths contribute to dryness of the skin. Supplemental lubrication of the skin decreases itching/flaking and reduces potential for breakdown. Massage improves circulation to the skin and skin tone. Involves client in monitoring and intervening in own therapy. |
| Discuss importance of adequate nutrition/fluid intake. | Improved nutrition will improve skin and oral condition, maintain electrolyte balance, and help clear thought processes. |
| Provide written information for MJB. | Helpful as reminder of and reinforcement for learning. |
| Encourage MJB to ask friends and coworkers to provide support for necessary changes. | Can serve as a support system to help client make necessary lifestyle changes. |
| Refer for dental consult/care. | Purging behavior (stomach acids) has damaged gum tissues and tooth enamel. |
| Refer to National Association of Anorexia Nervosa and Associated Disorders. | May be helpful source of support and information for client and significant other(s). |

# Sample Clinical Pathway of Care For MJB

Estimated Length of Stay: 28 days—Variations from Designated Pathway Should Be Documented in Progress Notes

| Nursing Diagnoses and Categories of Care | Time Dimension | Goals and/or Actions | Time Dimension | Goals and/or Actions | Time Dimension | Discharge Outcome |
|---|---|---|---|---|---|---|
| Altered nutrition: Less than body requires Fluid volume deficit | Ongoing | Client will establish adequate dietary pattern and maintain adequate state of hydration | | | Day 28 | Patient will exhibit no signs/symptoms of malnutrition or dehydration |
| Referrals | Day 1 and ongoing | Consult dietitian | Days 2–28 | Fulfill nutritional needs. Client will consume 80% of food provided and at least 2000 ml fluid/day | | |
| Diagnostic studies | Day 1 | Electrolytes Electrocardiogram Blood urea nitrogen/ creatine Urinalysis Complete blood count Thyroid function | Day 14 | Repeat of selected diagnostic studies | Day 28 | All laboratory values are within normal limits |
| Additional assessments | Daily; every shift | Vital signs | Day 3 | Vital signs within normal limits Appropriate balance is achieved | Days 22–28 | Client will refrain from self-induced vomiting and binging |
| | Daily; every shift | Input and output | | | | |
| | Day 1 | Weight | Days 2–28 | Client will maintain weight between 125 and 135 pounds | | |

*Continued*

# Sample Clinical Pathway of Care For MJB *(Continued)*

| Nursing Diagnoses and Categories of Care | Time Dimension | Goals and/or Actions | Time Dimension | Goals and/or Actions | Time Dimension | Discharge Outcome |
|---|---|---|---|---|---|---|
| | Day 1 | Monitor for purging following meals | Days 1–21 | Client bathroom is locked for 1 hour following meals | | |
| Patient education | Day 1 | Unit orientation; behavior modification plan | Days 7–14 | Principles of nutrition; foods for maintenance of wellness | Days 15–18 | Client will demonstrate ability to select appropriate foods for healthy diet 80% of time |
| Altered Thought Processes | Day 1 | Client will cooperate with orientation to unit and explanation of behavior modification plan | Days 2–28 | Client will cooperate with therapy to restore nutritional status; verbalizes understanding of relationship between nutritional status and thought processes | Days 18–28 | Client will acknowledge that eating behaviors are maladaptive and demonstrate improved ability to make decisions, problem-solve |
| Referrals | Day 7 (or when physical condition is stable) | Psychologist, social worker, psychodramatist | Days 8–28 | Client will attend group psychotherapies daily | Day 28 | Client will verbalize ways to gain control in life situation |
| Additional assessments | Days 1–17 | Assess client's ability to trust; set limits on manipulative behavior | Day 14 | Client will develop trusting relationship with at least one staff member each shift | Day 28 | Client will demonstrate decreased use of manipulation in interactions with others |
| Patient education | Day 1 and ongoing as required | Describe privileges and responsibilities of | Day 21 | Discuss role of support groups for individuals | Day 28 | Client and family will verbalize intention to |

| | | | | | | |
|---|---|---|---|---|---|---|
| | | behavior modification program; explain consequences of noncompliance | | with eating disorders | | attend community support group |
| Body Image/Self-Esteem chronic low | Day 7 | Client will acknowledge that attention will not be given to the discussion of body image and food, shift focus to other life interests | Days 14–21 | Client will acknowledge misperception of body image as fat and verbalize positive self-attributes | Day 28 | Client will verbalize more realistic body image and recognize areas of control within own life |
| Referrals | Day 1 (or when physical condition is stable) | Occupational therapy, recreational therapy, music | Days 2–28 | Client attends therapy sessions on a daily basis | Day 28 | Through self-expression, client has gained self-awareness, verbalizes positive attributes of self |
| Additional assessments | Day 7 | Compare specific measurements of client's body with client's perceived calculations; clarify discrepancies | Days 8–28 | Discuss strengths and weaknesses; client will strive to achieve self-acceptance | Day 28 | Client will verbalize acceptance of self, including "imperfections" |
| Patient education | Days 7–14 | Client will verbalize plans for lifestyle changes and assume responsibility for own learning | Days 14–28 | Discuss alternative coping strategies for dealing with feelings; have client keep diary of feelings, particularly when thinking about food | Day 28 | Client will demonstrate adaptive coping strategies unrelated to eating behaviors dealing with feelings |

## DOCUMENTATION AND EVALUATION

As nursing care is provided, ongoing assessments determine the client's response to therapy and progress toward accomplishing the desired outcomes. This activity serves as the feedback and control part of the nursing process, through which the status of the individual client diagnostic statement is judged to be resolved, continuing, or requiring revision.

This process is visualized in Figure 3–1. Discussion with MJB reveals she has reviewed dietary materials and completed the posttest (9 of 10 correct). She displays increased understanding of general dietary needs and is ready to progress to focusing on her individual needs as outlined in the

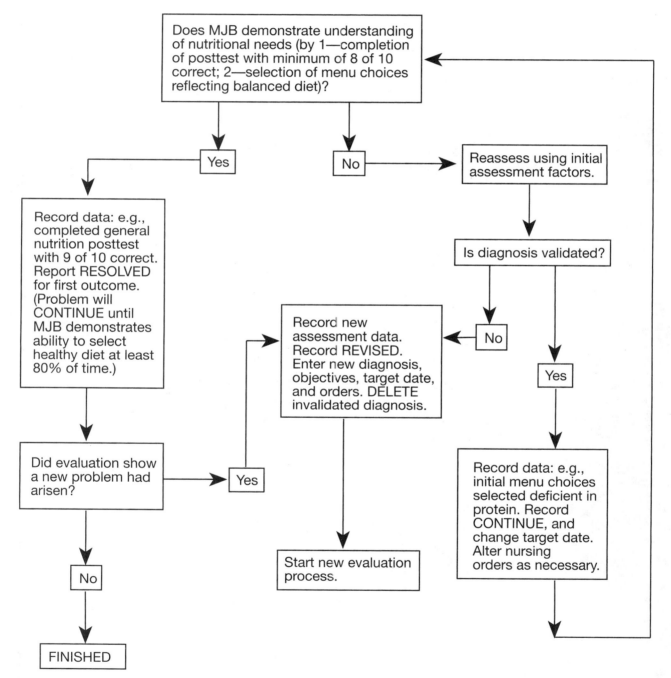

**Figure 3–1.** Outcome-based evaluation of the client's response to therapy. (Adapted from Cox, et al: Clinical Applications of Nursing Diagnosis: Adult, Child, Women's, Mental Health, Gerontic, and Home Health Considerations, ed 2. FA Favis, Philadelphia, 1993, p 544.)

plan of care. No revision in the treatment plan is required at this time.

There are several charting formats that have been used for documentation. These include block notes, with a single entry covering an entire shift (e.g., 7–3 PM); narrative timed notes (e.g., 9:30 AM, participated in group activity); and the problem-oriented record (POR) using the SOAP/SOAPIER approach, to name a few. The latter can provide thorough documentation, but it was designed by physicians for episodic care and requires that the entries be tied to a client problem identified from a problem list.

A new system format created by nurses for documentation of frequent/repetitive care is FOCUS® Charting. It was designed to encourage looking at the client from a positive rather than a negative (or problem-oriented) perspective by using precise documentation to record the nursing process. Recording of assessment, interventions, and evaluation information in a data, action, and response (DAR) format facilitates tracking and following what is happening to the client at any given moment. Charting focuses on client and nursing concerns. The focal point is client status and the associated nursing care. The focus is always stated in a way that reflects the *client's* concern/need rather than reflecting a nursing task or medical diagnosis.

Thus, the focus can be a client problem/concern or nursing diagnosis, signs/symptoms of potential importance (e.g., fever, blood pressure fluctuations), a significant event (e.g., use of "time out," seclusion, or application of restraints), a change in status, or specific standards of care/hospital policy. Based on the client situation of MJB, Table 3–3 provides examples of documentation.

## TABLE 3–3. Comparison of SOAP and FOCUS® Charting Formats Documenting Specific Client Situation

**SOAP/SOAPIER FORMAT**

| Problem-Oriented Charting | What Is Recorded | Nursing Process |
|---|---|---|
| S and O (Subjective and objective data) | Verbal reports to, and direct observation and examination by, the nurse | Assessment |
| A (Assessment) | Nurse's interpretation of S and O | Analysis |
| P (Plan) omitted in charting if written plan describes care to be given | Description of appropriate nursing actions to resolve the identified problem | Planning |
| I (Intervention) | Description of nursing actions actually carried out | Implementation |
| E (Evaluation) | A reassessment of the situation to determine results of nursing actions implemented | Evaluation |
| R (Revision) | Reflects change of plan of care to meet current needs | Planning |

| Date | Time | Number/Problem | Progress Note |
|---|---|---|---|
| 6/24/93 | 0900 | #4 (Self-Esteem) | S: "I see myself as a 'zero.' I'm not able to control my eating."<br>O: Sitting in group (3 members), shoulders hunched, looking down, fidgeting with hands.<br>A: Believes she is unable to control maladaptive eating behavior.<br>P: dentify individual strengths and encourage her to recognize positive characteristics related to self.<br>I: Have MJB start a list noting individual strengths, talents, abilities. List should be reviewed daily. Attend and participate in recreational/occupational therapy activities.<br>Signed: M Davis, RN |

*Continued*

## TABLE 3-3. Comparison of SOAP and FOCUS® Charting Formats Documenting Specific Client Situation *(Continued)*

| Date | Time | Focus | Progress Note |
|---|---|---|---|
| 7/6/93 | 1800 | #1 (Nutrition) | S: "I've seen the dietitian 3 times now and reviewed the material she gave me. I've finished this quiz and think I did well."<br>O: Appears tentative, slight smile, fidgeting with pencil. Postquiz, 9 out of 10 correct.<br>A: Following through with assignments. Displaying improved knowledge regarding dietary needs and achievement of outcome #2.<br>P: Continue teaching plan as outlined.<br>I: Select menu choices for next day, review with MJB.<br>E: Choices meet dietary guidelines formulated with dietician regarding fruits, vegetables, and grains. Protein deficiency noted. MJB added ½ cup 1% milk for breakfast and peanut butter with graham crackers for HS snack.<br>    Signed: M Sickus, RN |

**FORMAT**

| FOCUS®/Charting | What Is Recorded | Nursing Process |
|---|---|---|
| Focus | A nursing diagnosis: current client concern or behavior; significant change in client status; significant event in the client's therapy | Analysis of data |
| D (Data) | Information that supports the stated focus or describes pertinent observations about the client | Assessment |
| A (Action) | Immediate or future nursing actions that address the focus; evaluation of the plan of care along with any changes required | Plan/Implementation |
| R (Response) | Description of client responses to care provided | Evaluation |

| Date | Time | Focus | Progress Note |
|---|---|---|---|
| 7/6/93 | 1800 | Nutrition | D: Completed 3 sessions with dietician and posttest. Tentatively stated "Think I did well" while fidgeting with pencil.<br>A: Test reviewed, 9 of 10 correct. Applied learning to select individual menu choices for next day.<br>R: Choices met dietary guidelines formulated with dietician except for protein. MJB added ½ cup 1% milk to breakfast and peanut butter to HS snack of graham crackers. Demonstrated achievement of outcome #2.<br>    Signed: B Briner, RN |

The following is an example of documentation of a client need/concern that currently does not require identification as a client problem (nursing diagnosis) or inclusion in the plan of care and therefore is not easily documented in the SOAP format:

| Date | Time | Focus | Progress Note |
|---|---|---|---|
| 6/27/93 | 1920 | Gastric distress | D: Reports "indigestion/burning sensation" with hand over epigastric area. Skin warm/dry, color pink, vital signs unchanged. Noted she ate broccoli for dinner. |
| | | | A: Given Mylanta 30 ml PO. Head of bed elevated approximately 15 degrees. |
| | | | R: Reports pain relieved. Appears relaxed, resting quietly. |
| | | | B Briner, RN |

# CHAPTER 4

## CHILDHOOD AND ADOLESCENT DISORDERS

### PERVASIVE DEVELOPMENTAL DISORDERS: Autistic Disorder, Pervasive Developmental Disorder, and Childhood Disintegrative Disorder

#### DSM IV
299.00  Autistic Disorder
299.10  Childhood Disintegrative Disorder
299.80  Pervasive Developmental Disorder NOS (including Atypical Autism)

#### DSM III-R
299.00  Autistic Disorder (specify if childhood onset)
299.80  Pervasive Developmental Disorder NOS

### ETIOLOGIC THEORIES

#### Psychodynamics

The autistic child is described as fixed in the presymbiotic stage of development. These children do not achieve a symbiotic attachment, nor do they differentiate self from mother. Psychotic-like behaviors are based on abnormal primary development rather than on a regression from a higher level of functioning. Children with atypical development do not function beyond a primitive psychotic level of comprehension. They do not communicate or form relationships with others.

#### Biologic

It has been hypothesized that this severe psychiatric disorder of childhood is the result of a disturbance in central nervous system integration and in the biologic process of maturation. Predisposing organic factors that have been associated with this disorder are maternal rubella, phenylketonuria, encephalitis, meningitis, and tuberous sclerosis.

#### Family Dynamics

This disorder has been viewed in the past as a result of a severe disturbance in parent-child interaction. Lack of bonding and stimulation as well as maternal deprivation have been listed as causative factors. More recently, dysfunctional parenting has been seen less as contributing to the disorder and more as a response to the disturbed behavior.

## CLIENT ASSESSMENT DATABASE

### Activity/Rest

Problems in sleeping.

### Ego Integrity

Detached, separated from work, withdrawn, restive, may be passive.
Verbal/nonverbal communication may be incongruent.
Demonstrates repetitive stereotypical motor behaviors (hand flicking, head banging, complex whole-body movements).

### Elimination

Disturbances in bowel and bladder functioning.

### Food/Fluid

Disturbed eating patterns.

### Hygiene

Generally dependent.

### Neurosensory

Abnormalities may be noted in almost every sphere of development.
Delayed motor, perceptual, cognitive, and language development.
Soft neurologic signs are often seen, e.g., slight tremors, slowed responses.
Varied/bizarre responses to the environment with resistance or extreme behavioral reactions to minor occurrences, ritualistic behaviors. Extreme fascination with moving objects, special interest in music.
Alterations in mood.
Unreasonable insistence on following routines in precise detail; marked distress over changes in trivial aspects of environment.
Difficulty communicating verbally, with delays in/no development of speech; incorrect use of words, echolalia, inability to abstract terms.
May show periods of extreme agitation in which behavior becomes disruptive and unmanageable.
Does not initiate social imitative play appropriate for stage of development.

### Safety

Self-mutilative behaviors, e.g., head banging, hair pulling, may be noted.
Lack of appropriate fear/ignoring signs of danger, e.g., running into street with heavy traffic.

### Social Interactions

Poor eye contact, impaired responsiveness/communication when interacting with others.
Severely disturbed/impaired development in social relationships (characteristic of this disorder).
Marked impairment in use of nonverbal gestures associated with social interactions.
Lack of social or emotional reciprocity, does not express pleasure toward or in response to other people's happiness; indifference or aversion to physical contact.

### Teaching/Learning

High association with mental retardation.
Onset during infancy or early childhood before age 3 (autism), marked regression following at least 2 years of apparently normal development, and before age 10 (disintegrative disorder) predominantly males.

## DIAGNOSTIC STUDIES

Neurologic examination to determine presence and/or extent of organic impairment.

**BEAM/PET Scans:** May reveal abnormalities in cerebellum (regulates motion and some aspects of memory) and the limbic region (controls much of emotional life).

**EEG:** May be abnormal, reflecting presence/extent of organic impairment.

**Psychologic Testing/IQ:** Provides information about cognitive and personality functioning; IQ below 70 may be noted.

**Biochemical Studies:** Abnormalities have not been consistently noted.

**Laboratory Tests:** As indicated by antipsychotic drug therapy.

**Hearing Testing:** To rule out deafness as a cause of speech problems.

**Vision Testing:** To differentiate responses to auditory and visual stimuli as abnormal reactions versus distorted perceptions.

**Developmental Testing, e.g., Denver Developmental:** May reveal delays.

Determine physical causes for disturbances in age-appropriate functions and behaviors, e.g., toileting problems.

## NURSING PRIORITIES

1. Facilitate control/decrease of behavioral symptoms.
2. Enhance communication skills and social interaction.
3. Promote family involvement in treatment process and acceptance of child's disability.

## DISCHARGE GOALS

1. Current behavior problems or troublesome symptoms for which treatment is being sought are alleviated.
2. Treatment within the community is maintained, institutionalization is avoided, when possible.
3. Family verbalizes knowledge about resources to meet the need for a long-term structured therapeutic program.

| **NURSING DIAGNOSIS:** | **SOCIAL INTERACTION, IMPAIRED** |
|---|---|
| **May Be Related To:** | Disturbance in self-concept, lack of bonding and development of trust; inadequate sensory stimulation or abnormal response to sensory input, organic brain dysfunction. |
| **Possibly Evidenced By:** | Lack of responsiveness to others, lack of eye contact or facial responsiveness; treating persons as objects, lack of awareness of feelings in others; indifference or aversion to comfort, affection, or physical contact; failure to develop cooperative social play and peer friendships in childhood. |
| **Desired Outcomes/Evaluation Criteria— Client Will:** | Increase periods of eye contact. |
| | Tolerate short periods of physical contact with another person. |
| | Initiate interactions between self and others. |

| ACTIONS/INTERVENTIONS | RATIONALE |
|---|---|

### Independent

Assign limited number of caregivers to child.

Consistent approach by familiar persons increases chances for establishing trust.

Convey manner of warmth, acceptance, and availability.

These characteristics encourage nonthreatening interaction.

Have personal items (favorite toy, blanket) available and use in interactions as appropriate.

These items can provide sense of security when child feels distressed.

Reinforce eye contact with something acceptable to the child (food, object). Eventually replace with social reinforcement.

Establishing eye contact is essential to interventions for other symptoms.

Gradually increase proximity and planned intrusion into child's isolation, e.g., touch, smiling, hugging.

Client will likely feel threatened by onslaught of unaccustomed stimuli. Caregivers need to initiate interaction as avenue toward social response.

Be available as support during child's attempts to interact with others.

Presence of a trusted person provides a feeling of security.

Give careful directions, maintain reliable, consistent rules of behavior and constant checks on reality of child's thoughts and perceptions.

Provides structure to help child maintain control/ follow program. Feedback helps child differentiate between fantasy and reality.

Organize and plan time carefully. Manage tasks so child makes as few mistakes and suffers as few disappointments as possible.

Promotes successful experiences and encourages repetition of desired behaviors.

### Collaborative

Work with others who are involved, e.g., teachers, to maintain a structured environment.

Coordinated, consistent efforts are effective for helping the child to learn new behaviors.

Maintain contact with social services caseworker and involve in team conferences.

Provides continuity of care when child/family is involved with social services system.

---

| **NURSING DIAGNOSIS:** | **COMMUNICATION, IMPAIRED, VERBAL** |
|---|---|
| **May Be Related To:** | Inability to trust others. |
| | Withdrawal into self. |
| | Organic brain dysfunction. |
| | Inadequate sensory stimulation. |
| | Maternal deprivation. |
| **Possibly Evidenced By:** | Lack of interactive communication mode; does not use gestures or spoken language. |
| | Absent or abnormal nonverbal communication; lack of eye contact or facial expression. |
| | Peculiar patterns in form, content, or speech production, if speech is present. |
| | Impaired ability to initiate or sustain conversation despite adequate speech. |

| Desired Outcomes/Evaluation Criteria—Client Will: | Use sounds, words, or gestures in an interactive way with others.

Communicate needs/desires to significant others/caregivers.

Initiate verbal or nonverbal interaction with others. |
| --- | --- |

| ACTIONS/INTERVENTIONS | RATIONALE |
| --- | --- |

### Independent

| | |
| --- | --- |
| Maintain consistency in caregivers assigned to child. | Familiarity helps child to develop trust and caregivers to learn ways child attempts to communicate. |
| Anticipate and fulfill needs until communication can be established. | Reduces frustration while child is learning communication skills. Some therapists believe this process should be limited in order to force verbal requests for wants beyond basic needs. |
| Assess previously used words or sounds. Seek validation and clarification in order to decode communication attempts. | Facilitates recognition of speech efforts. These techniques are useful in determining accuracy of messages received. |
| Use face-to-face (eye-to-eye) approach to convey correct nonverbal expressions by example. | Expresses genuine interest in, and respect for, client. |
| Reinforce eye contact with something acceptable to the child, e.g., food, object. | Eye contact is essential to capture child's attention to successfully initiate conversation. |
| Repeat and reinforce approximations of sounds or words whenever used (shaping). | Response gives child information about the caregiver's expectations and may encourage attempts to communicate. |
| Teach deaf sign language as alternate communication tool for children with minimal language development. | Signing may produce less anxiety than verbal expression for some children. |

### Collaborative

| | |
| --- | --- |
| Refer for assessment and testing in cooperation with special education teachers and speech pathologists. | Provides for treatment planning with appropriate specialized interventions/techniques. |

| NURSING DIAGNOSIS:

Risk Factors May Include: | SELF-MUTILATION, HIGH RISK FOR

Organic brain dysfunction.

Inability to trust others.

Disturbance in self-concept.

Inadequate sensory stimulation or abnormal response to sensory input.

History of physical, emotional, or sexual abuse.

Response to demands of therapy, realization of severity of condition. |
| --- | --- |

| | |
|---|---|
| | History of self-injury/destructive behavior. |
| | Indifference to environment or marked distress over changes in environment. |
| **Possibly Evidenced By:** | [Not applicable; presence of signs and symptoms establishes an **actual** diagnosis]. |
| **Desired Outcomes/Evaluation Criteria— Client Will:** | Recognize angry feelings and underlying anxiety. |
| | Decrease incidence of self-mutilating behaviors by x times per day. |
| | Demonstrate alternative behavior (e.g., initiate interaction between self and nurse) in response to anxiety. |

| ACTIONS/INTERVENTIONS | RATIONALE |
|---|---|
| **Independent** | |
| Note prior history of violent behaviors and relationship to anxiety or stressful events. Identify events or stimuli that precipitate self-mutilating behavior, and intervene before these occur. | Useful in determining patterns and predicting and controlling violent behavior. Self-harm may be prevented if causes can be determined and averted. Note: May be first priority if this behavior is a prominent symptom. |
| Reinforce acceptable behavior; provide other satisfying activities (e.g., rocking, swinging, clapping hands to music). | Diversion or replacement activities may become substitutes for self-harm/destructive behaviors. |
| Apply protective devices (e.g., helmet, padded arm covers, bandages over sores or scabs). | Provides protection when potential for self-harm is present. |
| Stay with child during times of increasing anxiety. | Helps maintain feelings of trust and security, reducing frequency/severity of destructive behaviors. |
| Avoid physical restraint if possible, but hold child until agitation subsides as necessary. | Restriction of movement may increase anxiety. Protection from self-harm is essential for safety. Note: Some therapists advocate use of aversive conditioning to eliminate life-threatening behaviors. |
| **Collaborative** | |
| Administer antipsychotic medications or lithium as indicated. | May exert symptomatic control of agitated behaviors. Note: Current research indicates that medication may not extinguish behaviors and is not really helpful to change. |

| | |
|---|---|
| **NURSING DIAGNOSIS:** | **PERSONAL IDENTITY DISTURBANCE** |
| **May Be Related To:** | Organic brain dysfunction. |
| | Lack of development of trust. |
| | Maternal deprivation. |
| | Fixation at presymbiotic phase of development. |

| | |
|---|---|
| **Possibly Evidenced By:** | Lack of awareness of the feelings or existence of others. |
| | Increased anxiety resulting from physical contact with others. |
| | Absent or impaired imitation of others; repeats what others say. |
| | Persistent preoccupation with parts of objects; obsessive attachment to objects. |
| | Marked distress over changes in environment. |
| | Severe panic reactions to everyday events. |
| | Autoerotic, ritualistic behaviors; self-touching, rocking, swaying. |
| **Desired Outcomes/Evaluation Criteria— Client Will:** | Show signs of developing awareness of self as separate from others and environment (e.g., discontinuing echolalia, knows body boundaries). |
| | Tolerate separations and environmental changes without undue anxiety. |

| ACTIONS/INTERVENTIONS | RATIONALE |
|---|---|
| **Independent** | |
| Use positive reinforcement to encourage eye contact. | Eye contact focuses child on the recognition of another person. |
| Assist child in learning to name own body parts. Provide mirrors and pictures for self-identification. | This activity may increase awareness of self as separate from others. |
| Encourage appropriate exploratory touching of others and touching by caregivers. | If done gradually, child can feel the differences between self and others without excessive anxiety. |
| Encourage self-care activities that differentiate child from environment (self-feeding, washing, dressing, etc.). Divide activity into individual actions or steps and reinforce completion of each step. | Activities may help child to identify body boundaries. Reinforcement encourages learning. Behavior-modification techniques provide framework for learning. |

| | |
|---|---|
| **NURSING DIAGNOSIS:** | **FAMILY COPING, ineffective: compromised/disabling** |
| **May Be Related To:** | Family members unable to express feelings related to having a severely disturbed child. |
| | Excessive guilt, anger, or blaming among family members regarding child's condition. |
| | Ambivalent or dissonant family relationships; disagreements regarding treatment, coping strategies. |
| | Prolonged coping with problem exhausts supportive ability of family members. |

| | |
|---|---|
| **Possibly Evidenced By:** | Denial of existence or severity of disturbed behaviors. |
| | Preoccupation with personal emotional reaction to situation (anger, guilt). |
| | Persistent lack of acceptance of chronic nature of child's disorder; rationalization that problem is developmental and will eventually be outgrown. |
| | Attempts to intervene with child are achieving increasingly ineffective results. |
| | Withdraws from or becomes overly protective of child. |
| **Desired Outcomes/Evaluation Criteria—Family Will:** | Verbalize knowledge and appropriate understanding of child's disorder. |
| | Express feelings appropriately with decreased defensive behavior (denial, projection, rationalization). |
| | Demonstrate more consistent, effective methods of coping with child's behavior. |
| | Seek outside therapeutic support as needed. |

| ACTIONS/INTERVENTIONS | RATIONALE |
|---|---|
| **Independent** | |
| Meet regularly with family members to discuss feelings and attitudes. | Supportive counseling can help family members express feelings, explore own reactions to child's disorder. |
| Assess underlying circumstances that may be contributing to ineffective family coping (e.g., financial problems, health of other members, needs of other children). | Identification of stressors may help parents sort out feelings related to child and other issues. |
| Assist family to develop new methods for dealing with the child's behaviors. Reinforce effective parenting methods. (Refer to CP: Parenting.) | Effective intervention skills can assist family to regain self-esteem and control of their environment. |
| **Collaborative** | |
| Refer to other resources as necessary, e.g., psychotherapy, financial aid, respite care, clergy, support groups (National Society for Autistic Children). | Developing a support system can sustain family coping skills and integrity. |
| Encourage parental involvement in training program to serve as cotherapists as appropriate. | Promotes greater involvement and continuation of therapeutic milieu on a full-time basis. Allows for ongoing monitoring of therapy and child's development. |

# DISRUPTIVE BEHAVIOR DISORDERS:
## Attention-Deficit/Hyperactivity Disorders

### DSM IV
**ATTENTION-DEFICIT/HYPERACTIVITY DISORDER**
314.00 AD/HD Predominantly inattentive type
314.01 AD/HD Predominantly hyperactive-impulsive type
314.01 AD/HD Combined type
314.9 Attention-Deficit/Hyperactivity Disorder NOS (For other listings, consult DSM IV manual.)

### DSM III-R
314.01 Attention-Deficit Hyperactivity Disorder

Inattentive, impulsive, and hyperactive (ADHD) behavior that is maladaptive and inconsistent with developmental level. This behavior creates clinically significant impairment in social/academic functioning.

## ETIOLOGIC THEORIES
### Psychodynamics

The child with this disorder has impaired ego development. Ego development is retarded and impulsive behavior manifested represents id impulses unchecked, as in severe temper tantrums. Repeated performance failure, failure to attend to social cues, and limited impulse control reinforce low self-esteem. Some theories suggest that the child is fixed in the symbiotic phase of development and has not differentiated self from mother.

### Genetic/Biologic

The disorder may be gender-linked, since the incidence is higher in boys than in girls (3:1). ADHD is also more prevalent among children whose siblings have been diagnosed. Recent studies have established that the fathers of hyperactive children are more likely to be alcoholic or to have antisocial personality disorders. Studies have shown the presence of subtle chromosomal changes and mild neurologic deficits. Hyperactivity may result from Fetal Alcohol Syndrome, congenital infections, and brain damage resulting from birth trauma or hypoxia. Cognitive distractibility and impulsivity are associated with other disorders involving brain damage or dysfunction, such as mental retardation, seizure disorder, and brain lesions.

Physiologic conditions that can mimic the symptoms include constipation, hypoglycemia, lead toxicity, and thyroid and other metabolic diseases.

### Family Dynamics

This theory suggests that disruptive behavior is learned as a means for a child to gain adult attention. It is likely that whether or not the impulsive irritability seen in attention-deficit hyperactivity disorder was present from birth, some parental reactions tend to reinforce and thus maintain or increase its intensity. Anxiety generated by a dysfunctional family system, marital problems, etc., could also contribute to symptoms of this disorder. Parents become frustrated with the child's poor response to limit setting. Parenting interventions become overly sensitive or the reverse, with no external structure provided.

## CLIENT ASSESSMENT DATABASE
### Activity/Rest

Very active. "Always on the move," does not slow down when should/must.
Difficulty playing or engaging in leisure activities quietly.

## Ego Integrity

Emotional lability, hot temper, mood changes.

## Hygiene

Forgetful in daily activities.

## Neurosensory

Reports from parents and teachers of:
Being easily distracted, unable to sustain attention in order to remain on task or complete projects.
Having difficulty sitting still, sometimes physically overactive, fidgets with hands/feet, and may engage in disruptive behavior or dangerous activities without considering the consequences.
May have difficulty following instructions, organizing tasks/activities.

## Social Interactions

Reports that individuals do not seem to listen to what is being said to them.
Significant distress or impairment in social, academic, or occupational functioning.

## Teaching/Learning

Onset before age 7 (ADHD).
Family history of alcohol abuse.

## DIAGNOSTIC STUDIES

**Thyroid Studies:** May reveal hyper/hypothyroid conditions contributing to problems.
**Neurologic Testing, e.g., EEG, CT Scan:** Determines presence of organic brain disorders.
**Psychologic Testing as Indicated:** Rules out anxiety disorders; identifies gifted, borderline retarded, or learning disabled child; and assesses social responsiveness and language development.
Individual diagnostic studies dependent on presence of physical symptoms, e.g., rashes, upper respiratory illness, or other allergic symptoms, CNS infection (cerebritis).

## NURSING PRIORITIES

1. Facilitate child's achievement of more consistent behavioral self-control and improvement in self-esteem.
2. Promote parents' development of effective means of coping with and interventions for their child's behavioral symptoms.
3. Participate in the development of a comprehensive, ongoing treatment approach using family and community resources.

## DISCHARGE GOALS

1. Disruptive and/or dangerous behavior minimized or eliminated.
2. Child is able to function in a structured learning environment.
3. Parents have gained or regained the ability to cope with internal feelings and to intervene effectively with their child's behavioral problems.

**NURSING DIAGNOSIS:**

**COPING, INDIVIDUAL, INEFFECTIVE/COPING, DEFENSIVE**

**May Be Related To:**

Situational or maturational crisis; denial of obvious problems.

Mild neurologic deficits/retardation.

Retarded ego development; low self-esteem.

Projection of blame/responsibility; rationalization of failure.

Dysfunctional family system, negative role models; abuse/neglect.

**Possibly Evidenced By:**

Easily distracted by extraneous stimuli; shifts from one uncompleted activity to another; difficulty reality-testing perceptions.

Unable to meet age-appropriate role expectations.

Excessive motor activity; cannot sit still.

Unable to delay gratification.

Manipulation of others in environment for purpose of fulfilling own desires.

**Desired Outcomes/Evaluation Criteria— Client Will:**

Demonstrate a decrease in disruptive behaviors, expressing anger in socially acceptable manner.

Show improvements in attention span, concentration, and appropriate activity level.

Delay gratification without resorting to manipulation of others.

| ACTIONS/INTERVENTIONS | RATIONALE |
| --- | --- |

### Independent

| | |
| --- | --- |
| Provide quiet atmosphere; decrease amount of external stimuli. Maintain atmosphere of calm. | Reduction in environmental stimulation may decrease distractibility. Calm approach helps prevent transmission of anxiety between individuals. |
| Provide area and activities for gross motor movement, e.g., gym and/or outdoor area for running, large balls, climbing equipment. | Appropriate outlets are necessary to discharge motor activity. |
| Reinforce attending, concentrating, and completing tasks. | Desired behaviors will increase with positive reinforcement. |
| Set limits on disruptive behaviors (e.g., talking incessantly); suggest alternative competing behaviors such as playing quietly. | Child needs to know expectations and to learn competing acceptable behaviors, e.g., raising hand vs. shouting out, keeping hands to self vs. pushing others. |
| Encourage discussion of angry feelings and identity of true object of the hostility. | Dealing with the feelings honestly and directly helps discourage displacement of the anger onto others. |

| ACTIONS/INTERVENTIONS | RATIONALE |
|---|---|

### Independent

Explore alternative ways for handling frustration with client.

Promotes learning how to interact in society with others in more productive ways.

Provide positive feedback for trying new coping strategies.

Supports efforts and encourages use of acceptable behaviors.

Evaluate with client the effectiveness of new behaviors. Discuss modifications for improvement.

As client has limited problem-solving skills, assistance may be required to reassess and develop strategies.

Assist client to recognize signs of escalating anxiety. Explore ways client can intervene before behavior becomes disabling.

Helps client to recognize ineffective behaviors and develop new coping skills to effect positive change.

### Collaborative

Administer medication as indicated, e.g.,
Methylphenidate (Ritalin),
Imipramine (Tofranil),
Pemoline (Cylert),
Dextroamphetamine (Dexedrine);

Psychostimulants and antidepressants have been shown to improve attention and reduce impulsiveness in hyperactive children.

Diazepam (Valium),
Chlordiazepoxide (Librium),
Alprazolam (Xanax).

Antianxiety medications provide relief from immobilizing effects of anxiety, facilitating cooperation with therapy.

Investigate alternative treatments, e.g., diet, allergy.

Some children respond favorably to control of refined sugar, food dyes, and allergens.

| NURSING DIAGNOSIS: | SOCIAL INTERACTION, IMPAIRED |
|---|---|
| **May Be Related To:** | Retarded ego development; low self-esteem. |
| | Dysfunctional family system, negative role models; abuse/neglect. |
| | Neurologic impairment; mental retardation. |
| **Possibly Evidenced By:** | Discomfort in social situations. |
| | Difficulty waiting turn in games or group situations. |
| | Does not seem to listen to what is being said. |
| | Difficulty playing quietly, maintaining attention to task or play activity; often shifts from one activity to another. |
| | Interrupts or intrudes on others. |
| **Desired Outcomes/Evaluation Criteria— Client Will:** | Identify feelings that lead to poor social interactions. |
| | Participate appropriately in interactive play with another child or group of children. |
| | Develop a mutual relationship with another child or adult. |

| ACTIONS/INTERVENTIONS | RATIONALE |
|---|---|

### Independent

Develop trust relationship with child, show acceptance of child separate from unacceptable behavior.

Acceptance and trust encourage feelings of self-worth.

Encourage client to verbalize feelings of inadequacy and need for acceptance from others. Discuss how these feelings affect relationships by provoking defensive behaviors such as blaming and manipulating others.

Recognition of problem is first step toward resolution.

Offer positive reinforcement for appropriate social interaction. Ignore ineffective methods of relating to others; teach competing behaviors.

Behavior modification can be an effective method of reducing disruptive behaviors in children by encouraging repetition of desirable behaviors. Attention to unacceptable behavior may actually reinforce it.

Identify situations that provoke defensiveness and role-play more appropriate responses.

Provides confidence to deal with difficult situations when they occur.

Provide opportunities for group interaction and encourage a positive and negative peer feedback system.

Appropriate social behavior is often learned from age-mates.

### Collaborative

Arrange staffings with other professionals, e.g., social workers, teachers. Include parents and child when possible.

Cooperation and coordination among those working with these children will enhance the treatment program. Including the child and parents provides them with understanding of the total problem and proposed treatment program.

---

**NURSING DIAGNOSIS:**

**May Be Related To:**

**SELF-ESTEEM (specify)**

Retarded ego development.

Lack of positive feedback with repeated negative feedback.

Dysfunctional family system; abuse/neglect; negative role models.

Mild neurologic deficits.

**Possibly Evidenced By:**

Lack of eye contact.

Derogatory remarks about self.

Lack of self-confidence; hesitance to try new tasks.

Engagement in physically dangerous activity.

Distraction of others to cover up own deficits or failures, e.g., acting the clown.

Projection of blame/responsibility for problems; rationalization of personal failures, grandiosity.

| Desired Outcomes/Evaluation Criteria— Client Will: | Verbalize increasingly positive self-regard. |
| --- | --- |
| | Demonstrate beginning awareness and control of own behavior. |
| | Participate in new activities without extreme fear of failure. |

| ACTIONS/INTERVENTIONS | RATIONALE |
| --- | --- |
| **Independent** | |
| Convey acceptance and unconditional positive regard. | May help child to increase own sense of self-worth. |
| Assist child to identify basic ego strengths/positive aspects of self; give immediate feedback for acceptable behavior. | Focusing on positive aspects of personality may help improve self-concept. Positive reinforcement enhances self-esteem and increases desired behavior. |
| Spend time with client in 1:1 and group activities. | Conveys to client that you believe she or he is worthy of time and attention. |
| Provide opportunities for success; plan activities with short time span and appropriate ability level. | Repeated successes can help to improve self-esteem. |
| Discuss fears, encourage involvement of new activities/tasks. | Confronting concerns and engaging in new tasks promote personal growth and new skills. |
| Help client set realistic, concrete goals and determine appropriate actions to meet these goals. | Provides a structure to develop sense of hope for the future and framework for reaching desired goals. |
| **Collaborative** | |
| Provide learning opportunities, structured learning environment, e.g., self-contained classroom, individually planned educational program. | Successful school performance is essential to preserve a child's positive self-image. |

| NURSING DIAGNOSIS: | FAMILY COPING, ineffective: compromised/disabling |
| --- | --- |
| **May Be Related To:** | Excessive guilt, anger, or blaming among family members regarding child's behavior. |
| | Parental inconsistencies; disagreements regarding discipline, limit setting, and approaches. |
| | Exhaustion of parental resources due to prolonged coping with disruptive child. |
| **Possibly Evidenced By:** | Unrealistic parental expectations. |
| | Rejection or overprotection of child. |
| | Exaggerated expressions of anger, disappointment, or despair regarding child's behavior or ability to improve or change. |

| Desired Outcomes/Evaluation Criteria— Parent(s) Will: | Demonstrate more consistent, effective intervention methods in response to child's behavior. |
| --- | --- |
| | Express and resolve negative attitudes toward child. |
| | Identify and use support systems as needed. |

| ACTIONS/INTERVENTIONS | RATIONALE |
| --- | --- |

### Independent

| | |
| --- | --- |
| Provide information and materials related to child's disorder and effective parenting techniques. (Refer to CP: Parenting.) | Appropriate knowledge and skills may increase parental effectiveness. |
| Encourage parents to verbalize feelings and explore alternative methods of dealing with child. | Supportive counseling can assist parents in developing coping strategies. |
| Provide feedback and reinforce effective parenting methods. | Positive reinforcement can increase self-esteem and encourage continued efforts. |
| Involve siblings in family discussions and planning for more effective family interactions. | Family problems affect all members, and treatment is more effective when everyone is involved in therapy. |

### Collaborative

| | |
| --- | --- |
| Refer to community resources as indicated, e.g., psychotherapy, parent support groups, parenting classes (Parent Effectiveness). | Developing a support system can increase parental confidence and effectiveness. |

| NURSING DIAGNOSIS: | KNOWLEDGE DEFICIT [LEARNING NEED] regarding condition, prognosis, and treatment needs |
| --- | --- |
| May Be Related To: | Lack of knowledge; misinformation/misinterpretation. |
| | Mild neurologic deficits; associated developmental learning disabilities; inability to concentrate; cognitive deficits. |
| Possibly Evidenced By: | Verbalization of problem/misconceptions. |
| | Poor school performance; purposefully losing necessary articles to complete schoolwork, e.g., homework assignments, pencils, books. |
| | Shifting from one uncompleted activity to another. |
| | Unrealistic expectation of medication management. |
| Desired Outcomes/Evaluation Criteria— Client/Parent Will: | Verbalize understanding of reasons for behavioral problems, treatment needs within developmental ability. |

| Client Will: | Participate in learning and begin to ask questions and seek information.<br><br>Achieve cognitive goals consistent with level of temperament. |
| --- | --- |

| ACTIONS/INTERVENTIONS | RATIONALE |
| --- | --- |

## Independent

| | |
| --- | --- |
| Provide quiet environment, self-contained classrooms, small-group activities. Avoid overstimulating places, such as school bus, busy cafeteria, crowded hallways. | Reduction in environmental stimulation may decrease distractibility. Small groups may enhance ability to stay on task and help client learn appropriate interaction with others and avoiding sense of isolation. |
| Give instructional material in written and verbal form with step-by-step explanations. | Sequential learning skills will be enhanced. |
| Instruct child in problem-solving skills, practice situational examples. | Effective skills may increase performance levels. |
| Educate child and family on the use of psychostimulants and behavioral response anticipated. | Use of psychostimulants may not result in improved school grades without accompanying changes in child's study skills. |
| Coordinate overall treatment plan with schools, collateral personnel, the child, and the family. | Cognitive effectiveness will most likely be advanced when treatment is not fragmented, nor significant interventions missed because of lack of interdisciplinary communication. |

# DISRUPTIVE BEHAVIOR DISORDERS:
## Conduct Disorder

### DSM IV
312.8 Conduct Disorder

### DSM III-R
309.40 Adjustment Disorder with mixed disturbance of emotions and conduct (formerly Adolescent Adjustment Disorder)
312.90 Conduct Disorder

## ETIOLOGIC THEORIES
### Psychodynamics

According to psychoanalytic theory, these children are fixed in the separation-individuation phase of development. Ego development is retarded, and id behavior is prominent. The mother figure views separation/individuation as a "demand on her." The child incorporates an "overidealized" image of mother to compensate for her narcissistic need for gratification. There is a failure to build up identification, which is the core of a strong, sufficient superego.

### Biologic

Differences in temperament of infants at birth have been observed in relation to attention span, excitability, and adaptability. Correlations between these findings and the development of behavioral disorders in adolescence remain uncertain. Heredity also influences such traits as the tendency to seek risks or obey authority. One possibility is the biologic influence of high testosterone and heightened arousal of the central nervous system.

Current research suggests that negative experiences in infancy cause biologic and neurologic damage to the brain tissue itself. When persistent stress results in a constant state of perceived danger, the "fight-or-flight" hormones, adrenaline and cortisol, are constantly present, causing neurologic damage to the brain cells. These damaged brain cells react in unusual ways to stimuli, possibly resulting in epileptic seizures or depression. These children are often labeled as "behavior problems," and involvement with the legal system may be the precipitating factor that brings client into therapy.

### Family Dynamics

Certain family patterns contribute to the disruptive behavior. They include parental rejection; inconsistent or rigid, harsh discipline; unstable spousal relationship; and lack of feeling of security within the family system. The child initiates aggressive behavior at home and with peers in school. These children lack strong emotional bonds or reliable role models for responsible behavior.

## CLIENT ASSESSMENT DATABASE
### Ego Integrity

Has feelings of rejection, powerlessness.
Blames others for what happens to self.
Displays maladaptive coping behaviors.
Uses manipulation to get needs met.
May have responded to stressors by staying out at night, running away.

May have had frequent/recurrent life changes, e.g., multiple moves, change of schools, lifestyle changes, placement in foster homes.

### Food/Fluid

Skips meals, eats excessive amounts of junk foods.
Eats in response to external cues/stressors.
Reports nausea.
May have excessive weight for height; recent weight gain may be noted.

### Hygiene

Poor hygiene/personal habits.
Style of dress may reflect fashion trends or be atypical.

### Neurosensory

Nervousness, worry, and jitteriness/excessive psychomotor activity.
May be depressed, angry, or react with ambivalence or hostility.
Affect may be labile.
Physical characteristics/development may not be normal for age range.

### Sexuality

Early onset of sexual behavior, may have forced others into sexual activity.

### Social Interactions

Symptoms most often appear during prepubertal to pubertal period and may predispose the child to conduct or adjustment disorders in adolescence.
Family disharmony/disruption, little contact with absent parent/separation from extended family may be reported.
May have history of poor school/work performance.
Parents may report client isolates self, plays stereo loudly, does not participate in family activities; shows little empathy or concern for others.
Hostility toward authority figures, intimidates others.
May/may not participate in social activities.
Suicidal ideation, may have plan/means, may have attempted suicide.
May be involved with legal system/juvenile court, have record of antisocial behavior (e.g., fire setting, cruelty to people/animals, stealing, use of a weapon).

### Teaching/Learning

Onset usually between age 5 to early adolescence, rare after age 16.
May be involved in drug use/abuse, including cigarettes/chewing tobacco.
May have had previous psychiatric hospitalization for same or other problems.

## DIAGNOSTIC STUDIES

**Drug Screen:** To identify substance use/abuse.

## NURSING PRIORITIES

1. Provide a safe environment and protect client from self-harm.
2. Promote development of strategies that regulate impulse control, regain sense of self-

worth and security.

3. Facilitate learning of appropriate and satisfying methods of dealing with stressors/feelings.

4. Promote client's ability to engage in satisfying relationships with family members, peer group.

## DISCHARGE GOALS

1. Exhibits effective coping skills in dealing with problems.

2. Understands need and strategies for controlling negative impulses/acting-out behaviors.

3. Expresses anger in appropriate/nonviolent ways.

4. Family is involved in group therapy/participating in treatment program.

| NURSING DIAGNOSIS: | COPING, DEFENSIVE |
|---|---|
| **May Be Related To:** | Denial of obvious problems/weaknesses. |
| | Projection of blame/responsibility. |
| | Hypersensitivity to slight/criticism. |
| | Grandiosity; rationalizes failures. |
| | Inadequate coping strategies. |
| | Maturational crisis; multiple life changes. |
| | Lack of control of impulsive actions; personal vulnerability. |
| **Possibly Evidenced By:** | Inappropriate use of defense mechanisms; poor self-esteem; superior attitude toward others. |
| | Difficulty establishing/maintaining relationships; hostile laughter or ridicule of others. |
| | Difficulty in reality-testing perceptions. |
| | Inability to meet role expectations. |
| | Stealing and other acting-out behaviors; failure to assume responsibility for own actions. |
| | Verbalization of inability to cope. |
| | Excessive smoking/drinking. |
| **Desired Outcomes/Evaluation Criteria— Client Will:** | Express realistic view of the consequences of impulsive behavior. |
| | Verbalize understanding of the relationship between emotional needs and acting-out behaviors. |
| | Identify and demonstrate ways to meet own needs. |
| | Participate in treatment program/therapy. |

| ACTIONS/INTERVENTIONS | RATIONALE |
|---|---|

### Independent

Provide explanation of the rules of the treatment setting and develop consequences with the client for his or her lack of cooperation.

Clear explanation of the rules allows the client to make choices about participating. Involvement in setting of the consequences promotes an investment in which the client is more apt to comply.

Encourage client to express fears and concerns. Offer support and confront when appropriate.

Self-understanding and further exploration are enhanced when verbalizations of concern and anxiety are received in a nonjudgmental manner. Therapeutic confrontation can help client to look at incongruencies of behavior and own responsibility for actions.

Determine coping mechanisms used, e.g., projection, rationalization and how these affect current situation.

Provides a beginning point for client to see how use of ineffective coping methods causes problems in life/relationships.

Assist client to recognize the reality and nonproductivity of maladaptive behaviors (failing grades, trouble with the law, running away).

Old patterns of behavior tend to recur under stress. Continuous monitoring of behavior is necessary to avoid old, nonproductive methods of coping and problem-solving.

Describe all aspects of the problems through use of therapeutic communication skills (e.g., Active-listening).

Clarifies problems and promotes understanding by the client and nurse.

Focus on specific behaviors, e.g., poor academic performance, antisocial behavior, which are amenable to change.

Energy is best used when focus is on those areas that can be altered.

Set limits on manipulative behavior by telling the client what you will tolerate; be consistent in enforcing consequences when roles are broken and limits tested.

Being clear and confronting these behaviors in a consistent manner will help the client begin to change ways of getting needs met.

Reinforce client positively when change in behaviors indicates effective coping through behavior-modification system. Anticipate and accept occasional regressive behavior.

Adolescence is a time of stress and vulnerability because of a lack of well-developed coping skills. Positive reinforcement encourages continuing personal growth. Hospitalization may precipitate periodic regression.

Identify religious beliefs/affiliations. Encourage client to draw again on spiritual resources that had been useful in the past.

When these ties have been previously established, they may be helpful in providing resources for the adolescent to enhance inner controls.

Explore possible ways to rekindle relationships with former peers, influential adults, organizations/church youth group, as appropriate.

Attaining peer acceptance is of primary importance during adolescence. Peer groups that share common values promote the formation of belonging and identity.

| NURSING DIAGNOSIS: | VIOLENCE, HIGH RISK FOR, DIRECTED AT SELF/OTHERS |
|---|---|
| Risk Factors May Include: | Dysfunctional family system and loss of significant relationships. |
| | Retarded ego development. |

| | |
|---|---|
| **Possible Indicators:** | Behavior changes, e.g., absenteeism, poor grades, hostility toward authority figures, stealing. |
| | Poor impulse control; feelings of rejection. |
| | Powerlessness; loss of self-esteem. |
| | Overt aggressive acts directed at the environment. |
| | Self-destructive behavior and/or active suicidal threats/gestures. |
| **Desired Outcomes/Evaluation Criteria— Client Will:** | Verbalize understanding of behavior and factors that precipitate violent behavior. |
| | Express anger in appropriate ways, avoiding hostile or suicidal gestures/statements or harm to self or others. |
| | Identify and use resources and support systems in an effective manner. |

| ACTIONS/INTERVENTIONS | RATIONALE |
|---|---|
| **Independent** | |
| Monitor stressors and warning signals such as behavior changes, anger, anxiety, and recently disrupted family. | Impulsive reactions to stressful situations directed toward harm to self or others may be a cry for help. |
| Determine seriousness of suicidal tendency, gestures, threats, or previous attempts. (Use scale of 1–10 and prioritize according to severity of threat, availability of means.) | Knowledge of past and present behavior in reference to suicidal ideation will assist in assessing client's tolerance for stress, degree of concern. Note: May be no. 1 nursing diagnosis if suicide risk is rated 8–10. |
| Maintain a therapeutic milieu that includes a safe environment (e.g., suicide precautions). | Internal controls may be inadequate, requiring some external controls and interventions until internal control is learned. |
| Establish trusting relationship with client in order to allow exploration and verbalization of feelings related to suicide. | Client's expression of internal conflicts in words, rather than action, will more likely be made to knowledgeable and accepting staff. |
| Strike a balance in the intimacy of the therapeutic relationship. | Children who are more disturbed respond best to a less intrusive relationship in the beginning. |
| Observe client unobtrusively for signs of potential violence toward others. | Intervention before the onset of violence can prevent injury to the client and others. Overt monitoring may be interpreted negatively and potentiate acting-out behavior. |
| Have sufficient staff available to indicate a show of strength to client if it becomes necessary. | This conveys to client evidence of control over the situation and provides some sense of security for the client and staff. |
| Establish hierarchy of responses to aggressive behaviors, e.g., Time out. Explore and offer more satisfying alternatives to aggressive behavior, e.g., physical outlets for redirection of angry feelings; use of quiet room or "Soft Spot" with soft balls, pillows to pound. | Increased ability to discover satisfying alternatives in coping with stressors will decrease need for aggressive behavior. Physical outlets help to relieve pent-up tension and anxiety. |

| ACTIONS/INTERVENTIONS | RATIONALE |
|---|---|
| **Independent** | |
| Have staff member stay with client. Encourage client to choose own "Time out," going to room for alone time, taking medications, or choosing room schedules, use of seclusion and/or restraints. | Staff member can help client to express feelings and begin to recognize value of appropriate handling of anger. Adolescent may see "Time out" as punishment if staff imposes, but begins to take responsibility for own self by recognizing and choosing own quiet/alone time, other methods of control. |
| Encourage client to ask for time with staff, give permission to express angry feelings. Be alert to "acting out" to please peers or nursing staff. | Early interventions can interrupt the pattern prior to seriously escalating behavior. Recognizing feelings and taking responsibility by asking for time to discuss them helps the adolescent learn more effective ways of dealing with problems that can lead to anger and acting-out behaviors. |
| Include significant other(s) in discussions to educate regarding suicidal ideation/warnings. | May be unaware of/ignorant of meaning of warning signals when suicidal ideation exists. |
| Assess how unit functioning affects adolescent behaviors. | Milieu stressors, such as vacations, personnel changes, staff conflict, can affect client's own issues, e.g., abandonment. It is important to look at the psychodynamics as well as the unique meaning of individual behavior. |
| Engage in action-oriented recreational therapy, e.g., outdoor program, wall climbing, supervised sports activities. | Helps to relieve nervous, pent-up energy. Sustained activity stimulates release of endorphins, enhancing sense of well-being. |
| Include whole community/classroom in reinforcing positive behaviors. Use daily goal-setting group, problem-solving group. | Peer interaction is effective in this age group to help client control own behavior. |
| **Collaborative** | |
| Place in seclusion or apply restraints as necessary. | May need external restraints until client regains control of own behavior. |
| Administer, supervise, and monitor effects of medications. | Helps client to maintain impulse control. Neuroleptic medications will decrease aggressive outbursts and improve impulse control. |

| NURSING DIAGNOSIS: | ANXIETY [SPECIFY LEVEL] |
|---|---|
| **May Be Related To:** | Situational or maturational crises. |
| | Threat to physical integrity or self-concept. |
| | Dysfunctional family systems. |
| **Possibly Evidenced By:** | Somatic complaints. |
| | Excessive psychomotor activity. |
| | Poor attention to task. |
| | Poor impulse control. |

71

| **Desired Outcomes/Evaluation Criteria— Client Will:** | Verbalize awareness of propensity toward increased psychomotor activity, poor attention to task, and poor impulse control. |
| --- | --- |
| | Demonstrate self-initiated intervention strategies that facilitate more effective coping skills. |
| | Report absence of/demonstrate relief from somatic manifestations of anxiety. |

| ACTIONS/INTERVENTIONS | RATIONALE |
| --- | --- |

### Independent

| | |
| --- | --- |
| Assign primary nurse to foster a trusting relationship. | Continuity of care for client builds trust and clarifies expectation. |
| Observe/assist client to recognize manifestations of anxiety (e.g., nausea, compulsive eating). | Signs and symptoms of anxiety need to be identified before client can make constructive changes. |
| Identify factors that precede symptoms of anxiety. | Correct assessment and interpretation of premonitory conditions provide for timely intervention. |
| Support client's exploration to identify those behaviors or interventions that offer relief. | Connecting feelings of anxiety with behaviors that afford relief will encourage the development of more productive behaviors. |
| Channel excessive energy into physical activity such as exercises, noncompetitive games, jogging in gym, etc. | Discharge of physical energy tends to decrease built-up tensions that lead to manifestations of anxiety. Note: Competitive games may increase anxiety. |

| **NURSING DIAGNOSIS:** | **SELF-ESTEEM, CHRONIC LOW** |
| --- | --- |
| **May Be Related To:** | Life choices perpetuating failure (e.g., runaway behavior). |
| | Personal vulnerability (loss of family member/friends; poor school performance; relocation). |
| | Fixation in earlier level of development (lack of movement toward independence). |
| **Possibly Evidenced By:** | Self-negating verbalizations, self-blame, anger. |
| | Rationalizing away/rejecting of positive feedback and exaggeration of negative feedback about self; feelings of rejection. |
| | Frequent lack of success in school/other life events. |
| **Desired Outcomes/Evaluation Criteria— Client Will:** | Verbalize and recognize significance of losses in life. |
| | Verbalize beginning understanding of negative evaluation of self and reasons for problems. |

Participate positively in family/group/community activities.

Demonstrate behaviors/lifestyle changes to promote positive self-esteem.

| ACTIONS/INTERVENTIONS | RATIONALE |
|---|---|
| **Independent** | |
| Promote a trust relationship that is reliable, supportive, and reassuring. | Communication, growth, and insight flourish in an atmosphere of acceptance and trust. |
| Establish level of authority of primary nurse; monitor the need for nurturance and limit setting. | Consistent "parent figure" can uniformly reinforce consequence to behaviors of the client. |
| Review previous life situations and role changes, determining coping skills already developed. (Refer to ND: Family Coping, ineffective: compromised/disabling.) | Provides information about availability of skills for current use and direction for change. |
| Listen to client's perception of inability to adapt to situations presently occurring. | Provides clues to reality of these perceptions and avenues to assist in dealing with them. |
| Identify significant support systems past and present. | Reinforces availability of resources to aid the client to develop new coping skills. |
| Work with client to develop a plan of action to meet immediate needs, e.g., physical safety, hygiene, emotional support. | Provides opportunity for client to learn sense of control and fosters self-esteem. |
| Provide opportunities for client to make short-term attainable goals, e.g., crafts, activities. | Promotes feelings of self-worth, which can lead to increased risk taking and the development of more elaborate future-oriented goals. |
| Encourage client to recognize significance of losses and express feelings regarding these. | Grief work cannot begin until losses are acknowledged (e.g., divorce, relocation, loss of friends/extended family/support systems). |
| Encourage exploration of the relationship of behavior, anxiety, and somatic symptoms to the grief process. | Knowledge regarding possible psychologic and physiologic manifestations of the grief process aids in identifying etiology of existing symptoms and helps in the alleviation of denial. |
| Discuss appropriateness and desirability of the grief process as it relates to the loss(es). Discuss stages of the grief process and behaviors associated with each stage. | Grief work is necessary and a natural reaction to loss. A period of time is required (at least 6–12 months) to work through grief. The process gives the client permission to grieve and offers hope for eventual acclimation to the loss. |
| Encourage the development of a positive relationship with an adult. | A quality relationship with an adult (preferably a parent) reinforces the strength and supportive function of the relationship (family) and is a positive factor when setting limits with the adolescent. |

| NURSING DIAGNOSIS: | PERSONAL IDENTITY/BODY IMAGE DISTURBANCE/ROLE PERFORMANCE, ALTERED |
|---|---|
| May Be Related To: | Failure at life events (adolescence). |
| | Situational/developmental crisis, slow physical maturation. |
| | Disruption of family by divorce/death/absence of parent or other factors. |
| Possibly Evidenced By: | Behavioral signs, e.g., poor academic performance, stealing, loss of job, bragging about alleged sexual exploits. |
| | Rebellion against generally accepted fashion styles. |
| | Alteration in weight. |
| | Poor hygiene/personal habits. |
| | Difficulty accepting positive reinforcement. |
| | Not taking responsibility for self. |
| | Self-destructive behavior. |
| | Failure to assume role. |
| | Confusion about sense of self. |
| Desired Outcomes/Evaluation Criteria— Client Will: | Verbalize a sense of a more positive self-concept. |
| | Identify and appraise realistically what can be actively influenced by own actions. |
| | Develop ego strength sufficient to cope with inner impulses. |

## ACTIONS/INTERVENTIONS

### Independent

Explore and discuss feelings of rejection and anger related to individual situation.

Point out past academic success in order to assist in preserving self-esteem.

Assist client in understanding transient nature of poor academic performance related to current stressors.

Provide activities in areas of client's interest, tasks that can be completed successfully, and reinforce when these are accomplished.

Maintain positive attitude toward the client, providing opportunities for client to exercise control over as much as possible.

## RATIONALE

Recognition and expression of feelings eliminate need for displacement and denial. This directs focus of energy to problems and alternative solutions.

Past performance is a more accurate portrayal of ability than that indicated by recent grades.

High anxiety levels affect motivation, attention to task, and performance.

Success in accomplishing goals builds sense of self and diminishes need for disruptive acting-out behaviors.

Cooperation can be enhanced when client feels accepted and included in problem-solving and decision-making.

| ACTIONS/INTERVENTIONS | RATIONALE |
|---|---|

### Independent

Encourage participation in activities with peer group, e.g., outings, hikes, swimming.

Schedule time for one-to-one client/nurse interaction and communication.

Schedule regular exercise activities.

Involve in activities to improve personal appearance, e.g., makeup, hairstyling, clothing choices.

Use the techniques of role rehearsal to help the client develop new skills to cope with changes.

### Collaborative

Consult with resident educational therapist (teacher) regarding academic pursuits while client is hospitalized (residential treatment program).

Schedule staffings with home school counselors, social worker, teachers, and client/parents as possible.

---

Social interaction and peer acceptance are among the tasks of this developmental stage. Participation helps to develop social skills.

Individual attention conveys the importance of the individual. Communication skills are refined with frequent interaction.

Can enhance physical appearance and strength, aids in weight loss, lessens anxiety and stress, and builds positive self-esteem.

How an individual looks affects feelings about inner self and can improve sense of self.

Active participation in activity enhances learning.

Keeping up with class work while hospitalized can help to lessen further loss of self-concept. Can be an opportunity to form a positive relationship with teacher and experience learning successes fostering personal growth and improved self-esteem.

Maintains contact with own school setting, fosters continuity for return and sense of importance for the student.

---

| **NURSING DIAGNOSIS:** | **FAMILY COPING, ineffective: compromised/disabling** |
|---|---|
| **May Be Related To:** | Loss of significant relationship (parent/child). |
| | Highly ambivalent family relationships. |
| | Family disorganization/role changes. |
| | Presence of other situational/developmental crises affecting family members. |
| **Possibly Evidenced By:** | Client states feelings of abandonment, rejection and guilt about parent's response to adolescent's problems. |
| | Client expresses sense of powerlessness and lack of control. |
| | Parents describe preoccupation with own reactions, e.g., fear, guilt, anxiety. |
| | Parents withdraw or have limited communication with adolescent or display protective behavior disproportionate (too little or too much) to client's abilities or need for autonomy. |

| Desired Outcomes/Evaluation Criteria—Family Will: | Establish positive/amicable relationship with one another. |
|---|---|
| | Express feelings openly and honestly. |
| | Evaluate individual role in family problems. |
| | Identify factors and decisions that can be made and controlled. |
| | Explore possibility of positive changes in the family in the future. |
| | Identify need for/seek outside support as appropriate. |

| ACTIONS/INTERVENTIONS | RATIONALE |
|---|---|

### Independent

| ACTIONS/INTERVENTIONS | RATIONALE |
|---|---|
| Foster trust through 1:1 family/nurse relationship. | Basic trust and stability can be established through continuity and consistency of care. |
| Encourage client to identify and appropriately verbalize feelings of rejection, abandonment, and ambivalence related to individual situation. | Verbalizing feelings tends to alleviate tensions that may be internalized or somatized, e.g., reports of nausea. Client lacks emotional attachment to others and may be charming and engaging, which is a pretense to deceive others/facilitate exploitation. |
| Focus on specific behaviors that are amenable to change. | Changing of some behaviors can enhance feelings of self-esteem and encourage willingness to make other changes. |
| Identify underlying family dynamics and determine how they are operating in the present. | Established family patterns affect how the current situation has arisen as well as how the problems need to be resolved and changed now. |
| Guide client/family in correlating anger and feelings that are centered around lack of influence in family behavior. | Understanding internal dynamics of anger leads to acceptance of locus of control within self. |
| Encourage client and family to make as many decisions as are possible within the milieu. Example: Client decision to participate in choice of evening activity. | An increase in autonomy and decision-making enhances feelings of self-esteem and competency. |
| Explore feelings of self-blame and guilt related to problems/changes in the family system. Assist individual in realistic appraisal and verbalization of own role in situation. | Change or disruption in the family system affects all other parts of the system. Children may incorrectly assume that they were instrumental in family problems/marital disruption. |
| Encourage open communication between client and family when they visit. | Communication patterns affect the functional level of each family member. |
| Explore ways client and family can be mutually supportive without fostering overdependence on each other. | Security and trust provide a climate for growth and risk taking. |
| Give immediate, consistent, and positive reinforcement when desired behaviors are observed. Conversely, withhold reinforcement/ignore negative behaviors. | Consistent reinforcement of appropriate behaviors fosters continuation of those behaviors. Consequences for inappropriate behaviors and no reinforcement (ignoring) tend to extinguish undesired behaviors. |

## ACTIONS/INTERVENTIONS

### Independent

Discuss reasons for client behaviors.

### Collaborative

Explore potential sources of assistance available to meet needs. Refer to social services, other agencies as indicated.

Encourage family to participate in family therapy.

(Refer to CP: Parenting.)

## RATIONALE

Understanding of childhood/adolescent tasks, ambivalent feelings, etc., can help individual(s) accept and deal more appropriately with difficult behaviors. As a rule, client is easily bored and has a low frustration tolerance when desires are not immediately gratified. Emotional reactions can be erratic and demonstrate a lack of concern for others.

Knowledge of resources available in the event they are needed tends to decrease fears regarding postdischarge functioning.

Enables family to work on issues that affect all of the family system. Note: Family rift may be so severe that the most that can be expected is a neutral relationship where parties agree to disagree.

| NURSING DIAGNOSIS: | NUTRITION, ALTERED: LESS THAN/MORE THAN BODY REQUIREMENTS |
|---|---|
| May Be Related To: | Inadequate intake of balanced, nutritional meals. |
| Possibly Evidenced By: | Reported/observed inadequate food intake and lack of weight gain. |
| | Excessive intake in relation to metabolic need with subsequent weight gain. |
| | Satisfaction of hunger through consumption of excessive amounts of junk food. |
| Desired Outcomes/Evaluation Criteria— Client Will: | Verbalize understanding of the relationship of food intake, exercise, and metabolism. |
| | Demonstrate positive eating habits with appropriate nutritional intake. |
| | Achieve desired weight level. |

## ACTIONS/INTERVENTIONS

### Independent

Encourage client to eat well-balanced meals on a regular basis.

Provide information regarding nutritional intake and selection of appropriate foods that will encourage weight loss/gain as indicated.

## RATIONALE

Hunger can be satisfied with food intake, eliminating empty calories.

The correlation of food intake and weight gain/loss, if understood, can lead to food choices that result in achieving appropriate weight. Foods that are self-selected are more likely to be eaten and enjoyed.

77

## ACTIONS/INTERVENTIONS

## RATIONALE

### Independent

Assist client in developing insight into eating habits as they relate to feelings of anxiety. Encourage keeping a diary of food intake and related feeling(s).

Increased anxiety may lead to anorexia or frequent snacking as a response to feelings of tension.

### Collaborative

Refer to dietitian as needed.

Helps to determine individual caloric needs while considering child/adolescent dietary preferences.

| NURSING DIAGNOSIS: | SOCIAL INTERACTION, IMPAIRED |
|---|---|
| **May Be Related To:** | Lack of social skills. |
| | Developmental state (adolescence). |
| **Possibly Evidenced By:** | Verbalized or observed discomfort in social situations and use of unsuccessful social interaction behaviors. |
| | Dysfunctional interactions with peers, family, and/or others. |
| | Family report of change of style or pattern of interaction. |
| | Self-concept disturbance. |
| **Desired Outcomes/Evaluation Criteria— Client Will:** | Verbalize awareness of factors and identify feelings related to impaired social interactions. |
| | Be involved in achieving positive changes in social behaviors and interpersonal relationships. |
| | Develop effective social support systems. |

## ACTIONS/INTERVENTIONS

## RATIONALE

### Independent

Assess individual causes and contributing factors, e.g., disruption of the family, frequent moves during child's/adolescent's life, individual's poor coping, and adjustment to developmental stage.

While learning social skills is one of the maturational tasks, many factors can interfere with the client's ability to interact satisfactorily with others in social situations.

Review medical history.

Long-term illness/accident may have interfered with development of social skills at earlier stages.

Observe family patterns of relating and social behaviors. Explore possible family scripting of expectations of the child/adolescent. Note prevalent patterns.

Family may not have effective patterns of relating to others, and the child learns these skills in this setting. Often child is reflecting family expectations rather than own desires. Identification of patterns will help with plan for change.

Encourage client to verbalize feelings about discomfort, noting recurring factors or precipitating patterns.

Identifies areas of concern and suggests ways to learn new skills.

| ACTIONS/INTERVENTIONS | RATIONALE |
|---|---|

### Independent

Active-listen verbalizations indicating hopelessness, powerlessness, fear, anxiety, grief, anger, feeling unloved or unlovable, problems with sexual identity, and/or hate (directed or not).

Client may have belief that nothing can be done to change the way things are and that own actions do not make a difference. Active-listening client's words and feelings conveys a message of confidence in the individual's own abilities.

Assess client's coping skills and defense mechanisms.

May be effective for dealing with individual situation and/or provide a base for learning new skills.

Have client identify behaviors that cause discomfort and review negative behaviors others have identified.

Listing specific behaviors will help the client know where change is possible. Knowing what others see can assist the client to accept and effect change.

Explore with client and role-play new ways of handling identified behaviors/situations.

Active involvement is the most effective way to create change.

Provide reinforcement for positive social behaviors and interactions.

Promotes feelings of self-worth and helps to reinforce desired behaviors.

Work with client to correct basic negative self-concept. (Refer to ND: Personal Identity/Body Image disturbance; Role Performance, altered).

Negative self-concepts may be a major factor impeding positive social interactions.

Help client to identify responsibility for own behavior. Encourage keeping a daily journal of social interactions and feelings.

Enhances self-esteem and provides feedback to improve skills. Journal keeping can provide an ongoing record to note improvement and/or areas of need for change.

### Collaborative

Involve in group therapy as indicated.

Helpful arena to practice new social skills, receive feedback with support for efforts to improve.

Encourage reading, attendance at classes (e.g., Positive Image, Self-Help, Assertiveness), and community support groups.

Assists in alleviating negative self-concepts that lead to impaired social interactions.

| NURSING DIAGNOSIS: | KNOWLEDGE DEFICIT [LEARNING NEED] regarding behavioral changes, expected outcomes |
|---|---|
| May Be Related To: | Lack of information/misinterpretation of information; unfamiliarity with information resources. |
| Possibly Evidenced By: | Verbalization of the problem, request for information, statement of misconception. |
| | Inaccurate follow-through of instruction; inappropriate or exaggerated behaviors. |
| | Continuation/progression of problems. |

| Desired Outcomes/Evaluation Criteria— Client Will: | Describe a person with an antisocial personality. |
| --- | --- |
| | List characteristics of the antisocial personality that client sees in self. |
| | Explain the concept of thinking error, how it leads to antisocial behavior, and name those that personally apply. |
| | Maintain a thinking log with daily entry following the prescribed format. |
| | Identify how the knowledge of thinking errors has changed behavioral responses. |

| ACTIONS/INTERVENTIONS | RATIONALE |
| --- | --- |
| **Independent** | |
| Discuss characteristics of the antisocial personality with the client. Provide written handout and allow time for client to ask questions and clarify understanding. | Some common beliefs of the person with an antisocial personality are: does not have to conform to society's rules or norms; believes the world revolves around self and that others should meet client's needs, rather than client meeting society's expectations. |
| Discuss the concept of thinking errors in relation to client's behaviors. | A thinking error occurs when a person has a thought that is extremely different from the way most people under the same circumstances would think. If the person acts on the thought, the behavior will be outside of societal norms. |
| Have client read written handout, discuss information, and relate to own thinking errors and behavior. | Common thinking errors are: Victim stance: "He started it/I couldn't help it"; doesn't stop to think how actions will hurt others; lack of effort; unwilling to do anything perceived as boring or disagreeable; refusal to accept obligation, "I forgot/I don't have to"; power through anger; refusal to acknowledge fear; blames others when criticized; "I can't" attitude, statement of refusal, not inability. |
| Discuss thinking log, importance of writing actual thoughts and not trying to "con" the staff with what the client thinks they want to hear. Explain responsibility for daily entry and attendant consequence. | The entry consists of a brief statement of an incident when the client was angry or disagreed with another person, what the client thought about the incident (in own words), what the client thought about doing, what the client actually did, and the outcome. |
| Promote client responsibility for the review process and state clearly what the consequence is for failure to meet this responsibility. | Assists the client to begin to assume inner-directed self-control. |
| Review thinking log at specified time each day, identifying the thinking error and relating it to the client's pattern of thinking in everyday life. Reinforce that the thinking error is only the tip of the iceberg. | Promotes attention to content and conformity to process, allowing client to begin to identify ineffective methods of getting needs met. |
| Observe for shame reactions. Explain that the process is not judgmental, and discuss behavioral responses. | Log is a means for client to identify thinking errors and choose not to act on them. |

| ACTIONS/INTERVENTIONS | RATIONALE |
|---|---|

### Independent

Require attendance at Thinking Error Group. Facilitate honest noncritical feedback from group members. Continuously evaluate the group process and identify thinking errors as they occur in the group.

Sharing information from the log promotes awareness and opportunities to change behavior in safe environment of the group.

Review log with client before discharge. Provide feedback regarding improved behavioral responses and areas where continued work is needed. Encourage client to continue thinking log after discharge.

Provides opportunity for client to identify predominant pattern of thinking errors and recognize new ways to respond that have been learned in treatment.

# DISRUPTIVE BEHAVIOR AND ATTENTION-DEFICIT DISORDERS: Oppositional Defiant Disorders

## DSM IV
313.81   Oppositional Defiant Disorder
312.9     Disruptive Behavior Disorder NOS (For other listings, consult DSM IV manual.)

## DSM III-R
313.81   Oppositional Defiant Disorder

A pattern of negativistic, hostile, and defiant behavior lasting at least 6 months, in which the child loses temper, argues with adults, often actively defies or refuses adult requests or rules, blames others, deliberately does annoying things, and swears or uses obscene language. This behavior creates significant impairment in academic/social functioning but does not meet the criteria for Conduct Disorder. (Disruptive Behavior Disorder NOS reflects clinical features that are subthreshold for both Oppositional Defiant and Conduct Disorders.)

## ETIOLOGIC THEORIES

### Psychodynamics

The oppositional youth is fixed in the separation-individuation stage of development. The youth insists on autonomy by negative adaptive maneuvers in which he or she continually provokes adults or peers. As the youth develops internal controls, he or she will eventually grow out of these behaviors.

### Genetic/Biologic

Similar to the predisposition for conduct disorder, heredity contributes to individual temperament, frustration, tolerance, and the tendency to seek risks or disobey authority. The disorder may be gender-linked, since the incidence is higher in boys than in girls.

### Family Dynamics

Familial and cultural norms may prohibit the degree of individual differentiation among the family members. Attempts to maintain conformity are met by negativism, disobedience, and quarrelsome defiance. Parenting skills are ineffective and/or inconsistent with reactive and emotionally charged interchanges between parent and child. Some parents interpret average or increased levels of developmental oppositionalism as hostility and a deliberate effort on the part of the child to be in control. If power and control are issues for parents, or if they exercise authority for their own needs, a power struggle can be established between the parents and the child that sets the stage for the development of Oppositional Defiant Disorder.

A relationship between life events and the development of anxiety disorders has been identified.

This theory suggests that disruptive behavior is learned as a means for a child to gain adult attention. Anxiety generated by a dysfunctional family system, marital problems, etc., could also contribute to symptoms of this disorder. Parents become frustrated with the child's poor response to limit setting. Parenting interventions become oversensitive or the reverse, with no external structure provided.

## CLIENT ASSESSMENT DATABASE

### Activity/Rest

Difficulty playing or engaging in leisure activities quietly.

## Ego Integrity

Feelings of rejection, powerlessness, fear of abandonment.
Blames others for what happens to self; easily annoyed by others.
Passive-dependent or demanding attitude of entitlement.
Family may report emotional lability.

## Food/Fluid

Dawdling at mealtime.
Oppositional battles over food choices, mealtimes.

## Hygiene

Rebellious display of defiance in personal appearance, adherence to hygiene, and personal habits.

## Neurosensory

May be depressed, angry, or react with ambivalence or hostility.
Dawdling, passive resistance to following time schedules, missing school bus, etc.

## Social Interactions

Impaired social and academic functioning.
Provocative display of defiance of adult authority figures.
Deliberately engages in annoying behaviors; ignores verbal instructions/requests.
Often bullies or bosses others (peers, siblings).
Aggressive interruption in play activity of others; breaking toys, making up own rules for games, etc.
May/may not participate in social activities.
Impaired interpersonal relationships (e.g., loses temper, argues, refuses to comply with requests or rules, spiteful or vindictive, projects blame for own mistakes or misbehavior, interrupts or intrudes on others).

## Teaching/Learning

Onset usually before age 8 and not later than early adolescence.
Family history of alcohol abuse

## DIAGNOSTIC STUDIES

**Thyroid Studies:** May reveal hyper/hypothyroid conditions contributing to problems.
**Neurologic Testing, e.g., EEG, CT Scan:** Determines presence of organic brain disorders.
**Psychologic Testing as Indicated:** Rules out anxiety disorders; identifies gifted, borderline retarded, or learning disabled child; and assesses social responsiveness and language development.
Note presence of physical symptoms that might indicate the existence of physical illness, e.g., rashes, upper respiratory illness, or other allergic symptoms, CNS infection (cerebritis) requiring appropriate diagnostic studies.

## NURSING PRIORITIES

1. Promote client's ability to engage in satisfying relationships with family members, peer group.
2. Facilitate parents' development of effective means of coping with and interventions for their child's behavioral symptoms.
3. Participate in the development of a comprehensive, ongoing treatment approach using family and community resources.

# DISCHARGE GOALS

1. Demonstrates appropriate response to limits, rules, and consequences.
2. Parents have gained or regained the ability to cope with internal feelings and to intervene effectively with their child's behavioral problems.
3. Therapeutic plan in place, with family and client participating in treatment program.

| NURSING DIAGNOSIS: | COPING, INDIVIDUAL, INEFFECTIVE |
|---|---|
| **May Be Related To:** | Situational or maturational crisis. |
| | Mild neurologic deficits/retardation. |
| | Retarded ego development; low self-esteem. |
| | Family system with dysfunctional coping methods, negative role models; abuse/neglect. |
| **Possibly Evidenced By:** | Unable to meet age-appropriate role expectations. |
| | Hostility toward others, defiant response to requests/rules. |
| | Unable to delay gratification; manipulation of others in environment for purpose of fulfilling own desires. |
| **Desired Outcomes/Evaluation Criteria— Client Will:** | Demonstrate appropriate ways to assert self and establish self-worth. |
| | Identify adaptive coping skills that will achieve a healthy balance between independence and dependence. |
| | Delay gratification without resorting to manipulation of others. |

| ACTIONS/INTERVENTIONS | RATIONALE |
|---|---|

### Independent

| | |
|---|---|
| Allow flexibility in shifting from one activity to another, particularly transitioning at bedtime for younger children. | Recognizing the onset of anxiety and providing flexibility will decrease likelihood of child taking an oppositional stance. |
| Reinforce all efforts of the child when displaying appropriate efforts to establish autonomy. | Decreases pattern of negative attention-seeking behavior. |
| Provide opportunities for imaginary play, including use of puppets, clay, sand. | The medium of play materials provides physical displacement of feelings and visualization of dynamics. |
| Set limits on disruptive behaviors (e.g., talking incessantly); suggest alternative competing behaviors such as playing quietly. | Child needs to know expectations and to learn competing acceptable behaviors, e.g., raising hand vs. shouting out, keeping hands to self vs. pushing others. |
| Encourage discussion of angry feelings and identity of true object of the hostility. | Dealing with the feelings honestly and directly helps discourage displacement of the anger onto others. |
| Explore with client alternative ways for handling frustration. | Promotes learning how to interact in society with others in more productive ways. |

| ACTIONS/INTERVENTIONS | RATIONALE |
|---|---|

### Independent

Provide positive feedback for trying new coping strategies.

Evaluate with client the effectiveness of new behaviors. Discuss modifications for improvement.

Assist client to recognize signs of escalating anxiety. Explore ways client can intervene before behavior becomes disabling.

Supports efforts and encourages use of acceptable behaviors.

Because client has limited problem-solving skills, assistance may be required to reassess and develop strategies.

Helps client to recognize ineffective behaviors and develop new coping skills to effect positive change.

### Collaborative

Administer medication as indicated, e.g.:
Imipramine (Tofranil),
Paroxetine (Paxal),
Sertraline (Zoloft);

Diazepam (Valium),
Chlordiazepoxide (Librium),
Alprazolam (Xanax).

Antidepressants may be used when depression is a factor in the disorder.

Antianxiety medications provide relief from effects of anxiety, facilitating cooperation with therapy.

| NURSING DIAGNOSIS: | SOCIAL INTERACTION, IMPAIRED |
|---|---|
| **May Be Related To:** | Retarded ego development; low self-esteem. |
| | Family system with dysfunctional coping methods, negative role models; abuse/neglect. |
| | Neurologic impairment; mental retardation. |
| **Possibly Evidenced By:** | Discomfort in social situations. |
| | Difficulty playing with others; interactions, aggressive, loses temper, argues, bullies/bosses others. |
| | Interrupts or intrudes on others; refuses to comply with requests or rules. |
| **Desired Outcomes/Evaluation Criteria— Client Will:** | Identify feelings that lead to poor social interactions. |
| | Participate appropriately in interactive play with another child or group of children. |
| | Develop a mutual relationship with another child or adult. |

| ACTIONS/INTERVENTIONS | RATIONALE |
|---|---|

### Independent

Develop trust relationship with child, show acceptance of child separate from unacceptable behavior.

Acceptance and trust encourage feelings of self-worth.

| ACTIONS/INTERVENTIONS | RATIONALE |
|---|---|
| **Independent** | |
| Encourage client to verbalize feelings of inadequacy and need for acceptance from others. Discuss how these feelings affect relationships by provoking defensive behaviors such as blaming and manipulating others. | Recognition of problem is first step toward resolution. |
| Engage in play activities, board games, sports, team-building exercises. | Learning appropriate cooperative play activities provides outlet for healthy cooperation, leadership skills. |
| Offer positive reinforcement for appropriate social interaction. Ignore ineffective methods of relating to others; teach competing behaviors. | Behavior modification can be an effective method of reducing disruptive behaviors in children by encouraging repetition of desirable behaviors. Attention to unacceptable behavior may actually reinforce it. |
| Identify situations that provoke defensiveness, and role-play more appropriate responses. | Provides confidence to deal with difficult situations when they occur. |
| Provide opportunities for group interaction, and encourage a positive and negative peer feedback system. | Appropriate social behavior is often learned from age-mates. |
| **Collaborative** | |
| Participate in psychoeducation groups on assertiveness training, problem-solving, social skills. | Helpful arena to practice new social skills, receive feedback with the support for efforts to improve. |
| Arrange staffings with other professionals, e.g., social workers, teachers. Include parents and child when possible. | Cooperation and coordination among those working with these children will enhance the treatment program. Including the child and parents provides them with understanding of the total problem and proposed treatment program. |

| | |
|---|---|
| **NURSING DIAGNOSIS:** | **SELF-ESTEEM DISTURBANCE** |
| **May Be Related To:** | Retarded ego development. |
| | Lack of positive feedback with repeated negative feedback. |
| | Family system with dysfunctional coping methods; abuse/neglect; negative role models. |
| | Mild neurologic deficits. |
| **Possibly Evidenced By:** | Lack of eye contact. |
| | Lack of self-confidence. |
| | Engagement in physically dangerous activity. |
| | Refusal to engage in activities or involvement without consideration of consequences. |
| | Derogatory remarks about self and/or bragging about self. |

| **Desired Outcomes/Evaluation Criteria— Client Will:** | Distraction of others to cover up own deficits or failures, e.g., acting the clown. |
| | Projection of blame/responsibility for problems; rationalization of personal failures, grandiosity. |
| | Verbalize increasingly positive self-regard. |
| | Demonstrate beginning awareness and control of own behavior. |
| | Participate in new activities without extreme fear of failure. |

| ACTIONS/INTERVENTIONS | RATIONALE |
| --- | --- |

### Independent

| | |
| --- | --- |
| Convey acceptance and unconditional positive regard. | May help child to increase own sense of self-worth. |
| Assist child to identify basic ego strengths/ positive aspects of self; give immediate feedback for acceptable behavior. | Focusing on positive aspects of personality may help improve self-concept. Positive reinforcement enhances self-esteem and increases desired behavior. |
| Spend time with client in 1:1 and group activities. | Conveys to client that you believe she or he is worthy of time and attention. |
| Provide opportunities for success; plan activities based on ability level (including noncompetitive and team building), set agreed-upon time limits for task completion. | Repeated successes can help to improve self-esteem. |
| Discuss fears, encourage involvement in new activities/tasks. | Confronting concerns and engaging in new tasks promotes personal growth and new skills. |
| Identify possible consequences of actions, e.g., refusal to follow rules, engaging in activities/ high-risk behaviors without forethought. | Helps client begin to recognize own responsibility for consequences of behavior and provides opportunity to consider alternatives. |
| Help client set realistic, concrete goals and determine appropriate actions to meet these goals. | Provides a structure to develop sense of hope for the future and framework for reaching desired goals. |

### Collaborative

| | |
| --- | --- |
| Provide learning opportunities, structured learning environment, e.g., self-contained classroom, individually planned educational program. | Successful school performance is essential to preserve a child's positive self-image. |

| **NURSING DIAGNOSIS:** | **FAMILY COPING, ineffective: compromised/disabling** |
| --- | --- |
| **May Be Related To:** | Excessive guilt, anger, or blaming among family members regarding child's behavior. |
| | Parental inconsistencies; disagreements regarding discipline, limit setting, and approaches. |
| | Exhaustion of parental resources due to prolonged coping with disruptive child. |

| Possibly Evidenced By: | Unrealistic parental expectations. |
| | Rejection or overprotection of child. |
| | Exaggerated expressions of anger, disappointment, or despair regarding child's behavior or ability to improve or change. |
| Desired Outcomes/Evaluation Criteria— Parent(s) Will: | Demonstrate more consistent, effective intervention methods in response to child's behavior. |
| | Express and resolve negative attitudes toward child. |
| | Identify and use support systems as needed. |

| ACTIONS/INTERVENTIONS | RATIONALE |
| --- | --- |

### Independent

| Provide information and materials related to child's disorder and effective parenting techniques. (Refer to CP: Parenting.) | Appropriate knowledge and skills may increase parental effectiveness |
| Encourage parents to verbalize feelings and explore alternative methods of dealing with child. | Supportive counseling can assist parents in developing coping strategies. |
| Provide feedback and reinforce effective parenting methods. | Positive reinforcement can increase self-esteem and encourage continued efforts. |
| Involve siblings in family discussions and planning for more effective family interactions. | Family problems affect all members, and treatment is more effective when everyone is involved in therapy. |

### Collaborative

| Refer to community resources as indicated, e.g., psychotherapy, parent support groups, parenting classes (Parent Effectiveness). | Developing a support system can increase parental confidence and effectiveness. |

| NURSING DIAGNOSIS: | **KNOWLEDGE DEFICIT [LEARNING NEED] regarding condition, prognosis, and treatment needs** |
| May Be Related To: | Lack of knowledge; misinformation/misinterpretation. |
| | Mild neurologic deficits; associated developmental learning disabilities; inability to concentrate; cognitive deficits. |
| Possibly Evidenced By: | Verbalization of problem/misconceptions. |
| | Poor school performance; repeated school suspensions. |
| | Inappropriate or exaggerated behaviors. |
| | Development of untoward consequences of behavior. |

| Desired Outcomes/Evaluation Criteria—Client/Parent Will: | Verbalize understanding of reasons for behavioral problems, treatment needs within developmental ability. |
| | Participate in learning and begin to ask questions and seek information. |
| Client Will: | Achieve cognitive goals consistent with level of temperament. |

| ACTIONS/INTERVENTIONS | RATIONALE |
| --- | --- |

### Independent

| | |
| --- | --- |
| Provide quiet environment, self-contained classrooms, small-group activities. Avoid overstimulating places, such as school bus, busy cafeteria, crowded hallways. | Reduction in environmental stimulation may decrease distractibility and diminish onset of temper tantrums. Small groups may prevent opportunity for power struggles/control, enhancing ability to stay on task and helping client learn appropriate interaction with others, avoiding sense of isolation. |
| Give instructional material in written and verbal form with step-by-step explanations. | Sequential learning skills will be enhanced. |
| Instruct child in problem-solving skills, practice situational examples. | Effective skills may increase performance levels. |
| Educate child and family on the use of medications and response anticipated. | Lessening of depression and/or anxiety may promote cooperation in therapy, resulting in more acceptable behavior. |
| Coordinate overall treatment plan with schools, collateral personnel, the child and family. | Cognitive effectiveness will most likely be advanced when treatment is not fragmented, nor significant interventions missed because of lack of interdisciplinary communication. |

# ELIMINATION DISORDERS:
## Enuresis/Encopresis

### DSM IV
307.6 Enuresis (not due to a general medical condition)
307.7 Encopresis without Constipation and Overflow Incontinence
787.6 Encopresis with Constipation and Overflow Incontinence

### DSM III-R
307.70 Functional Encopresis
307.60 Functional Enuresis

DSM IV defines enuresis/encopresis as repeated involuntary (or much more rarely intentional) voiding/passage of feces into places not appropriate for that purpose, after attaining the developmental level at which continence is expected. If continence is not achieved, the condition can be termed functional or primary. The period of continence necessary to differentiate between primary and secondary enuresis/encopresis is now considered to be 1 year. There does seem to be a significant relationship between enuresis and encopresis, although neither condition can be the direct effect of a general medical condition (e.g., diabetes, spina bifida, seizure activity) to be included in this category.

## ETIOLOGIC FACTORS
### Psychodynamics

Numerous psychologic interpretations exist speculating on the dynamics of toilet training and the significance of flushing bodily fluids down the toilet. Freudian theory places the fixation at the anal stage of development whereby the child fails to neutralize libidinal urges and the aggressive impulses are fused with the pleasure of controlling bodily functions. Expulsion of feces or urination and untimed feces or urination or intentionally placing the feces in inappropriate places elicits hostility from parents. Loss of bodily functions leads to loss of self-respect, loss of friends, and feelings of shame and isolation.

### Biologic

Learning to control urination/defecation is a developmental task most likely achieved by age 4 or 5 and requires a mechanically effective anatomy. In some enuretic children, abnormalities in regulation of vasopressor/antidiuretic hormone (ADH) have been evidenced with ADH regulation being linked to both the dopaminergic and serotonergic systems. A theory of developmental delay suggests there is a common underlying maturational factor that predisposes children to manifest both enuresis and behavioral disturbances. Enuresis and encopresis are normal responses to environmental stress such as a child separated from his or her family or abuse. In both cases, as the child matures and when the environmental stressors are alleviated, normal bodily control is resumed. Children who are hyperactive may have occasional accidents as they do not attend to the sensory stimuli until it is too late.

Enuresis, and its relationship to bladder capacity and urinary tract infections, has been explored as well as sleep studies in which nocturnal enuresis occurred during deep sleep with no response to arousal signals. In addition, research has been conducted to investigate the physiologic basis for encopresis. These studies indicate that the act of bearing down led to decreased anal sphincter control in almost all cases.

Soiling may result from excessive fluid buildup caused by diarrhea, anxiety, or the retention overflow process, whereby leakage occurs around a retentive fecal mass. This mechanism is responsible for 75% of encopretic children.

Genetically, a child is at risk for enuresis if the parent has a history of enuresis after the age of 4.

## Family Dynamics

As mentioned previously, the parental attitude toward cleanliness and the rigidity with which this behavior is controlled may perpetuate the fear associated with loss of bodily control. Parents often get caught up in the volitional aspects, blaming the child for "acting like a baby." Further social embarrassment ensues when school personnel target the problem in terms of "the dirty child from a dirty family." Attempts to deny the problem lead to covert behaviors such as hiding soiled clothing in lockers, under the bed, or in the trash. The child may in fact be using the only weapon available, as in the case of severe neglect and/or sexual assault.

## CLIENT ASSESSMENT DATABASE

### Activity/Rest

May/may not be awakened when bedwetting occurs.
Unusual sleep habits, increased incidence of sleepwalking or Sleep Terror disorders.

### Ego Integrity

Expressions of poor self-esteem, e.g., "I am bad."
Shy, withdrawn, feelings of isolation, shame.
Overly anxious around adult figures.
Stressors may include family conflicts/change in structure (e.g., divorce, birth of a sibling).

### Elimination

History of delayed or difficult toilet training.
Inattention to cues of need for elimination.
Episodes of urinary incontinence twice a week for at least 3 consecutive months in child of at least 5 years of age (or equivalent developmental level).
Pattern of diurnal and/or nocturnal enuresis.
One episode of soiling per month, over 3-month period in child at least 4 years of age (or equivalent developmental level).
Fecal incontinence; seepage secondary to fecal retention/colorectal loading.
Anal self-stimulation may be noted in nocturnal pattern of soiling.

### Hygiene

Deliberate attempts to hide evidence of soiled clothing.

### Neurosensory

May have developmental delays; neuromuscular or gross motor.
Less than 1/3 of enuretic children have documented emotional disorders (regression is rarely reason for problem).
Acting-out behaviors (e.g., placing feces or defecating in inappropriate places for retaliation).

### Safety

History/evidence of abuse may be present (condition may be related to abuse and/or the cause of abuse).

### Sexuality

Avoidance of sexual activity in older adolescents.

### Social Interactions

Impaired social, academic functioning.
Power struggles with family/school to maintain personal hygiene, change bed linens.

Reluctance to engage in peer activities; social rejection (body odor).
Uncomfortable spending the night with friends either in own home or away.

### Teaching/Learning

Usual age of onset 5–7, developmental age of at least 4 (encopresis) or 5 (enuresis).
Prevalence as high as 22% of 5-year-olds, 10% of 10-year-olds.
Boys more often affected than girls (3:1).
History of parental enuresis.
Bedwetting suppressed only as long as medication is taken; relapse usually occurring within 3 months.

## DIAGNOSTIC STUDIES

**Urinalysis:** Rule out UTI.
**Electrolytes:** Identify imbalance in presence of chronic diarrhea.
**Abdominal, Lower GI X-Rays:** Evaluate anatomic abnormalities such as anal fissure, obstruction.
**Cystometrogram (CMG):** Test for bladder capacity when in question.
**Detailed Toilet Training History:** Baseline continence data clarifying problem and evaluating for secondary vs. primary enuresis/encopresis.
**ECG:** Baseline when starting antidepressant medication.

## NURSING PRIORITIES

1. Promote understanding of condition.
2. Identify and support change in parent/child patterns of interaction.
3. Enhance self-esteem.
4. Assist client in achieving continence.

## DISCHARGE GOALS

1. Condition/therapy needs are understood.
2. All parties are participating in therapeutic regimen.
3. As near a normal pattern of bowel/bladder functioning as individually possible is achieved.

| NURSING DIAGNOSIS: | URINARY ELIMINATION, ALTERED/BOWEL INCONTINENCE |
|---|---|
| **May Be Related To:** | Situational/maturational crisis. |
| | Psychogenic factors: predisposing vulnerability; threat to physical integrity (child/sexual abuse). |
| | Constipation. |
| **Possibly Evidenced By:** | Nocturnal and/or diurnal enuresis. |
| | Involuntary passage of stool at least once monthly. |
| | Strong odor of urine/feces on client. |
| | Hiding fecal material/soiled clothing in inappropriate places. |

| Desired Outcomes/Evaluation Criteria—Client/Family Will: | Verbalize understanding of contributing factors and appropriate interventions. |
|---|---|
| | Participate in appropriate toileting program. |
| Client Will: | Achieve continence. |

## ACTIONS/INTERVENTIONS

### Independent

Identify times of occurrence, preceding/precipitating events, amounts of oral fluids, and family/client response to incontinence.

Check for fecal impaction.

Discuss measures client/family have tried and successes/failures to date.

Suggest use of bladder stretching exercises, e.g., ask child to drink favorite beverage and wait to urinate until the urge becomes very strong, then measure the amount of urine voided. Gradually increase amount of liquid and waiting period.

Discuss use of conditioning programs and ask parents/caregivers to maintain a record of occurrences for a specified period before either program begins.

Instruct client/family in use of electronic nighttime (bell and pad) monitoring device, e.g., Wet-Stop®.

Instruct parents/caregiver initially to get child up each time the urine alarm buzzer sounds, shifting the responsibility gradually to child by stating, "I want you to know you can do this all by yourself." Keep a record of how often the alarm sounds and how sound the child's sleep is.

Institute a system of positive reinforcement. Active-listen and involve client in developing the plan for remaining dry/clean. Use rewards that the child would like or agrees to. Use the previously determined baseline data to determine parameters of the reward system and when to increase schedule.

## RATIONALE

Baseline data will help identify patterns and document improvement after treatment begins.

May be contributing factor.

Typically parents/caregivers have tried various methods, usually getting child up periodically at night, limiting fluids before bedtime, and having older children change the bed linens. These methods are not very effective and usually lead to frustration, power struggles/battles.

Although this method can have good results, the length of time needed may be discouraging and result in the family stopping the program.

The use of conditioning therapy and/or behavior modification usually does not begin until the child is 7 or older. The child needs to make a commitment to be involved for the program to succeed. Information regarding the current individual pattern provides a baseline for future evaluation.

Urine alarms have been found to have an effective cure rate of 75%–90%. Once treatment is started, the alarm should be used every night.

The client may be fearful at first because of previous family interactions. In the beginning, the parents will probably waken before the child and take the child to the bathroom. However, as the program progresses, the child will waken more quickly and assume control. Empowerment promotes feelings of being in control.

Establishing a plan to which the client agrees has more chance of success than using aversive operant behavioral interventions (e.g., bell alarm) alone. Behavioral therapy may be useful when client is included in the planning, with rewards such as tokens having value if client agrees to their use. Note: If client is not involved in planning/vested in behavioral program, then therapy becomes an external control manipulating the client rather than promoting internal control and growth.

| ACTIONS/INTERVENTIONS | RATIONALE |
|---|---|

### Independent

Establish toileting routine with positive reinforcement for "sitting time" and depositing urine/feces in lavatory appropriately.

Client may begin to establish bowel/bladder habits often missing prior to treatment.

Treat occasional relapses with matter-of-fact attitude and follow through with procedures for self-hygiene.

Relapse (whether intentional or not) is to be expected, but may be minimized when the client does not feel pressured/blamed for lack of cooperation.

Discuss length of treatment with parents/client and make plans for maintaining dry status.

Knowing that treatment is ongoing prevents becoming discouraged and giving up treatment.

### Collaborative

Administer medications as appropriate, e.g.:
Imipramine (Tofranil);

May be used after age 7 for enuresis. However, drug therapy is only a temporary treatment, not a cure, as condition recurs within 3 months after medication is discontinued. Pharmacologic studies indicate improvement in encopresis with relatively low doses over 2-week period. Note: Factors such as child's age, duration of problem, and child's motivation to change are factors that affect decision to include pharmacologic agents in combination with behavioral interventions.

Desmopressin acetate (DDAVP);

Used for enuresis that has been intractable to other approaches.

Amphetamines;

Lightens sleep; therefore, client is more likely to awaken to arousal signals.

Laxatives and/or mineral oil.

Given daily for a specified period of time, these agents may promote bowel motility.

Refer for evaluation of the use of hypnosis.

Used alone or in conjunction with conditioning, the use of hypnosis can help the child develop positive suggestions that she or he has good muscle control and will be dry in the morning.

| NURSING DIAGNOSIS: | BODY IMAGE DISTURBANCE/SELF-ESTEEM, CHRONIC LOW |
|---|---|
| **May Be Related To:** | Negative view of self, maturational expectations. |
| | Social factors; stigma attached to loss of bodily functions in public. |
| | Belief of family that soiling/enuresis is volitional. |
| | Shame related to body odor. |
| **Possibly Evidenced By:** | Angry outbursts/oppositional behavior. |
| | Verbalization of powerlessness to change/control bodily functions. |
| | Reluctance to take social risks with friends (e.g., overnights, dancing). |

| Desired Outcomes/Evaluation Criteria— Client Will: | Verbalize acceptance of self in situation. |
| --- | --- |
| | Acknowledge own responsibility and control over situation. |
| | Participate in treatment program to effect change. |
| | Engage in social activities. |

| ACTIONS/INTERVENTIONS | RATIONALE |
| --- | --- |

**Independent**

| | |
| --- | --- |
| Establish a therapeutic nurse/client relationship. | Within a helping relationship, the individual will begin to trust and try out new thinking and behaviors. |
| Promote self-concept without moral judgment by use of therapeutic communication skills. Discuss how elimination habits are formed and fact that new habits can be learned. | Individual may see self as weak, even though he or she acts as if in control. Age-appropriate information can help the child/family understand there is nothing wrong with the child and the problem can be solved. |
| Explain to child/family that many children have this problem. Suggest stories child can read, e.g., *Clouds and Clock*, by M. Galvin (1989). | There is an increased risk for poor self-esteem/isolation when client views self as being "the only one." Use of bibliotherapy can help child to identify with others. |
| Promote active problem-solving and self-hygiene behaviors around some of the disagreeable aspects of enuresis/encopresis, e.g., control of odor, management of laundry, and successful overnight visits with friends. | Gives sense of control, supports ability to overcome stigma, enhancing self-esteem. |
| Be aware of own reaction to the client's behavior. Avoid controlling attitude or arguing with child around hygiene, toileting routine. | Feelings of disgust, hostility, and wanting distance from these clients are not uncommon. The child may in fact be projecting his or her own negative feelings onto the caretaker. The nurse needs to deal with own response/feelings so they do not interfere with care of the child. |
| Give positive reinforcement and encouragement for all attempts to join in peer activities or take additional risks in social situations, e.g., invite friend over. | Promotes repetition of desired behaviors, strengthens client's willingness to change, and enhances self-esteem. |

| NURSING DIAGNOSIS: | FAMILY COPING: ineffective (specify) |
| --- | --- |
| May Be Related To: | Inadequate/incorrect information or understanding by primary person; belief that behavior is volitional. |
| | Disagreement regarding treatment, coping strategies. |

| **Possibly Evidenced By:** | Attempts to intervene with child are increasingly ineffective. |
| | Significant person describes preoccupation with personal reaction (e.g., excessive guilt, anger, blame regarding child's condition/behavior). |
| | Significant person displays protective behavior disproportionate (too little or too much) to client's abilities or need for autonomy. |
| **Desired Outcomes/Evaluation Criteria— Family Will:** | Express feelings openly and honestly. |
| | Identify resources within self to deal with situation. |
| | Verbalize realistic understanding and expectations of client. |
| | Provide opportunity for client to deal with situation in own way as appropriate. |

| ACTIONS/INTERVENTIONS | RATIONALE |
|---|---|
| **Independent** | |
| Identify behaviors of/interactions between family members. | Withdrawal, anger/hostility toward client/others, ways of touching between family members, expressions of guilt provide clues to problems within family related or contributing to problem. |
| Assess for signs of child/sexual abuse. | These issues may be contributing factors to this problem. (Refer to CP: Problems Related to Abuse or Neglect). |
| Note verbal/nonverbal expressions of frustration, guilt/blame. | Problems of enuresis/encopresis are difficult for family members to deal with because of the long-term aspect of the problem. Uncommitted member may sabotage the program. |
| Determine willingness of family members to be involved in treatment program. | Success of any program will be dependent on all members being positively committed to therapy. |
| Encourage expression of feelings openly and honestly. | Feelings of frustration and fear are common and unless discussed can interfere with progress of therapy. |
| Discuss with the parents/caregivers the importance of not being too strict or permissive in dealing with this problem. | Effective use of Win-Win methods, e.g., Active-listening, I-messages, and problem-solving, can enhance the parent/child relationship, promote good feelings about selves and others. (Refer to CP: Parenting). |
| Avoid the use of spanking or other harsh punishment. | The use of harsh discipline usually results in power struggles where no one wins, making the problem worse and damaging the relationship between adult and child. |

| ACTIONS/INTERVENTIONS | RATIONALE |
|---|---|
| **Independent** | |
| Help parents recognize they are not responsible for and to separate themselves from the child's behavior. | Often, parents believe they have been "bad" parents and are responsible for the child's failure to achieve what they view as a "natural" behavior. When they see the child as a separate individual who has responsibility for own self, they can let go and be more comfortable in resolving the problem. |

# OTHER DISORDERS OF CHILDHOOD AND ADOLESCENCE: Anxiety Disorders

**DSM IV**
309.21  Separation Anxiety Disorder
313.23  Selective Mutism (Elective Mutism)
313.89  Reactive Attachment Disorder of Infancy or Early Childhood
309.24  Adjustment Disorder with Anxiety
307.3    Stereotypic Movement Disorder (Stereotypy/Habit Disorder)

**DSM III-R**
309.21  Separation Anxiety Disorder
313.21  Avoidant Disorder of Childhood or Adolescence
313.00  Overanxious Disorder
309.24  Adjustment Disorder with Anxious Mood

Anxiety is distinguished from fear, in that the emotional response to dangers is not within conscious awareness, although the anxiety may be focused on specific situations. Anxiety disorders are diagnosed when the anxiety symptoms cause significant distress or impairment. The more chronic and generalized anxiety states are called Generalized Anxiety Disorder (see CP). Nonphobic anxiety reactions to specific stressors are included under the diagnosis of Adjustment Disorder with Anxiety for children and adolescents. In the very young, the diagnosis would include Reactive Attachment Disorder of Infancy. Separation anxiety is the most frequent diagnosis.

## ETIOLOGIC THEORIES

### Psychodynamics

Anxiety arises from the unconscious as internalized conflicts are brought into awareness. By the 8th month of infancy, the infant displays separation distress, an indication of the capacity for a healthy infant to differentiate self from significant others and strangers. Clinging behavior and mild separation distress are seen as appropriate and adaptive responses to stressful situations throughout childhood. When the child experiences intense and diffuse symptoms in anticipation of separation, the immature ego is not strong enough to resolve the conflict.

### Biologic

Anticipatory anxiety is generated physiologically within the limbic system of the brain. Several neurotransmitters including serotonin and norepinephrine are associated with the anxiety response within the central nervous system. There is some evidence that children who meet behavioral criteria for anxiety disorders may not manifest panic symptoms because of the immaturity of the norepinephrine system. Should this be proved, panic disorders may emerge in latter stages of childhood or adolescence. The biologic response can be elicited and maintained by modifying external events. Current research indicates an increased risk for children in families with a history of anxiety disorders (panic disorder, agoraphobia, etc.) to develop these disorders themselves. The genetic mode of transmission has not been determined. Temperamental characteristics may be related to the acquisition of fear and anxiety disorders in childhood, referred to as anxiety proneness or vulnerability and may indicate inherited "disposition."

Anxiety disorders are often associated with physical complaints of "stomachaches" and "chest pains" or palpitations. On average the child will exhibit up to 8 somatic complaints. Medical causes for the pain should not be overlooked. However, often a pattern of physical symptoms coincides with attendance at school or other anticipated events. Stereotypic behaviors may also develop in an attempt to deal with overwhelming feelings of anxiety.

### Family Dynamics

The child with separation anxiety is seen as the contagion or compensation for anxiety within the family system. The child experiences distress/anxiety in response to family events, such as life-threatening illness or change in family home (divorce, move). The parents will, in turn, become distressed by the clinging behavior, and a vicious cycle begins. Often the child refuses to go to school or sleep alone. Mutism may be a conscious or unconscious response to these stressors.

Parents may instill anxiety in their children by overprotecting them from expectable dangers or by exaggerating the dangers of the present and the future. Role modeling may also transfer fears and anxiety to children. Eldest children, those in small families or upper-socioeconomic groups, and families in which there is a concern about achievement, as well as children who come from single-parent homes and a slightly lower socioeconomic class, may be at increased risk.

## CLIENT ASSESSMENT DATABASE

### Activity/Rest

Reluctance to sleep alone or to go to sleep away from home.
Frequent reports of nightmares involving theme of separation.
Insomnia.
Reluctant to engage in activities with any possible danger or may engage in excessive risk taking (counterphobic).

## EGO INTEGRITY

Acute behavioral expression of distress, crying loudly, shakes, tantrum, anxious mood, fretful.
Feels "different" or left out when social inhibition is present.
Described as nervous or "high strung" by others.
Fears losing (e.g., getting lost, being kidnapped, dying) or that harm will befall major attachment figure.

### Elimination

Frequent urination.
Diarrhea.

### Food/Fluid

Nausea, vomiting.
Stomachaches.
May be malnourished (reactive attachment).

### Neurosensory

Dizziness, fainting with panic attacks.
Headaches.
Startles easily.
Repetitive, driven, nonfunctional motor behavior, e.g., body rocking, head banging, mouthing of objects (stereotypic movement).
Responses inhibited, hypervigilant or highly ambivalent and contradictory (reactive attachment).
Depressed mood.

## Safety

Self-destructive behaviors, e.g., head banging, self-biting, picking at skin, hitting own body (stereotypic movement).
Evidence of bodily injury, e.g., bruising (stereotypic movement), physical abuse (reactive attachment).

## Social Interactions

Difficulty being alone or participating in activities without significant adult.
Appears clingy, needy, dependent (leading to parental frustration/family conflict); displays indiscriminate sociability, excessive familiarity with relative strangers (reactive attachment).
May be shy, withdrawn, avoidant of social contact; fail to speak in specific situations.
Impairment in social, academic/occupational, or other important areas of functioning.
Family displays grossly negligent caretaking; repeated changes of primary caregiver.

## Teaching/Learning

Early age onset before 18 years (before age of 6 in separation anxiety) or age 5 for reactive attachment disorder), with equal gender distribution.
Behaviors persist for 4 weeks or more.
Reluctance/refusal to go to school out of fear of separation.
Frequent visits to school nurse for somatic complaints.
Persistent failure to initiate or respond in a developmentally appropriate fashion; growth delayed (reactive attachment).

## DIAGNOSTIC STUDIES

**Dexamethasone Suppression Tests:** Children with severe separation anxiety are nearly as likely as severely depressed children to have an abnormal test result.
**Laboratory Tests:** As indicated by antidepressant drug therapy, nutritional state.
**Neurologic Testing (EEG, CT/Other Scans):** Rules out presence of organic brain disorders.

## NURSING PRIORITIES

1. Facilitate reduction in symptoms and relieve distress.
2. Prevent injury associated with the disorder, particularly with the presence of panic attacks.

## DISCHARGE GOALS

1. Somatic complaints/physical symptoms decreased or alleviated as a response to distressful activities or thoughts.
2. Age-appropriate activities are engaged in without fear or distress in the absence of the parent.
3. Understanding of the contagion effect of anxiety verbalized and using effective coping skills.
4. Parent(s) enforce regular school attendance/sleeping alone while providing positive feedback and encouragement.

| NURSING DIAGNOSIS: | ANXIETY [severe/panic] |
| --- | --- |
| May Be Related To: | Situational/maturational crisis; internal transmission/contagion. |

| | |
|---|---|
| | Threat to physical integrity or self-concept; unmet needs. |
| | Dysfunctional family system; independence conflicts. |
| **Possibly Evidenced By:** | Somatic complaints; nightmares; excessive psychomotor activity. |
| | Refusal to attend school; reluctance to engage in activities without presence of specific adult figure. |
| | Persistent worry/fear of catastrophic doom to family or self. |
| **Desired Outcomes/Evaluation Criteria— Client Will:** | Appear relaxed and report/demonstrate relief from somatic manifestations of anxiety. |
| | Engage in age-appropriate activities in absence of parent/primary caregiver without fear or distress noted. |
| | Demonstrate a decrease in somatic complaints and physical symptoms when faced with impending separation from significant other. |

| ACTIONS/INTERVENTIONS | RATIONALE |
|---|---|
| **Independent** | |
| Establish an atmosphere of calmness, trust, and genuine positive regard. | Trust and unconditional acceptance are necessary for satisfactory nurse/client relationship. Calmness is important because anxiety is easily transmitted from one person to another. |
| Identify a primary nurse for client/family. | Often the caregiver will experience separation anxiety at the same level as the child, and trust is necessary to begin to deal with these issues. Note: Disorder may be related to loss of family of origin/frequent moves and/or foster care. |
| Ensure client of his or her safety and security, e.g., listen to client, identify needs, be available for support. | Symptoms of panic anxiety are very frightening and providing information regarding safety can be reassuring. |
| Discuss with family members contagious nature of anxious feelings. | Understanding of this contagion allows the participants to begin to recognize and deal with anxiety other is exhibiting. |
| Explore the child/adolescent's fears of separating from the parent(s)/caregiver. Explore with the adults possible fears they may have of separation from the child. | Some parents may have an underlying fear of separation from the child of which they are unaware and which they are unconsciously transferring to the child. |
| Observe/assist client to recognize manifestations of anxiety (e.g., stomachaches, dizziness, frequent urination). | Identifies relationship of symptoms so client can make constructive changes. |
| Explain to child that feelings are normal bodily reactions to stress, not harmful or dangerous, just unpleasant. | Prevents adding to panic with overexaggeration or misconception about the consequences of acknowledging feeling state. |

101

| ACTIONS/INTERVENTIONS | RATIONALE |
|---|---|

### Independent

| | |
|---|---|
| Identify factors that precede symptoms of anxiety. | Allows client to plan coping strategy and assess level of self-control. |
| Encourage child to bring transitional object from home, e.g., familiar toys, special pillow or blanket, pictures, posters, or music. | Use of age-appropriate object when child or adolescent is hospitalized enhances sense of security. |
| Use play materials, e.g., puppets, doll house, doctor/nurse kits, fairytale stories, clay, sand tray. | Play therapy enables child to explore conflicts, express fears, and release tension. |
| Encourage family visitation while structuring length and frequency of contact when child is hospitalized. | Repeated reunions and separations without disastrous consequences will help to desensitize the child to separation. |
| Stress the importance of staff/family giving verbal prompts in anticipation of absences. Maintain honest information about when the caregiver will leave and when he or she will return. | Avoidance of discussion around impending separation only increases likelihood of anxiety response. |
| Provide information for family/siblings regarding the typical responses of childhood anxiety during critical stages of development. | Knowledge of "anticipatory anxiety state" will decrease guilt experienced by other family members while they are entering school/separating from home/family. |
| Help adults and child initiate realistic goals (e.g., child to stay with sitter for 2 hours with minimal anxiety, or child to stay at friend's house without own parents until 6 PM without experiencing panic anxiety). | Parents may be so frustrated with child's clinging and demanding behaviors that a different perspective and assistance with problem-solving may be helpful. |
| Give, and encourage parent(s)/caregiver to give, positive reinforcement for desired behaviors. | Positive reinforcement encourages repetition of desirable behaviors. |

### Collaboration

| | |
|---|---|
| Administer medications as appropriate:<br>Tricyclic antidepressants, e.g., imipramine (Tofranil);<br>Antihistamines: diphenhydramine (Benadryl);<br>Antianxiety agents: benzodiazepines such as alpraxzolam (Xanax), clonazepam (Clonopin). | Use of medication is effective in ameliorating symptoms of anxiety. |

| NURSING DIAGNOSIS: | COPING INDIVIDUAL, INEFFECTIVE |
|---|---|
| **May Be Related To:** | Maturational crisis; multiple life changes and/or losses. |
| | Personal vulnerability. |
| | Inadequate coping strategies. |
| **Possibly Evidenced By:** | Inability to cope/problem-solve. |
| | Persistent, overwhelming fears and anxieties. |
| | Inability to meet role expectations; refusal to attend school. |

| Desired Outcomes/Evaluation Criteria—Client Will: | Social inhibition; shy, withdrawn demeanor. |
| --- | --- |
| | Panic attacks. |
| | Demonstrate use of more effective coping techniques in response to stressful situations. |
| | Verbalize understanding of the need for strategies to control frightening thoughts. |
| | Demonstrate level of autonomy to maximize developmental potential. |

| ACTIONS/INTERVENTIONS | RATIONALE |
| --- | --- |
| **Independent** | |
| Encourage child/adolescent to discuss specific situations in life that produce the most distress and describe his or her response to these situations. Include parent(s)/caregiver(s) in the discussion. | Client and family may be unaware of the correlation between stressful situations and the exacerbation of physical symptoms. |
| Encourage client to express fears and concerns. Avoid arguing about client's perception of situation. | Self-understanding and further explanation are enhanced when verbalizations of anxiety and distress are received in a nonjudgmental manner. |
| Have client envision situation in which fear commonly occurs. Assist client to accept fear, listening to bodily reactions, giving the fear time to pass. | Allows client to recognize that fears are not catastrophic or harmful. Practicing in nonstressful situation will enhance ability to deal with separation/other stressors. |
| Help the child/adolescent who is perfectionistic to recognize that self-expectations may be unrealistic. Connect times of unmet self-expectations to the exacerbation of physical symptoms. | Recognition of maladaptive patterns is the first step in the change process. |
| Assist client to learn relaxation techniques, e.g., breathing exercise, visualization and guided imagery skills. | Enables client to manage fears/anxiety, increasing self-reliance. |
| Encourage parent(s)/caregiver(s) and child to identify more adaptive coping strategies that the child could use in the face of anxiety that feels overwhelming. Practice through role-playing. | Practice facilitates the use of the desired behavior when the individual is actually faced with the stressful situation. |
| Reinforce client positively when change in behavior indicates effective coping. Anticipate and accept occasional set-backs. | Positive reinforcement encourages personal growth. Consistency in effective coping is a maturational process requiring time and patience. |

| NURSING DIAGNOSIS: | **SOCIAL INTERACTION, IMPAIRED** |
| --- | --- |
| **May Be Related To:** | Excessive self-consciousness. |
| | Inability to interact with unfamiliar people. |
| | Self-concept disturbance; altered thought processes. |
| **Possibly Evidenced By:** | Verbalized/observed discomfort in social situations. |

103

| | Verbalized/observed inability to receive or communicate a satisfying sense of belonging, caring, interest, or shared history. |
|---|---|
| | Observed use of unsuccessful social interaction behaviors. |
| **Desired Outcomes/Evaluation Criteria— Client Will:** | Identify feelings that lead to poor social interactions. |
| | Interact within therapy peer group. |
| | Verbalize intention of attending school and follow through with action. |
| | Give self positive reinforcement for changes that are achieved. |

| ACTIONS/INTERVENTIONS | RATIONALE |
|---|---|
| **Independent** | |
| Develop trusting relationship with client. | This is the first step in helping the client learn to interact with others. |
| Attend group with the child and support efforts to interact with others. Give positive feedback. | Presence of a trusted individual provides security during times of distress. Positive feedback encourages repetition. |
| Convey to the child the acceptability of his or her not participating in contributions until he or she is able to participate more fully. | Small successes will gradually increase self-confidence and decrease self-consciousness, so that client will feel less anxious in the group situation. |
| Help client set small personal goals, e.g., "Today I will speak to one person I don't know." | Simple, realistic goals provide opportunities for success that increase self-confidence and may encourage the client to attempt more difficult objectives in the future. |

| NURSING DIAGNOSIS: | VIOLENCE/SELF-MUTILATION, HIGH RISK FOR |
|---|---|
| **Risk Factors May Include:** | Panic states. |
| | Emotionally disturbed child; presence of separation anxiety. |
| | Dysfunctional family. |
| **Possible Indicators:** | Increasing anxiety level. |
| | Increased motor activity (e.g., excitement, agitation). |
| | Self-destructive behaviors (e.g., head banging, self-biting, picking at skin, hitting own body). |
| **Desired Outcomes/Evaluation Criteria— Client Will:** | Identify precipitating factors/awareness of arousal state that occurs prior to incident. |
| | Express increased self-concept/esteem. |
| | Demonstrate self-control as evidenced by lessened episodes of acting out/self-mutilation, use of alternate methods of management of feelings. |

| ACTIONS/INTERVENTIONS | RATIONALE |
|---|---|

### Independent

| | |
|---|---|
| Determine underlying dynamics of individual situation. Review previous episodes of acting out/self-destructive behavior. | Information necessary to promote individualized planning of care. |
| Identify situations that interfere with ability to control own behavior, e.g., panic state. | May need additional restraints to control behavior until self-control is regained. |
| Observe for early signs of distress/increasing anxiety. (Refer to ND: Anxiety [severe/panic]/Fear.) | Allows for early interventions to prevent exacerbation of situation. |
| Provide external controls/limit setting. Hold client, speak in low commanding voice, tell client to STOP behavior. | Helps client to regain self-control in a safe setting, maintains dignity, promoting self-esteem. |
| Assist client to identify feelings that precede negative behaviors. | Provides opportunity for client to institute controls/ask for help before losing control. |
| Assist client to learn assertive/healthy behavior rather that use of aggression. Role-play situations and responses. | Promotes positive ways of responding to stress, lessening need for anxious/nonproductive behaviors. |
| Provide protective headgear as indicated. Use restraints with caution. | May need this additional protection when behavior is severe/persists. Restraints may result in injury when client fights against them. |

| | |
|---|---|
| **NURSING DIAGNOSIS:** | **FAMILY COPING, ineffective: compromised/disabling** |
| **May Be Related To:** | Presence of other situational/developmental crises affecting family members (e.g., divorce, addition/loss of family member, midlife crisis). |
| | Frequent disruptions in living arrangements. |
| | Unrealistic parental expectations for child's achievement in areas of sports, academics, etc. |
| | High-risk family situations, e.g., history of neglect/abuse, substance abuse, panic disorder, depression. |
| **Possibly Evidenced By:** | SO reports frustration with clinging behaviors; colludes with truancy. |
| | SO displays emotional lability; harsh or punitive response to tyrannical behaviors. |
| | Neglectful care of child in regard to basic human needs. |
| | SO displays protective behavior disproportionate (too little or too much) to child's abilities or need for autonomy. |
| **Desired Outcomes/Evaluation Criteria— Family/Caregiver Will:** | Verbalize knowledge and understanding of child's condition. |

105

Verbalize more realistic understanding and expectations of client.

Develop strategies to help child begin to deal with stressful situations, e.g., attending school, sleeping alone, etc.

Provide opportunity for child to deal with situation in own way.

| ACTIONS/INTERVENTIONS | RATIONALE |
| --- | --- |

### Independent

| | |
| --- | --- |
| Establish rapport with family members/caregivers. Acknowledge difficulty of the situation for the family by Active-listening. | Promotes trust, opens lines of communication and provides feeling of being understood. |
| Identify current and past behaviors of family member(s) (e.g., overprotectiveness, withdrawal, anger toward child, neglect of emotional/physical needs). | Provides beginning point to create plan of care for individual client and family/caregiver. |
| Provide information and materials related to child's disorder including discussion of developmental stages and growth. | Promotes knowledge and skills that help parents understand and may increase parental effectiveness. |
| Encourage parents/caregivers to verbalize feelings and explore alternative methods of dealing with child. | Supportive counseling can assist adults in developing coping strategies. |
| Provide feedback and reinforce effective parenting methods. (Refer to CP: Parenting.) | Positive reinforcement can increase self-esteem and encourages continued efforts. |
| Formulate plan for regular school attendance/sleeping alone. | Provides specific interventions to help family resolve problem and goals to measure effectiveness of actions/additional needs. |
| Involve siblings in family discussions and planning for more effective family interactions. | Family problems affect all members, and treatment is more effective when everyone is involved in therapy. |

### Collaborative

| | |
| --- | --- |
| Refer to community resources as indicated, e.g., psychotherapy, parent support groups, parenting classes (Parent Effectiveness). | Developing a support system, learning new skills can increase parental confidence and effectiveness. |

# PARENTING (GROWTH PROMOTING RELATIONSHIP)

**DSM IV**
V61.20 Parent-Child Relational Problem

**DSM III-R**
No listing.

Many parents are concerned about how to raise responsible children who have high self-esteem, demonstrate self-control, and display skills of cooperation and consideration of others. Most people believe that we somehow know how to "parent" instinctively. Usually, this attitude results in parenting the same way we were parented. However, it is clear that the traditional authoritarian or permissive methods of parenting create inner conflict for most parents, and praise, punishment, and rewards do not have the desired effects of positive relationships with children. Conflicts in the parent/child relationship can lead to dysfunctional/abusive relationship patterns. In addition, when children are experiencing mental health crises requiring therapeutic intervention, learning different ways of parenting becomes essential to developing positive relationships between parent and child.

## ETIOLOGIC THEORIES

### Psychodynamics

Effective parenting is a learned skill and is not a set of instinctive behaviors. Parental roles are derived from many factors, e.g., the family of origin, family myths and scripts, parental skills, knowledge and level of differentiation, socioeconomic and cultural factors, and the marital relationship.

### Biologic

There is a genetic plan for the growth and development of the physical body. In the same way, there is a biologic plan for intelligence that is genetically encoded within the individual and drives the child from within. At the same time, parents provide an anxiety-conditioned view of the world that is in conflict with the child's nature. Many of the problems of parenting are caused by people, brought about by ignoring this plan of nature.

### Family Dynamics

A family is seen as a natural social system, with its own set of rules, definition of roles, power structure, and methods of communicating, negotiating, and problem-solving that provide a means of dealing with the process of daily living. These family patterns are largely unconscious and set the emotional tone. These systems are multigenerational, with underlying family dynamics affecting all members in some way. These patterns may be functional or dysfunctional.

## PARENT ASSESSMENT DATABASE

### Activity/Rest

Difficulty sleeping.
Exhaustion.

### Ego Integrity

Broad range of feelings (e.g., calm to hysterical) may be noted.
May display increasing tension and disorganization, e.g., anger, frustration, crying, depression; may repeat the same question over and over.

Defense mechanisms, e.g., denial, rationalization, defensiveness, intellectualization, projection.

Multiple stress factors, changes in relationships.

Feelings of helplessness, hopelessness, powerlessness.

## Food/Fluid

Difficulty eating, loss of appetite.

## Hygiene

General appearance of family members (neat or disheveled; clean or odious) may be indicators of coping ability, state of denial, presence of crisis.

## Neurosensory

**Behavior:** Upset, anxious, rapid speech or quiet and withdrawn; appropriate or inappropriate.

## Social Interactions

Family structure may be traditional 2-parent, single-parent (mother or father as head), or blended (stepfamily).

**Family Genogram:** Notes patterns between family members and generations.

Lack of limited support (presence of/geographic distance, and degree of involvement of extended family).

Some family member(s) may not appear to be experiencing symptoms of stress or may have changed their usual patterns of interacting.

Varied socioeconomic/cultural factors, e.g., financial status, inclusion of extended family, family myths and beliefs, sense of community.

Multiple losses/crises, e.g., death, divorce, other separations, frequent relocation.

History of period of family disorganization often present.

Child-rearing practices may be ineffective; dysfunctional/ineffective communication patterns.

History of child abuse/sexual abuse.

## NURSING PRIORITIES

1. Promote positive feelings about parenting abilities.
2. Involve parents in problem-solving solutions for current situation.
3. Provide assistance to enable family to develop skills to deal with present situation.
4. Facilitate learning of new parenting skills.

## DISCHARGE GOALS

1. Understands parenting role, expectations, and responsibilities.
2. Aware of own strengths, individual needs, and methods/resources to meet them.
3. Appropriate attachment/parenting behaviors demonstrated.
4. Involved in activities directed at family growth.

| NURSING DIAGNOSIS: | PARENTING, ALTERED, ACTUAL (OR HIGH RISK FOR) |
|---|---|
| **May Be Related To:** | Lack of/ineffective role model; lack of support between or from significant other(s). |
| | Interruption in bonding process. |

**Possibly Evidenced By:**

Lack of knowledge; unrealistic expectations for self, child, partner.

Presence of stressors: recent crisis, financial, legal, household move, change in family structure.

Physical/psychosocial abuse by nurturing figure.

Lack of appropriate response of child to parent/parent to child.

Frequent verbalization of disappointment in child; resentment toward child; inability to care for/discipline child.

Lack of parental attachment behaviors, e.g., negative characterizations of child; lack of touching; inattention to child's needs.

Inappropriate or inconsistent discipline practices and/or caretaking behaviors.

Growth and/or developmental lag in child.

Presence of child abuse or abandonment.

**Desired Outcomes/Evaluation Criteria—Parent(s) Will:**

Verbalize realistic information and expectations of parenting role and acceptance of situation.

Identify own needs, strengths, and methods/resources to meet them.

Demonstrate appropriate attachment and effective parenting behaviors.

| ACTIONS/INTERVENTIONS | RATIONALE |
|---|---|
| **Independent** | |
| Determine existing situation and parent(s)' perception of the problems, noting presence of specific factors such as psychiatric/physical illness, disabilities of child or parent. | Identification of the individual factors will aid in establishing the plan of care. |
| Determine developmental stage of the family, e.g., first child/new infant, school-age/adolescent children, stepfamily. | These factors affect how family members view current problems and how they will solve them. |
| Assess parenting skill level, considering intellectual, emotional, and physical strengths and limitations. | Identifies areas of need for further information, skill training, and factors that might interfere with ability to assimilate new information. |
| Note attachment behaviors between parent and child(ren). Encourage the parent(s) to hold and spend time with the child, particularly the newborn/infant. | Lack of eye contact, touching may be indicative of problems of bonding. Behaviors such as eye-to-eye contact, use of en face position, talking to the infant in a high-pitched voice are indicative of attachment behaviors in American culture. Failure to bond effectively is thought to affect subsequent parent-child interaction. |
| Observe interactions between parent(s) and child(ren). | Identifies relationships, communication skills, feelings about one another. |

109

| ACTIONS/INTERVENTIONS | RATIONALE |
|---|---|

### Independent

Note presence/effectiveness of extended family/support systems.

Provides role models for parent(s) to help them develop own style of parenting. Note: Role models may be negative and/or controlling.

Stress the positive aspects of the situation, maintaining a positive attitude toward the parents' capabilities and potential for improving.

Helping the parent(s) to feel accepting about self and individual capabilities will promote growth.

Involve all members of the family in learning activities.

Learning new skills is enhanced when everyone is is interacting.

Provide specific information about limit setting, time management, and conflict resolution.

Helpful in managing parenting responsibilities.

Encourage parent(s) to identify positive outlets for meeting own needs, e.g., going to a movie, out to dinner. (Refer to ND: Self-Esteem disturbance/Role Performance, altered.)

Parent often believes it is "selfish" to do things for own self, that children are primary. However, parents are important, children are important, and the family is important. As a rule, when parents take care of themselves, they are better parents.

Discuss issues of stepparenting and ways to achieve positive relationships in a blended family. Refer to resources such as books, classes for stepfamilies.

Blending two families can be a very demanding task. Providing information can help people learn to negotiate and develop skills for living together in a new configuration.

| NURSING DIAGNOSIS: | SELF-ESTEEM DISTURBANCE [specify]/ROLE PERFORMANCE, ALTERED |
|---|---|
| May Be Related To: | View of self as "poor," ineffective parent(s). |
| | Problems of child(ren), psychiatric/physical illness of the child. |
| | Belief that seeking help is an admission of defeat/failure. |
| Possibly Evidenced By: | Change in usual patterns/responsibility. |
| | Expressions of lack of information about parenting skills. |
| | Lack of follow-through of therapy. |
| | Not keeping appointments. |
| | Nonparticipation in therapy. |
| Desired Outcomes/Evaluation Criteria— Parent(s) Will: | Verbalize acceptance of selves as parents who are not perfect. |
| | Verbalize understanding of role expectations/obligations. |
| | Demonstrate personal growth as evidenced by seeking information, setting of realistic goals, and active participation in improving parent/child relationship. |

| ACTIONS/INTERVENTIONS | RATIONALE |
| --- | --- |

### Independent

| | |
| --- | --- |
| Assess level of parent's anxiety, and determine the parent's perception and reality of the situation. | Identification of how family members view the situation and their role in what is happening is essential to the development of the plan of care. The difference between what is actually happening and individual perception can provide helpful clues to family problems and defense mechanisms. |
| Discuss parental perceptions of their skills and roles as parents. Give information as needs are identified. | Parent may see self as a "bad parent" when children have problems and do not live up to expectations of either the parents or society. Information can be given and may be more readily accepted in casual learning environment. |
| Listen to expressions of concern about others' reactions to child's behavior/problems, sense of control over self/situations. | Parent(s) may allow themselves to be influenced by "what others think" rather than establishing their own actions, beliefs, and control. |
| Note previous and current level of adaptive behaviors/defense mechanisms. | Identifies positive/negative skills and establishes baseline for assisting parents to identify things they already do well and to learn new ways of parenting. |
| Encourage open discussion of situation/expression of feelings. | Assists individuals to identify areas of concern, hear own ideas, and share with other members of the family. |
| Acknowledge and accept feelings of anger and hostility. | May believe that expression of negative feelings is not acceptable. |
| Set limits on maladaptive behaviors and suggest alternative actions, such as hitting pillows, pounding mattress. | Anger may be expressed by unacceptable actions such as hitting/breaking objects in the environment or in violence toward themselves or others. |
| Have parents identify positive behaviors they demonstrate, e.g., the use of positive I-messages, hugging one another, use of listening skills. | Improves feelings of self-worth and increases sense of self-esteem when parents recognize that they do have strengths on which to build/establish more positive family interactions. |
| Encourage individuals to become aware of own responsibility for dealing with what is happening. | Each person only has control over own self and cannot control or make another do anything. |
| Assist parent(s) to look at own role(s) as actor/reactor to what has been happening in the family. | May limit own options by reacting to situations rather than taking action to make things better. |
| Help parent(s) to avoid comparisons with others. | Each family and the individuals involved have unique ways of dealing with own problems, and comparisons are usually used in a negative way to prove own lack of self-worth. |
| Assist parents to learn therapeutic communication skills, e.g., I-messages, Active-listening. Discuss the use of positive I-messages instead of praise. | Improving skills for talking to others offers the opportunity to enhance relationships. Positive I-messages help the individual to develop own internal sense of self-worth, self-esteem. |
| Provide empathy, not sympathy. | Empathy is objective and communicates an understanding of the other's problems as viewed by that individual, promoting the "I-Thou" relationship. Sympathy is subjective and expresses concern for the nurse's own feelings. |

| ACTIONS/INTERVENTIONS | RATIONALE |
|---|---|
| **Independent** | |
| Use positive words of encouragement for improvements noted. | Reinforces developing positive coping behaviors. |
| Discuss inaccuracies in perception as they become apparent. | Helps parents to identify areas of needed action. |
| **Collaborative** | |
| Encourage attendance at group therapy (family and multifamily), assertiveness training, and positive self-esteem classes. | Learning new skills helps individuals develop an improved sense of self-esteem. |

| NURSING DIAGNOSIS: | FAMILY PROCESSES, ALTERED |
|---|---|
| **May Be Related To:** | Situational crisis of child/adolescent, e.g., illness/hospitalization, delinquency. |
| | Maturational crisis, e.g., adolescence, midlife. |
| **Possibly Evidenced By:** | Expressions of confusion and difficulty coping with situation. |
| | Family system not meeting physical/emotional/security needs of members. |
| | Having difficulty accepting help, not dealing with traumatic experiences constructively. |
| | Parents not respecting each other's parenting practices. |
| **Desired Outcomes/Evaluation Criteria— Family Will:** | Express feelings appropriately. |
| | Demonstrate individual involvement in problem-solving. |
| | Verbalize understanding of child/family problems. |

| ACTIONS/INTERVENTIONS | RATIONALE |
|---|---|
| **Independent** | |
| Assess family components, roles, dynamics, developmental stage (e.g., young/adolescent children, divorced with stepparents, children leaving home), and cultural influences. | Information essential to development of plan of care. |
| Identify patterns of communication within family. | Helps to establish areas of positive and negative patterns. |
| Determine boundaries within the family system. | Boundaries need to be clear so individual family members are free to be responsible for themselves. |
| Assess use of addictive substances by members of the family. | Alcoholism and other drug use may be a critical issue in the interacting of the family as well as in developing a treatment plan. (Note: Individuals may be reluctant to share this information until they feel safe within the therapeutic relationship.) |

| ACTIONS/INTERVENTIONS | RATIONALE |
|---|---|
| **Independent** | |
| Identify patterns of communication between individual members and the family as a whole. | May be ineffective to accomplish family tasks. These patterns may be maintaining the maladaptive behaviors/relationships. |
| Identify and encourage previously successful coping mechanisms. | Using these behaviors will be comfortable for the individual, and a sense of competence and assurance will be gained. |
| Acknowledge differences among family members with open dialogue about how these differences have been derived. | Conveys an acceptance of these differences among individuals and helps to look at how the differences can be used to facilitate the family process. |
| Identify effective parenting skills already being used and suggest new ways of handling difficult behaviors. | Allows the individual to realize that some of what has been done already has been helpful and assists in learning new skills to manage the situation in a more effective manner. |
| Encourage participation in role-reversal activities. | Helps to gain insight and understanding of the other person's feelings and point of view. |

| NURSING DIAGNOSIS: | **FAMILY COPING, ineffective: compromised/disabling** |
|---|---|
| **May Be Related To:** | Individual preoccupation with own emotional conflicts and personal suffering/anxiety about the crisis. |
| | Temporary family disorganization. |
| | Situational crisis. |
| | Exhausted supportive capacities of family members. |
| | Chronically unexpressed feelings of guilt, anger, etc. |
| | Highly ambivalent family relationships. |
| | Arbitrary handling of a family's resistance, which solidifies defensiveness. |
| **Possibly Evidenced By:** | Expressions of concern. |
| | Complaints about SO(s)' response to problem; expressions of despair about family reactions. |
| | Withdrawal and/or display of protective behavior; distortion of reality about problems; denial. |
| | Intolerance, agitation, depression, hostility, aggression. |
| | Neglecting relationships. |
| | Decisions/actions that are detrimental. |
| **Desired Outcomes/Evaluation Criteria— Family Will:** | Express more realistic expectations of themselves and situation. |

113

Identify internal and external resources.

Interact with each other realistically and with understanding.

Participate in activities to promote improved coping.

| ACTIONS/INTERVENTIONS | RATIONALE |
|---|---|
| **Independent** | |
| Establish rapport with family members. | Helps family members to feel comfortable and talk freely about the problems they are experiencing. |
| Identify premorbid behaviors and interactions. Compare with current behaviors. | Necessary baseline to establish treatment goals. Family members may be withdrawn, angry, hostile, and ignoring each other (or one specific member). |
| Note readiness of family to be involved in treatment. | Readiness is necessary for the success of therapy. |
| Encourage communication, free expression of feelings without judgment. | Promotes understanding of how others are feeling, perceiving what is happening. |
| Note other stressors impacting the family, e.g., financial, legal, physical illness. | May need assistance with these factors before the family can begin to deal with the issues at hand. |
| Encourage questions, provide accurate information, involving family in treatment planning. (Refer to ND: Knowledge Deficit.) | Personal involvement by client and family enhances learning and promotes cooperation with/ success of therapy. |
| Reframe individual's negative statements when possible. | Provides a different way of looking at the problem/ situation. |
| Encourage dealing with the problems in small increments. | One moment at a time can seem more manageable than looking at the whole picture. |
| **Collaborative** | |
| Refer to social services, support group, marriage counselor, community/spiritual resources as indicated. | Family may need additional help and support to resolve issues, incorporating new techniques and problem-solving. |

| **NURSING DIAGNOSIS:** | **FAMILY COPING, POTENTIAL FOR GROWTH** |
|---|---|
| **May Be Related To:** | Surfacing of self-actualization goals. |
| **Possibly Evidenced By:** | Expressing interest in making contact with another person experiencing a similar situation. |
| | Moving in direction of health promoting/enriching lifestyle, auditing/negotiating therapy program, generally choosing experiences that optimize growth. |
| **Desired Outcomes/Evaluation Criteria— Family Will:** | Express willingness to look at own role in the problem. |
| | Verbalize desire to change, feelings of self-confidence, satisfaction with progress. |
| | Identify/use resources appropriately. |

| ACTIONS/INTERVENTIONS | RATIONALE |
|---|---|

## Independent

Determine situation and stage of growth family is experiencing. Note verbalizations of awareness of the growth, impact of the crisis, and expressed interest in learning opportunity.

Baseline data required to establish plan of assistance.

Listen to expressions of hope, planning, etc.

Acknowledgment by the nurse provides reinforcement of hopes and desires for positive change for the future.

Note expression of change of values, discussion of values/beliefs.

Willingness to look at own values, discuss meanings, and make decisions about own beliefs is helpful to growth of family members.

Provide role model for parent(s) to be involved with and observe.

Role model provides opportunity for individual members to learn new behaviors.

Provide opportunities to role-play new ways of interacting.

Role-play allows client and family to "practice" how they will respond in stressful situations, in an effort to prevent future crises.

Encourage open communication within the family (no "family secrets") and use of effective communication skills, e.g., I-messages, Active-listening.

Open acceptance of a variety of feelings and attitudes is necessary for growth within the family system.

Assist individuals to learn new effective ways of dealing with feelings.

Learning to identify and express feelings provides opportunity to act in different ways.

## Collaborative

Involve with others who have had similar experiences, e.g., multifamily group therapy, support groups, stepfamily group.

Sharing of experiences provides opportunities to develop empathy and understanding of parenting roles.

Identify/refer to resources, e.g., group therapy, parenting classes, etc.

Involvement with others helps individuals to see how they and others solve problems, effectively or ineffectively, and provides opportunities to learn new skills.

| | |
|---|---|
| **NURSING DIAGNOSIS:** | **KNOWLEDGE DEFICIT [LEARNING NEED] regarding parenting skills, developmental stages** |
| **May Be Related To:** | Lack of information/unfamiliarity with resources about child growth and development; information misinterpretation. |
| | Ineffective parenting skills. |
| **Possibly Evidenced By:** | Angry expressions about parenting role. |
| | Verbalization of problems in dealing with child(ren). |
| | Statements of misconceptions about how to parent. |
| | Inappropriate or exaggerated behaviors, e.g., hostile, agitated, apathetic. |

| Desired Outcomes/Evaluation Criteria—Family Will: | Participate in learning process. |
| --- | --- |
| | Assume responsibility for learning new parenting skills. |
| | Identify stressors and actions to deal effectively with them. |
| | Initiate necessary lifestyle changes and participate in learning activities. |

## ACTIONS/INTERVENTIONS

### Independent

Determine level of knowledge of parenting skills and beliefs.

Note level of anxiety and signs of avoidance; cultural beliefs about parents and children; feelings about self as a parent.

Review information about developmental level of child(ren), expected maturational progression, and individual nature of process. Discuss parental expectations.

Provide information and help parent(s) learn new communication skills of Active-listening and declarative, responsive, preventive, and positive I-messages.

Discuss conflict-resolution concepts of "who owns the problem," problem-solving and resolving of value collisions.

Be aware of "teachable moments" that occur during interaction with the family and/or individual members.

Promote active participation in learning by the use of role-play, participant discussion, and other activities.

Provide positive reinforcement for attempts to learn new behaviors/communication skills.

Provide information about additional resources, e.g., books on related topics, tapes.

Refer to social workers, clergy, psychotherapy, and/or classes such as Parent Effectiveness, assertiveness training.

## RATIONALE

Individual needs are based on current information and/or beliefs and misconceptions.

Moderate to severe anxiety, level of self-esteem, cultural beliefs can interfere with desire/ability to learn new information.

This knowledge helps parents to recognize and accept behavior related to growth process and promotes realistic individual expectations.

Learning new methods of interaction promotes improved relationships among family members and helps to resolve current situation.

Conflict is inevitable in relationships with others, and learning to understand the other person's point of view and effective ways to deal with differences can strengthen and enhance the relationship between family members.

Taking advantage of opportunities as they present themselves can enhance the learning situation.

Learning is enhanced when the individual is actively engaged in the process.

Parent frequently feels guilty and critical of self when a child has difficulties, and positive feedback can help individual to be more realistic about own self, the child, and the situation.

Bibliotherapy can be a helpful adjunct to information given by other means as well as providing a continuation of learning in informal/home setting.

Additional resources may help with resolution of other, deeper problems/concerns, e.g., divorce, stepfamily issues.

# CHAPTER 5

# DEMENTIA, AMNESTIC, AND OTHER COGNITIVE DISORDERS

## DEMENTIA OF THE ALZHEIMER'S TYPE/ VASCULAR DEMENTIA

### DSM IV
**DEMENTIA OF THE ALZHEIMER'S TYPE (CODE 331.0 ON AXIS III)**
**Early Onset: At or Below Age 65:**
290.10  Uncomplicated
290.11  With Delirium
290.12  With Delusions
290.13  With Depressed Mood
**Late Onset: After Age 65:**
290.0  Uncomplicated
290.3  With Delirium
290.20  With Delusions
290.21  With Depressed Mood
(For dementias due to other general medical conditions, refer to DSM IV for specific code listing.)
**VASCULAR DEMENTIA**
290.40  Uncomplicated
290.41  With Delirium
290.42  With Delusions
290.43  With Depressed Mood

### DSM III-R
290.1x  Primary Degenerative Dementia
290.4x  Multi-infarct Dementia

### ETIOLOGIC THEORIES

#### Psychodynamics

A chronic organic mental disorder that has an insidious onset and runs a uniform, gradual, progressive course. Presenile onset occurs before age 65 (e.g., Alzheimer's, Pick's). Symptoms of senile onset appear after age 65 (e.g., senile dementia of the Alzheimer's type [SDAT]); however, the pathophysiologic process is the same.

### Biologic Theories

Vascular dementia reflects a pattern of intermittent deterioration in the brain. Symptoms fluctuate and are determined by the area of the brain that is affected. Deterioration is thought to occur in response to repeated infarcts of the brain. Predisposing factors include cerebral and systemic vascular disease, hypertension, cerebral hypoxia, hypoglycemia, and cerebral embolism.

Although the exact cause of Alzheimer's is unknown, several hypotheses have been supported by varying amounts and quality of supporting data. Research indicates that the enzyme required to produce acetylcholine is dramatically reduced, especially in the areas of the brain where the senile plaques and neurofibrillary tangles occur in the greatest numbers. This decrease in acetylcholine production reduces the amount of neurotransmitter that is released to cells in the cortex and hippocampus and nucleus basalis, resulting in a disruption of memory processes.

Several studies have shown that antibodies are produced in the brain of the person with Alzheimer's disease. Although it is not known what the antibodies are produced in response to, the reactions are actually autoantibody production, suggesting a possible alteration in the body's immune system.

Genetics may also be a factor. Studies reveal a familial pattern of transmission that is 4 times greater than in the general population. Some families exhibit a pattern of inheritance that suggests possible autosomal-dominant gene transmission. Down syndrome may have some relationship to Alzheimer's disease. At autopsy, both have many of the same pathophysiologic changes. A high percentage of clients with Down syndrome who survive to adulthood eventually develop Alzheimer's lesions, which has led researchers to theorize that the extra chromosome of Down might be related to the cause of Alzheimer's.

Serious head injury may be a predisposing factor. No evidence of environmental causes, such as the ingestion of aluminum, has been found.

## CLIENT ASSESSMENT DATABASE

Incidence of primary degenerative dementia is more common in women (who live longer) than in men; vascular dementia occurs more often in men than in women.

### Activity/Rest

Feeling tired; fatigue may increase severity of symptoms, especially as evening approaches.
Day/night reversal; wakefulness/aimless wandering, disturbance of sleep rhythms.
Lethargy; decreased interest in usual activities, hobbies; inability to recall what is read/follow plot of television program.
Impaired motor skills; inability to carry out familiar, purposeful movements.
Content sitting and watching others.
Main activity may be hoarding inanimate objects, repetitive motions (fold-unfold-refold linen), hiding articles, or wandering.

### Ego Integrity

Behavior often inconsistent, and verbal/nonverbal behavior may be incongruent.
Suspicious or fearful of imaginary people/situations.
Misperception of environment, misidentification of objects and people, hoarding objects; clinging to significant other(s); belief that misplaced objects are stolen.
Multiple losses, changes in body image, self-esteem, may show strong, depressive overlay.
Emotional lability; cry easily, laugh inappropriately; variable mood changes (apathy, lethargy, restlessness, short attention span, irritability); sudden angry outbursts (catastrophic reactions).
May deny symptoms, especially cognitive changes, and/or describe vague, hypochondriacal reports of fatigue, diarrhea, dizziness, or occasional headaches.
Strong, depressive overlay; delusions; paranoia.

### Elimination

Urgency (may indicate loss of muscle tone).
Incontinence of urine/feces; prone to constipation.

### Food/Fluid

Hypoglycemic episodes (predisposing factor).
Lack of interest in/forgetting of mealtime; dependence on others for food cooking and preparation at table, feeding, using utensils.
Changes in taste; appetite, denial of hunger/need to eat.
Loss of ability to chew (silent aspiration).
Avoidance/refusal to eat (may be trying to conceal lost skills).
Weight loss.
Emaciation (advanced stage).

### Hygiene

May be dependent on SO to meet basic hygiene needs.
Appearance disheveled, unkempt, body odor.
Clothing may be inappropriate for situation/weather conditions.
May forget to go to bathroom, forget steps involved in toileting self, or be unable to find the bathroom.

### Neurosensory

May present a total healthy picture except for memory/behavioral changes.
Family members may report a gradual decrease in cognitive abilities, impaired judgment/inappropriate decisions, impaired recent memory but good remote memory, behavioral changes/individual personality traits altered or exaggerated.
Concealing inabilities (makes excuses not to perform task, may thumb through a book without reading it).
Seizure activity, secondary to the brain damage in Alzheimer's disease, may be reported/noted.
Neurologic status:
    May laugh at or feel threatened by exams.
    Disoriented to time initially, then place; usually oriented to person until late in disease process.
    Impaired recent memory, progressive loss of remote memory.
    May change answers during the interview.
    Unable to do simple calculations or repeat the names of three objects, short attention span.
    Primitive reflexes (e.g., positive snout, suck, palmar) may be present.
    May have impaired communication: difficulty with finding correct words, especially nouns, conversation repetitive or scattered with substituted meaningless words, speech may become inaudible; gradual loss of ability to write or read (fine motor skills).
Facial signs/symptoms dependent on degree of vascular insults.

### Safety

History of recent viral illness or head trauma, drug toxicity, stress, nutritional deficits may be associated with confusion.
Disturbance of gait.

### Social Interactions

Speech may be fragmented; aphasia and dysphasia may be present.
May ignore rules of social conduct/inappropriate behavior.
Family roles may be altered/reversed as individual becomes more dependent.

### Teaching/Learning

May have been forced to retire.

Prior psychosocial factors, individuality, and personality influence present altered behavioral patterns.

## DIAGNOSTIC STUDIES

Note: While no diagnostic studies are specific for Alzheimer's, they are used to rule out reversible problems that may be confused with these dementias.

**Antibodies:** Abnormally high levels may be found (leading to a theory of an immunologic defect).

**CBC, RPR, Electrolytes, Thyroid Studies:** May determine and/or eliminate treatable/reversible dysfunctions, e.g., metabolic disease processes, fluid/electrolyte imbalance, neurosyphilis.

**$B_{12}$:** May disclose a nutritional deficit if low.

**Folate Levels:** Low level can affect memory function.

**Dexamethasone Suppression Test (DST):** To rule out treatable depression.

**ECG:** May be normal; need to rule out cardiac insufficiency.

**EEG:** May be normal or show some slowing (aids in establishing treatable brain dysfunctions), reveal focal lesions (vascular).

**Skull X-Rays:** Usually normal.

**Vision/Hearing Tests:** To rule out deficits that may be the cause of or contribute to disorientation, mood swings, altered sensory perceptions (rather than cognitive impairment).

**Positron-Emission Tomography (PET) Scan, Brain Electrical Activity Mapping (BEAM), Magnetic Resonance Imaging (MRI):** May show areas of decreased brain metabolism characteristic of Alzheimer's.

**CT Scan:** May show widening of ventricles, cortical atrophy.

**CSF:** Presence of abnormal protein from the brain cells is 90% indicative of DAT.

**Alzheimer Disease-Associated Protein (ADAP):** Postmortem studies have been positive in more than 80% of DAT patients. Adaptation for live testing is being investigated.

## NURSING PRIORITIES

1. Provide safe environment, prevent injury.
2. Promote socially acceptable responses, limit inappropriate behavior.
3. Maintain reality orientation/prevent sensory deprivation/overload.
4. Encourage participation in self-care within individual limitations.
5. Facilitate communication with client/significant other(s).
6. Promote coping mechanisms of client/significant other(s).
7. Support client/family in grieving process.

## DISCHARGE GOALS

1. Adequate supervision/support systems are available.
2. Maximal level of independent functioning achieved.
3. Family/SO(s) verbalize understanding of disease process/prognosis and client expectations/needs.
4. Family/SO(s) developing/strengthening coping skills and using available resources.

| NURSING DIAGNOSIS: | INJURY/TRAUMA, HIGH RISK FOR |
|---|---|
| **Risk Factors May Include:** | Inability to recognize/identify danger in environment, impaired judgment. |
| | Disorientation, confusion. |

| | Weakness, muscular incoordination, balancing difficulties, altered perception (missing chairs, steps, etc.). |
|---|---|
| | Seizure activity. |
| **Possibly Evidenced By:** | [Not applicable; presence of signs and symptoms establishes an **actual** diagnosis.] |
| **Desired Outcomes/Evaluation Criteria—Family/Caregiver(s) Will:** | Recognize potential risks in the environment. |
| | Identify/implement steps to correct/compensate for individual factors. |
| **Client Will:** | Be free of injury. |

## ACTIONS/INTERVENTIONS

## RATIONALE

### Independent

| ACTIONS/INTERVENTIONS | RATIONALE |
|---|---|
| Assess degree of impairment in ability/competence. Assist SO to identify risks/potential hazards that may cause harm. | Identifies potential risks in the environment and heightens awareness of risks so caregivers are more alert to dangers. Clients demonstrating impulsive behavior are at increased risk of injury because they are less able to control their own behavior/actions. Visual-perceptual deficits increase the risk of falls. |
| Eliminate/minimize identified hazards in the environment. | A person with cognitive impairment and perceptual disturbances is prone to accidental injury, because of the inability to take responsibility for basic safety needs or to evaluate the unforeseen consequences, e.g., may light a stove/cigarette and forget it, mistake plastic fruit and eat it, misjudge chairs, stairs. |
| Monitor behavior routinely. Initiate least restrictive interventions before behavior escalates. | Early identification of negative behaviors with appropriate action can prevent need for more stringent measures. |
| Distract/redirect client's attention when behavior is agitated or dangerous, e.g., climbing out of bed. | Maintains safety while avoiding a confrontation that could escalate behavior/increase risk of injury. |
| Provide with an identification bracelet showing name, phone number, and diagnosis. Do not allow access to stairwell or exit. | Facilitates safe return of client if lost. Because of poor verbal ability and confusion, these persons may be unable to state address, phone number, etc. It is likely that they may be detained by police for confused, wandering, irritable/violent outbursts and poor judgment. |
| Lock outside doors as appropriate, especially in evening/night. Provide supervision and activities for client who is regularly awake during night. | Preventive measures can contain client without constant supervision. Activities promote involvement and keep client occupied. |
| Dress according to physical environment/individual need. | The general slowing of metabolic processes results in lowered body heat. The hypothalamic gland is affected by the disease process, causing person to feel cold. Client may have seasonal disorientation and may wander out in the cold. Note: Leading causes of death are pneumonia/accidents. |

121

| ACTIONS/INTERVENTIONS | RATIONALE |
|---|---|
| **Independent** | |
| Inspect skin during self-care activities. | Presence of ecchymosis, lacerations, rashes, etc., may require treatment as well as signal need for closer monitoring/protective interventions. |
| Be attentive to nonverbal physiologic symptoms. | Because of sensory loss and language dysfunction, may express needs in nonverbal manner, e.g., thirst by panting; pain by sweating, doubling over. |
| Be alert to underlying meaning of verbal statements. | May direct a question to another, such as, "Are you cold/tired?" meaning *client* is cold/tired. |
| Monitor for medication side effects, signs of over-medication, e.g., extrapyramidal signs, ortho-static hypotension, visual disturbances, GI upsets. | Client may not be able to report signs/symptoms, and drugs can easily build up to toxic levels in the elderly. Dosages/drug choice may need to be altered. |
| Recommend child-proof locks; lock up medications, poisonous substances, tools, sharp objects, etc. Remove stove knobs, burners. | As the disease worsens, the client may fidget with objects/locks (hypermetamorphosis) or put small items in mouth (hyperorality), which potentiates accidental injury/death. |
| Avoid continuous use of restraints. Have SO/others stay with client during periods of acute agitation. | Endangers the individual who succeeds in partial removal of restraints. May increase agitation and potentiate fractures in the elderly, who have reduced calcium in the bones. |

| **NURSING DIAGNOSIS:** | **THOUGHT PROCESSES, ALTERED** |
|---|---|
| **May Be Related To:** | Irreversible neuronal degeneration. |
| | Loss of memory. |
| | Sleep deprivation. |
| | Psychologic conflicts. |
| **Possibly Evidenced By:** | Inability to interpret stimuli accurately and evaluate reality. |
| | Disorientation and difficulty in grasping ideas/commands. |
| | Paranoia, delusions, confusion/frustration, and changes in behavioral responses. |
| **Desired Outcomes/Evaluation Criteria—Client Will:** | Recognize changes in thinking/behavior and causative factors when able. |
| | Demonstrate a decrease in undesired behaviors, threats, and confusion. |

| ACTIONS/INTERVENTIONS | RATIONALE |
| --- | --- |

### Independent

| | |
| --- | --- |
| Assess degree of cognitive impairment, e.g., changes in orientation to person, place, time; attention span; thinking ability. Talk with SO about changes from usual behavior/length of time problem has existed. | Provides accurate information on which to base care. |
| Maintain a pleasant, quiet environment. | Reduces distorted input, whereas crowds, clutter, noise generate sensory overload that stresses the impaired neurons. |
| Approach in a slow, calm manner. | This nonverbal gesture lessens the chance of misinterpretation and potential agitation. Hurried approaches can startle and threaten the confused client who misinterprets or feels threatened by imaginary people and/or situations. |
| Face the individual when conversing. | Maintains reality, expresses interest, and arouses attention, particularly in persons with perceptual disturbances, e.g., unable to focus or perceive by sound. |
| Address client by name. | Names are the basis of self-identity, establish reality and individual recognition. Client may respond to own name long after failing to recognize SO. |
| Use lower voice register and speak slowly to client. | Increases the chance for comprehension. High-pitched, loud tones convey stress and anger, which may trigger memory of previous confrontations and provoke an angry response. |
| Give simple directions, 1 at a time, or step-by-step instructions, using short words and simple sentences. | As the disease progresses, the communication centers in the brain become impaired, hindering the individual's ability to process and comprehend complex messages. Simplicity is the key to communicating (both verbally and nonverbally) with the cognitively impaired person. |
| Pause between phrases or questions, give hints, and use open-ended phrases when possible. | Invites a verbal response and may increase comprehension. Hints stimulate communication and give the person a chance for a positive experience. |
| Listen with regard despite content of client's speech. | Conveys interest and worth to the individual, who has difficulty processing and decoding messages. |
| Interpret statements, meanings, and words. If possible, supply the correct word. | Assisting the client with word processing aids in decreasing frustration. |
| Reduce provocative stimuli: negative criticism, arguments, confrontations. | Any provocation decreases self-esteem and may be interpreted as a threat, which may trigger agitation or increase inappropriate behavior. |
| Use distraction. Talk about real people and real events when client begins ruminating about false ideas, unless it increases anxiety/agitation. | Rumination serves to promote disorientation. Reality orientation increases client's sense of reality, self-worth, and personal dignity. |

123

| ACTIONS/INTERVENTIONS | RATIONALE |
|---|---|

### Independent

| | |
|---|---|
| Refrain from forcing activities and communications. Change activity if client loses interest in present activity. | Force decreases cooperation and may increase suspiciousness, delusions. Changing activity maintains interest, reduces restlessness and possibility of confrontation. |
| Use humor with interactions. | Laughter can assist in communication and help reverse emotional lability. |
| Focus on appropriate behavior. Give positive reinforcement, e.g., a pat on the back, positive feedback, applause. Use touch judiciously. Respect individual's personal space/response. | Reinforces correctness, appropriate behavior. A focus on inappropriate behavior can stimulate that kind of behavior. While touch frequently transcends verbal interchange, conveying warmth, acceptance, and reality, the individual may misinterpret the meaning of touch. Intrusion into personal space may threaten the client's distorted world. |
| Respect individuality and evaluate individual needs. | Persons experiencing a cognitive decline deserve respect, dignity, and worth as an individual. Client's past and background are important in maintaining self-concept, planning activities, communicating, etc. |
| Allow personal belongings. | Familiarity enhances security, sense of self, and avoids increased feelings of loss/deprivation. |
| Permit hoarding of safe objects. | An activity that preserves security and counterbalances irrevocable losses. |
| Create simple, noncompetitive activities paced to the individual's abilities. | Motivates client in ways that will reinforce usefulness and self-worth and stimulate reality. |
| Make useful activities out of hoarding and repetitive motions, e.g., collecting junk mail, creating scrapbook, folding/unfolding linen, bouncing balls, dusting, sweeping floors. | May decrease restlessness and provide option for pleasurable activity. |
| Label drawers/assist with finding misplaced items. Do not challenge client. | Decreases defensiveness when client believes she or he is being accused of stealing a misplaced, hoarded, or hidden item. Refuting the accusation will not change the belief and may invite anger. |
| Monitor phone use closely. Post significant phone numbers in prominent place. Secure long-distance numbers. | Can be used as reality orientation. However, impaired judgment does not allow for distinguishing long-distance numbers and makes client easy prey for phone sales pitches. Clients may call dead relative, forget time of day when making calls, etc. |
| Evaluate sleep/rest pattern and adequacy. Note lethargy, increasing irritability/confusion, frequent yawning, dark circles under eyes. | Lack of sleep can impair thought processes and coping abilities. (Refer to ND: Sleep Pattern disturbance). |
| Monitor for medication side effects, signs of overmedication. | Drugs can easily build up to toxic levels in the elderly, aggravating confusion. Dosages/drug choice may need to be altered. |

| ACTIONS/INTERVENTIONS | RATIONALE |
|---|---|
| **Collaborative** | |
| Administer medications as individually indicated:<br>Antipsychotic: e.g., haloperidol (Haldol), thioridazine (Mellaril); | Small dosages may be used to control agitation, delusions, hallucinations. Mellaril is being used widely because there are fewer extrapyramidal side effects (e.g., dystonia, akathisia), visual problems, and especially gait disturbances. Note: Phenathiazines may cause oversedation, excitation, or bizarre reactions. Presence of postural hypotension increases the risk of falls and development of constipation, requiring inclusion of a bowel program. |
| Vasodilators: e.g., cyclandelate (Cyclospasmol); | May improve mental function but requires further research. |
| ergoloid mesylates (Hydergine LC); | A metabolic enhancer (increases brain's ability to metabolize glucose and use oxygen) that has few side effects. Although it does not increase cognition and memory, it may make client more alert and less anxious/depressed. However, it may be of little value in dementia therapy because there is usually only a limited degree of improvement. Note: This is an expensive drug, and families need accurate information to make informed therapy decisions and avoid false hopes and disappointment, because of lack of dramatic results. |
| tacrine (Cognex); | Elevates acetylcholine levels in the cerebral cortex to improve cognition and functional autonomy in mild to moderate dementia. Does not appear to alter the course of the disease, and the effects may lessen as the disease advances. |
| Anxiolytic agents: diazepam (Valium), chlordiazepoxide (Librium), oxazepam (Serax); | More useful in early/mild stages for relief of anxiety. Can increase confusion/paranoia in the elderly. Note: Serax may be preferred because it is shorter acting. |
| thiamine. | Studies are currently underway to verify the usefulness of high doses of thiamine during the early phase of the disease to slow progression of impairment/slightly improve cognition. |

| NURSING DIAGNOSIS: | **SENSORY/PERCEPTUAL ALTERATIONS (SPECIFY)** |
|---|---|
| **May Be Related To:** | Altered sensory reception, transmission, and/or integration (neurologic disease/deficit). |
| | Socially restricted environment (homebound/institutionalization). |
| | Sleep deprivation. |

| **Possibly Evidenced By:** | Change in problem-solving abilities; altered abstraction/conceptualization. |
| | Changes in usual response to stimuli, e.g., spatial disorientation, confusion, rapid mood swings. |
| | Exaggerated emotional responses, e.g., anxiety, paranoia, and hallucinations. |
| | Inability to tell position of body parts. |
| | Diminished/altered sense of taste. |
| **Desired Outcomes/Evaluation Criteria— Client Will:** | Demonstrate improved/appropriate response to stimuli. |
| **Caregiver(s) Will:** | Identify/control external factors that contribute to alterations in sensory/perceptual abilities. |

| ACTIONS/INTERVENTIONS | RATIONALE |
|---|---|
| **Independent** | |
| Assess degree of impairment and how it affects the individual, including hearing/visual deficits. | While brain involvement is usually global, a small percentage may exhibit asymmetric involvement, which may cause the client to neglect one side of the body (unilateral neglect). May not be able to locate internal cues, recognize hunger/thirst, perceive external pain, or locate body within the environment. |
| Encourage use of corrective lenses, hearing aids as appropriate. | May enhance sensory input, limit/reduce misinterpretation of stimuli. |
| Maintain a reality-oriented relationship and environment. | Reduces confusion and promotes coping with the frustrating struggles of misperception and being disoriented/confused. |
| Provide clues for 24-hour reality orientation with calendars, clocks, notes, cards, signs, music, seasonal hues, color-code rooms, scenic pictures. | Dysfunction in visual-spatial perception interferes with the ability to recognize directions and patterns, and the client may become lost, even in familiar surroundings. Clues are tangible reminders that aid recognition and may permeate memory gaps, increasing independence. |
| Provide quiet, nondistracting environment when indicated, e.g., soft music, plain but colorful wallpaper/paint, etc. | Helps to avoid visual/auditory overload, by emphasizing qualities of calmness, consistency. (Note: Patterened wallpaper may be disturbing to the client.) |
| Provide touch in a caring way. | May enhance perception of self/body boundaries. |
| Engage in individually meaningful activities, supporting remaining abilities and minimizing failures, e.g., daily living skills including meal preparation, setup/cleaning activities, making bed, gardening/watering plants. | Supports client's dignity, familiarizes them with home/community events and enables them to experience satisfaction and pleasure. |
| Use sensory games to stimulate reality, e.g., smell Vick's and tell of the time mother used it on client; use of spring/fall nature boxes. | Communicates reality through multiple channels. |

| ACTIONS/INTERVENTIONS | RATIONALE |
|---|---|

### Independent

Indulge in periods of reminiscence (old music, historic events, photos, mementoes).

Stimulates recollections, awakens memories, aids in the preservation of self/individuality via past accomplishments, increases feelings of security, while easing adaptation to a changed environment.

Provide intellectual activities, e.g., word games, review of current events, storytime, travel discussions.

Stimulate remaining cognitive abilities, provides sense of normalcy.

Include in Bible study group, church activities, television services for shut-ins, or arrange for visitation by clergy/spiritual advisor as appropriate.

Provides opportunity to meet spiritual needs, maintains connection with religious beliefs, may help reduce sense of isolation from humanity.

Encourage simple outings, short walks. Monitor activity.

Outings refresh reality and provide pleasurable sensory stimuli, which may reduce suspiciousness/hallucinations caused by feelings of imprisonment. Motor functioning may be decreased, because nerve degeneration results in weakness, decreasing stamina.

Promote balanced physiologic functions using colorful Nerf/beach balls/bean bags for toss; target games; marching, dancing, or arm dancing with music.

Preserves mobility (reducing the potential for bone and muscle atrophy) and provides diversional opportunity for interaction with others.

Involve in activities with others as dictated by individual situation, e.g., 1:1 visitors, animal visitation, socialization groups at Alzhemier center, occupational therapy to include crafts, painting/finger paints, modeling clay, etc.

Provides opportunity for participation with others and may maintain some level of socialization.

| NURSING DIAGNOSIS: | FEAR |
|---|---|
| May Be Related To: | Decreased ability in function. |
| | Public disclosure of disabilities. |
| | Further mental/physical deterioration. |
| Possibly Evidenced By: | Social isolation. |
| | Aggressive behavior. |
| | Apprehension. |
| | Irritability; defensiveness; suspiciousness. |
| Desired Outcomes/Evaluation Criteria— Client Will: | Demonstrate more appropriate range of feelings and lessened fear. |

| ACTIONS/INTERVENTIONS | RATIONALE |
|---|---|

### Independent

Note change of behavior, suspiciousness, irritability, defensiveness.

Change in moods may be one of the first signs of cognitive decline, and the client, fearing helplessness, tries to hide the increasing inability to remember and do normal activities.

| ACTIONS/INTERVENTIONS | RATIONALE |
|---|---|

### Independent

| | |
|---|---|
| Identify strengths the individual had previously. | Facilitates assistance with communication and management of current deficits. |
| Deal with aggressive behavior by imposing calm, firm limits. | Acceptance can reduce fear and aggressive behavior. |
| Provide clear, honest information about actions/events. | Assists in maintaining trust and orientation as long as possible. When the client knows the truth about what is happening, coping is often enhanced, and guilt over what is imagined is decreased. |

| | |
|---|---|
| **NURSING DIAGNOSIS:** | **GRIEVING, ANTICIPATORY** |
| **May Be Related To:** | Client awareness of something "being wrong" with changes in memory/family reaction, physiopsychosocial well-being. |
| | Family perception of potential loss of loved one. |
| **Possibly Evidenced By:** | Expressions of distress/anger at potential loss. |
| | Choked feelings, crying. |
| | Alteration in activity level, communication patterns, eating habits, and sleep patterns. |
| **Desired Outcomes/Evaluation Criteria—Client/Family Will:** | Express concerns openly. |
| | Discuss loss and participate in planning for the future. |

| ACTIONS/INTERVENTIONS | RATIONALE |
|---|---|

### Independent

| | |
|---|---|
| Assess degree of deterioration/level of coping. | Information is helpful to understand how much the client is capable of doing to maintain highest level of independence and to provide encouragement to help individuals deal with losses. |
| Provide open environment for discussion. Use therapeutic communication skills of Active-listening, acknowledgment, etc. | Encourages client/SOs to discuss feelings and concerns realistically. |
| Note statements of despair, hopelessness, "nothing to live for," expressions of anger. | May be indicative of suicidal ideation. Angry behavior may be client's way of dealing with feelings of despair. |
| Respect desire not to talk. | May not be ready to deal with or share grief. |
| Be honest; do not give false reassurances or dire predictions about the future. | Honesty promotes a trusting relationship. Expressions of gloom, such as, "You'll spend the rest of your life in a nursing home," are not helpful. (No one knows what the future holds.) |
| Discuss with client/SOs ways they can plan together for the future. | Having a part in problem-solving/planning can provide a sense of control over anticipated events. |

| ACTIONS/INTERVENTIONS | RATIONALE |
|---|---|

### Independent

Assist client/SO to identify positive aspects of the situation.

Identify strengths client/SO see in self/situation and support systems available.

Ongoing research, possibility of slow progression may offer some hope for the future.

Recognizing these resources provides opportunity to work through feelings of grief.

### Collaborative

Refer to other resources, counseling, clergy, etc.

May need additional support/assistance to resolve feelings.

| NURSING DIAGNOSIS: | SLEEP PATTERN DISTURBANCE |
|---|---|
| May Be Related To: | Sensory impairments: psychologic stress, changes in activity pattern, environmental changes, inability to interpret social cues. |
| Possibly Evidenced By: | Changes in behavior and performance. |
| | Disorientation (day/night reversal). |
| | Irritability. |
| | Wakefulness/interrupted sleep, increased aimless wandering; inability to identify need/time for sleeping. |
| | Lethargy, dark circles under eyes, frequent yawning. |
| Desired Outcomes/Evaluation Criteria— Client Will: | Establish adequate sleep pattern, with wandering reduced. |
| | Report/appear rested. |

| ACTIONS/INTERVENTIONS | RATIONALE |
|---|---|

### Independent

Provide for rest/naps; reduce mental activity late in the day.

While prolonged physical and mental activity results in fatigue, which can increase confusion, programmed activity without overstimulation promotes sleep.

Avoid use of continuous restraints (particularly when in room alone).

Potentiates sensory deprivation, increases agitation, and restricts rest.

Evaluate level of stress/orientation as day progresses.

Increasing confusion, disorientation, and uncooperative behaviors (Sundowner's syndrome) may interfere with attaining restful sleep pattern.

Adhere to regular bedtime schedule and rituals. Tell client that it is time to sleep.

Reinforces that it is bedtime and maintains stability of environment. Note: Later than normal bedtime may be indicated to allow client to dissipate excess energy and facilitate falling asleep.

| ACTIONS/INTERVENTIONS | RATIONALE |
|---|---|

### Independent

Provide evening snack, warm milk, bath, and back rub/general massage with lotion.

Promotes relaxation and drowsiness. Also helps address skin care needs.

Reduce fluid intake in the evening. Toilet before retiring.

Decreases need to get up to go to the bathroom during the night.

Provide soft music or "white noise."

Reduces sensory stimulation by blocking out other environmental sounds that could interfere with restful sleep.

### Collaborative

Administer medications as indicated for sleep:
   Antidepressants: e.g., amitriptyline (Elavil), doxepin (Seneguan), and trazodone (Desyrel);

May be effective in treating pseudodementia or depression, improving ability to sleep. However, the anticholinergic properties can induce confusion or worsen cognition. Orthostatic hypotension and other side effects (e.g., constipation) limit their usefulness.

   Sedative-Hypnotics, e.g., chloral hydrate, oxazepam (Serax), triazolam (Halcyon).

Used sparingly, low-dose hypnotics may be effective in treating insomnia or Sundowner's syndrome.

Avoid use of diphenhydramine (Benadryl).

Once used for sleep, this drug is now contraindicated because it interferes with the production of acetylcholine, which is already inhibited in the brains of clients with DAT.

---

| NURSING DIAGNOSIS: | SELF-CARE DEFICIT (SPECIFY LEVEL) |
|---|---|
| **May Be Related To:** | Cognitive decline, physical limitations. |
| | Frustration over loss of independence, depression. |
| **Possibly Evidenced By:** | Impaired ability to perform ADLs, e.g., frustration, forgetfulness, misuse/misidentification of objects, inability to bring food from receptacle to mouth; inability to wash body part(s), regulate temperature of water; impaired ability to put on/take off clothing; difficulty completing toileting tasks. |
| **Desired Outcomes/Evaluation Criteria— Client Will:** | Perform self-care activities within level of own ability. |
| | Identify and use personal/community resources that can provide assistance. |

| ACTIONS/INTERVENTIONS | RATIONALE |
|---|---|
| **Independent** | |
| Identify reason for difficulty in self-care, e.g., physical limitations in motion, apathy/depression, cognitive decline (such as apraxia), or room temperature ("too cold to get dressed"). | Underlying cause affects choice of interventions/ strategies. Problem may be minimized by changes in environment or adaptation of clothing, etc; or may be more complex, requiring consultation from other specialists. |
| Determine individual hygienic needs and provide assistance as needed with activities including care of hair/nails/skin, cleaning glasses, brushing teeth. | As the disease progresses, basic hygienic needs may be forgotten. Infection, gum disease, disheveled appearance, or harm may occur when client/ caregivers become frustrated, irritated, or intimidated by degree of care required. |
| Incorporate usual routine into activity schedule as possible. | Maintaining routine may prevent worsening of confusion and enhance cooperation. |
| Be attentive to nonverbal physiologic symptoms. | Sensory loss and language dysfunction may cause client to express self-care needs in nonverbal manner, e.g., thirst by panting; need to void by holding self/fidgeting. |
| Be alert to underlying meaning of verbal statements. | May direct a question to another, such as "Are you cold?" meaning, "I am cold and need additional clothing." |
| Supervise but allow as much autonomy as possible. | Eases the frustration over lost independence. |
| Allot plenty of time to perform tasks. | Tasks that were once easy (e.g., dressing, bathing) are now complicated by decreased motor skills or cognitive and physical change. Time and patience can reduce chaos resulting from trying to hasten this process. |
| Assist with neat dressing/provide colorful clothes. | Enhances esteem, may diminish sense of sensory loss and convey aliveness. |
| Offer 1 item of clothing at a time, in sequential order. | Simplicity reduces frustration and the potential for rage and despair. |
| Talk through each step of the task 1 at a time. | Guidance reduces confusion and allows autonomy. |
| Wait and/or change the time to approach dressing/ hygiene if a problem arises. | Because anger is quickly forgotten, another time or approach may be successful. |
| Provide reminders for elimination needs. Involve in bowel/bladder program as appropriate. | Loss of control/independence in this self-care activity can greatly impact self-esteem and limit socialization. (Refer to ND: Constipation.) |
| Assist with and provide reminders for pericare after toileting/incontinence. | Good hygiene promotes cleanliness and reduces risks of skin irritation and infection. |
| Allow to sleep in shoes/clothing or wear 2 sets of clothing if client demands. | Providing no harm is done, altering the "normal" lessens the rebellion and allows rest. |

131

| NURSING DIAGNOSIS: | NUTRITION, ALTERED, LESS/MORE THAN BODY REQUIREMENTS, HIGH RISK FOR |
|---|---|
| Risk Factors May Include: | Sensory changes. |
| | Impaired judgment and coordination. |
| | Agitation. |
| | Forgetfulness, regressed habits, and concealment. |
| Possibly Evidenced By: | [Not applicable; presence of signs and symptoms establishes an **actual** diagnosis.] |
| Desired Outcomes/Evaluation Criteria— Client Will: | Ingest nutritionally balanced diet. |
| | Maintain/regain appropriate weight. |

| ACTIONS/INTERVENTIONS | RATIONALE |
|---|---|
| **Independent** | |
| Assess SO/client's knowledge of nutrition. | Identifies needs to assist in formulating individual teaching plan. A role-reversal situation can occur (e.g., child now cooking for parent, husband taking over "duties" of wife), increasing the need for information. |
| Determine amount of exercise/pacing client does. | Nutritional intake may need to be adjusted to meet needs related to individual energy expenditure. |
| Offer/provide assistance in menu selection. | Poor judgment may lead to poor choices or client may be indecisive/overwhelmed by choices and/or unaware of the need to maintain elemental nutrition. In general, metabolic rate decreases with age, requiring caloric adjustment that must be balanced with activity. |
| Provide privacy when eating habits become an insoluble problem. Accept eating with hands, spills, and whimsical mixtures, e.g., salad dressing in milk, salt and pepper on ice cream. (Note: Avoid solo dining or separating client from other people too early in the disease process.) | Socially unacceptable and embarrassing eating habits develop as the disease progresses. Acceptance preserves esteem, decreases irritability or refusal to eat as a result of anger, frustration. Early separation can result in client feeling upset and rejected and can actually result in decreased food intake. |
| Offer small feedings and/or snacks of 1 or 2 foods around the clock as indicated. | Large feedings may overwhelm the client, resulting either in complete abstinence or gorging. |
| Simplify steps of eating, e.g., serve food in courses. Anticipate needs, cut foods, provide soft/finger foods. | Promotes autonomy and independence. Decreases potential frustration/anger over lost abilities. Small feedings may enhance appropriate intake. Limiting number of foods offered at a single time reduces confusion regarding which food to choose. |
| Provide ample time for eating. | Coordination decreases with the progression of the disease process, and the ability to chew and handle utensils becomes impaired. A leisurely approach aids digestion and decreases the chance of anger precipitated by rushing. |

132

## ACTIONS/INTERVENTIONS

### Independent

Place food items in pita bread/paper sack for the client who paces.

Avoid baby food and excessively hot foods.

Stimulate oral-suck reflex by gentle stroking of the cheeks or stimulating the mouth with a spoon.

### Collaborative

Refer to dietitian.

## RATIONALE

Carrying food may encourage client to eat.

Baby foods lack adequate nutritional content, fiber, and taste for adults and can add to client's humiliation. Hot foods may result in mouth burns and/or refusal to eat.

As the disease progresses, the client may clench teeth and refuse to eat. Stimulating the reflex may increase cooperation/intake.

Assistance may be needed to develop nutritionally balanced diet individualized to meet client needs/food preferences.

| NURSING DIAGNOSIS: | CONSTIPATION/URINARY ELIMINATION, ALTERED |
|---|---|
| May Be Related To: | Disorientation. |
| | Lost neurologic functioning/muscle tone. |
| | Inability to locate the bathroom/recognize need. |
| | Changes in dietary/fluid intake. |
| Possibly Evidenced By: | Urgency/inappropriate toileting behaviors. |
| | Incontinence/constipation. |
| Desired Outcomes/Evaluation Criteria— Client Will: | Establish adequate/appropriate pattern of elimination. |

## ACTIONS/INTERVENTIONS

### Independent

Assess prior pattern and compare with current situation.

Locate bed near a bathroom when possible; make signs for/color-code door. Provide adequate lighting, particularly at night.

Take to the toilet at regular intervals. Dictate each step 1 at a time and use positive reinforcement.

Encourage adequate fluid intake during the day (at least 2 liters, as appropriate), diet high in fiber and fruit juices. Limit intake during the late evening and at bedtime.

## RATIONALE

Provides information about changes that may require further assessment/intervention.

Promotes orientation/finding bathroom. Incontinence may be attributed to inability to find a toilet.

Adherence to a daily and regular schedule may prevent accidents. Frequently the problem is forgetting how to do, e.g., pushing pants down, positioning.

Essential for bodily functions and prevents potential dehydration/constipation. Restricting intake in evening may reduce frequency/incontinence during the night.

| ACTIONS/INTERVENTIONS | RATIONALE |
|---|---|

### Independent

| | |
|---|---|
| Avoid a sense of hurrying/being rushed. | Hurrying may be perceived as intrusion, which leads to anger and lack of cooperation with activity. |
| Be alert to nonverbal cues, e.g., restlessness, holding self, or picking at clothes. | May signal urgency/inattention to cues, and/or inability to locate bathroom. |
| Be discreet and respect person's privacy. | Although the client is confused, a sense of modesty is often retained. |
| Convey acceptance when incontinence occurs. Change promptly, provide good skin care. | Acceptance is important to decrease the embarrassment and feelings of helplessness that may occur during the changing process. Reduces risk of skin irritation/breakdown. |
| Record frequency of voidings/bowel movements. | Provides visual reminder of elimination and may indicate need for intervention. |
| Monitor appearance/color of urine; note consistency of stool. | Detection of changes provides opportunity to alter interventions to prevent complications or acquire treatment as indicated (e.g., constipation/urinary infection). |

### Collaborative

| | |
|---|---|
| Administer stool softeners, Metamucil, glycerin suppository, as indicated. | May be necessary to facilitate/stimulate regular bowel movement. |

| NURSING DIAGNOSIS: | SEXUAL DYSFUNCTION, high risk for |
|---|---|
| **Risk Factors May Include:** | Confusion; forgetfulness and disorientation to place or person. |
| | Altered body function, decrease in habit/control of behavior. |
| | Lack of intimacy/sexual rejection by SO. |
| | Lack of privacy. |
| **Possibly Evidenced By:** | [Not applicable; presence of signs and symptoms establishes an **actual** diagnosis.] |
| **Desired Outcomes/Evaluation Criteria— Client Will:** | Meet sexuality needs in an acceptable manner. |
| | Experience fewer/no episodes of inappropriate behavior. |

| ACTIONS/INTERVENTIONS | RATIONALE |
|---|---|

### Independent

| | |
|---|---|
| Assess individual needs/desires/abilities. | Alternative methods need to be designed for the individual situation to fulfill the need for intimacy and closeness. |

| ACTIONS/INTERVENTIONS | RATIONALE |
|---|---|
| **Independent** | |
| Encourage partner to show affection/acceptance. | The cognitively impaired person retains the basic needs for affection, love, acceptance, and sexual expression. |
| Assure privacy. | Sexual expression or behavior may differ. The individual may masturbate, expose self. Privacy allows sexual expression without embarrassment and the objections of others. |
| Use distraction, as indicated. Remind client that this is a public area and current behavior is unacceptable. | Useful tool when there is inappropriate/objectionable behavior, e.g., self-exposure. |
| Provide time to listen/discuss concerns of SO. | May need information and/or counseling about alternatives for sexual activity/aggression. |

| NURSING DIAGNOSIS: | FAMILY COPING, ineffective: compromised/disabling |
|---|---|
| **May Be Related To:** | Disruptive behavior of client. |
| | Family grief about their helplessness watching loved one deteriorate. |
| | Prolonged disease/disability progression that exhausts the supportive capacity of SO. |
| | Highly ambivalent family relationships. |
| **Possibly Evidenced By:** | Family becoming embarrassed and socially immobilized. |
| | Home maintenance becoming extremely difficult and leading to difficult decisions with legal/financial considerations. |
| **Desired Outcomes/Evaluation Criteria— Family Will:** | Identify/verbalize resources within themselves to deal with the situation. |
| | Acknowledge loved one's condition and demonstrate positive coping behaviors in dealing with situation. |
| | Use outside support systems effectively. |

| ACTIONS/INTERVENTIONS | RATIONALE |
|---|---|
| **Independent** | |
| Include SOs in teaching and planning for home care. | Can ease the burden of home management and increase adaptation. Comfortable and familiar lifestyle at home is helpful in preserving the affected individual's need for belonging. |

| ACTIONS/INTERVENTIONS | RATIONALE |
|---|---|

### Independent

| | |
|---|---|
| Review past life experiences, role changes, and coping skills. | Opportunity to identify skills that may help individuals cope with grief of current situation more effectively. |
| Encourage unlimited visitation as tolerated by client. | Contact with familiarity forms a base of reality and can provide a reassuring freedom from loneliness. Recurrent contact helps family members realize and accept situation. |
| Focus on specific problems as they occur, the "here and now." | Disease progression follows no set pattern. A premature focus on the possibility of long-term care or possible incontinence, for example, impairs the ability to cope with present issues. |
| Establish priorities. | Helps to create a sense of order and facilitates problem-solving. |
| Be realistic and honest in all matters. | Decreases stress that surrounds false hopes, e.g., that individual may regain past level of functioning from advertised or unproven medication. |
| Reassess family's ability to care for client at home on an ongoing basis. | Behaviors like hoarding, clinging, unjust accusations, angry outbursts, etc., can precipitate family burnout and interfere with ability to provide effective care. |
| Help caregiver/family understand the importance of maintaining psychosocial functioning. | Embarrassing behavior, the demands of care, etc., may cause withdrawal from social contact. |
| Provide time/listen with regard to concerns/anxieties. | The self-sacrificing, painful nature of the care required in this disease necessitates constant support for SOs in order to deal effectively with the multifaceted problems arising during the course of this illness and to ease the process of adaptation and grieving. |
| Discuss possibility of isolation. Reinforce need for support system. | The belief that a single individual can meet all the needs of the client increases the potential for physical/mental illness (caregiver role strain). Note: Mortality rate for primary caregivers is actually higher than for the client with DAT. |
| Provide positive feedback for efforts. | Reassures individuals that they are doing their best. |
| Support concerns generated by consideration/decision to place in LTC facility. | Constant care requirements may be more than can be managed by SO. Support is needed for this difficult guilt-producing decision, which may create a financial burden as well as family disruption/dissension. |

| ACTIONS/INTERVENTIONS | RATIONALE |
|---|---|

### Collaborative

Refer to local resources, e.g. adult day care, respite care, homemaker services, or a local chapter of Alzheimer's Disease and Related Disorders Association (ADRDA).

Coping with this individual is a full-time, frustrating task. Respite/day care may lighten the burden, reduce potential social isolation, and prevent family burnout/caregiver role strain. ADRDA provides group support and family teaching and promotes research. Local groups provide a social outlet for sharing grief and promote problem-solving with such matters as financial/legal advice, home care, etc.

| NURSING DIAGNOSIS: | HOME MAINTENANCE MANAGEMENT, IMPAIRED/HEALTH MAINTENANCE, ALTERED |
|---|---|
| **May Be Related To:** | Progressively impaired cognitive functioning. |
| | Complete or partial lack of gross and/or fine motor skills. |
| | Significant alteration in communication skills. |
| | Ineffective individual/family coping. |
| | Insufficient family organization or planning. |
| | Unfamiliarity with resources; inadequate support systems. |
| **Possibly Evidenced By:** | Overtaxed family members, e.g., exhausted, anxious. |
| | Household members express difficulty and request help in maintaining home in safe/comfortable fashion. |
| | Home surroundings appear disorderly/unsafe. |
| | Reported or observed inability to take responsibility for meeting basic health practices. |
| | Reported or observed lack of equipment, financial, or other resources; impairment of personal support system. |
| **Desired Outcomes/Evaluation Criteria—Family/Caregiver(s) Will:** | Identify and correct factors related to difficulty in maintaining a safe environment for the client. |
| | Demonstrate appropriate, effective use of resources, e.g., respite care, homemakers, Alzheimer groups. |
| | Assume responsibility for and adopt lifestyle changes supporting client health-care goals. |
| | Verbalize ability to cope adequately with existing situation. |

| ACTIONS/INTERVENTIONS | RATIONALE |
|---|---|

### Independent

| | |
|---|---|
| Evaluate level of cognitive/emotional/physical functioning (level of independence). | Identifies strengths, areas of need and how much responsibility the client may be expected to assume. (Refer to ND: Self-Care deficit.) |
| Assess environment, noting unsafe factors and ability of client to care for self. | Determines what changes need to be made to accommodate disabilities. (Refer to ND: Injury/Trauma, high risk for). |
| Assist client to develop plan for keeping track of/dealing with health needs. | Schedule can be helpful to maintain system for managing routine health care. |
| Identify support systems available to client/SO, e.g., other family members, friends, respite care services. | Planning and constant care is necessary to maintain this client at home. If family system is unavailable/unaware, client needs, e.g., nutrition, dental care, eye exams, can be neglected. Primary caregiver may benefit from someone to come in and provide relief/respite from constant care to reduce risk of caregiver role strain. |
| Evaluate coping abilities, effectiveness, commitment of caregiver(s)/support persons. | Progressive debilitation taxes caregiver(s) and may alter ability to meet client/own needs. (Refer to ND: Family Coping, ineffective, compromised/disabling.) |

### Collaborative

| | |
|---|---|
| Identify alternate care sources (such as sitter/day care facility), senior care services, e.g., Meals on Wheels/respite care, home care agency. | As client's condition worsens, SO may need additional help from several sources or may eventually be unable to maintain client at home. |
| Refer to supportive services as need indicates. | Medical and social services consultant may be needed to develop ongoing plan/identify resources as needs change. |

| | |
|---|---|
| **NURSING DIAGNOSIS:** | **CAREGIVER ROLE STRAIN, HIGH RISK FOR** |
| **Risk Factors May Include:** | Illness severity of the care receiver; duration of caregiving required; complexity/amount of caregiving tasks. |
| | Caregiver is female; spouse. |
| | Care receiver exhibits deviant, bizarre behavior. |
| | Family/caregiver isolation; lack of respite and recreation for caregiver. |
| **Possibly Evidenced By:** | [Not applicable; presence of signs/symptoms establishes an **actual** diagnosis.] |
| **Desired Outcomes/Evaluation Criteria— Caregiver Will:** | Identify individual risk factors and appropriate interventions. |

Demonstrate/initiate behaviors or lifestyle changes to prevent development of impaired function.

Use available resources appropriately.

Report satisfaction with current situation.

| ACTIONS/INTERVENTIONS | RATIONALE |
|---|---|

### Independent

| | |
|---|---|
| Note physical/mental condition, therapeutic regimen of care receiver. | Determines individual needs for planning care. |
| Determine caregiver's level of responsibility, involvement in and anticipated length of care. Use assessment tool, such as Burden Interview, to further determine caregiver's abilities, when appropriate. | Allows caregiver to realistically look at what is involved in commitment to provide care. |
| Identify strengths of caregiver and care receiver. | Helps to use positive aspects of each individual to the best of abilities in daily activities. |
| Discuss caregiver's view of and concerns about situation. | Allows ventilation and clarification of concerns, promoting understanding. |
| Determine available supports and resources currently used. | Provides information regarding adequacy of supports/current needs. |
| Facilitate family conference to share information and develop plan for involvement in care activities as appropriate. | When others are involved in care, the risk of one person becoming overloaded is lessened. |
| Identify additional resources to include financial, legal, respite care. | These areas of concern can add to burden of caregiving if not adequately resolved. |
| Identify equipment needs/resources, adaptive aids. | Enhances independence and safety of the care receiver. |
| Provide information and/or demonstrate techniques for dealing with acting-out/violent or disoriented behavior. | Helps caregiver to maintain sense of control and competency. Enhances safety for care receiver and giver. |
| Stress importance of self-nurturing, e.g., pursuing self-development interests, personal needs, hobbies, and social activities. | Taking time for self can prevent caregiver role strain/burnout. |
| Assist caregiver to plan for changes that may be necessary for the care receiver (e.g., home care providers, eventual placement in long-term care facility). | Planning for this eventuality is important for the time when burden of care becomes too great for one person. |

# DEMENTIAS DUE TO OTHER GENERAL MEDICAL CONDITIONS: Dementia Due to HIV Disease

### DSM IV
294.9 Dementia Due to HIV Disease (Code 043.1 on Axis III)

### DSM III-R
294.10 Dementia Associated with Axis III Physical Disorders or Conditions

Dementia is defined as impairment of short- and long-term memory, abstract thinking, and judgment with personality changes, severe enough to interfere with work, normal social activities, and relationships.

HIV has been shown to directly affect the brain by crossing the blood-brain barrier on two types of immune cells, monocytes and macrophages. Cells within the CNS have been found to have express CD4 receptor sites for HIV entry into cells. However, although several hypotheses have been proposed, it is not known exactly by what mechanism neurologic dysfunction occurs. The immune dysfunction of AIDS can lead to brain infections by other organisms, and the AIDS virus also appears to cause dementia directly. Neuropsychiatric symptoms may range from barely perceptible changes in a person's normal psychologic presentation to acute delirium to profound dementia.

Three people in 10 who are HIV symptomatic will exhibit symptoms of dementia, although recent studies suggest symptoms can occur prior to an AIDS diagnosis, being the first clinical symptoms of progression. A retrospective study (1979–1984) revealed CNS abnormalities in 73% of 49 AIDS clients.

## CLIENT ASSESSMENT DATABASE

### Activity/Rest

Low energy level, constant fatigue.
Insomnia, change in sleep patterns.
Irritability, yawning frequently.
Wakefulness at night.

### Ego Integrity

Emotional lability, e.g., agitation, combativeness, and panic attacks.
Reports feeling like she or he is losing his or her mind.
Feelings of powerlessness, worthlessness.
Increased anxiety; panic attacks.
Increased irritability, decreased concentration.

### Elimination

Constipation.
Increasing frequency of incontinence.

### Food/Fluid

Decreased interest in food.
Apraxia (inability to carry out motor functions of chewing and swallowing despite intact sensory function).
Agnosia (failure to recognize foods despite intact sensory function).
Weight loss.

## Hygiene

Unable to do simple/difficult tasks of ADL.
Deficits in many or all personal care areas.
No concern for hygiene; disheveled, unkempt appearance.

## Neurosensory

Changes in mental status, loss of mental acuity/ability to problem-solve, forgetfulness, poor concentration/decreased alertness, apathy; impaired impulse control.
Paranoid ideation, free-floating anxiety, unrealistic expectations.
Organic psychosis (hallucinations, delusions).
Psychomotor retardation/slowed responses, decreased grip strength, decreased pinprick sensation, ataxic gait.
Impaired sensation or sense of position.
Numbness, tingling of feet (paresthesias).
Decreased verbal comprehension, aphasia, mutism; deterioration in handwriting.
History of seizure activity.
Antisocial personalities (drug users).

## PAIN/DISCOMFORT

Headache.
Pain in lower extremities, burning in feet.
Guarding behavior (posturing, withdrawal), request not to be touched.

## SAFETY

Decline in general strength; muscle tremors, sense of lack of balance; spastic weakness, changes in gait/ataxia, hemiparesis.
History of falls.
Not completing tasks, e.g., not turning off stove/burning food.
Bruises, burns/lesions.
Needle marks on skin may indicate IV drug use.

## SEXUALITY

Decreased interest in sexual activity; withdrawal from others (intimacy).
Decreased ability/inability to obtain arousal.
Unsafe sexual practices related to drug abuse.

## Social Interactions

Disinterest in friends/social interaction; loss of social responsiveness; withdrawal.
Labile personality, increased anger.
Slurred speech/aphasia, mutism (late).
Disorganized activities.
Chaotic lives due to drug use, e.g., homeless, unemployed.

## DIAGNOSTIC STUDIES

(Choice of studies is dependent on individual situation to rule out conditions with symptoms mimicking HIV dementia, especially depression.)
**Wechsler Adult Intelligence Scale (WAIS-R):** Used to screen for the presence of HIV-induced brain damage; a low score may indicate memory loss or sensorimotor deficit (may be influenced by depression, anxiety, and hostile states).
**Minnesota Multiphasic Personality Inventory (MMPI):** Identify degree of depression, presence of personality disorders.

**Picture Drawing:** Differentiates depression from dementia (depressed person can draw, demented person cannot).

**TNF:** Elevated levels may account for white matter pallor.

**Mental Status Examinations, e.g., Galveston Orientation and Amnesia Scale (GOAT); Neurobehavioral Rating Scale (NRS, Freeman); Self-Rating Depression Scale; Cognitive Evaluation:** Identifies specific deficits.

**CBC:** May show anemia, affecting cerebral oxygenation/mentation.

**Blood Chemistries:** Rule out metabolic causes (e.g., diabetes mellitus, hypoglycemia, hypothyroid) and electrolyte deficiencies.

**$B_{12}$:** Identifies diminished levels (affects synaptic responses and biochemical interactions).

**Albumin:** Provides a measure of nutritional status.

**ABGs:** Rule out effect of hypoxia on mentation (presence of anemia, pneumonitis).

**Serology (RPR)/Screens:** May reveal infection (STD) requiring treatment.

**Alcohol/Drug Screen:** Rule out acute drug intoxication, drug or alcohol withdrawal.

**CT/MRI/PET:** Determine changes in brain mass (lesions or atrophy) and activity (expect to find cerebral atrophy mainly in the subcortical regions, white matter pallor, and ventricular enlargement).

**Lumbar Puncture:** Rule out tumors, identify infections of CNS. May show increased protein (60%), glucose, WBC (can culture for HIV).

## NURSING PRIORITIES

1. Promote socially acceptable responses, limit inappropriate behavior.
2. Prevent injury/complications.
3. Provide information about condition, prognosis, and treatment.

## DISCHARGE GOALS

1. Maximal level of independent functioning achieved.
2. Injury prevented/minimized, complications resolved.
3. Condition, prognosis, and therapeutic regimen understood.

| NURSING DIAGNOSIS: | THOUGHT PROCESSES, ALTERED |
|---|---|
| **May Be Related To:** | Direct CNS infection by HIV, disseminated systemic opportunistic infection, hypoxemia, brain malignancies, and/or CVA/hemorrhage; vasculitis. |
| | Alteration of drug metabolism/excretion, accumulation of toxic elements; renal failure, severe electrolyte imbalance, hepatic insufficiency. |
| | Sleep deprivation. |
| | Psychologic conflicts; inappropriate non–reality-based thinking. |
| **Possibly Evidenced By:** | Altered attention span; distractibility; memory deficit. |
| | Disorientation; cognitive dissonance; delusional thinking. |

| | Impaired ability to make decisions/problem-solve; inability to follow complex commands/mental tasks, loss of impulse control. |
|---|---|
| | Sleep disturbances. |
| **Client Outcomes/Evaluation Criteria—Client Will:** | Maintain optimum reality orientation and cognitive functioning. |
| | Demonstrate a decrease in undesired behaviors, threats, and confusion. |

| ACTIONS/INTERVENTIONS | RATIONALE |
|---|---|

### Independent

| ACTIONS/INTERVENTIONS | RATIONALE |
|---|---|
| Assess mental and neurologic status using appropriate tools, e.g., Neurobehavioral Rating Scale (Freeman). Note changes in orientation, response to stimuli, ability to problem-solve, anxiety, altered sleep patterns, hallucinations, paranoid ideation. Repeat serial/periodic evaluation every 2–4 months. | Establishes functional level at time of admission. Serial evaluations alert the nurse to changes in status that may be associated with progression of HIV dementia, exacerbation of CNS infection/opportunistic disease, environmental stressors, psychologic stress, or side effects of drug therapy. |
| Consider effects of emotional distress, e.g., anxiety, grief, anger, depression. | May contribute to reduced alertness, confusion, withdrawal, hypoactivity and require further evaluation and intervention. |
| Monitor medication regimen and usage. | Actions and interactions of various medications, prolonged drug half-life/altered excretion results in cumulative effects, potentiating risk of toxic reactions. Some drugs may have adverse side effects; e.g., haloperidol (Haldol) can seriously impair motor function in clients with AIDS dementia complex. |
| Note signs of acute CNS infection, e.g., headache, nuchal rigidity, vomiting, fever. | CNS symptoms associated with disseminated meningitis/encephalitis may range from subtle personality changes to confusion, irritability, drowsiness, stupor, seizures, and dementia. |
| Approach in a slow, calm manner. | Hurried approaches can startle/threaten the confused client who misinterprets or feels threatened by imaginary people and/or situations. |
| Maintain a pleasant environment with appropriate auditory, visual, and cognitive stimuli. | Providing normal environmental stimuli can help in maintaining some sense of reality orientation. |
| Decrease noise, especially at night. | Promotes sleep, reducing cognitive symptoms and sleep deprivation. |
| Maintain safe environment: e.g., excess furniture out of the way, call bell within client's reach, bed in low position/rails up; restriction of smoking (unless monitored by caregiver/SO), seizure precautions, soft restraints if indicated. | Decreases the possibility of client injury. |
| Provide information about care/answer questions simply and honestly without negating hope. Repeat explanations as needed and supplement with written materials as appropriate. | Can reduce anxiety and fear of unknown; may enhance client's understanding and involvement/cooperation in treatment and maintain hope in the context of the individual situation. |

| ACTIONS/INTERVENTIONS | RATIONALE |
|---|---|

### Independent

Provide cues for reorientation, e.g., radio, television, calendars, clocks, room with an outside view. Use client's name; identify yourself.

Frequent reorientation to place, time, and person may be necessary, especially during fever/acute CNS involvement.

Maintain consistent personnel and structured schedules matching home routines as appropriate.

Sense of continuity may help limit confusion and reduce associated anxiety.

Suggest use of datebooks, lists, alarm watch/pill box, other devices to keep track of activities.

These techniques help client to manage problems of forgetfulness.

Encourage client to do as much as is able (e.g., dress and groom daily, sit in chair, see friends). Allow adequate time to complete ADLs, provide step-by-step directions for activities, as appropriate.

Can help to maintain sense of normalcy and mental abilities for longer period.

Encourage family/SO to socialize and provide re-orientation with current news, family events.

Familiar contacts are often helpful in maintaining reality orientation, especially if client is halluci-nating.

Reduce provocative/noxious stimuli. Maintain bed rest in quiet room with subdued light, if indicated.

If the client is prone to agitation, violent behavior, or seizures, reducing external stimuli may be help-ful. Note: Darkened room can create unusual shadows that are hard for client to identify and may increase confusion.

Redirect attention, set limits on maladaptive/abusive behavior; avoid open-ended choices.

Provides sense of security/stability in an otherwise confusing situation.

Provide support for SO/family. Encourage discus-sion of concerns/fears.

Bizarre behavior/deterioration of abilities may be very frightening for loved ones and makes man-agement of care/dealing with situation difficult. SO may feel a loss of control as stress, anxiety, burnout, and anticipatory grieving impair usual coping abilities.

Discuss causes/future expectations and treatment if dementia is diagnosed. Use concrete terms.

Obtaining information that AZT has been shown to improve cognition can provide hope and control for losses.

### Collaborative

Assist with diagnostic studies, e.g., MRI/CT scan, spinal tap. Monitor laboratory studies as indicated, e.g., BUN/Cr, electrolytes, ABGs.

Choice of tests/studies is dependent on clinical manifestations and index of suspicion, as changes in mental status may reflect a wide variety of causative factors, e.g., CMV meningitis/encephalitis, drug toxicity, electrolyte imbalances, and altered organ function.

Administer medications as indicated:
  AZT (Retrovir);

Shown to improve neurologic and mental function-ing.

  Amphotericin B (Fungizone);

Antifungal useful in treatment of cryptococcosis meningitis.

  Antipsychotics, e.g., haloperidol (Haldol), and/or antianxiety agents, e.g., lorazepam (Ativan);

Cautious use may help with problems of sleep-lessness, emotional lability, hallucinations, suspiciousness, and agitation.

| ACTIONS/INTERVENTIONS | RATIONALE |
| --- | --- |
| **Collaborative** | |
| dextroamphetamine (Dexedrine) and methyl-phenidate (Ritalin). | These stimulants may be effective in improving mood and intellectual functioning. |
| Provide controlled environment/behavioral management. | Team approach may be required to protect client when mental impairment (e.g., delusions) threatens client safety. |
| Refer to counseling as indicated. | May help client gain control in presence of thought disturbances or psychotic symptomatology. |

| | |
| --- | --- |
| **NURSING DIAGNOSIS:** | **ANXIETY (specify level)** |
| **May Be Related To:** | Threat to self–concept. |
| | Perceived threat or change in health status; threat of death. |
| | Interpersonal transmission/contagion. |
| | Unmet needs. |
| **Possibly Evidenced By:** | Reports feeling scared, shaky, increased tension, apprehension, "feel like I'm going crazy." |
| | Increased somatic complaints; increased wariness. |
| | Extraneous movements, tremors. |
| **Desired Outcomes/Evaluation Criteria— Client Will:** | Verbalize awareness of feelings. |
| | Identify healthy ways to deal with anxiety and underlying causative factors. |
| | Use support systems effectively. |
| | Experience reduction in frequency and duration of episodes of anxiety. |
| | Direct energies to maintaining optimal level of functioning. |

| ACTIONS/INTERVENTIONS | RATIONALE |
| --- | --- |
| **Independent** | |
| Assure client of confidentiality within limits of situation. | Provides reassurance and opportunity for client to problem-solve solutions to anticipated situations. |
| Establish a therapeutic relationship, conveying empathy and caring. | Promotes openness and opportunity for client to talk freely about concerns and fears. |
| Ascertain client's perception of the threat represented by the situation. | The client may be aware of cognitive changes, thus increasing the sense of anxiety. The potential for suicide may be worsened if client perceives the situation as hopeless. |

| ACTIONS/INTERVENTIONS | RATIONALE |
|---|---|

### Independent

| | |
|---|---|
| Encourage client to acknowledge and express feelings. | Although an underlying medical cause for cognitive impairment may be present, the symptoms can increase anxiety. |
| Permit expressions of anger, fear, despair without confrontation. Give information that feelings are normal and are to be appropriately expressed. | Acceptance of feelings allows client to begin to deal with situation. |
| Assist the client to develop own awareness of verbal and nonverbal behaviors. | Being aware of self-behaviors brings increased understanding of responses of others. |
| Identify coping skills the individual is using. Review additional strategies when repertoire is limited. | Assists the client to identify coping techniques and draw on past and current styles that may be helpful in the situation. |
| Maintain frequent contact with client. Talk with and touch client. Limit use of isolation clothing/masks, restrictive environment. | Provides assurance that the client is not alone or rejected. Conveys respect for and acceptance of the person, fostering trust. Avoiding unnecessary use of "protective clothing/restrictions" promotes positive social contact and general sense of normalcy. |
| Identify and encourage client interaction with support systems. Encourage verbalization/interaction with family/SO. | Reduces feeling of isolation. If family support systems are not available, outside sources may be needed immediately, e.g., local AIDS task force. |
| Provide accurate, consistent information regarding prognosis. Encourage cooperation with medical evaluation to rule out conditions requiring medical intervention. | Can reduce anxiety and enable client to make decisions/choices based on realities. Some causative factors for cognitive impairment are treatable/reversible. |
| Explain procedures, providing opportunity for questions. Stay with client during procedures and consultations. | Accurate information allows the client a sense of control. Client may be calmer when she or he understands procedure and expectations. |
| Review medication regimen for evidence of interactions between OTC and prescribed medications. | Certain drug interactions can induce anxiety. |
| Be alert to signs of denial/depression (e.g., withdrawal; angry, inappropriate remarks). Determine presence of suicidal ideation and assess potential on a scale of 1–10. | Client may use defense mechanism of denial and continue to hope that diagnosis is inaccurate. Feelings of guilt and spiritual distress may cause the client to become withdrawn. The individual may believe that suicide is a viable alternative. |
| Include SO as indicated when major decisions are to be made. | Ensures a support system for the client and allows the SO the chance to participate in client's life. Note: If client, family, and SO are in conflict, separate care consultations and visiting times may be needed. |

### Collaborative

| | |
|---|---|
| Monitor results of diagnostic studies. | Identification/treatment of underlying conditions (e.g., opportunistic infections, chemical imbalances, or lymphomas) may limit progression/reverse cognitive impairment and corresponding anxiety. |

| ACTIONS/INTERVENTIONS | RATIONALE |
|---|---|

### Collaborative

Administer antianxiety medications with caution. Begin with low doses and increase slowly.

While these medications may be useful in individual situations, they may have increased untoward effects because these clients are sensitive to side effects.

Refer for ongoing individual/family psychiatric therapy as indicated. Identify available resources/support groups.

May require further assistance in dealing with diagnosis/prognosis, especially when suicidal thoughts are present.

| NURSING DIAGNOSIS: | SLEEP PATTERN DISTURBANCE |
|---|---|
| May Be Related To: | Psychologic stress, e.g., anxiety, depression. |
| | HIV neurologic impairment (neurotransmitter impairment). |
| | Inactivity/changes in activity patterns. |
| Possibly Evidenced By: | Verbalization of not feeling rested. |
| | Difficulty falling asleep; frequent awakening. |
| | Increasing irritability, disorientation, restlessness, or lethargy. |
| Desired Outcomes/Evaluation Criteria—Client Will: | Identify appropriate interventions to promote sleep. |
| | Report improved sleep pattern, sense of being rested. |

| ACTIONS/INTERVENTIONS | RATIONALE |
|---|---|

### Independent

Identify factors contributing to insomnia and problem-solve solutions.

Chronic pain of neuropathy, cough of pneumonias and other URI, medication interactions can interfere with sleep.

Evaluate use of caffeine and alcohol.

Overindulgence in these substances reduces REM sleep.

Reduce environmental stimulation. Provide soft music.

Reduces sensory stimulation; soft music can block out disturbing sounds. If stage IV sleep is not reached, there is increased risk of psychologic symptoms.

Provide evening snack, warm milk, back rub, straighten sheets (no wrinkles).

Promotes relaxation. L-Tryptophan (found in milk) is believed to induce drowsiness.

Reduce fluid intake after 5 PM.

Prevents wakefulness related to sensation of bladder fullness and episodes of incontinency.

Administer pain medications when indicated, 30–60 minutes before bedtime.

Alleviating pain can help client to relax, fall asleep more quickly, and sleep better.

147

| ACTIONS/INTERVENTIONS | RATIONALE |
|---|---|

**Collaborative**

| | |
|---|---|
| Administer medications as needed, e.g., amyltriptyline (Elavil). | May reduce depression, pain of peripheral neuropathy and promote sleep. |

| NURSING DIAGNOSIS: | INJURY/TRAUMA, HIGH RISK FOR |
|---|---|
| Risk Factors May Include: | Weakness, balancing difficulties, reduced tactile sensation. |
| | Cognitive deficits, inability to recognize/identify danger in environment. |
| | Smoking unattended. |
| | Seizure activity. |
| Possibly Evidenced By: | [Not applicable; presence of signs/symptoms establishes an **actual** diagnosis.] |
| Desired Outcomes/Evaluation Criteria— Client Will: | Remain safe, without injury to person or damage to environment. |
| Client/Caregiver Will: | Recognize potential risks in the environment. |
| | Identify/implement steps to correct/compensate for individual factors. |

| ACTIONS/INTERVENTIONS | RATIONALE |
|---|---|

**Independent**

| | |
|---|---|
| Assess degree of impairment in cognitive and functional abilities. Assist client/SO to identify risks and potential hazards. | Increases awareness of dangers and provides opportunity to implement anticipatory interventions. |
| Assist client/SO to plan for activities and safety measures to be considered, e.g., direct monitoring of cigarette use, use of cane/walker for ambulation, seizure precautions. | Involving client in planning may reduce frustration and increase client sense of control and self-worth. |
| Inspect skin during self-care activities. | Presence of ecchymosis, lacerations, rashes, etc., may require treatment as well as signal need for closer monitoring/protective interventions. |
| Investigate availability of/evaluate client's ability to use home emergency call system. | Allows for periodic monitoring and prompt response as needed, enhancing safety in home setting. |
| Provide for protective environment when indicated, someone to stay with client on a full-time basis, use of restraints, admission to long-term care facility. | Near end stage the client may no longer be able to recognize safety factors and may wander. This is not likely to be a prolonged period of time for the client with HIV dementia. |

| NURSING DIAGNOSIS: | FAMILY COPING, ineffective: compromised/disabling/CAREGIVER ROLE STRAIN |
|---|---|
| May Be Related To: | Situational conflict (parent–adult-child conflict, adult/child returning home with terminal illness; financial difficulties/insufficient resources). |
| | Disruptive/bizarre behavior of client. |
| | Unpredictable illness course or instability in the care receiver's health. |
| | Individual helplessness/grief about watching loved one deteriorate. |
| | Sense of shame surrounding a diagnosis of AIDS (regardless of how contracted). |
| | Prolonged disease/disability progression that exhausts the supportive capacity of SO. |
| | Highly ambivalent family relationships. |
| | Difficulty with acceptance of/adaptation to client's sexual orientation/lifestyle/behaviors previous to caregiving situation. |
| Possibly Evidenced By: | Family becoming embarrassed and socially immobilized. |
| | Family feeling stress or nervousness in relationship with the care receiver; conflict around issues of providing care. |
| | Lack of resources/inability to provide level of care indicated; difficult decisions with legal/financial considerations. |
| | Feelings of loss because care receiver is like a different person compared to before caregiving began. |
| Desired Outcomes/Evaluation Criteria— Family/Caregiver Will: | Identify/verbalize resources within themselves to deal with the situation. |
| | Verbalize realistic understanding/expectations of client. |
| | Demonstrate positive coping behaviors in dealing with situation. |
| | Use outside support systems effectively. |

| ACTIONS/INTERVENTIONS | RATIONALE |
|---|---|

### Independent

| | |
|---|---|
| Review past life experiences, role changes, and coping skills. | Opportunity to identify skills that may help individuals cope with grief of current situation more effectively. |

| ACTIONS/INTERVENTIONS | RATIONALE |
|---|---|

### Independent

| | |
|---|---|
| Encourage unlimited visitation as tolerated by client. | Contact with family forms a base of reality and can provide a reassuring freedom from loneliness. Recurrent contact helps family members realize and accept situation. |
| Provide time/listen with regard to concerns/anxieties. | The self-sacrificing, painful nature of the care required in this disease necessitates constant support for SOs in order to deal effectively with the multifaceted problems arising during the course of this illness and to ease the process of adaptation and grieving. |
| Determine family's/SO's ability to care for client at home; reevaluate periodically. | Behaviors like hoarding, clinging, unjust accusations, angry outbursts, etc., can precipitate family/caregiver burnout and interfere with ability to provide effective care. |
| Include SOs in teaching and planning for home care. | Can ease the burden of home management and increase adaptation. Comfortable and familiar lifestyle at home is helpful in preserving the affected individual's need for belonging. |
| Focus on specific problems as they occur, the "here and now." | Disease progression follows no set pattern. A premature focus on the possibility of long-term care or possible incontinence, for example, impairs the ability to cope with present issues. |
| Establish priorities. | Helps to create a sense of order and facilitates problem-solving. |
| Be realistic and honest in all matters. | Decreases stress that surrounds false hopes, e.g., that individual may regain past level of functioning from advertised or unproven medication/herbal preparations. |
| Help caregiver/family understand the importance of maintaining psychosocial functioning. | Embarrassing behavior, the demands of care, etc., may cause withdrawal from social contact. |
| Discuss possibility of isolation. Reinforce need for support system. | The belief that a single individual can meet all the needs of the client increases the potential for physical/mental illness (caregiver role strain). |
| Provide positive feedback for efforts. | Reassures individuals that they are doing as well as they can and encourages continued efforts. |
| Support concerns generated by consideration/decision to place in LTC facility. | Constant care requirements may be more than can be managed by SO. Support is needed for this difficult, guilt-producing decision, which may create a financial burden as well as family disruption/dissension. |

| ACTIONS/INTERVENTIONS | RATIONALE |
|---|---|
| **Collaborative** | |
| Refer to local resources, e.g. adult day care (if available), respite care, homemaker services, or AIDS support organizations. | Coping with this individual is a full-time, frustrating task. Respite/day care may lighten the burden, reduce potential social isolation, and prevent family/caregiver burnout. AIDS organizations provide group support and family teaching and promote research. Local groups provide a social outlet for sharing grief and promote problem-solving with such matters as financial/legal advice, home care, etc. |
| Refer to CPs: Dementia of the Alzheimer's Type; Major Depression regarding issues of self-care, urinary elimination, nutrition, sensory-perceptual alterations, health maintenance, home maintenance management, etc. | |

# CHAPTER 6

# SUBSTANCE-RELATED DISORDERS

## ALCOHOL-RELATED DISORDERS

**DSM IV**
**ALCOHOL-INDUCED DISORDERS**
303.00 Alcohol Intoxication
291.8 Alcohol Withdrawal
291.8 Alcohol-Induced Mood Disorder
291.8 Alcohol-Induced Anxiety Disorder
**ALCOHOL USE DISORDERS**
303.90 Alcohol Dependence
305.00 Alcohol Abuse
(Refer to DSM IV for further listings.)

**DSM III-R**
303.00 Intoxication
291.40 Idiosyncratic Intoxication
291.80 Uncomplicated Alcohol Withdrawal

Alcohol is a CNS depressant drug that is used socially in our society for many reasons, e.g., to enhance the flavor of food, to encourage relaxation and conviviality, for feelings of celebration, and as a sacred ritual in some religious ceremonies. Therapeutically, it is the major ingredient in many OTC/prescription medications. It can be harmless, enjoyable, and sometimes beneficial when used responsibly and in moderation. Like other mind-altering drugs, however, it has the potential for abuse and, in fact, is the most widely abused drug in the United States. Frequently, the client who is in a residential setting has been using alcohol in conjunction with other drugs. It is believed that alcohol is often used by clients who have other mental illnesses to assuage the pain they feel. The term "dual diagnosis" is used to mean an association between the use/abuse of drugs (including alcohol) and other psychiatric diagnoses. It may be difficult to determine cause and effect in any given situation to determine an accurate diagnosis. However, it is important to recognize when both conditions are present so that the often overwhelming problems of treatment are instituted for both conditions.

This plan of care is to be used in conjunction with CP: Substance Dependence/Abuse Rehabilitation.

## ETIOLOGIC THEORIES

### Psychodynamics

The individual remains fixed in a lower level of development, with retarded ego and weak superego. The person retains a highly dependent nature, with characteristics of poor impulse control, low frustration tolerance, and low self-esteem.

### Biologic

Enzymes, genes, brain chemistry, and hormones create and contribute to an individual's response to alcohol. There are two types: (1) familial, which is largely inherited, and (2) acquired. A childhood history of Attention-Deficit Disorder or Conduct Disorder also increases a child's risk of becoming alcoholic. There are physiologic changes that cause addiction to alcohol, or alcoholism.

### Family Dynamics

One in 12–15 persons has serious problems from drinking. In a dysfunctional family system, alcohol may be viewed as the primary method of relieving stress. Children of alcoholics are 4 times more likely to develop alcoholism than children of nonalcoholics. The child has negative role models and learns to respond to stressful situations in like manner. The use of alcohol is cultural, and many factors influence one's decision to drink, how much, and how often. Denial of the illness can be a major barrier to identification and treatment of alcoholism and alcohol abuse.

## CLIENT ASSESSMENT DATABASE

Data are dependent on the duration/extent of use of alcohol, concurrent use of other drugs, and degree of organ involvement.

### Activity/Rest

Difficulty sleeping, not feeling well rested.

### Circulation

Peripheral pulses weak, irregular, or rapid.
Hypertension common in early withdrawal stage but may become labile/progress to hypotension.
Tachycardia common during acute withdrawal; numerous dysrhythmias may be identified; other abnormalities depend on underlying heart disease/concurrent drug use.

### Ego Integrity

Feelings of guilt/shame; defensiveness about drinking.
Denial, rationalization.
Reports of multiple stressors; problems with relationships.
Multiple losses, e.g., relationships, jobs, financial, etc.
Use of substances to deal with life stressors, boredom, etc.

### Elimination

Diarrhea.
Bowel sounds varied, related to gastric complications such as gastric hemorrhage or distension.

### Food/Fluid

Nausea/vomiting, food intolerance.
Difficulty chewing/swallowing food.
Muscle wasting, dry/dull hair, swollen salivary glands, inflamed buccal cavity, capillary fragility (malnutrition).
Generalized tissue edema may be noted (protein deficiencies).
Gastric distension; ascites, liver enlargement (seen in cirrhosis with long-term use).

## Neurosensory

"Internal shakes."

Headache, dizziness, blurred vision, "blackouts."

Psychopathology, e.g., paranoid schizophrenia, major depression (dual diagnosis).

**Level of Consciousness/Orientation:** Confusion, stupor, hyperactivity, distorted thought processes, slurred/incoherent speech.

Memory loss/confabulation.

**Affect/Mood/Behavior:** May be fearful, anxious, easily startled, inappropriate, silly, euphoric, irritable, physically/verbally abusive, depressed, and/or paranoid.

**Hallucinations:** Visual, tactile, olfactory, and auditory, e.g., picking items out of air or responding verbally to unseen person/voices.

Nystagmus (associated with cranial nerve palsy).

Pupil constriction (may indicate CNS depression).

Arcus senilis, a ringlike opacity of the cornea (normal in aging populations, suggests alcohol-related changes in younger clients).

Fine motor tremors of face, tongue, and hands; seizure activity (commonly grand mal).

Gait unsteady (ataxia), may be due to thiamine deficiency or cerebellar degeneration (Wernicke's encephalopathy).

## Pain/Discomfort

May report constant upper abdominal pain and tenderness radiating to the back (pancreatic inflammation).

## Respiration

History of tobacco use, recurrent/chronic respiratory problems.

Tachypnea (hyperactive state of alcohol withdrawal).

Cheyne-Stokes respirations or respiratory depression.

**Breath Sounds:** Diminished/adventitious sounds (suggests pulmonary complications, e.g., respiratory depression, pneumonia).

## Safety

History of recurrent accidents, such as falls, fractures, lacerations, burns, blackouts, or automobile accidents.

**Skin:** Flushed face/palms of hands, scars, ecchymotic areas, cigarette burns on fingers, spider nevi (impaired portal circulation); fissures at corners of mouth (vitamin deficiency).

Fractures—healed or new (signs of recent/recurrent trauma).

Temperature elevation (dehydration and sympathetic stimulation); flushing/diaphoresis (suggests presence of infection).

Suicidal ideation/attempts (some research suggests alcoholic suicide attempts are 30% higher than national average for general population).

## Social Interactions

Frequent sick days off work/school, fighting with others, arrests (disorderly conduct, motor vehicle violations/DUIs).

Denial that alcohol intake has any significant effect on the present condition.

Dysfunctional family system of origin; problems in current relationships.

Mood changes.

## Teaching/Learning

History of alcohol and/or drug use/abuse.

Ignorance and/or denial of addiction to alcohol or inability to cut down or stop drinking despite repeated efforts.

Large amount of alcohol consumed in last 24–48 hours, previous periods of abstinence/withdrawal.

Previous hospitalizations for alcoholism/alcohol-related diseases, e.g., cirrhosis, esophageal varices.

Family history of alcoholism/substance use.

## DIAGNOSTIC STUDIES

**Blood Alcohol/Drug Levels:** Alcohol level may/may not be severely elevated depending on amount consumed and length of time between consumption and testing. In addition to alcohol, numerous controlled/illicit substances, e.g., amphetamine, cocaine, morphine, Percodan, Quaalude, may be identified in a polydrug screen.

**CBC:** Decreased Hb/Hct may reflect such problems as iron-deficiency anemia or acute/chronic gastrointestinal (GI) bleeding. White blood cell count may be increased with infection or decreased, if immunosuppressed.

**Glucose:** Hyperglycemia/hypoglycemia may be present, related to pancreatitis, malnutrition, or depletion of liver glycogen stores.

**Electrolytes:** Hypokalemia and hypomagnesemia are common.

**Liver Function Tests:** CPK, LDH, AST, ALT, and amylase may be elevated, reflecting liver or pancreatic damage.

**Nutritional Tests:** Albumin is low and total protein decreased, vitamin deficiencies are usually present, reflecting malnutrition/malabsorption.

**Urinalysis:** Infection may be identified; ketones may be present related to breakdown of fatty acids in malnutrition (pseudodiabetic condition).

**Chest X-Ray:** May reveal right lower lobe pneumonia (malnutrition, depressed immune system, aspiration) or chronic lung disorders associated with tobacco use.

**ECG:** Dysrhythmias, cardiomyopathies, and/or ischemia may be present owing to direct effect of alcohol on the cardiac muscle and/or conduction system, as well as effects of electrolyte imbalance.

**Addiction Severity Index (ASI):** An assessment tool that produces a "problem severity profile" of the client, including chemical, medical, psychologic, legal, family/social, and employment/support aspects, indicating areas of treatment needs.

## NURSING PRIORITIES

1. Maintain physiologic stability during withdrawal phase.
2. Promote client safety.
3. Encourage/support SO involvement in "Intervention" (confrontation) process.

## DISCHARGE GOALS

1. Homeostasis achieved.
2. Complications prevented/resolved.
3. Sobriety maintained on a day-to-day basis.
4. Participation in a rehabilitation program/attendance at group therapy, e.g., Alcoholics Anonymous, ongoing.

| NURSING DIAGNOSIS: | BREATHING PATTERN, INEFFECTIVE, high risk for |
| --- | --- |
| Risk Factors May Include: | Direct effect of alcohol toxicity on respiratory center and/or sedative drugs given to decrease alcohol withdrawal symptoms. |
| | Tracheobronchial obstruction. |

| | |
|---|---|
| | Presence of chronic respiratory problems, inflammatory process. |
| | Decreased energy/fatigue. |
| **Possibly Evidenced By:** | [Not applicable; presence of signs and symptoms establishes an **actual** diagnosis.] |
| **Desired Outcomes/Evaluation Criteria— Client Will:** | Maintain effective respiratory pattern with respiratory rate within normal range, free of cyanosis and other signs/symptoms of hypoxia. |

## ACTIONS/INTERVENTIONS

## RATIONALE

### Independent

| ACTIONS/INTERVENTIONS | RATIONALE |
|---|---|
| Monitor respiratory rate/depth and pattern as indicated. Note periods of apnea, Cheyne-Stokes respirations. | Frequent assessment is important because toxicity levels may change rapidly. Hyperventilation is common during acute withdrawal phase. Kussmaul respirations are sometimes present because of acidotic state associated with vomiting and malnutrition. However, marked respiratory depression can occur because of CNS depressant effects from alcohol. This may be compounded by drugs used to control alcohol withdrawal symptoms. |
| Elevate head of bed. | Decreases possibility of aspiration; lowers diaphragm, enhancing lung inflation. |
| Encourage cough/deep breathing exercises and frequent position changes. | Facilitates lung expansion and mobilization of secretions to reduce risk of atelectasis/pneumonia. |
| Auscultate breath sounds. Note presence of adventitious sounds, e.g., rhonchi, wheezes. | Client is at risk for atelectasis related to hypoventilation and pneumonia. Right lower lobe pneumonia is common in alcohol-debilitated clients and is often due to aspiration. Chronic lung diseases are also common, e.g., emphysema, chronic bronchitis. |
| Have suction equipment, airway adjuncts available. | Sedative effects of alcohol/drugs potentiates risk of aspiration, relaxation of oropharyngeal muscles, and respiratory depression, requiring intervention to prevent respiratory arrest. |

### Collaborative

| ACTIONS/INTERVENTIONS | RATIONALE |
|---|---|
| Administer supplemental oxygen if necessary. | Hypoxia may occur with CNS/respiratory depression. |
| Review chest x-rays, pulse oximetry as indicated. | Monitors presence of secondary complications such as atelectasis/pneumonia; evaluates effectiveness of respiratory effort, identifies therapy needs. |

| | |
|---|---|
| **NURSING DIAGNOSIS:** | **CARDIAC OUTPUT, DECREASED, high risk for** |
| **Risk Factors May Include:** | Direct effect of alcohol on the heart muscle. |

| **Possibly Evidenced By:** | Altered systemic vascular resistance. |
| | Electrical alterations in rate, rhythm, conduction. |
| | [Not applicable; presence of signs and symptoms establishes an **actual** diagnosis.] |
| **Desired Outcomes/Evaluation Criteria—Client Will:** | Display vital signs within client's normal range; absence of/reduced frequency of dysrhythmias. |
| | Demonstrate an increase in activity tolerance. |
| | Verbalize understanding of the effect of alcohol on the heart |

| ACTIONS/INTERVENTIONS | RATIONALE |
|---|---|
| **Independent** | |
| Monitor vital signs frequently during acute withdrawal. | Hypertension frequently occurs in acute withdrawal phase. Extreme hyperexcitability accompanied by catecholamine release and increased peripheral vascular resistance raises blood pressure (and heart rate). However, BP may become labile/progress to hypotension. Note: May have underlying cardiovascular disease that is compounded by substance withdrawal. |
| Monitor cardiac rate/rhythm. Document dysrhythmias. | Long-term alcohol abuse may result in cardiomyopathy/congestive heart failure. Tachycardia is common due to sympathetic response to increased circulating catecholamines. Irregularities/dysrhythmias may develop with electrolyte shifts/imbalance. All of these may have an adverse effect on cardiac function/output. |
| Monitor body temperature. | Elevation may occur because of sympathetic stimulation, dehydration, and/or infections, causing vasodilation and compromising venous return/cardiac output. |
| Monitor intake/output. Note 24-hour fluid balance. | Preexisting dehydration, vomiting, fever, and diaphoresis may result in decreased cirulating volume, which can compromise cardiovascular function. Note: Hydration is difficult to assess in the alcoholic because the usual indicators are not reliable, and overhydration is a risk in the presence of compromised cardiac function. |
| Be prepared for/assist in cardiopulmonary resuscitation. | Causes of death during acute withdrawal stages include cardiac dysrhythmias, respiratory depression/arrest, oversedation, excessive psychomotor activity, severe dehydration or overhydration, and massive infections. Mortality for unrecognized/untreated delirium tremens (DTs) may be as high as 15%–25%. |

157

| ACTIONS/INTERVENTIONS | RATIONALE |
|---|---|

## Collaborative

| | |
|---|---|
| Note initial serum electrolyte levels. | Electrolyte imbalance, e.g., potassium/magnesium, potentiates risk of cardiac dysrhythmias and CNS excitability. |
| Administer medications as indicated, e.g.:<br>clonidine (Catapres); | Provides for greater mean reductions in heart rate and systolic blood pressure with less nausea and vomiting. |
| potassium. | Corrects deficits that can result in life-threatening dysrhythmias. |

| NURSING DIAGNOSIS: | INJURY, HIGH RISK FOR (specify) |
|---|---|
| Risk Factors May Include: | Cessation of alcohol intake with varied autonomic nervous system responses to the system's suddenly altered state. |
| | Involuntary clonic/tonic muscle activity (convulsions). |
| | Equilibrium/balancing difficulties, reduced muscle and hand/eye coordination. |
| Possibly Evidenced By: | [Not applicable; presence of signs and symptoms establishes an **actual** diagnosis.] |
| Desired Outcomes/Evaluation Criteria— Client Will: | Demonstrate absence of untoward effects of withdrawal. |
| | Experience no physical injury. |

| ACTIONS/INTERVENTIONS | RATIONALE |
|---|---|

## Independent

| | |
|---|---|
| Identify stage of alcohol withdrawal, i.e.:<br>Stage I is associated with signs/symptoms of hyperactivity (e.g., tremors, sleeplessness, nausea/vomiting, diaphoresis, tachycardia, hypertension).<br>Stage-II is manifested by increased hyperactivity plus hallucinations and/or seizure activity.<br>Stage-III symptoms include delirium tremens (DTs) and extreme autonomic hyperactivity with profound confusion, anxiety, insomnia, fever. | Prompt recognition and intervention may halt progression of symptoms and enhance recovery/improve prognosis. In addition, reoccurrence/progression of symptoms indicates need for changes in drug therapy/more intense treatment. |
| Monitor/document seizure activity. Maintain client airway. Provide environmental safety, e.g., padded side rails, bed in low position. | Grand mal seizures are most common and may be related to decreased magnesium levels, hypoglycemia, elevated blood alcohol, or history of head trauma. Note: In absence of previous history of other pathology causing seizure activity, seizures usually stop spontaneously, requiring only symptomatic treatment. |

| ACTIONS/INTERVENTIONS | RATIONALE |
|---|---|
| **Independent** | |
| Check deep-tendon reflexes. Assess gait, if possible. | Reflexes may be depressed, absent, or hyperactive. Peripheral neuropathies are common, especially in malnourished clients. Ataxia (gait disturbance) is associated with Wernicke's syndrome (thiamine deficiency) and cerebellar degeneration. |
| Assist with ambulation and self-care activities as needed. | Prevents falls with resultant injury. |
| Provide for environmental safety when indicated. (Refer to ND: Sensory/Perceptual alteration [specify].) | May be required when equilibrium, hand/eye co-ordination problems exist. |
| **Collaborative** | |
| Administer IV/PO fluids with caution, as indicated. | Cautious replacement corrects dehydration and promotes renal clearance of toxins while reducing risk of overhydration. |
| Administer medications as indicated: benzodiazepines, e.g.: chlordiazepoxide (Librium), diazepam (Valium), clonazepam (Klonopin); | Commonly used to control neuronal hyperactivity that occurs as alcohol is detoxified. IV/oral administration is the route preferred, as intramuscular absorption is unpredictable. Muscle-relaxant qualities are particularly helpful to the client in controlling the "shakes," trembling, and ataxic quality of movements. Clients may initially require large doses to achieve desired effect, and then the drug(s) may be tapered and discontinued, usually within 96 hours. Note: These agents must be used cautiously in clients with hepatic disease, as the agents are metabolized by the liver. |
| oxazepam (Serax); | Although less dramatic for control of withdrawal symptoms, may be drug of choice in client with liver disease because of its shorter half-life. |
| phenobarbital; | Useful in suppressing withdrawal symptoms and is an effective anticonvulsant. Use must be monitored to prevent exacerbation of respiratory depression. |
| magnesium sulfate. | Reduces tremors and seizure activity by decreasing neuromuscular excitability. |

| | |
|---|---|
| **NURSING DIAGNOSIS:** | **SENSORY/PERCEPTUAL ALTERATIONS (SPECIFY)** |
| **May Be Related To:** | Chemical alteration: Exogenous (e.g., alcohol consumption/sudden cessation) and endogenous (e.g., electrolyte imbalance, elevated ammonia and BUN). |

| | |
|---|---|
| **Possibly Evidenced By:** | Sleep deprivation. |
| | Psychologic stress (anxiety/fear). |
| | Disorientation in time, place, or person. |
| | Changes in usual response to stimuli; exaggerated emotional responses, change in behavior. |
| | Bizarre thinking. |
| | Anxiety, restlessness, irritability. |
| **Desired Outcomes/Evaluation Criteria— Client Will:** | Regain/maintain usual level of consciousness. |
| | Report absence of auditory/visual hallucinations. |
| | Identify external factors that affect sensory-perceptual abilities. |

## ACTIONS/INTERVENTIONS

## RATIONALE

### Independent

Assess level of consciousness, ability to speak, response to stimuli/commands.

Speech may be garbled, confused, or slurred. Response to commands may reveal inability to concentrate, impaired judgment, or muscle coordination deficits.

Observe behavioral responses, e.g., hyperactivity, disorientation, confusion, sleeplessness, irritability.

Hyperactivity related to CNS disturbances may escalate rapidly. Sleeplessness is common due to loss of sedative effect gained from alcohol usually consumed prior to bedtime. Sleep deprivation may aggravate disorientation/confusion. Progression of symptoms may indicate impending hallucinations (Stage II) or DTs (Stage III).

Note onset of hallucinations. Document as auditory, visual, and/or tactile.

Auditory hallucinations are reported to be more frightening/threatening to client. Visual hallucinations occur more at night and often include insects, animals, or faces of friends/enemies. Clients are frequently observed picking the air. Yelling may occur if client is calling for help from perceived threat (usually seen in Stage III).

Provide quiet environment. Speak in calm, quiet voice. Regulate lighting as indicated. Turn off radio/TV during sleep.

Reduces external stimuli during hyperactive stage. Client may become more delirious when surroundings cannot be seen, although some respond better to quiet, darkened room.

Provide care by same personnel whenever possible.

Promotes recognition of caregivers and a sense of consistency that may reduce fear.

Provide frequent reality orientation to person, place, time, and surrounding environment as indicated.

May reduce confusion/misinterpretation of external stimuli.

Avoid bedside discussion about client or topics unrelated to the client that do not include the client.

Client may hear and misinterpret conversation, which can aggravate hallucinations.

| ACTIONS/INTERVENTIONS | RATIONALE |
|---|---|
| **Independent** | |
| Provide environmental safety, e.g., place bed in low position, leave doors in full open or closed position, observe frequently, place call light/bell within reach, remove articles that can harm client. | Client may have distorted sense of reality, be fearful, or be suicidal, requiring protection from self-harm. |
| **Collaborative** | |
| Provide seclusion, restraints as necessary. | Clients with excessive psychomotor activity, severe hallucinations, violent behavior, and/or suicidal gestures may respond better to seclusion. Restraints are usually ineffective and add to client's agitation but occasionally may be required for short periods to prevent self-harm. |
| Monitor laboratory studies: e.g., electrolytes, liver function studies, BUN, ABGs, glucose, magnesium levels, ammonia. | Changes in organ function may precipitate or potentiate sensory-perceptual deficits. Electrolyte imbalance is common. Liver function is often impaired in the chronic alcoholic. Ammonia intoxication can occur if the liver is unable to convert ammonia to urea. Ketoacidosis is sometimes present without glycosuria; however, hyperglycemia or hypoglycemia may occur, suggesting pancreatitis or impaired gluconeogenesis in the liver. Hypoxemia and hypercarbia are common manifestations in chronic alcoholics who are also heavy smokers. |
| Administer medications as indicated, e.g.: minor tranquilizers as indicated (refer to ND: Anxiety [severe/panic]/Fear); | Reduces hyperactivity, promoting relaxation/sleep. Drugs that have little effect on dreaming may be desired to allow dream recovery (REM rebound) to occur, which has been suppressed by alcohol use. |
| thiamine; multivitamins high in C/B complex; Stresstabs. | Vitamins are depleted because of insufficient intake and malabsorption. Vitamin deficiency (especially thiamine) is associated with ataxia, loss of eye movement and pupillary response, palpitations, postural hypotension, and exertional dyspnea. |

| | |
|---|---|
| **NURSING DIAGNOSIS:** | **NUTRITION, ALTERED, LESS THAN BODY REQUIREMENTS** |
| **May Be Related To:** | Poor dietary intake (replaced by alcohol consumption). |
| | Effects of alcohol on organs involved in digestion, e.g., pancreas/liver; interference with absorption and metabolism of nutrients and amino acids; and increased loss of vitamins in the urine. |
| **Possibly Evidenced By:** | Reports of inadequate food intake, altered taste sensation, lack of interest in food, abdominal pain. |

|  | Body weight 20% or more under ideal. |
|  | Pale conjunctiva and mucous membranes; sore, inflammed buccal cavity/cheilosis. |
|  | Poor muscle tone, skin turgor. |
|  | Hyperactive bowel sounds, diarrhea. |
|  | Third spacing of circulating blood volume (e.g., edema of extremities, ascites). |
|  | Presence of neuropathies. |
|  | Laboratory evidence of decreased red cell count (anemias), vitamin deficiencies, reduced serum albumin, or electrolyte imbalance. |
| **Desired Outcomes/Evaluation Criteria— Client Will:** | Demonstrate stable weight or progressive weight gain toward goal with normalization of laboratory values and absence of signs of malnutrition. |
|  | Verbalize understanding of effects of alcohol ingestion and reduced dietary intake on nutritional status. |
|  | Demonstrate behaviors, lifestyle changes to regain/maintain appropriate weight. |

| ACTIONS/INTERVENTIONS | RATIONALE |
|---|---|

### Independent

| Evaluate presence/quality of bowel sounds. Note abdominal distension, tenderness. | Irritation of gastric mucosa is common and may result in epigastric pain, nausea, and hyperactive bowel sounds. More serious effects of GI system may occur secondary to cirrhosis and hepatitis. |
| Note presence of nausea/vomiting, diarrhea. | Nausea and vomiting are often among the first signs of alcohol withdrawal and may interfere with achieving adequate nutritional intake. |
| Assess ability to feed self. | Tremors, altered mentation/hallucinations may interfere with ingestion of nutrients and indicate need for assistance. |
| Provide small, easily digested, frequent feedings/snacks and advance as tolerated. | May limit gastric distress and enhance intake and toleration of nutrients. As appetite and ability to tolerate food increase, diet should be adjusted to provide the necessary calories and nutrition for cellular repair and restoration of energy. |

### Collaborative

| Review laboratory tests, e.g., AST, ALT, LDH, serum albumin, transferrin. | Assesses liver function, adequacy of nutritional intake; influences choice of diet and need for/effectiveness of supplemental therapy. |
| Refer to dietitian/nutritional support team. | Useful in coordinating individual nutritional regimen. |

| ACTIONS/INTERVENTIONS | RATIONALE |
|---|---|
| **Collaborative** | |
| Provide diet high in protein with at least half of calories obtained from carbohydrates. | Stabilizes blood sugar, thereby reducing risk of hypoglycemia while providing for energy needs and cellular regeneration. |
| Administer medications as indicated; e.g.: antacids, antiemetics, antidiarrheals; | Reduces gastric irritation and effects of sympathetic stimulation. |
| vitamins, thiamine. | Replace losses. Note: All clients should receive thiamine and vitamins, because deficiencies (clinical or subclinical) exist in most if not all chronic substance abusers. |
| Institute/maintain NPO status as indicated. | Provides gastrointestinal rest to reduce harmful effects of gastric/pancreatic stimulation in presence of GI bleeding or excessive vomiting. |

| NURSING DIAGNOSIS: | ANXIETY [severe/panic]/FEAR |
|---|---|
| **May Be Related To:** | Cessation of alcohol intake/physiologic withdrawal. |
| | Situational crisis (hospitalization). |
| | Threat to self-concept, perceived threat of death. |
| **Possibly Evidenced By:** | Feelings of inadequacy, shame, self-disgust, and remorse. |
| | Increased helplessness/hopelessness with loss of control of own life. |
| | Increased tension, apprehension. |
| | Fear of unspecified consequences; identifies object of fear. |
| **Desired Outcomes/Evaluation Criteria— Client Will:** | Verbalize reduction of fear and anxiety to an acceptable and manageable level. |
| | Express sense of regaining some control of situation/life. |
| | Demonstrate problem-solving skills and use resources effectively. |

| ACTIONS/INTERVENTIONS | RATIONALE |
|---|---|
| **Independent** | |
| Identify cause of anxiety, involving client in the process. Explain that alcohol withdrawal increases anxiety and uneasiness. Reassess level of anxiety on an ongoing basis. | Person in acute phase of withdrawal may be unable to identify and/or accept what is happening. Anxiety may be physiologically/environmentally caused. Continued alcohol toxicity will be manifested by increased anxiety and agitation as effects of tranquilizers wear off. |

163

| ACTIONS/INTERVENTIONS | RATIONALE |
|---|---|

### Independent

Develop a trusting relationship through frequent contact, honesty, and nonjudgmental attitude.

Provides client with a sense of humanness, helping to decrease paranoia and distrust. Client will be able to detect biased or condescending attitude of caregivers.

Inform client what you plan to do and why. Include client in planning process/provide choices when possible.

Enhances sense of trust, and explanation may increase cooperation/reduce anxiety. Feelings of self-worth are intensified when one is treated as a worthwhile person. Provides sense of control over self in circumstances where loss of control is a significant factor.

Reorient frequently. (Refer to ND: Sensory/Perceptual alteration [specify].)

Client may experience periods of confusion, resulting in increased anxiety.

### Collaborative

Administer medications as indicated; e.g.:
    benzodiazepines: chlordiazepoxide (Librium), diazepam (Valium);

Minor tranquilizers are given during acute withdrawal to help client relax, be less hyperactive, and feel more in control.

    barbiturates: phenobarbital, or possibly secobarbital (Seconal), pentobarbital (Nembutal).

These drugs suppress alcohol withdrawal but need to be used with caution as they are respiratory depressants and REM sleep cycle inhibitors.

Arrange "Intervention" (confrontation) in controlled group setting.

Process of "Intervention," wherein family members, supported by staff, provide information about how the client's drinking and behavior have affected each one of them, helps the client to acknowledge that drinking is a problem and has resulted in current situational crisis.

Discuss need for ongoing treatment program.

Client is more likely to contract for treatment while still hurting and experiencing fear and anxiety from most recent episode of intoxication. Motivation decreases as well-being increases and person again feels able to control the problem. Direct contact with available treatment resources provides realistic picture of help. Decreases time for client to think about it/change mind or restructure and strengthen denial systems.

# STIMULANT- (AMPHETAMINES, CAFFEINE, COCAINE AND NICOTINE) AND INHALANT-RELATED DISORDERS

## DMS IV

### AMPHETAMINE-INDUCED DISORDERS
292.89 Amphetamine Intoxication
292.0   Amphetamine Withdrawal
292.11 Psychotic Disorders with Delusions
292.12 Psychotic Disorders with Hallucinations

### CAFFEINE-INDUCED DISORDERS
305.90 Caffeine Intoxication
292.89 Caffeine-Induced Anxiety Disorder
292.89 Caffeine-Induced Sleep Disorder

### COCAINE-INDUCED DISORDERS
292.89 Cocaine Intoxication
292.0   Cocaine Withdrawal
292.81 Intoxication Delirium

### INHALANT-INDUCED DISORDERS
292.89 Inhalant Intoxication
292.81 Inhalant Intoxication Delirium
292.84 Inhalant-Induced Mood Disorder
292.89 Inhalant-Induced Anxiety Disorder

### NICOTINE-INDUCED DISORDER
292.0   Nicotine Withdrawal
(For additional listings, consult DSM IV.)

## DSM III-R

### AMPHETAMINE OR SIMILARLY ACTING SYMPATHOMIMETIC
305.70 Amphetamine or Similarly Acting Sympathomimetic Abuse/Intoxication
305.60 Cocaine Abuse/Intoxication
305.90 Caffeine Intoxication

Stimulants are natural and manufactured drugs that speed up the nervous system. They can be swallowed, injected, inhaled, or smoked. These substances are identified by the behavioral stimulation and psychomotor agitation that they induce. They differ widely in their molecular structures and in their mechanisms of action. The most prevalent and widely used stimulants are caffeine and nicotine. Caffeine is readily available as a common ingredient in coffee, tea, colas, and chocolate. Nicotine is a primary substance in tobacco products. These are generally accepted as a part of our culture and are not usually seen in overdose situations. Other more potent stimulants (e.g., cocaine, amphetamines, and non-amphetamine stimulants) are regulated by the Controlled Substance Act. They are available for therapeutic purposes by prescription only but are also widely available on the illicit drug market. The potential for overdose and even death is high.

Inhalant substances include gasoline, glue, paint, paint thinners, spray paints, and cleaning compounds. Although this group is not technically classified as stimulants, the intoxicating effects and therapeutic interventions are similar and therefore included here.

This plan of care is to be used in conjunction with CP: Substance Dependence/Abuse Rehabilitation.

## ETIOLOGIC THEORIES

### Psychodynamics

Individuals who abuse substances fail to complete tasks of separation-individuation, resulting in underdeveloped egos. The person retains a highly dependent nature, with char- 165 acteristics of poor impulse control, low frustration tolerance, and low self-esteem, low social conformity, neuroticism, and introversion. The superego is weak, resulting in absence of guilt feelings for behavior. Underlying psychiatric status must be assessed, as these individuals may use stimulants for varying self-medication reasons (dual diagnosis).

### Biologic

An apparent genetic link is involved in the development of substance use disorders. However, the statistics are currently inconclusive regarding abuse of stimulant drugs.

### Family Dynamics

Predisposition to substance use disorders occurs in a dysfunctional family system. There is often one parent who is absent or who is an overpowering tyrant and/or one who is weak and ineffectual. Substance abuse may be evident as the primary method of relieving stress. The child has negative role models and learns to respond to stressful situations in like manner.

## CLIENT ASSESSMENT DATABASE

May present with intoxication or in various stages of withdrawal, affecting data gathered. Data are dependent on stage of withdrawal, concurrent use of alcohol/other drugs, or contaminants in drug "cut."

### Activity/Rest

Insomnia; hypersomnia; nightmares.
Anxiety.
Hyperactivity, increased alertness, or falling asleep during activities; lethargy (inhalants).
Inability to tolerate or to correct chronic fatigue (depression and/or loneliness may be a factor).
General muscle weakness, incoordination, unsteady gait (inhalants).

### Circulation

Elevated or lowered BP, tachycardia, cardiac dysrhythmias.
Diaphoresis.

### Ego Integrity

Underdeveloped ego; highly dependent nature, with characteristics of poor impulse control, low frustration tolerance, and low self-esteem; weak superego; reckless/rebellious, craving for excitement.
May be seen or view self as susceptible to influence by others, having an inability to say "no"; need to feel elated, sociable, happy with self; desire to prove self-worth, improve self-esteem.
Absence of guilt feelings for behavior; compulsion regarding stimulant use, or denial of powerlessness over the stimulant (use of drug for celebration or crisis, believing drug can be used in regulated quantities, often resulting in binge use).
May think of recovery process as notion of willpower, subject to impulse control.
Feelings of helplessness, hopelessness, powerlessness.
Emotional status: Anxious, evasive, irritable, may be angry/hostile, belligerent.

### Food/Fluid

Nausea/vomiting, anorexia; increased appetite (withdrawal).
Weight loss; thin, cachectic appearance.
Compulsiveness with food (especially sugars).

## Neurosensory

Dizziness.

Hypersensitive to sound, light, touch.

Numbness in hands and feet; twitching, jerking in face, neck, arms, hands; dyskinesias; dystonias.

Psychomotor retardation, depressed reflexes, unsteady gait (inhalants).

Stereotyped compulsive motor behavior, e.g., sorting, taking things apart and putting them back together, moving mouth from side to side in a stereotypic grimacing pattern.

Delirium with tactile and olfactory hallucinations, as well as hallucinations of insects or vermin crawling in/under the skin (formication); labile affect, violent or aggressive behavior, symptoms of a paranoid delusional disorder (amphetamine or similarly acting substances).

Pupillary dilation; blurred vision or diplopia, nystagmus (inhalants).

Apathy, stupor, coma, or euphoria (inhalants).

Anxiety; impaired judgment and perception.

Aggressiveness, hostility, violence, quick response to anger; psychomotor agitation/hyperactivity.

Emotional/psychologic symptoms, e.g., elation, grandiosity, loquacity, hypervigilance.

Ideas of reference.

Fixed delusional system of a persecutory nature, lasting weeks to 1 year or more.

Psychosis can occur with a 1-time high dose of amphetamine (especially with IV administration) or with long-term use at moderate or high dose.

## Pain/Discomfort

Bone pain, chest pain.

## Respiration

Tachypnea, coughing.

Nasal rhinitis (chronic cocaine use).

Chronic/recurrent bronchiolitis; pneumonia.

Pulmonary hemorrhage.

## Safety

History of accidents, involvement with legal system.

Exposure to STDs, including HIV.

Elevated temperature.

Fever/chills, diaphoresis.

Nasal damage (if drug is snorted).

Evidence of trauma, e.g., bruises, lacerations, burns.

Acute allergic/anaphylactic reaction may have occurred in response to contaminants in drug cut.

Assaultive behavior (inhalants).

## Sexuality

Male use of stimulants 2:1 over female.

Primary use is in the age range of 21–44.

Diminished/enhanced sexual desire; disinhibition regarding sexual behavior (promiscuity/prostitution).

Increased likelihood of pregnancy/abortion.

## Social Interactions

Impairment in relationship, social or occupational functioning.

Encounters with the legal system; expulsion from school.

Dysfunctional family system (family of origin).

## Teaching/Learning

Learning difficulties, e.g., attention-deficit hyperactivity disorder.

Family history of substance abuse (especially alcohol).

Concurrent use of alcohol/other drugs (compounds symptoms/reactions).

Pattern of habitual use of the particular drug or pathologic abuse, with inability to reduce or to stop use, occurring for at least 1 month.

Intoxication throughout the day, sometimes with daily involvement.

Previous hospitalizations or having been in residential treatment program for substance use/dual diagnosis.

During period of abstinence, may report drug hunger, display delayed reemergence of withdrawal symptoms (reemergence may occur at 3 months, between 9 and 12 months, and perhaps as late as 18 months after abstinence).

Health beliefs about use of drugs, e.g., "diet pills are OK to use to lose weight."

History of attendance at recovery groups, e.g., Narcotics/Alcoholics Anonymous or other drug-specific recovery groups.

## DIAGNOSTIC STUDIES

**Blood and Urine Screens:** Determines presence/type of drug(s).

**Tests for Hepatitis and HIV:** May be routine in known IV drug users or when client has identified risk factors.

**Addiction Severity Index (ASI):** Produces a "problem severity profile," which indicates areas of treatment needs.

## NURSING PRIORITIES

1. Maintain physiologic stability.
2. Promote safety and security.
3. Prevent complications.
4. Support client's acceptance of reality of situation.
5. Promote family involvement in "Intervention"/treatment process.

## DISCHARGE GOALS

1. Homeostasis maintained.
2. Complications prevented/resolved.
3. Client is dealing with situation realistically/planning for the future.
4. Abstinence from drug(s) maintained on a day-to-day basis.
5. Attending rehabilitation program/therapy group.

| NURSING DIAGNOSIS: | CARDIAC OUTPUT, DECREASED, high risk for |
|---|---|
| Risk Factors May Include: | Drug (e.g., cocaine) effect on myocardium (dependent on drug purity/quantity used). |
| | Preexisting myocardiopathy (with or without previous prolonged drug abuse). |
| | Alterations in electric rate/rhythm/conduction. |
| Possibly Evidenced By: | [Not applicable; presence of signs/symptoms establishes an **actual** diagnosis.] |

| Desired Outcomes/Evaluation Criteria—Client Will: | Report absence of chest pain. |
|---|---|
| | Demonstrate adequate cardiac output free of signs of dysrhythmias, shock. |

| ACTIONS/INTERVENTIONS | RATIONALE |
|---|---|
| **Independent** | |
| Monitor BP. | BP fluctuations can be extreme, with both hypertension and hypotension affecting cardiac output. |
| Monitor cardiac rate and rhythm. Document dysrhythmias. | Ventricular dysrhythmias/cardiac arrest may occur at any time, especially with toxic levels of certain drugs, e.g., cocaine, crack, ice, and amphetamine cogeners. |
| Investigate reports of chest pain, indigestion/heartburn. | Incidence of myocardial infarction increased in cocaine users. |
| Have emergency equipment/medications available. | Prompt treatment of dysrhythmias may prevent cardiac arrest. |
| **Collaborative** | |
| Administer supplemental oxygen as needed. | Tachycardia and other cardiac dysrhythmias may be improved/decreased with increased oxygen delivery to tissues. |
| Administer emergency medications as indicated. | Abort life-threatening dysrhythmia/maintain cardiac function. |
| Transfer to medical setting as appropriate. | Will require closer observation and more aggressive interventions. |

| NURSING DIAGNOSIS: | VIOLENCE, HIGH RISK FOR, DIRECTED AT SELF/OTHERS |
|---|---|
| **Risk Factors May Include:** | Toxic reaction to drug, withdrawal from drug. |
| | Panic state, profound depression/suicidal behavior. |
| | Organic brain syndrome. |
| **Possible Indicators:** | Overt and aggressive acts. |
| | Increased motor activity. |
| | Possession of destructive means. |
| | Suspicion of others, paranoid ideation, delusions and hallucinations. |
| | Expressed intent directly/indirectly. |
| **Desired Outcomes/Evaluation Criteria—Client Will:** | Acknowledge fearfulness and realities of situation. |

169

Verbalize understanding of behavior and precipitating factors.

Demonstrate self-control as evidenced by use of problem-solving skills in usually precipitating situations.

| ACTIONS/INTERVENTIONS | RATIONALE |
|---|---|

### Independent

| | |
|---|---|
| Obtain information specific to pattern of drug use over past month, what drugs have been used together, in addition to immunization history, allergies, medications used for other purposes. | Initial factual history can reveal information essential to treatment needs. Where person obtained drug could assist in investigating possible "cut" with other drugs. |
| Decrease stimuli; provide quiet in own room or place in stimulus-reduction room with supervision. | Reduces reactivity, enhances calm feelings. Observation enhances client safety, allowing for timely intervention. |
| Remove potentially harmful objects from environment. | Reduces opportunity for client to carry out suicidal ideas. Client may be suicidal when/if rebound CNS depression occurs secondary to stimulant withdrawal. |
| Explain consistent rules of unit, e.g., no violence, no threats. | Secure environment enhances sense of safety, which can decrease perceived threat. Enhances opportunity for client to learn ways to cope with aggressive feelings before reacting. |
| Maintain high staff profile in situations where potential violence can occur. | May prevent onset of violence, allows quick response if violence does occur. |
| Provide opportunities for verbal expression of aggressive feelings in acceptable ways. | Encouragement of new avenue of expression helps client learn new coping skills. |
| Assist client in identifying what provokes anger. | Awareness of reaction is the first step in learning change. |
| Provide outlets for expression that involve physical activity, e.g., stationary bicycle, racquetball/basketball/volleyball. | Physical activity in protected environment can lessen aggressive drive. |
| Discuss consequences of aggressive behavior. | Learning choices assists client to gain control of situation and self. |
| Be alert to violence potential, e.g., increased pacing, verbalization of delusional persecutory content, hypervigilance regarding specific persons in the milieu, gesturing aggressively, threatening others verbally or physically. | Recognizing potential and assisting client to gain control can be more effective prior to violent outbreak. |
| Isolate immediately if client becomes violent, using adequate staff trained in assaultive management to separate client from other individuals. Maintain calm, nonpunitive attitude. | Client will feel safer if others take control until internal locus of control can be regained. An attitude of acceptance is important while refusing to tolerate the violent behavior. Note: Use of seclusion and restraints may exacerbate hyperactivity. |
| Negotiate conditions for coming out of isolation/"quiet time" when the client is calm, based on agreement of social appropriateness. | Clear expectations aid client in feeling secure about own control. |

| ACTIONS/INTERVENTIONS | RATIONALE |
|---|---|
| **Independent** | |
| Build trust: follow through on commitments/ agreements, maintain consistent staff and frequent brief contact with client. | Trust is essential to working with all clients. Brief contacts can prevent overstimulation. |
| **Collaborative** | |
| Administer medications as indicated, e.g.: chlorpromazine (Thorazine), haloperidol (Haldol); | Short-term use of major tranquilizers during acute intoxication/psychosis assists client in gaining self-control; promotes sedation/rest when agitated, assaultive, overstimulated. Note: Thorazine may cause postural hypotension, and Haldol may provoke acute extrapyramidal reaction, requiring additional evaluation/medication. |
| diazepam (Valium), chlordiazepoxide (Librium). | Occasionally useful for treatment of acute cocaine intoxication. Either drug is useful for preventing delirium tremens when substance use is combined with alcohol. |

| NURSING DIAGNOSIS: | SENSORY/PERCEPTUAL ALTERATIONS (SPECIFY) |
|---|---|
| **May Be Related To:** | Chemical alteration: exogenous (CNS stimulants or depressants, mind-altering drugs). |
| | Altered sensory reception, transmission and/or integration: altered status of sense organs. |
| **Possibly Evidenced By:** | Bizarre thinking, anxiety/panic. |
| | Preoccupation with/appears to be responding to internal stimuli from hallucinatory experiences, e.g., assumes "listening pose," laughs and talks to self, stops in midsentence and listens, "picks" at self and clothing, tries to "get away from bugs." |
| | Changes in sensory acuity, decreased pain perception. |
| **Desired Outcomes/Evaluation Criteria— Client Will:** | Distinguish reality from altered perceptions. |
| | State awareness that hallucinations may result from stimulant use. |

| ACTIONS/INTERVENTIONS | RATIONALE |
|---|---|
| **Independent** | |
| Notice client's preoccupation, responses, gesturing, social skill. | Helps assess whether or not client is hallucinating without overstimulating verbally. |

171

| ACTIONS/INTERVENTIONS | RATIONALE |
|---|---|

### Independent

| | |
|---|---|
| Assist client in checking perceptions verbally, provide reality information. | Can calm the client and provide reassurance of safety and that formication (illusion of insects crawling on the body) or other misperceptions are not occurring. |
| Acknowledge client's emotional state; reassure regarding safety. | Empathetic response can diminish intensity of fear. |
| Explore ways of calming client. Encourage use of relaxation techniques. | May enhance clarity of perception. Relaxation can promote positive outlook, distracting from negativity of perceptions. |
| Be aware that altered sensation and perception may cause injury, e.g., be alert for client burning self with cigarette, excessive scratching at skin to rid self of bugs or drug (which may feel as though it is in the skin), accidentally harming self through poor judgment or misperceptions. (Refer to ND: Violence, high risk for, directed at self/others) | Amphetamine use causes impaired judgment, increasing risk of injury/self-harm. Overdose of many stimulants causes frightening hallucinations, often of large insects crawling on skin. |
| Inform client (if calm enough) of temporary nature of hallucinations that have resulted from stimulant use. | Learning cause, effect, and possible temporary nature of misperceptions may reduce fear, anxiety, and negativity. May inject hope and positive attitude. |

| | |
|---|---|
| **NURSING DIAGNOSIS:** | **FEAR/ANXIETY [specify level]** |
| **May Be Related To:** | Paranoid delusions associated with stimulant use. |
| **Possibly Evidenced By:** | Feelings/beliefs that others are conspiring against or are about to attack/kill client. |
| **Desired Outcomes/Evaluation Criteria— Client Will:** | Recognize frightening feelings before preoccupying self with fears or becoming violent. |
| | Discuss reality base of persecutory fears with staff. |
| | Report fear/anxiety reduced to manageable level. |
| | Demonstrate appropriate range of feelings and appear relaxed. |

| ACTIONS/INTERVENTIONS | RATIONALE |
|---|---|

### Independent

| | |
|---|---|
| Establish consistent staff. Build trust by being reliable, honest, genuine, prompt. | Trust and rapport are necessary for overcoming fear. |
| Acknowledge awareness of client's feelings, e.g., fear, terror, overwhelmed, panic, anxiety, confusion. | Empathy can assist client to tolerate/deal with own feelings. |

| ACTIONS/INTERVENTIONS | RATIONALE |
|---|---|
| **Independent** | |
| Be concrete, clear in communication. Assess client's readiness for humor and/or touch. | Fear negatively influences one's ability to laugh. Fear is serious to the perceiver and must be respected. Touch can be misinterpreted/increase anxiety. |
| Encourage verbalization of fears/anxieties. | Ventilating feelings to trusted staff can lessen intensity of fearfulness. Provides opportunity to clarify misunderstandings and comforts client. |
| Assist client in reality-checking fears. Use gentle confrontation. | Client can reduce fear if he or she understands difference between reality and delusions. Should be used cautiously, as reality-checking a delusional system puts trust at risk. |

| NURSING DIAGNOSIS: | NUTRITION, ALTERED, LESS THAN BODY REQUIREMENTS |
|---|---|
| **May Be Related To:** | Anorexia (stimulant use). |
| | Insufficient/inappropriate use of financial resources. |
| **Possibly Evidenced By:** | Reported/observed inadequate intake. |
| | Lack of interest in food; weight loss. |
| | Poor muscle tone. |
| | Signs/laboratory evidence of vitamin deficiencies. |
| **Desired Outcomes/Evaluation Criteria— Client Will:** | Demonstrate progressive weight gain toward goal. |
| | Verbalize understanding of causative factors and individual needs. |
| | Identify appropriate dietary choices, lifestyle changes to regain/maintain desired weight. |

| ACTIONS/INTERVENTIONS | RATIONALE |
|---|---|
| **Independent** | |
| Ascertain intake pattern over past several weeks. | Stimulants cause decreased appetite and impaired judgment regarding body needs. |
| Discuss needs/likes/dislikes about food choices. | Will be more likely to maintain desired intake if individual preferences are considered. |
| Anticipate hyperphagia and weigh every other day. | Overeating may be a consequence of stimulant withdrawal and may result in sudden/inappropriate weight gain. |
| Provide meals in a relaxed, nonstimulating environment. | Stimulus reduction aids relaxation and ability to focus on eating. |

| ACTIONS/INTERVENTIONS | RATIONALE |
|---|---|

### Independent

Encourage frequent nutritional snacks, small nutritious meals.

Small amounts of food frequently can prevent/reduce GI distress.

### Collaborative

Obtain/review routine lab work, e.g., CBC, UA; protein, vitamin levels.

Assessment of nutritional state is necessary to treat preexisting deficiencies and rule out anemia, dehydration, or ketosis.

Consult with dietitian.

Useful in establishing individual nutritional needs/dietary program.

Administer multivitamins as indicated.

Supplementation enhances correction of deficiencies.

| NURSING DIAGNOSIS: | INFECTION, HIGH RISK FOR |
|---|---|
| Risk Factors May Include: | IV drug-use techniques; impurities of injected drugs. |
| | Localized trauma; nasal septum damage (snorting cocaine). |
| | Malnutrition; altered immune state. |
| Possibly Evidenced By: | [Not applicable; presence of signs and symptoms establishes an **actual** diagnosis.] |
| Desired Outcomes/Evaluation Criteria— Client Will: | Verbalize understanding of individual risk factors. |
| | Identify interventions to prevent/reduce risk factors. |
| | Demonstrate lifestyle changes to promote safe environment. |
| | Achieve timely healing of infectious process if present/develops and is afebrile. |

| ACTIONS/INTERVENTIONS | RATIONALE |
|---|---|

### Independent

Obtain information specific to pattern of drug use over past month, immunization history, allergies, medications used for other purposes.

Helps identify risk factors, can reveal information essential to need for further evaluation/specific physical treatment.

Assess skin integrity and character. Assist as needed with body and oral hygiene; obtain clean clothes, properly fitting shoes.

Maintaining skin integrity requires cleanliness. Sores may need care to prevent infection.

174 Use blood/body fluid precautions as appropriate.

Protects caregivers from possible contamination by infectious disease viruses, e.g., hepatitis/HIV.

| ACTIONS/INTERVENTIONS | RATIONALE |
|---|---|
| **Independent** | |
| Monitor vital signs. Assess level of consciousness. | Abnormal signs, including fever, can indicate presence of infection. Cerebral complications, e.g., meningitis, brain abscess, may occur, affecting mentation. Note: Fever is also a symptom of toxic CNS effect. |
| Review physical assessment on a regular basis. | Can reveal daily changes and problematic areas. Provides recognition of pathology, identifies areas for providing information for health promotion and problem prevention. |
| Investigate recurrent cough; note characteristics of sputum. Auscultate breath sounds. | These clients are at increased risk for development of pulmonary infections. |
| Observe for nasal stuffiness, pain, bleeding, abnormal mucus production. | Cocaine snorting can cause erosion of the nasal septum, requiring additional therapy/interventions. |
| Investigate reports of acute/chronic bone pain, tenderness, guarding with movement, regional muscle spasm. | Occasionally, osteomyelitis may develop because of hematogenous spread of bacteria, most often affecting lumbar vertebrae. |
| Ascertain health status of family members/SO(s) currently in contact with client. | May have exposed client to diseases such as colds, tuberculosis, hepatitis, HIV, which could be problematic for client. |
| **Collaborative** | |
| Review laboratory studies, e.g., UA, CBC, Bio-chem screen, RPR, ESR, ELISA/Western Blot test. | May identify complications of IV cocaine and amphetamine use such as hepatitis, nephritis, tetanus, vasculitis, septicemia, subacute bacterial endocarditis, embolic phenomena, malaria. Toxic allergic reactions may result from other substances in the cut, and immunologic abnormalities may occur because of repreated antigenic stimulation. Note: IV needle drug users are at high risk for contamination with HIV and hepatitis viruses. |

| | |
|---|---|
| **NURSING DIAGNOSIS:** | **SLEEP PATTERN DISTURBANCE** |
| **May Be Related To:** | CNS sensory alterations: External factor (stimulant use), internal factor (psychologic stress). |
| **Possibly Evidenced By:** | Altered sleep cycle; initial signs of insomnia and then hypersomnia. |
| | Constant alertness; racing thoughts that prevent rest. |
| | Denial of need to sleep or report of inability to stay awake. |
| **Desired Outcomes/Evaluation Criteria— Client Will:** | Sleep 6–8 hours at night. |
| | Rest minimally, appropriately, during the day. |
| | Verbalize feeling rested when awakens. |

175

| ACTIONS/INTERVENTIONS | RATIONALE |
| --- | --- |
| **Independent** | |
| Establish sleep cycle in which client sleeps at night, is awake during day with only brief rest periods as needed. | Adequate rest and sleep can improve emotional state; restoration of regular pattern is a priority in a sleep-deprived stimulant user. |
| Decrease stimuli and enhance relaxation prior to bedtime; encourage use of presleep routines, e.g., hot bath, warm milk, stretching. | Client may need calming in order to attempt rest. |
| Provide opportunities for fresh air, mild exercise, noncaffeinated beverages, quiet environment as client can tolerate. | Promotes drowsiness/desire for sleep. |

# DEPRESSANT- (BENZODIAZEPINES, BARBITURATES, OPIOIDS) RELATED DISORDERS

## DSM IV
### SEDATIVE, HYPNOTIC, OR ANXIOLYTIC INDUCED DISORDERS
292.89 Sedative, Hypnotic, or Anxiolytic Intoxication
292.0   Sedative, Hypnotic, or Anxiolytic Withdrawal
292.81 Withdrawal Delirium
292.84 Induced Mood Disorder
### OPIOID-RELATED DISORDERS
292.89 Opioid Intoxication
292.81 Intoxication Delirium
292.0   Opioid Withdrawal
(For further listings, consult DSM IV.)

## DSM III-R
305.40 Sedative, Hypnotic, or Anxiolytic Intoxication
292.00 Uncomplicated Sedative, Hypnotic, or Anxiolytic Withdrawal/Delirium
305.50 Opioid Intoxication
292.00 Opioid Withdrawal

CNS depressants are drugs that slow down the central nervous system. They are usually divided into four types: barbiturates, tranquilizers, sedative-hypnotics, and narcotics (e.g., morphine, heroin).

CNS depressants prescribed for symptoms of anxiety, depression, and sleep disturbances are among the most widely used and abused drugs. These drugs are very likely to be abused when the underlying conditions remain untreated. Sometimes these drugs are used in conjunction with stimulants, with the user developing a pattern of taking a stimulant to be "up," then needing the depressant drug to "come down."

Several principles apply to all CNS depressants: (1) The effects are interactive and cumulative with one another and with the behavioral state of the user, (2) there is no specific antagonist that will block the action of these drugs, (3) low doses produce an initial excitatory response, (4) they are capable of producing physiologic and psychologic dependency, and (5) cross-tolerance and cross-dependence may exist between various CNS depressants. While the margin of safety of these drugs is great, they have a characteristic syndrome of withdrawal that can be very severe.

This plan of care is to be used in conjunction with CP: Substance Dependence/Abuse Rehabilitation.

## ETIOLOGIC THEORIES

### Psychodynamics

Individuals who abuse substances fail to complete tasks of separation-individuation, resulting in underdeveloped egos. The person has a highly dependent nature, with characteristics of poor impulse control, low frustration tolerance, and low self-esteem. The superego is weak, resulting in absence of guilt feelings. Underlying psychiatric status must be assessed, as these individuals may use stimulants for varying self-medication reasons.

### Biologic

A genetic link is thought to be involved in the development of substance use disorders. Although statistics are currently inconclusive, hereditary factors are generally accepted to be a factor in the abuse of substances.

Psychostructural factors (e.g., personality) are seen as significant. The defect is believed **177** to precede the addiction, with the ego structure breaking down and the substance being used as a maladaptive coping mechanism. Characteristics that have been identified include impulsivity, negative self-concept, weak ego, low social conformity, neuroticism, and introversion.

### Family Dynamics

There is an apparent predisposition to substance abuse disorders in the dysfunctional family system. Factors such as the absence of a parent or one who is an overpowering tyrant or weak and ineffectual and the use of substances as the primary method of relieving stress appear to contribute to this dysfunction. These role models have a negative influence, and the child learns to handle stress in like manner. However, parents may be average, normal individuals with children who succumb to overwhelming peer pressure and become involved with drugs. Cultural factors such as acceptance of the use of alcohol and other drugs may also influence the individual's choice.

## CLIENT ASSESSMENT DATABASE

### Activity/Rest

General malaise.
Interference with sleep pattern, insomnia (withdrawal).
Lethargy, drowsiness, somnolence.
Yawning.

### Circulation

**Pulse:** Tachycardia suggests withdrawal syndrome; atrial fibrillation, ventricular dysrhythmias.
Hypotension.

### Ego Integrity

Uses substance for stress management.
Feelings of helplessness, hopelessness, powerlessness.
Underdeveloped ego; highly dependent nature, with characteristics of poor impulse control, low frustration tolerance, and low self-esteem.
Weak superego, with absence of guilt feelings.
Psychostructural factors (e.g., personality) are seen as significant with substance use/abuse (maladaptive coping mechanisms).

### Elimination

Diarrhea, occasionally constipation.

### Food/Fluid

Nausea/vomiting.

### Neurosensory

Twitching.
Temporary psychosis with acute onset of auditory hallucinations and paranoid delusions (unexplained neuropsychiatric presentation may be indicative of drug use).
**Mental Status:** Confusion, concentration and memory problems, impaired judgment with some affective change; alterations in consciousness may exist, from extreme agitation to coma; speech may be slurred.
**Behavior:** Mood swings, lack of motivation, aggression, combativeness (related to general

disinhibiting effect of the drug, loss of impulse control), dysphoric mood (withdrawal).
Psychomotor activity may be increased.
Hypersensitivity, e.g., anxiety, tremors, hypotension, irritability, restlessness, and seizure activity may be noted.
**Pupils:** Small/pinpoint constriction (opiates), dilated (barbiturates).
**Gait:** Unsteady/staggering, loss of coordination, positive Romberg sign.

### Pain/Discomfort

Muscle aches.

### Respiration

Continuous rhinorrhea, excessive lacrimation, sneezing.
Respiratory depression (noted in overdose).
Increased rate (withdrawal syndrome).

### Safety

Hot/cold flashes, diaphoresis.
Thermoregulation instability with hyperpyrexia, hypothermia.
**Skin:** Piloerection ("gooseflesh"); puncture wounds on arms, hands, legs, under tongue, indicating IV drug use.

### Social Interactions

Dysfunctional family of origin system.
History from family member/significant other(s) may reveal dysfunctional patterns of interaction.

### Teaching/Learning

Preexisting physical/psychologic conditions.
May present with mild intoxication, overdose, or in various stages of withdrawal, affecting data gathered.
Family history of substance use/abuse.
History of chronic condition/disease process.
Concurrent use of other drugs, including alcohol.

## DIAGNOSTIC STUDIES

**Drug Screen:** Identifies drug(s) being used.
**STD Screening:** To determine presence of HIV, hepatitis B, etc.
**Addiction Severity Index (ASI):** Produces a problem severity profile, which indicates areas of treatment needs.

## NURSING PRIORITIES

1. Achieve physiologic stability.
2. Protect client from injury.
3. Provide appropriate referral and follow-up.

## DISCHARGE GOALS

1. Homeostasis achieved.
2. Complications prevented/resolved.
3. Maintains abstinence from drug(s) on a day-to-day basis.
4. Attends rehabilitation program, group therapy, e.g., Narcotics Anonymous.

| NURSING DIAGNOSIS: | TRAUMA/SUFFOCATION/POISONING, HIGH RISK FOR |
| --- | --- |
| Risk Factors May Include: | CNS depression (effect of overdose). |
| | CNS agitation (effect of abrupt withdrawal). |
| | Hypersensitivity to the drug(s). |
| | Psychologic stress (narrowed perceptual fields seen with anxiety). |
| Possibly Evidenced By: | [Not applicable; presence of signs and symptoms establishes an **actual** diagnosis.] |
| Desired Outcomes/Evaluation Criteria— Client Will: | Verbalize understanding of risks of taking drugs. |
| | Refrain from acting on hallucinations/impaired judgment. |
| | Complete withdrawal without injury to self/ development of complications. |

| ACTIONS/INTERVENTIONS | RATIONALE |
| --- | --- |

### Independent

| ACTIONS/INTERVENTIONS | RATIONALE |
| --- | --- |
| Determine degree of impairment by talking to client/SO, noting when person was last seen well; also note sleep patterns, history/duration of health problems, and prescriptions used. | Information provides an approximate time frame for impairment, with sleep disruption often the first observable sign of problem. Ongoing health problems (e.g., chronic pain conditions) potentiate substance use. Prescription information provides clues to identify drug(s) and amount taken. |
| Identify drug(s) taken, when taken, and route used, if possible. | Helpful to identify interventions for specific drug. Determining drug(s) taken may be difficult outside of blood/urine testing as the client may not feel free to tell because of embarrassment or for legal reasons or may not know what has been ingested. |
| Assess level of consciousness, e.g., agitated, stuporous, lethargic, confused. Note pinpoint pupils. | May be indicator of degree of intoxication and level of intervention required. Constricted pupils are a classic sign of opioid (heroin) use. |
| Evaluate for evidence of head trauma. | Important to note for differential diagnosis to prevent incorrect treatment/interventions. |
| Determine when food was last eaten. Note reports of nausea. | Presence of food in stomach may slow absorption of drug(s) into the bloodstream; however, if level of consciousness is depressed, the risk of vomiting and aspiration is increased. |
| Monitor temperature as indicated. Observe for signs of dehydration. | Hypothermia may be seen in intoxication, while hyperpyrexia may occur with withdrawal or indicate infectious process. Note: Dehydration often accompanies hyperpyrexia, requiring additional intervention/fluid replacement. |
| Monitor BP, pulse, respirations. | Changes depend on drug taken, e.g., diazepam (Valium) may be evidenced by hypotension, tachycardia. |

| ACTIONS/INTERVENTIONS | RATIONALE |
|---|---|

### Independent

Provide quiet, lighted room, e.g., an isolation room with simple furniture.

Reduces stimuli, internal or external, which may lead to injury as the client responds.

Observe client at all times; use staff or family member as available.

Client with varying levels of consciousness should not be left alone because of the danger of accidental injury.

Reorient to surroundings and circumstances as needed.

Maintaining contact provides reassurance, reduces anxiety when sensorium clears.

Note presence of tremors.

Involuntary movements of one or more parts of the body may result from abrupt removal of drug.

Provide seizure precautions, e.g., padded side rails, bed in low position, airway adjunct/suction at bedside.

Precautions can prevent injury if convulsions occur during withdrawal.

Note changes in behavior indicative of psychosis, e.g., distorted reality, altered mood, impaired language and memory.

Drug intoxication can precipitate an alteration in perceptions/psychotic behavior.

Assess emotional state, noting psychiatric history and suicide gestures/attempts. Note use/abuse of other substances.

Patterns of drug use will indicate likelihood of intentional or accidental overdose. Substance abuse/suicidal attempts may be symptom of, or response to, underlying psychiatric illness or to hallucinations caused by sensitivity to drug.

Determine history/characteristics of hallucinations.

May be auditory, visual, or tactile and be very frightening. May also trigger suicidal/homicidal behavior.

Institute suicide precautions, as indicated.

May need environmental restraints to protect client until own coping abilities improve and internal locus of control is attained/regained.

### Collaborative

Administer medication per current treatment/protocol, e.g.:

    phenobarbital;

Prolonged effect provides smoother sedation with "high" of more rapidly acting drugs. Also has an anticonvulsant effect.

    methadone;

Replaces heroin or other narcotic analgesics in detoxification program, reducing/minimizing withdrawal symptoms.

    clonidine (Catapres);

Can suppress/reverse symptoms of opioid withdrawal and has lesser likelihood of abuse than methadone. Drug may be used instead of or in combination with methadone during detoxification. Note: May be contraindicated for some clients because of high degree of sedation and hypotension.

    buprenorphine (Buprenex).

Current research suggests low doses of this drug may block opioid withdrawal symptoms.

| ACTIONS/INTERVENTIONS | RATIONALE |
|---|---|

**Independent**

| | |
|---|---|
| Assist with barbiturate detoxification program. | Reintoxication should be done before drug withdrawal is attempted. This establishes an independent estimate of prior drug use and provides a baseline to begin the detox schedule. The reintoxication should begin as soon as there are signs of intoxication, e.g., nystagmus, slurred speech, ataxia on backward and forward tandem gait. |
| Involve in "Intervention" (confrontation) and/or therapy as indicated. | Client will need ongoing assistance to acknowledge and maintain drug-free existence. |
| Transfer to medical setting as indicated. | Severe CNS depression/deterioration of condition (physiologic instability) requires more aggressive intervention than that generally provided in psychiatric setting. |

| NURSING DIAGNOSIS: | BREATHING PATTERN, INEFFECTIVE/GAS EXCHANGE, IMPAIRED, high risk for |
|---|---|
| Risk Factors May Include: | Neuromuscular impairment. |
| | Decreased energy/fatigue. |
| | Inflammatory process. |
| | Decreased lung expansion. |
| Possibly Evidenced By: | [Not applicable; presence of signs/symptoms establishes an **actual** diagnosis.] |
| Desired Outcomes/Evaluation Criteria— Client Will: | Maintain normal/effective breathing pattern with absence of cyanosis/symptoms of respiratory distress. |

| ACTIONS/INTERVENTIONS | RATIONALE |
|---|---|

**Independent**

| | |
|---|---|
| Monitor respiratory rate/depth/rhythm and breath sounds. | Sedative/depressant effects on CNS may result in loss of airway patency and/or respiratory depression. Prompt treatment is necessary to prevent respiratory arrest. Note: Acute pulmonary edema is a common complication in heroin overdose/intoxication. |
| Have suction equipment/airway adjuncts available. | Sedative effects of drugs, increased salivation, vomiting potentiate risk of aspiration. Relaxation of oropharyngeal muscles and respiratory depression requires prompt intervention to prevent respiratory compromise. |

| ACTIONS/INTERVENTIONS | RATIONALE |
|---|---|
| **Collaborative** | |
| Review chest x-ray. | Common complications of depressant (opiate) abuse include pneumonia, aspiration pneumonitis, lung abscess, atelectasis, which will require specific treatment. |
| Monitor pulse oximetry, when indicated. | Chronic addiction may result in decreased vital capacity and pulmonary diffusion affecting gas exchange. Presence of septic pulmonary emboli or pulmonary fibrosis (from talc granulomatosis occurring in IV drug abuse) may further compromise respiratory function. |
| Provide supplemental oxygen. | May be necessary to improve oxygen intake in presence of respiratory depression. |
| Administer medications, as indicated, e.g., naloxone (Narcan), and transfer to medical setting. | Narcotic antagonist that may reverse effects of respiratory depression in opioid intoxication. Note: May trigger acute withdrawal syndrome, requiring more aggressive intervention. |

| NURSING DIAGNOSIS: | INFECTION, HIGH RISK FOR |
|---|---|
| **Risk Factors May Include:** | IV drug use techniques, impurities in injected drugs. |
| | Localized trauma. |
| | Malnutrition; altered immune state. |
| **Possibly Evidenced By:** | [Not applicable; presence of signs/symptoms establishes an **actual** diagnosis.] |
| **Desired Outcomes/Evaluation Criteria— Client Will:** | Verbalize understanding of and demonstrate lifestyle changes to reduce risk factor(s). |
| | Achieve timely healing of infectious process if present/develops; be afebrile. |

## ACTIONS/INTERVENTIONS

### Independent

Refer to CP: Stimulants, ND: Infection, high risk for, for interventions specific to this nursing diagnosis.

# HALLUCINOGEN-, PHENCYCLIDINE-, AND CANNABIS-RELATED DISORDERS

## DSM IV
### HALLUCINOGEN-RELATED DISORDERS
**Hallucinogen-Induced Disorders**
292.89 Hallucinogen Intoxication
292.89 Hallucinogen Persisting Perception Disorder (Flashbacks)
292.89 Hallucinogen-Induced Anxiety Disorder
292.84 Hallucinogen-Induced Mood Disorder
### PHENCYCLIDINE (OR PHENCYCLIDINE-LIKE) DISORDERS
**Phencyclidine-Induced Disorders**
292.89 Phencyclidine Intoxication
292.81 Intoxication Delirium
292.11 Induced Psychotic Disorder with Delusions
292.12 Induced Psychotic Disorder with Hallucinations
### CANNABIS-RELATED DISORDERS
**Cannabis-Induced Disorders**
292.89 Cannabis Intoxication
292.89 Cannabis-Induced Anxiety Disorder

## DSM III-R
### HALLUCINOGEN
(Includes substances structurally related to 5-hydroxytryptamine, e.g., lysergic acid diethylamide [LSD] and dimethyltryptamine [DMT] and substances related to catecholamine [e.g., mescaline])
305.30 Hallucinosis
292.11 Delusional Disorder
292.84 Mood Disorder
### PHENCYCLIDINE (PCP) OR SIMILARLY ACTING ARYLCYCLOHEXYLAMINE
292.90 Organic Mental Disorder
305.90 Intoxication
292.81 Delirium
292.11 Delusional Disorder
### CANNABIS
305.20 Intoxication
292.11 Delusional Disorder

Hallucinogenic substances are capable of distorting an individual's perception of reality, altering sensory perception, and inducing hallucinations. For this reason, they are referred to as "mind expanding." They are highly unpredictable in the effects they may induce each time they are used, and adverse reactions, including "flashbacks," can recur at any time, even without current use of the drug. Hallucinogens have been used as part of religious ceremonies and at social gatherings by Native Americans for more than 2000 years. Therapeutic uses for LSD have been proposed; however, more research is required. At this time, no real evidence speaks to the safety and efficacy of the drug in humans.

The three major groups of hallucinogens are (1) indolealkylamines (LSD, DMT), resembling serotonin; (2) phenylethylamines (mescaline, DOM ["STP"]), related to dopamine, norepinephrine, and amphetamines; and (3) "designer drugs" (MDMA ["ecstasy"], MDEA ["Eve"]) with some amphetamine-like sympathomimetic effects. Although PCP ("angel dust") has an entirely different chemical structure from the above hallucinogenic drugs, PCP use results in similar behaviors and therefore is included here.

Additionally, cannabis (marijuana, hashish, synthetic THC) also produces an altered state of awareness accompanied by feelings of relaxation and mild euphoria and is often used in conjunction with other substances.

This plan of care is to be used in conjunction with CP: Substance Dependence/Abuse Rehabilitation.

## ETIOLOGIC THEORIES

### Psychodynamics

Individuals who abuse substances fail to complete tasks of separation-individuation, resulting in underdeveloped egos. The person is thought to have a highly dependent nature, with characteristics of poor impulse control, low frustration tolerance, and low self-esteem. The superego is weak, and this results in absence of guilt feelings for their behavior.

Certain personality traits may play an important part in the development and maintenance of dependence. Characteristics that have been identified include impulsivity, negative self-concept, weak ego, low social conformity, neuroticism, and introversion. Substance abuse has also been associated with antisocial personality and depressive response styles.

### Biologic

A genetic link is thought to be involved in the development of substance use disorders. Although statistics are currently inconclusive, hereditary factors are generally accepted to be a factor in the abuse of substances. Research is currently being done into the role biochemical factors play in the problems of substance abuse.

### Family Dynamics

A predisposition to substance use disorders is found in the dysfunctional family system. There is often one parent who is absent or who is an overpowering tyrant, and/or one who is weak and ineffectual. Substance abuse may be evident as the primary method of relieving stress. The child has negative role models and learns to respond to stressful situations in like manner. However, parents may be average, normal individuals with children who succumb to overwhelming peer pressure and become involved with drugs.

In the family the effects of modeling, imitation, and identification on behavior can be observed from early childhood onward. Peer influence may exert a great deal of influence also.

Cultural factors may help to establish patterns of substance use by attitudes of acceptance of such use as a part of daily or recreational life.

## CLIENT ASSESSMENT DATABASE

Factors that can affect the kind of reaction (positive or negative) experienced by the hallucinogen user include individual circadian rhythms (fatigue), previous drug-taking experience, personality, mood, and expectations. One's educational level can also cause different perceptions.

### Activity/Rest

Insomnia, fatigue.
Disturbances of sleep/wakefulness.
Hyperactivity (LSD, mescaline, PCP).

### Circulation

**Blood Pressure:** Decreased diastolic (cannabis, high-dose PCP); hypertension, hypertensive crisis (low- to moderate-dose PCP).
Tachycardia/palpitations; possible dysrhythmias (high-dose PCP).

### Ego Integrity

Euphoria, anxiety, suspiciousness, paranoia (PCP psychosis).
Highly dependent nature, with characteristics of poor impulse control, low frustration toler-

ance, low self-esteem; depersonalization, weak superego, possibly resulting in absence of guilt feelings for behavior *or* self-reproach, excessive guilt, fearfulness.

Moods reflect depression or anxiety.

Preoccupation with the idea that brain is destroyed and/or will not return to a normal state.

### Food/Fluid

Increased appetite (cannabis).

Nausea/vomiting, increased salivation.

### Neurosensory

Blurred vision, altered depth perception.

Dizziness, headache (LSD).

Flashback (spontaneous transitory recurrence of a drug-induced expereince [LSD] in a drug-free state) often associated with fatigue, emotional stress, and other drug use (especially alcohol, marijuana).

"Bad trips" (self-limiting and confined to period of intoxication):
   1. **LSD:** 3 kinds: (1) bad body trip, e.g., my body is purple; (2) bad environment trip, e.g., visual distortions so real the person thinks he or she is going crazy; (3) bad mind trip, e.g., unexpected subconscious material bursts forth into consciousness, as in, "I'm responsible for my mother's death."
   2. **PCP:** Aggravates any underlying psychopathology.
   3. **Cannabis:** Rare; however, when occurs, panic attacks are usually seen.

Pupil constriction, vertical and horizontal nystagmus (PCP); pupillary dilation, catatonic staring (LSD, PCP, mescaline).

Muscle incoordination/tremors, spasms or increased muscle strength may be noted with PCP because of the anesthetic effect that deadens pain perception, deep-tendon reflexes increased (low- to moderate-dose PCP) or depressed (high-dose PCP), opisthotonos (body-arching spasm).

**Level of Consciousness:** Usually responsive; coma may be noted (especially if intracranial hemorrhage occurs with PCP); slurred speech, mutism.

**Mental Status:** Perceptual changes, e.g., sensation of slowed time, perceptions enhanced (colors richer, music more profound, smells and tastes heightened), synesthesia (merging of senses, colors are "heard" or sounds are "seen"), changes in body image, hallucinations (usually visual), and depersonalization.

Delirium with clouded state of consciousness (sensory misperception, disorientation, memory impairment, difficulty in sustaining attention, disordered stream of thought, psychomotor activity; delusions, illusions, hallucinations (rare with cannabis intoxication). May occur within 24 hours after use or following recovery days after PCP has been taken.

Delusions occurring in a normal state of consciousness; may persist beyond 24 hours after cessation of hallucinogen use. Persecutory delusions can follow cannabis use immediately or may occur during the course of cannabis intoxication.

**Mood:** Euphoria/dysphoria, anxiety, emotional lability, apathy, grandiosity.

**Behavioral Findings:** May include assaultiveness, bizarre behavior, impulsivity, unpredictability, belligerence, impaired judgment, paranoid ideation, panic attacks.

Convulsions (high-dose PCP).

### Pain/Discomfort

Decreased awareness of pain.

Sudden intense chest pain or persistent chest discomfort (if drug is smoked).

### Respiration

Decreased rate/depth of respiration (PCP, heavy cannabis use).

Rhonchi, gurgling sounds.

### Safety

Diaphoretic.
Conjunctival redness/infection (cannabis).
Assaultive behavior (PCP psychosis), risk to self (impaired judgment/acting on altered perceptions).

### Social Interactions

Sense of "happy sociability," friendliness (intoxication).
Dysfunctional family system; one parent who is absent or who is an overbearing tyrant and/or one who is weak and ineffectual.
Substance abuse as the primary coping method.
Overwhelming peer pressure leading to involvement with drugs.
Social or occupational functioning impairment (fights, loss of friends, absence from work, loss of job, or legal difficulties) may be seen with drug use/tolerance.

### Teaching/Learning

Concurrent use of other drugs including alcohol.
Family history of substance abuse.

## DIAGNOSTIC STUDIES

**Drug Screen/Urinalysis:** To identify drug(s) being used.
**Addictive Severity Index (ASI):** To assess substance abuse and determine treatment needs.

## NURSING PRIORITIES

1. Protect client/others from injury.
2. Promote physiologic/psychologic stability.
3. Support client/family in "Intervention" (confrontation) process for decision to stop using drugs.

## DISCHARGE GOALS

1. Homeostasis achieved.
2. Complications prevented/resolved.
3. Abstinence from drug(s) maintained on a day-to-day basis.
4. Participation in drug rehabilitation program.

| NURSING DIAGNOSIS: | VIOLENCE, HIGH RISK FOR, DIRECTED AT SELF/OTHERS |
|---|---|
| Risk Factors May Include: | Chemical alteration, exogenous (CNS stimulants/mind-altering drug), toxic reactions to drug(s). |
| | Organic brain syndrome (drug anesthetizes mind and body). |
| | Psychologic state (narrowed perceptual field). |
| Possible Indicators: | Synesthesias, hallucinations, illusions, visual/auditory distortions; panic state; suspiciousness of others, paranoid ideation, delusions. |

| | Hostile, threatening verbalizations; unpredictable behavior. |
|---|---|
| | Change in behavior pattern; exaggerated emotional response. |
| | Increased motor activity, pacing, excitement, irritability, agitation. |
| | Overt and aggressive acts; self-destructive behavior. |
| | Increasing anxiety, fear, and feelings of loss of control. |
| | Decreased response to pain. |
| **Desired Outcomes/Evaluation Criteria— Client Will:** | Demonstrate self-control, as evidenced by relaxed posture, free of violent behavior. |
| | Acknowledge reality of situation and understanding of relationship of behavior to drug use. |

| ACTIONS/INTERVENTIONS | RATIONALE |
|---|---|
| **Independent** | |
| Place in darkened, quiet, nonthreatening environment with a nonintrusive observer. | Lowered stimulation decreases the likelihood of confusion and fear, thus there is less chance of violent behavior. Use of the observer promotes safety. Note: PCP users seek help only after the situation has gotten out of hand, and it is therefore important to take safe action immediately. |
| Speak in a soft, nonthreatening voice. Use "Talk-downs" when LSD has been taken. If technique is tried with other drugs (PCP) and agitation increases, stop immediately. | Nonthreatening communication may have a calming effect. However, "Talk-downs" (the use of orientation, support, and reassuring words/touch) may be deleterious in the presence of PCP intoxication, resulting in an increase in the user's agitation level. |
| Observe for escalating anxiety, fear, irritability, and agitation. | May indicate potential for progression to violent behavior. Note: Client is not in complete control of self because of drug use. |
| Accept and deal with client's anger without reacting emotionally. | Responding emotionally on a personal level is not constructive and may escalate reactions. |
| Provide protection within the environment via constant observation and removal of objects that may be used to hurt self or others. | Reduces risk of injury to client and/or staff. Client may not feel pain and may not be able to follow directions because of the drug. |
| Observe behavior without administering medications. | A period of drug-free observation should precede any decision to administer medications (e.g., tranquilizers), so that a clear clinical picture can develop. In addition, because it is not known what other drugs may also have been ingested, it is not generally advisable to add another drug. |

| ACTIONS/INTERVENTIONS | RATIONALE |
|---|---|

### Collaborative

| | |
|---|---|
| Administer medications as necessary, e.g.:<br>  diazepam (Valium); | Used to reduce muscle spasms and/or restlessness in PCP user. |
|   haloperidol (Haldol). | Preferred to control psychosis and assaultive behavior. |
| Avoid use of phenothiazine neuroleptics. | Drugs such as chlorpromazine (Thorazine) should probably be avoided because of the possibility of potentiating PCP anticholinergic effects. |
| Apply restraints, if needed, and document reason(s) for use. | Restraints should be avoided in a frightened, hallucinating client but may be necessary because of potential injury to self or others, or when other dangerous drugs have been taken. PCP users are unpredictable, so it is best to err on the side of safety (using restraints with sufficient documentation) rather than risking injury. |

| | |
|---|---|
| **NURSING DIAGNOSIS:** | **TRAUMA/SUFFOCATION/POISONING, HIGH RISK FOR** |
| **Risk Factors May Include:** | Muscle incoordination; reduced hand/eye coordination. |
| | Decreased response to/perception of pain, reduced temperature/tactile sensation. |
| | Clouded sensorium and impaired judgment; unfamiliar environment, fear. |
| | Clonic movements, muscle rigidity (may precede/occur with generalized seizure activity). |
| | Internal factors, host: psychologic perception (hallucinations). |
| | Interactive conditions between individual and environment that impose a risk to the defensive and adaptive resources of the individual, e.g., placing hand in open flame, "flying out of window." |
| **Possibly Evidenced By:** | [Not applicable; presence of signs/symptoms establishes an **actual** diagnosis.] |
| **Desired Outcomes/Evaluation Criteria— Client Will:** | Verbalize understanding of factors (e.g., drug use) that contribute to possibility of injury and take steps to correct situation. |
| | Demonstrate behaviors and lifestyle changes necessary to minimize and/or prevent injury. |
| | Maintain/achieve physiologic stability evidenced by patent airway and adequate respiratory/cardiac function. |

| ACTIONS/INTERVENTIONS | RATIONALE |
|---|---|

**Independent**

| | |
|---|---|
| Ascertain what drugs have been taken. | Necessary for appropriate intervention/anticipation of needs. Lethal overdoses of hallucinogenic drugs (except for MDA, PCP) are rare; however, caution must be taken because adulterants such as sedative/hypnotics, anticholinergics, and strychnine are often used for "cutting" the drug. Note: Two reasons one might not know what drug was taken are (1) the individual lies for legal reasons or may feel embarrassed and (2) the person who sold the drugs to the client either did not know what was in them or lied about the drug. In either case, the nurse needs to listen to the client but be aware that the information the client gives may not be accurate. |
| Anticipate some form of unpredictability and be prepared for the unexpected, including physiologic as well as psychologic emergencies. | These drugs are dangerous and they do lead to bizarre thinking/harmful behavior. |
| Maintain client under close observation. Note precursors that might indicate increasing agitation, e.g., body tension, rising voice tone, quickening movements. | These drugs alter thinking, and many are anesthetic; therefore, the client may hurt self because of bizarre thinking, e.g., attempt to jump out window or escape from restraints. |
| Provide a hockey/bicycle helmet as indicated. | If client is banging head against hard objects, a helmet can decrease the potential for/severity of injury. |
| Remove objects that may be used to hurt self or others, and observe client constantly. | Provides protection within the environment. (Refer to ND: Violence, high risk for, directed at self/others.) |
| Monitor vital signs, respiratory rate/depth and rhythm. | Decreased diastolic blood pressure (cannabis) or hypertensive crisis (PCP) may develop. Bradypnea/respiratory arrest can occur, especially with PCP or heavy cannabis use. |
| Assess gag/swallow response and character of respirations. | Hypersalivation and vomiting, especially in the presence of ineffective cough and/or loss of muscle tone, may result in occlusion of airway, crowing/gurgling/choked respirations, leading to respiratory arrest. |
| Position client on side, or with head to the side, as indicated. | Facilitates drainage of vomitus and buildup of saliva and prevents aspiration in sedated/comatose client. |
| Encourage fluid intake frequently, if able to swallow safely. | Increased hydration keeps secretions loose and easier to expectorate and enhances renal clearance of drugs. |
| Have emergency equipment (including airway adjunct/suction) and medications available. | Toxic effects of several of these drugs on the heart and respiratory system may result in cardiac/respiratory arrest, requiring prompt intervention to prevent death. |

| ACTIONS/INTERVENTIONS | RATIONALE |
|---|---|
| **Collaborative** | |
| Administer medications as indicated, e.g., diazepam (Valium). | May be useful to reduce agitation and hyperactivity once drug(s) used are identified. |
| Transfer to medical setting as indicated. | Provides closer monitoring and more aggressive therapy, e.g., IV fluids with ammonium chloride or ascorbic acid for forced diuresis and acidifying of urine to enhance renal clearance of PCP. Note: Drug effects are dose related: >5 mg = low dose; >10 mg = high dose; >20 mg can lead to hypertensive crisis, coma/death due to respiratory/cardiac failure. |
| Apply restraints with caution when used. | May prevent injury to self or others. However, restraints should be avoided, if possible, in a frightened, hallucinating client because they can increase agitation. |

| NURSING DIAGNOSIS: | TISSUE PERFUSION, ALTERED, cerebral, high risk for |
|---|---|
| **Risk Factors May Include:** | Alterations in blood flow (hypertensive crisis). |
| **Possibly Evidenced By:** | [Not applicable; presence of signs and symptoms establishes an **actual** diagnosis.] |
| **Desired Outcomes/Evaluation Criteria— Client Will:** | Maintain usual level of consciousness free of adverse neurologic symptoms/complications. |

| ACTIONS/INTERVENTIONS | RATIONALE |
|---|---|
| **Independent** | |
| Elevate head of the bed; keep head in midline position. | Enhances venous drainage, thereby reducing risk of vascular congestion, which increases intracranial pressure and possibility of hemorrhage in PCP intoxication. |
| Observe for pupillary or vital sign changes, decreased level of consciousness and/or motor function. | Provides for early detection and intervention to minimize intracranial pressure/injury. |
| Encourage rest and quiet. Reduce environmental stimuli. | Promotes relaxation and may assist with lowering of the blood pressure. |
| Monitor BP. | Evaluates need for/effectiveness of interventions. |
| **Collaborative** | |
| Administer antihypertensive medications, e.g., diazoxide (Hyperstat) and hydralazine (Apresoline). | Effective in lowering blood pressure to prevent hypertensive crisis, which can be associated with PCP intoxication. |

| NURSING DIAGNOSIS: | THOUGHT PROCESSES, ALTERED |
|---|---|
| **May Be Related To:** | Physiologic changes (use of hallucinogenic substance). |
| | Impaired judgment with loss of memory. |
| **Possibly Evidenced By:** | Inaccurate interpretation of environment, memory impairment, bizarre thinking, disorientation. |
| | Inability to make decisions; unpredictable behavior. |
| | Cognitive dissonance; distractibility. |
| | Inappropriate/non–reality-based thinking. |
| | Sleep deprivation. |
| | Inability to communicate needs/desires effectively (mutism or confusion). |
| **Desired Outcomes/Evaluation Criteria— Client Will:** | Exhibit return of memory and ability to function. |
| | Communicate effectively. |
| | Report absence of visual/auditory distortions. |
| | Verbalize understanding that the drug is the cause of/contributes to alteration in perception. |

| ACTIONS/INTERVENTIONS | RATIONALE |
|---|---|

### Independent

| | |
|---|---|
| Observe closely; do not leave unattended; make sure restraints are secure when used. Remove objects from the environment that client could use to harm self and others. (Refer to ND: Violence, high risk for, directed at self/others.) | PCP is an anesthetic that alters thinking, and client may hurt self via attempt to jump out window, jump in front of cars, escape from restraints, and so forth. Removal of potentially harmful objects provides for protection and safety. |
| Anticipate some form of unpredictable behavior, and be prepared for the unexpected. | Use of hallucinogens can lead to bizarre thinking/harmful responses. |
| Tell client that current thoughts and feelings are a result of the drug if indicated. | This information may be helpful to the client who can accept it; however, it may cause agitation. |
| Allow client to sleep whenever possible. | Sleep cycle is disturbed by PCP. Client will need sleep after being agitated and expending excessive amounts of energy; sleeping also provides time for drug(s) to clear system. |
| Observe for behavioral indicators of psychosis, e.g., delusions, hallucinations. | Overdose may precipitate a psychotic episode that will clear within hours to days. When psychosis remains, preexisting condition (schizophrenia) may have been precipitated. |
| Note altered speech ability/patterns. Refer to loss of speech as temporary. | Mutism and confusion may occur, and information may reassure client that problem is drug-induced and that it will improve with time. Note: "Talk-down" approach may agitate the client and should be used with caution. |

| ACTIONS/INTERVENTIONS | RATIONALE |
|---|---|

### Independent

Anticipate client's needs and allow more time for client to respond to any necessary questions and/or comments.

May reduce need to communicate in presence of confusion/interference with memory. Adequate time allows full expression. Note: Be aware that touching and/or physical closeness may increase anxiety and agitation.

### Collaborative

Administer medications as indicated, e.g., diazepam (Valium) or chlordiazepoxide (Librium).

Chronic PCP users in whom psychiatric conditions develop/coexist may require further treatment for the thought disorder or depressive illness. The response may be very slow because of the persistence of PCP in the body tissues, sometimes for a period of several months.

| NURSING DIAGNOSIS: | ANXIETY [specify level]/FEAR |
|---|---|
| May Be Related To: | Situational crisis; threat to/change in health status. |
| | Perceived threat of death. |
| | Inexperience or unfamiliarity with the effect of drug(s) (e.g., PCP, LSD). |
| | Impaired thought processes; sensory impairment. |
| Possibly Evidenced By: | Assumptions of "losing my mind, losing control"; verbalized concern of unknown consequences/outcomes. |
| | Sympathetic stimulation, e.g., cardiovascular excitation, superficial vasoconstriction, pupil dilation, vomiting/diarrhea, restlessness, trembling. |
| | Preoccupation with feelings of impending doom; apprehension. |
| | Attack behavior. |
| Desired Outcomes/Evaluation Criteria—Client Will: | Verbalize awareness/cause of feelings of anxiety. |
| | Report anxiety reduced to a manageable level. |
| | Appear relaxed. |
| | Identify the fear and verbalize feelings of control of self and situation. |

| ACTIONS/INTERVENTIONS | RATIONALE |
|---|---|

### Independent

Assess level of anxiety on an ongoing basis.

Increased anxiety may lead to agitation and violent behavior as client is not in complete control of actions/responses.

193

| ACTIONS/INTERVENTIONS | RATIONALE |
|---|---|

### Independent

| | |
|---|---|
| Place in darkened, quiet, nonthreatening environment with a nonintrusive observer. | Lowered stimulation decreases the likelihood of confusion and fear. Observer is used for safety (with other personnel available to help if needed). |
| Orient clients to surroundings, time, and who is with them. Speak in soft voice, in a nonthreatening manner. | Knowing where one is can increase the feeling of security when experiencing a bad trip. |
| Use "Talk-down" with caution, telling the client that the ingested drug is the cause of feelings of anxiety, the effects are only temporary, and permanent damage should not occur. | Reassurance can be the single most important therapeutic intervention. "Talk-downs" are effective with persons who have taken LSD or similar substances. If the client can realize that the perceptions are drug-related, then an increase in control can take place. However, in some situations (e.g., PCP) "Talk-downs" can result in an increase in fear and agitation. |
| Encourage verbal expression of changes in perception that are occurring. | Can be used for assessment and provides guidance on direction for support. |

### Collaborative

| | |
|---|---|
| Administer sedatives if necessary, e.g., diazepam (Valium) or chlordiazepoxide (Librium). | These are drugs of choice to be used in extreme cases in order to calm client. Note: Medications are often discouraged because bad trips are usually self-limiting, and time is the best remedy for treating the negative effects. |

| | |
|---|---|
| **NURSING DIAGNOSIS:** | **SELF-CARE DEFICIT (specify)** |
| **May Be Related To:** | Perceptual/cognitive impairment. |
| | Therapeutic management (restraints). |
| **Possibly Evidenced By:** | Inability to meet own physical needs. |
| **Desired Outcomes/Evaluation Criteria— Client Will:** | Resume/perform self-care activities within level of own ability. |
| | Verbalize commitment to lifestyle changes to meet self-care needs. |

| ACTIONS/INTERVENTIONS | RATIONALE |
|---|---|

### Independent

| | |
|---|---|
| Provide care as needed/permitted. | Client may be agitated, and care will need to be postponed until control is regained. |
| Involve client in formulation of plan of care, as possible. | Enables client to participate at level of ability and enhances sense of control. Note: PCP user is often unable to interact without becoming agitated. |
| Work with client's present abilities. Do not pressure to perform beyond capabilities. | Failure can produce discouragement, depression, and agitation. |

| ACTIONS/INTERVENTIONS | RATIONALE |
|---|---|

### Independent

Provide and promote privacy within limits of safety needs.

Important to enhance self-esteem.

### Collaborative

Include client in team meeting/staffing as indicated. Problem-solve particulars of self-care needs.

Multidisciplinary approach with involvement of everyone who is caring for the client, along with the client, increases probability of plan being effective/successful.

# SUBSTANCE DEPENDENCE/ ABUSE REHABILITATION

**DSM IV**
**ALCOHOL USE DISORDERS**
303.90  Alcohol Dependence
305.00  Alcohol Abuse
**AMPHETAMINE (OR AMPHETAMINE-LIKE) USE DISORDERS**
304.40  Amphetamine Dependence
305.70  Amphetamine Abuse
**CANNABIS USE DISORDERS**
304.30  Cannabis Dependence
305.20  Cannabis Abuse
**COCAINE USE DISORDERS**
304.20  Cocaine Dependence
305.60  Cocaine Abuse
**HALLUCINOGEN USE DISORDERS**
304.50  Hallucinogen Dependence
305.30  Hallucinogen Abuse
**INHALANT USE DISORDERS**
304.60  Inhalant Dependence
305.90  Inhalant Abuse
**NICOTINE USE DISORDER**
305.10  Nicotine Dependence
**PHENCYCLIDINE USE DISORDERS**
304.90  Phencyclidine Dependence
305.90  Phencyclidine Abuse
**OPIOID USE DISORDERS**
304.00  Opioid Dependence
305.50  Opioid Abuse
**SEDATIVE, HYPNOTIC, OR ANXIOLYTIC SUBSTANCE USE DISORDERS**
304.10  Sedative, Hypnotic, or Anxiolytic Dependence
305.40  Sedative, Hypnotic, or Anxiolytic Abuse
**POLYSUBSTANCE USE DISORDER**
304.80  Polysubstance Dependence
(For other listings, consult DSM IV manual.)

**DSM III-R**
**PSYCHOACTIVE SUBSTANCE USE DISORDERS**
Alcohol: 303.90  Dependence; 305.00  Abuse
Amphetamine or similarly acting sympathomimetic: 304.40 Dependence; 305.70  Abuse
Cannabis: 304.30 Dependence; 305.20 Abuse
Cocaine: 304.20 Dependence; 305.60 Abuse
Hallucinogen: 304.50 Dependence; 305.30 Abuse
Opioid: 304.00 Dependence; 305.50 Abuse
Sedative/Hypnotic/Anxiolytic: 304.10 Dependence; 305.40 Abuse

This disorder is a continuum of phases incorporating a cluster of cognitive, behavioral, and physiologic symptoms that include loss of control over use of the substance and a continued use of the substance despite adverse consequences. A number of factors have been implicated in the predisposition to abuse a substance, e.g., biologic, biochemical, psychologic (including developmental), personality, sociocultural and conditioning, cultural and ethnic influences. However, no single theory adequately explains the etiology of this problem.

Alcohol; amphetamines or similar acting sympathomimetics; cannabis, cocaine, hallucinogens, opioids; sedatives/hypnotics/anxiolytics are drugs that are subject to abuse.

## CLIENT ASSESSMENT DATABASE

Refer to appropriate plans of care: Alcohol, Stimulants, Hallucinogens, Depressants.

## DIAGNOSTIC STUDIES

**Drug Screen:** Identifies drug(s) being used.

**Addiction Severity Index (ASI) Assessment:** Produces a "problem severity profile" of the client, including chemical, medical, psychologic, legal, family/social, and employment/support aspects indicating areas of treatment needs.

Additional tests dependent on specific drug(s) used and individual risk factors.

## NURSING PRIORITIES

1. Provide support for decision to stop substance abuse.
2. Strengthen individual coping skills.
3. Facilitate learning of new ways to reduce anxiety.
4. Promote family involvement in rehabilitation program.
5. Facilitate family growth/development.
6. Provide information about condition, prognosis, and treatment needs.

## DISCHARGE GOALS

1. Responsibility for own life and behavior assumed.
2. Plan to maintain substance-free life formulated.
3. Family relationships/codependency issues being addressed.
4. Treatment program successfully begun.
5. Condition, prognosis, and therapeutic regimen understood.

| **NURSING DIAGNOSIS:** | **DENIAL, INEFFECTIVE** |
| --- | --- |
| **May Be Related To:** | Personal vulnerability; fear; difficulty handling new situations. |
| | Learned response patterns; cultural factors, personal/family value systems. |
| **Possibly Evidenced By:** | Delays seeking or refuses health-care attention to the detriment of health/life situation. |
| | Does not perceive personal relevance of symptoms or danger, unable to admit impact of disease on life pattern. |
| | Uses manipulation to avoid responsibility for self. |
| **Desired Outcomes/Evaluation Criteria— Client Will:** | Verbalize awareness of relationship of substance abuse to current situation. |
| | Engage in therapeutic program. |
| | Verbalize acceptance of responsibility for own behavior. |
| | Attend support group (e.g., Cocaine/Narcotics/ Alcoholics Anonymous) regularly. |

| ACTIONS/INTERVENTIONS | RATIONALE |
|---|---|
| **Independent** | |
| Ascertain by what name client would like to be addressed. | Shows courtesy and respect. Gives sense of orientation and control. |
| Convey attitude of acceptance of client, separating individual from unacceptable behavior. | Promotes feelings of dignity and self-worth. |
| Review definition of drug dependence and categories of symptoms (e.g., patterns of use, impairment caused by use, tolerance to substance.) | Provides information to help client make decisions regarding acceptance of problem and treatment choices. |
| Answer questions honestly, provide factual information. Keep all promises. | Creates trust, which is the basis of the therapeutic relationship. |
| Provide information about addictive use vs. experimental, occasional use; biochemical/genetic disorder theory (genetic predisposition); use activated by environment; pharmacology of stimulant; compulsive desire as a lifelong occurrence. | Progression of use continuum in the addict is from experimental/recreational to addictive use. Comprehending this process is important in combating denial. Education may relieve client of blame, may help awareness of recurring addictive characteristics. |
| Discuss current life situation and impact of substance use. | First step in decreasing use of denial is for client to see the relationship between substance use and personal problems. |
| Confront and examine denial in peer group. Use confrontation with caring. | Because denial is the major defense mechanism in addictive disease, confrontation by peers can help the client accept the reality of what is happening and that drug use is a major problem. Caring attitude preserves self-esteem and helps decrease defensive responses. |
| Provide information regarding effects of addiction on mood/personality. | Individuals often mistake effects of addiction on mood/personality for its cause and use this to justify or excuse drug use. |
| Confront use of anger, rationalization, or projection. | Anger is often a response of defensiveness, and pointing this out to the client can help him or her to accept feelings underlying anger. These defense mechanisms prolong the stage of denial that problems exist in client's life because of substance use. |
| Remain nonjudgmental. Be alert to changes in behavior, e.g., restlessness, increased tension. | Confrontation can lead to an increase in agitation that may compromise safety of client/staff. |
| Provide positive feedback for expressing awareness of denial in self/others. | Positive feedback is necessary to enhance self-esteem and to reinforce insight into behavior. |
| Maintain firm expectation that client attend recovery support/therapy groups regularly. | Attendance is related to admitting need for help, working with denial, and maintaining a long-term drug-free existence. |
| Encourage and support client's taking responsibility for own recovery (e.g., development of alternative behaviors to drug urge). Assist client to learn own responsibility for recovering. | Denial can be replaced with responsible action when client accepts the reality of own responsibility. |

**NURSING DIAGNOSIS:**

**COPING, INDIVIDUAL, INEFFECTIVE**

**May Be Related To:**

Personal vulnerability.

Negative role modeling; inadequate support systems.

Previous ineffective/inadequate coping skills with substitution of drug(s).

**Possibly Evidenced By:**

Altered social patterns/participation.

Impaired adaptive behavior and problem-solving skills.

Decreased ability to handle stress of illness/hospitalization.

Financial affairs in disarray; employment difficulties, e.g., losing time on job/not maintaining steady employment, poor work performance, on-the-job injuries.

Verbalization of inability to cope/ask for help.

**Desired Outcomes/Evaluation Criteria— Client Will:**

Identify ineffective coping behaviors/consequences, including use of substance as a method of coping.

Use effective coping skills/problem-solving.

Initiate necessary lifestyle changes.

Attend support group (e.g., Cocaine/Narcotics/Alcoholics Anonymous) regularly.

| ACTIONS/INTERVENTIONS | RATIONALE |
|---|---|
| **Independent** | |
| Review unit rules, philosophy, expectations. | Having information provides opportunity for client to cooperate and function as member of group/milieu, enhancing sense of control and sense of success. |
| Determine understanding of current situation and previous methods of coping with life's problems. | Provides information about degree of denial, identifies coping skills that can be used in present plan of care. |
| Set limits and confront efforts to get caregiver to grant special privileges, making excuses for not following through on behaviors agreed on and attempting to continue drug use. | Client has learned manipulative behavior throughout life and needs to learn a new way of getting needs met. Following through on consequences of failure to maintain limits can help the client to change ineffective behaviors. |
| Be aware of staff enabling behaviors and feelings. | Lack of understanding of enabling and codependence can result in nontherapeutic approaches to addicts. |
| Encourage verbalization of feelings, fears, anxieties. | May help client begin to come to terms with long-unresolved issues. |

199

| ACTIONS/INTERVENTIONS | RATIONALE |
|---|---|

### Independent

| | |
|---|---|
| Explore alternative coping strategies. | Client may have little or no knowledge of adaptive responses to stress. |
| Assist client to learn/encourage use of relaxation skills, imagery, visualizations. | Helps client to relax, develop new ways to deal with stress, problem-solve. |
| Structure diversional activity that relates to recovery (e.g., social activity within support group) wherein issues of being chemical-free are examined. | Discovery of alternative methods for coping with drug hunger can remind client that addiction is a life-long process, and opportunity for changing patterns is available. |
| Use peer support to examine ways of coping with drug hunger. | Self-help groups are valuable for learning and promoting abstinence in each member using understanding, support, and peer pressure. |
| Have client begin to write autobiography. | This activity provides an opportunity for the client to remember and identify sequence of events in his or her life that relate to current situation. |

### Collaborative

| | |
|---|---|
| Administer medications as indicated, e.g.:<br>    disulfiram (Antabuse); | This drug can be helpful in maintaining abstinence from alcohol while other therapy is undertaken. By inhibiting alcohol oxidation, the drug leads to an accumulation of acetaldehyde, with a highly unpleasant reaction if alcohol is consumed (or even absorbed through the skin via colognes or shaving preparations). |
|     methadone; | This drug is thought to blunt the craving for/diminish the effects of heroin and is used to assist in withdrawal and long-term maintenance programs. It has fewer side effects and allows the individual to maintain daily activities and ultimately withdraw from drug use. |
|     naltrexone (Trexan). | Used to suppress craving for heroin and may help prevent relapse in alcoholics. Current research suggests that naltrexone suppresses urge to continue drinking by interfering with alcohol-induced release of endorphins. |
| Encourage involvement with self-help associations, e.g., Alcoholics/Narcotics Anonymous. | Puts client in direct contact with support systems necessary for continued sobriety/drug-free life. |

| NURSING DIAGNOSIS: | POWERLESSNESS |
|---|---|
| **May Be Related To:** | Substance addiction with/without periods of abstinence. |
| | Episodic compulsive indulgence; attempts at recovery. |
| | Lifestyle of helplessness. |

| **Possibly Evidenced By:** | Ineffective recovery attempts; statements of inability to stop behavior/requests for help. |
| | Continuous/constant thinking about drug and/or obtaining drug. |
| | Alteration in personal, occupational, and social life. |
| **Desired Outcomes/Evaluation Criteria—Client Will:** | Admit inability to control drug habit, surrender to powerlessness over addiction. |
| | Verbalize awareness of need for treatment and awareness that willpower alone cannot control abstinence. |
| | Engage in peer support. |
| | Demonstrate active participation in program. |
| | Regain and maintain healthful status with a drug-free lifestyle. |

| ACTIONS/INTERVENTIONS | RATIONALE |
| --- | --- |
| **Independent** | |
| Use crisis intervention techniques, e.g.: | Client is more amenable to acceptance of need for treatment at this time. |
| Assist client to recognize problem exists; | While client is hurting, it is easier to admit the drug(s) is a problem. |
| Identify goals for change; | Helpful in planning direction for care, promoting belief that change can occur. |
| Discuss alternative solutions; | Brainstorming helps creatively identify possibilities and provides sense of control. |
| Assist in selecting most appropriate alternative; | As possibilities are discussed, the most useful solution becomes clear. |
| Support decision and implementation of selected alternative(s). | Helps the client to persevere in process of change. |
| Discuss need for help in a caring, nonjudgmental way. | A caring, confrontive manner is more therapeutic because the client may respond defensively to a moralistic attitude, blocking recovery. |
| Identify ways in which drug has interfered with life, occupation, personal/interpersonal relationships. | Awareness of how the drug has controlled life is important in combatting denial/sense of powerlessness. |
| Have client list areas of life that could be affected by continued drug use. | Facing reality of further losses (e.g., job, relationship, family) may provide motivation for change. Note: Success of recovery efforts is enhanced when individual has a stake in something besides the drug. Individuals who are reasonably satisfied with their career, family lives, and/or community standing have something to lose and are more likely to sustain recovery. |

201

| ACTIONS/INTERVENTIONS | RATIONALE |
|---|---|

### Independent

Explore support in peer group. Encourage sharing of drug hunger, situations that increase the desire to indulge, ways that substance has influenced life.

May need assistance in expressing self, speaking about powerlessness, and admitting need for help in order to face up to problem and begin resolution.

Assist client to learn ways to enhance health and structure healthy diversion from drug use, e.g., a balanced diet, adequate rest, acupuncture, biofeedback, deep meditative techniques, exercise (walking, slow/long-distance running, etc.).

Learning to empower self in constructive areas can strengthen ability to continue recovery. These activities help restore natural biochemical balance; aid detoxification; and manage stress, anxiety, use of free time. These diversions can increase self-confidence, thereby improving self-esteem. Note: Release of endorphins from lengthy exercise can create a feeling of well-being.

Involve client in development of treatment plan using problem-solving process in which client agrees to desired outcomes.

The client is committed to the outcomes when the decision-making process involves solutions that are promulgated by the individual.

Provide information regarding understanding of human behavior and interactions with others, e.g., Transactional Analysis.

Understanding these concepts can help the client to begin to deal with past problems/losses and prevent repeating ineffective coping behaviors and self-fulfilling prophecies.

Assist client in self-examination of spirituality, faith.

Surrendering to and faith in a power greater than oneself has been found effective in substance recovery; may decrease sense of powerlessness.

Assist client to learn assertive communication.

Effective in assisting in ability to refuse use, to stop relationships with users and dealers, to build healthy relationships, regain control of own life.

Provide treatment information on an ongoing basis.

Helps client know what to expect. Creates opportunity for client to be a part of what is happening and make informed choices about participation/outcomes.

### Collaborative

Refer to/assist with making appointment to treatment program for continuation after discharge, e.g., outpatient/day and partial hospitalization drug treatment programs; Narcotics/Alcoholics Anonymous groups.

Follow-through on appointments may be easier than making the initial contact, and continuing treatment is essential to positive outcome.

| NURSING DIAGNOSIS: | NUTRITION, ALTERED, LESS THAN BODY REQUIREMENTS |
|---|---|
| May Be Related To: | Insufficient dietary intake to meet metabolic needs (psychologic, physiologic, or economic reasons). |
| Possibly Evidenced By: | Weight loss; weight below norm for height/body build; decreased subcutaneous fat/muscle mass. |

**Desired Outcomes/Evaluation Criteria—
Client Will:**

Reported altered taste sensation; lack of interest in food.

Poor muscle tone.

Sore, inflamed buccal cavity.

Laboratory evidence of protein/vitamin deficiencies.

Demonstrate progressive weight gain toward goal, with normalization of laboratory values and absence of signs of malnutrition.

Verbalize understanding of effects of substance abuse and reduced dietary intake on nutritional status.

Demonstrate behaviors and lifestyle changes to regain and maintain appropriate weight.

| ACTIONS/INTERVENTIONS | RATIONALE |
|---|---|
| **Independent** | |
| Assess height/weight, age, body build, strength, activity/rest level. Note condition of oral cavity. | Provides information about individual on which to base dietary plan. Type of diet/foods may be affected by condition of mucous membranes and teeth. |
| Take anthropometric measurements, e.g., triceps skinfold. | Calculates subcutaneous fat and muscle mass to aid in determining dietary needs. |
| Note total daily calorie intake; maintain a diary of intake, times, and patterns of eating. | Information about client's dietary pattern will identify nutritional needs/deficiencies. |
| Evaluate energy expenditure (e.g., pacing versus sedentary) and establish an individualized exercise program. | Activity level affects nutritional needs. Exercise enhances muscle tone, may stimulate appetite. |
| Provide opportunity to choose foods/snacks to meet dietary plan. | Enhances participation/sense of control and may promote resolution of nutritional deficiencies. |
| Weigh weekly and record. | Provides information regarding effectiveness of dietary plan. |
| **Collaborative** | |
| Consult with dietitian. | Useful in establishing individual dietary needs. Provides additional source for learning. |
| Review lab work as indicated, e.g., glucose, serum, albumin, electrolytes. | Identifies anemias, electrolyte imbalances, other abnormalities that may be present, requiring specific therapy. |
| Refer for dental consultation as necessary. | Teeth are essential to good nutritional intake, and dental hygiene/care is often a neglected area in this population. |

| NURSING DIAGNOSIS: | SELF-ESTEEM DISTURBANCE [specify] |
| --- | --- |
| May Be Related To: | Negative role models; abuse/neglect, dysfunctional family system. |
| | Extreme poverty. |
| | Life choices perpetuating failure; situational crisis with loss of control over life events. |
| | Social stigma attached to substance abuse, social expectation that one control behavior. |
| | Biochemical body change (e.g., withdrawal from alcohol/drugs). |
| Possibly Evidenced By: | Confusion about self, purpose, or direction in life. |
| | Change in usual patterns or responsibility (family, job, legal). |
| | Denial that substance use is a problem; projection of blame/responsibility for problems. |
| | Self-negating verbalization, expressions of shame/guilt. |
| | Not taking responsibility for self/self-care; lack of follow-through; self-destructive behavior. |
| Desired Outcomes/Evaluation Criteria— Client Will: | Identify feelings and underlying dynamics for negative perception of self. |
| | Verbalize acceptance of self as is and an increased sense of self-esteem. |
| | Set goals and participate in realistic planning for lifestyle changes necessary to live without drugs. |

| ACTIONS/INTERVENTIONS | RATIONALE |
| --- | --- |
| **Independent** | |
| Provide opportunity for and encourage verbalization/discussion of individual situation. | Client often has difficulty expressing self, even more difficulty accepting the degree of importance that substance has assumed in life and the relationship it has to the present situation. |
| Assess mental status. Note the presence of other psychiatric disorders (dual diagnosis). | Many clients use substances (alcohol and other drugs) to seek relief from depression or anxiety, which can be preexisting or a result of the substance abuse. Note: Approximately 60% of substance-dependent clients also have mental illness problems, and treatment for both is imperative. |
| Spend time with client. Discuss client's behavior/use of substance in a nonjudgmental way. | Presence of the nurse conveys acceptance of the individual as a worthwhile person. Discussion provides opportunity for insight into the problems abuse has created for the client. |

| ACTIONS/INTERVENTIONS | RATIONALE |
|---|---|
| **Independent** | |
| Provide reinforcement for positive actions, and encourage client to accept this input. | Failure and lack of self-esteem have been problems for this client, who needs to learn to accept self as an individual with positive attributes. |
| Observe family/significant other(s) dynamics/ support. | Substance abuse is a family disease, and how the members act and react to the client's behavior affects the course of the disease and how the client sees self. Many members unconsciously become enablers, helping the individual to cover up the consequences of the abuse. (Refer to ND: Family Coping, ineffective, compromised/disabling/Caregiver Role Strain.) |
| Encourage expression of feelings of guilt, shame, and anger. | The client often has lost respect for self and believes that the situation is hopeless. Expression of these feelings helps the client to begin to accept responsibility for own self and take steps to make changes. |
| Help the client to acknowledge that substance use is the problem and that problems can be dealt with without the use of drugs. Confront the use of defenses, e.g., denial, projection, rationalization. | When drugs can no longer be blamed for the problems that exist, the client can begin to deal with the problems and live without substance use. Confrontation helps the client accept the reality of the problems as they exist. |
| Ask the client to list past accomplishments and positive happenings. | There are things in everyone's life that have been successful. Often when self-esteem is low, it is difficult to remember these successes or to view them as successes. |
| Use techniques of role rehearsal. | Assists client to practice the development of skills to cope with new role as a person who no longer uses or needs drugs to handle life's problems. |
| **Collaborative** | |
| Involve in group therapy. | Group sharing helps encourage verbalization, as other members of group are in various stages of abstinence from drugs and can address the client's concerns/denial. The client can gain new skills, hope, and a sense of family/community from group participation. |
| Refer to other resources, such as Narcotics/ Alcoholics Anonymous. | One of the oldest and most popular forms of group treatment, which uses a basic strategy known as the "12 steps." The client admits powerlessness over drug and, although not necessary, may seek help from a "higher power." Members help one another, and meetings are available at many different times and places in most communities. The philosophy of "1 day at a time" helps attain the goal of abstinence. |

| ACTIONS/INTERVENTIONS | RATIONALE |
|---|---|
| **Collaborative** | |
| Formulate plan to treat other mental illness problems. (Refer to appropriate CP as indicated.) | Clients who seek relief for other mental health problems through drugs will continue to do so once discharged. Both the substance use and the mental health problems need to be treated together to maximize abstinence potential. |
| Administer antipsychotic medications as necessary. | Prolonged/profound psychosis following LSD or PCP use can be treated with these drugs, as it is probably the result of an underlying functional psychosis that has now emerged. Note: Avoid the use of phenothiazines as they may decrease seizure threshold and cause hypotension in the presence of LSD/PCP. |

| NURSING DIAGNOSIS: | FAMILY COPING, ineffective: compromised/dysfunctional/CAREGIVER ROLE STRAIN |
|---|---|
| **May Be Related To:** | Personal vulnerability of individual family members; codependency issues. |
| | Situational crises. |
| | Compromised social systems; family disorganization/role changes. |
| | Prolonged disease progression that exhausts supportive capability of family members. |
| | Significant person(s) with chronically unexpressed feelings of guilt, anger, hostility, despair. |
| **Possibly Evidenced By:** | Denial (one of the strongest and most resistant symptoms); lack of acceptance that drinking/drug use is causing the present situation or belief that all problems are due to substance use. |
| | Severely dysfunctional family, e.g., family violence, spouse/child abuse, separation/divorce, children displaying acting-out behaviors. |
| | Financial affairs in disarray; employment difficulties. |
| | Altered social patterns/participation. |
| | Significant other(s) demonstrating enabling or codependent behaviors, e.g., avoiding and shielding, attempting to take control, taking over responsibilities, rationalizing and accepting, cooperating and collaborating, rescuing and subserving. |

| Desired Outcomes/Evaluation Criteria— Family Will: | Verbalize understanding of dynamics of codependence and participate in individual and family programs. |
| --- | --- |
| | Identify ineffective coping behaviors/consequences. |
| | Demonstrate/plan for necessary lifestyle changes. |
| | Take action to change self-destructive behaviors/alter behaviors that contribute to partner's/SO's addiction. |

| ACTIONS/INTERVENTIONS | RATIONALE |
| --- | --- |

### Independent

| | |
| --- | --- |
| Assess family history; explore roles of family members, circumstances involving drug use, strengths, areas for growth. | Determines areas for focus, potential for change. |
| Explore how the significant other has coped with the addict's habit, e.g., denial, repression, rationalization, projection. | Codependent also suffers from the same feelings as the client (e.g., anxiety, self-hatred, helplessness, hurt, loneliness, low self-worth, guilt) and needs help in learning new/effective coping skills. |
| Determine understanding of current situation and previous methods of coping with life's problems. | Provides information on which to base present plan of care. |
| Assess current level of functioning of family members. | Affects individual's ability to cope with situation. |
| Determine extent of enabling behaviors being evidenced by family members; explore with individual and client. | "Enabling" is doing for the client what she or he needs to do for own self. People want to be helpful and do not want to feel powerless to help their loved one to stop substance use and change the behavior that is so destructive. However, the substance abuser often relies on others to cover up own inability to cope with daily responsibilities. |
| Identify and discuss sabotage behaviors of family members. | Even though family member(s) may verbalize a desire for the individual to become substance free, the reality of interactive dynamics is that they may unconsciously not want the individual to recover as this would impact the family member(s), own role in the relationship. For example, family member(s) may feel in control, needed, or that their existence is "justified" by taking care of the substance abuser. Additionally, they may receive sympathy/attention from others (secondary gain). |
| Provide information about enabling behavior, addictive disease characteristics for both user/non-user who is codependent. | Awareness and knowledge provide opportunity for individuals to begin the process of change. |
| Provide factual information to client and family about the effects of addictive behaviors on the family and what to expect after discharge. | Many clients/families are not aware of the nature of addiction. If client is using legally obtained drugs, may believe this does not constitute abuse. |

207

| ACTIONS/INTERVENTIONS | RATIONALE |
|---|---|

### Independent

Encourage family members to be aware of their own feelings and to look at the situation with perspective and objectivity. They can ask themselves, "Am I being conned? Am I acting out of fear, shame, guilt, or anger? Do I have a need to control?"

When the codependent family members become aware of their own actions that perpetuate the addict's problems, they need to decide to change themselves. If they change, the client can then face the consequences of his or her own actions and may choose to get well.

Provide support for codependent partner(s). Encourage group work.

Families/significant others need support as much as addicts to produce change.

Assist the codependent partner to become aware that client's abstinence or drug use is not the partner's responsibility.

Partners need to learn that user's habit may or may not change despite partner's involvement in treatment.

Help the recovering (former user) codependent to distinguish between destructive aspects of enabling behavior and genuine motivation to aid the user.

Enabling behavior can be partner's attempts at personal survival.

Note how the codependent partner relates to the treatment team/staff.

Determines enabling style. A parallel exists between how partner relates to user and to staff, based on partner's feelings about self and situation.

Assess conflicting feelings the person who is codependent may have, e.g., feelings similar to those of abuser (blend of anger, guilt, fear, exhaustion, embarrassment, loneliness, distrust, grief, and possibly relief).

Useful in establishing therapeutic needs of codependent person(s). The individual's own identity may have been lost; he or she may fear self-disclosure to staff and may have difficulty giving up the dependent relationship.

Involve family in discharge referral plans.

Drug abuse is a family illness. Because family members have been so involved in dealing with the substance abuse behavior, they need help adjusting to the new behavior of sobriety/abstinence. Incidence of recovery is almost doubled when the family is treated along with the client.

Be aware of staff enabling behaviors and feelings about particular clients and codependent partners.

Lack of understanding of enabling and codependence can create nontherapeutic approaches to clients and their families.

### Collaborative

Encourage involvement with self-help associations, Alcoholics/Narcotics Anonymous, Al-Anon, Alateen, and professional family therapy.

Puts client/family in direct contact with support systems necessary for continued sobriety and assists with problem resolution.

| **NURSING DIAGNOSIS:** | **SEXUAL DYSFUNCTION** |
|---|---|
| **May Be Related To:** | Altered body function: neurologic damage and debilitating effects of drug use (particularly alcohol and opiates). |
| **Possibly Evidenced By:** | Progressive interference with sexual functioning. |

| Desired Outcomes/Evaluation Criteria—Client Will: | In men a significant degree of testicular atrophy is noted (testes are smaller and softer than normal); gynecomastia (breast enlargement); impotence/decreased sperm counts. |
| | In women loss of body hair, thin soft skin, and spider angiomas (elevated estrogen) are noted; amenorrhea/increase in miscarriages. |
| | Verbally acknowledge effects of drug use on sexual functioning/reproduction. |
| | Identify interventions to correct/overcome individual situation. |

| ACTIONS/INTERVENTIONS | RATIONALE |
| --- | --- |
| **Independent** | |
| Have client describe problem in own words. | Determines level of knowledge, client's perception of needs. |
| Encourage and accept individual expressions of concern. | Most people find it difficult to talk about this sensitive subject and may not ask directly for information. |
| Provide education opportunity (e.g., pamphlets, consultation from appropriate persons) for patient to learn effects of drug on sexual functioning. | Much of denial and hesitancy to seek treatment may be decreased with sufficient and appropriate information. |
| Provide information about individual's condition. | Sexual functioning may have been affected by drug (alcohol) intake or physiologic and/or psychologic factors (such as stress). Information will assist client to understand own situation and identify actions to be taken. |
| Provide information about effects of drugs on the reproductive system/fetus (e.g., increased risk of premature birth, brain damage, and fetal malformation). Assess drinking/drug history of pregnant client. | Awareness of the negative effects of alcohol/other drugs on reproduction may motivate client to stop using drug(s). When client is pregnant, identification of potential problems aids in planning for future fetal needs/concerns. |
| Discuss prognosis for sexual dysfunction, e.g., impotence/low sexual desire. | In about 50% of cases, impotence is reversed with abstinence from drug(s); in 25%, the return to normal functioning is delayed; approximately 25% remain impotent. |
| **Collaborative** | |
| Refer for sexual counseling, if indicated. | Client may need additional assistance to resolve more severe problems/situations. Client may have difficulty adjusting, if drug has improved sexual experience (heroin decreases dyspareunia in women/premature ejaculation in men). Further, the client may have engaged enjoyably in bizarre, erotic sexual behavior under influence of the stimulant drug; client may have found no substitute for the drug, may have driven a partner away, and may have no motivation to adjust to sexual experience without drugs. |

| ACTIONS/INTERVENTIONS | RATIONALE |
|---|---|

### Collaborative

| | |
|---|---|
| Review results of sonogram, if pregnant. | Assesses fetal growth and development to identify possibility of fetal alcohol syndrome (FAS) and future needs. |

| | |
|---|---|
| **NURSING DIAGNOSIS:** | **KNOWLEDGE DEFICIT [LEARNING NEED] regarding condition, prognosis, and treatment needs** |
| **May Be Related To:** | Lack of information; misinterpretation. |
| | Cognitive limitations/interference with learning (other mental illness problems/organic brain syndrome); lack of recall. |
| **Possibly Evidenced By:** | Statements of concern; questions/misconceptions. |
| | Inaccurate follow-through of instructions/development of preventable complications. |
| | Continued use in spite of complications/bad trips. |
| **Desired Outcomes/Evaluation Criteria— Client Will:** | Verbalize understanding of own condition/disease process, prognosis, and treatment plan. |
| | Identify/initiate necessary lifestyle changes to remain drug-free. |
| | Participate in treatment program. |

| ACTIONS/INTERVENTIONS | RATIONALE |
|---|---|

### Independent

| | |
|---|---|
| Be aware of and deal with anxiety of client and family members. | Anxiety can interfere with ability to hear and assimilate information. |
| Provide an active role for the client and family members in the learning process, e.g., discussions, group participation, role-play. | Learning is enhanced when people are actively involved. |
| Provide written and verbal information as indicated. Include list of articles and books related to client/family needs, and encourage reading and discussing what they learn. | Helps client and family to make informed choices about future. Bibliotherapy can be a useful addition to other therapeutic approaches. |
| Time activities to individual needs. | Facilitates learning, as information is more rapidly assimilated when pacing is considered. |
| Assess client's knowledge of own situation, e.g., condition, complications and needed changes in lifestyle. | Assists in planning for long-range changes necessary for maintaining sobriety/drug-free status. Client may have street knowledge of the drug but be ignorant of medical facts. |

| ACTIONS/INTERVENTIONS | RATIONALE |
|---|---|

**Independent**

| | |
|---|---|
| Review condition and prognosis/future expectations. | Provides knowledge base on which client can make informed choices. |
| Discuss relationship of drug use to current situation. | Often client has misperception (denial) about real reason for admission to the psychiatric setting. |
| Discuss effects of drug(s) used, e.g., PCP is deposited in body fat and may reactivate (causing flashbacks) even after long interval of abstinence; alcohol use may result in mental deterioration/liver involvement/damage; cocaine can damage postcapillary vessels and increase platelet aggregation, promoting thromboses and infarction of skin/internal organs, causing localized atrophie blanche or sclerodermatous lesions. | Information will help client understand possible long-term effects of drug use. |
| Discuss potential for reemergence of withdrawal symptoms in stimulant abuse as early as 3 months or as late as 9–12 months. | While symptoms of intoxication may have passed, client may manifest denial, drug hunger, periods of "flare up" wherein there is a delayed recurrence of withdrawal symptoms, e.g., anxiety, depression, irritability, sleep disturbance, compulsiveness with food (especially sugars). |
| Inform client of effects of Antabuse with alcohol intake and importance of avoiding use of alcohol-containing products, e.g., cough syrups or foods/candy, colognes. | Interaction of alcohol and Antabuse results in nausea and hypotension, which may produce fatal shock. Individuals on Antabuse are sensitive to alcohol on a continuum: some are able to drink on the drug, whereas others have a reaction with only slight exposure, e.g., alcohol-containing foods or products such as aftershave. Reactions appear to be dose-related as well. |
| Review specific aftercare needs, e.g., PCP user should drink cranberry juice and continue use of ascorbic acid; alcohol abuser with liver damage should refrain from drugs/anesthesias/household cleaning products that are detoxified in the liver. | Promotes individualized care related to specific situation. Cranberry juice and ascorbic acid enhance clearance of PCP from the system. Substances that have potential for liver damage are more dangerous in presence of already damaged liver. |
| Review drug laws/consequences, potential for relapse. | Helps client to think about the possibility of legal problems of drug use. Clients often believe they will not go back to using the drug(s), and it is important to talk about this issue. |
| Discuss variety of helpful organizations and programs that are available for assistance/referral. | Long-term support is necessary to maintain optimal recovery. Psychosocial needs as well as other issues may require addressing. |

# CHAPTER 7

---

# SCHIZOPHRENIC AND OTHER PSYCHOTIC DISORDERS

## SCHIZOPHRENIA

### DSM IV
**SCHIZOPHRENIA**
295.30 Paranoid Type
295.10 Disorganized Type
295.20 Catatonic Type
295.90 Undifferentiated Type
295.60 Residual Type
(Refer to DSM IV for other listings.)

### DSM III-R
295.1x Disorganized Type
295.2x Catatonic Type
295.3x Paranoid Type
295.9x Undifferentiated Type
295.6x Residual Type

The term "schizophrenia" describes a psychotic state that at some point in time is characterized by apathy, avolition, asociality, affective blunting, and alogia. The client has alterations in thoughts, percepts, mood, and behavior. Subjective experiences of disordered thought are manifested in disturbances of concept formation that sometimes lead to misinterpretations of reality, delusions (particularly delusions of influence and ideas of reference), and hallucinations. Mood changes include ambivalence, constriction or inappropriateness of feeling, and loss of empathy with others. Behavior may be withdrawn, regressive, or bizarre (Shader, 1994).

## ETIOLOGIC THEORIES

### Psychodynamics

Psychosis is the result of a weak ego. The development of the ego has been inhibited by a symbiotic parent/child relationship. Because the ego is weak, the use of ego defense mechanisms in times of extreme anxiety is maladaptive, and behaviors are often representations of the id segment of the personality.

## Biologic

Certain genetic factors may be involved in the development of this psychotic disorder. Individuals are at higher risk for the disorder if there is a familial pattern of involvement (parents, siblings, other relatives). Schizophrenia has been determined to be a sporadic illness (meaning you cannot currently follow genes from generation to generation). It is an autosomal dominant trait. However, most scientists agree that what is inherited is a vulnerability or predisposition, which may be due to an enzyme defect or some other biochemical abnormality, a subtle neurologic deficit, or some other factor or combination of factors. This predisposition, in combination with environmental factors, results in development of the disease.

Some research implies that these disorders may be a birth defect, occurring in the hippocampus region of the brain. The studies show a disordering of the pyramidal cells in the brains of schizophrenics, while the cells in the brains of nonschizophrenic individuals appear to be arranged in an orderly fashion. Ventricular brain ratio (VBR) or disproportionately small brain (or specific areas of the brain) may be inherited and/or congenital. The cause can be a virus, lack of oxygen, or birth trauma.

A biochemical theory suggests the involvement of elevated levels of the neurotransmitter dopamine, which is thought to produce the symptoms of overactivity and fragmentation of associations that are commonly observed in psychoses.

Although occurrence is relatively equal between males and females, resources report a predominant male bias with 2/3 of young adults with serious mental illnesses being male. It has been demonstrated that boys react more strongly than girls to stress and conflicts in the family home and are more vulnerable to infantile autism. A significantly larger number of males than females exhibit obsessive and suicidal behaviors, fetishism, and schizophrenia. Schizophrenia develops earlier in males, and they respond less well to treatment and have less chance of recovery and return to normal life than females. The incidence in females may have more familial origins. It is becoming clearer that the different brain organization of men and women, and the effect of sex hormones on brain growth are likely to result in subtle differences that define the "scope and range of sex differences in the incidence, clinical presentation, and course of specific psychiatric diseases" (Moir & Jessel, 1991).

## Family Dynamics

Family systems theory describes the development of schizophrenia as it evolves out of a dysfunctional family system. Conflict between spouses drives one parent to attach to the child. This overinvestment in the child redirects the focus of anxiety in the family, and a more stable condition results. A symbiotic relationship develops between parent and child; the child remains totally dependent on the parent into adulthood and is unable to respond to the demands of adult functioning.

Interpersonal theory relates that the psychotic person is the product of a parent/child relationship fraught with intense anxiety. The child receives confusing and conflicting messages from the parent and is unable to establish trust. High levels of anxiety are maintained, and the child's concept of self is one of ambiguity. A retreat into psychosis offers relief from anxiety and security from intimate relatedness. Some research indicates that clients who live with families high in expressed emotion (e.g., hostility, criticism, disappointment, overprotectiveness, and overinvolvement) show more frequent relapses than clients who live with families who are low in expressed emotion.

Current research into genetic and biologic influences suggests that these family interactions are more likely to be contributing factors rather than the cause of the disorder.

## CLIENT ASSESSMENT DATABASE

## General

### ACTIVITY/REST

Interruption of sleep by hallucinations and delusional thoughts, early awakening, insomnia, and hyperactivity (e.g., pacing).

213

## HYGIENE

Poor personal hygiene, unkempt/disheveled appearance.

## NEUROSENSORY

History of alteration in functioning for at least 6 months, including an active phase of at least 2 weeks in which psychotic symptoms were evident.

Family reports presence of psychologic symptoms (primarily in thought and perception) and deterioration from previous level of adaptive functioning.

## MENTAL STATUS

**Thought:** Delusions, loose association.
**Perception:** Hallucinations, illusions.
**Affect:** Blunted, flat, inappropriate, incongruous, or silly.
**Volition:** Cannot self-initiate or participate in goal-oriented activity.
**Capacity to Relate to Environment:** Mental/emotional withdrawal and isolation (autism) and/or psychomotor activity ranging from marked reduction to stereotypic, purposeless activity.
**Speech:** Frequently incoherent, echolalia may be noted /alogia (inability to speak) may occur.
**Delusions:**
  **Disorganized Type:** Systematized delusions are absent; however, fragmentary delusions or hallucinations (disorganized, unthematized [without theme] content) are common.
  **Paranoid Type:** One or more systematized delusions with prominent persecutory or grandiose content; delusional jealousy may be observed.
  **Undifferentiated Type:** Delusions are prominent.
**Behaviors:** Grimaces, mannerisms, hypochondriac complaints, extreme social withdrawal, as well as other odd behaviors.
**Negativism:** Resistance to all directions or attempts to move without apparent motive.
**Rigidity:** Rigid posture, maintained despite attempts to move client.
**Excitement:** Purposeless motor activity not caused by external stimuli.
**Posturing:** Voluntarily assuming inappropriate or bizarre posture.
**Emotions:** Unfocused anxiety, anger, argumentativeness, and violence may be observed.

## TEACHING/LEARNING

Affects women and men equally, although symptoms in men are usually more severe and require higher doses of medication.

May have had previous acute episodes with impairment ranging from none to severe deterioration requiring institutionalization; onset of symptoms most commonly occurring between late teens and mid-30s.

Correlations with family history of psychiatric illness; lower socioeconomic groups, higher stressors, and premorbid personality described as suspicious, introverted, withdrawn, or eccentric have been noted.

## Disorganized

### NEUROSENSORY

Speech disorganized; communication consistently incoherent.
Behavior is regressive/primitive, incoherent, and grossly disorganized.
**Psychomotor:** Stupor, markedly decreased reactivity to milieu, and/or reduced spontaneity of movement/activity or mutism.
Incoherence: flat, incongruous, silly affect.

### SOCIAL INTERACTIONS

Usually correlated with extreme social impairment/withdrawal; odd mannerisms.
Poor premorbid personality.

### TEACHING/LEARNING

Chronic course with no significant remissions.

## Catatonic

The incidence of this type is rare in the western hemisphere, although it was common several decades ago.

### ACTIVITY/REST

Marked psychomotor retardation or excessive/purposeless motor activity.
Exhaustion (extreme agitation).

### FOOD/FLUID

Weight below norms, other signs of malnutrition.

### NEUROSENSORY

Marked psychomotor disturbance, e.g., stupor, rigidity, mutism or excitement, negativism, waxy flexibility, and/or posturing.
Speech: Echolalia or echopraxia.

### SAFETY

Potential for violence to self/others exists during catatonic stupor or excitement.

### TEACHING/LEARNING

Hypochondriacal complaints or oddities of behavior may be noted.

## Paranoid

Symptoms characteristic of disorganized and catatonic types are absent.

### NEUROSENSORY

Systematized delusions and/or auditory hallucinations of a persecutory or grandiose nature, usually related to a single theme.

### SAFETY

Easily agitated, assaultive, and violent (if delusions are acted on).
Impairment in functioning may be minimal, with gross disorganization of behavior relatively rare.

### SOCIAL INTERACTIONS

Significant impairment may be noted in social/marital areas.
Affective responsiveness may be preserved but with a stilted, formal quality or extreme intensity in interpersonal interactions often observed.

### SEXUALITY

May express doubts about gender identity (e.g., fear of being thought of as, or approached by, a homosexual).

### TEACHING/LEARNING

Onset usually late 20s to 40s.
Other family members may have had paranoid problems.

## Undifferentiated

This category is used when illness does not meet the criteria for the other specific types of schizophrenias, meets the criteria for more than one, or when the course of the last episode is unknown.

### NEUROSENSORY

Prominent delusions/hallucinations, incoherence, and grossly disorganized behaviors.

215

### Residual

NEUROSENSORY

Inappropriate affect.

SOCIAL INTERACTIONS

Social withdrawal, eccentric behavior.

TEACHING/LEARNING

History of at least 1 episode of schizophrenia in which psychotic symptoms were evident, but the current clinical picture presents no psychotic symptoms.

## DIAGNOSTIC STUDIES

(Usually done to rule out physical illness, which may be cause of reversible symptomatology, e.g., toxic/deficiency states, infections, neurologic disease, endocrine/metabolic disorders.)

**Computed Axial Tomography (CT) Scan:** May show subtle abnormalities of brain structures in some schizophrenics, e.g., atrophy of temporal lobes; enlarged ventricles with increased ventricle-brain ratio may correlate with degree of symptoms displayed.

**Positron Emission Tomography (PET) Scan:** Measures the metabolic activity of specific areas of the brain and may reveal low metabolic activity in the frontal lobes, especially in prefrontal area of cerebral cortex.

**Magnetic Resonance Imaging (MRI):** Provides a three-dimensional image of the brain; may reveal smaller than average frontal lobes, atrophy of left temporal lobe (specifically anterior hippocampus, parahippocampogyrus, and superior temporal gyrus).

**Regional Cerebral Blood Flow (RCBF):** Maps blood flow and implies the intensity of activity in various brain regions.

**Brain Electrical Activity Mapping (BEAM):** Shows brain wave responses to various stimuli with delayed and decreased response noted, particularly in left temporal lobe and associated limbic system.

**Addiction Severity Index (ASI):** Determines problems of addiction (substance abuse), which may be associated with mental illness, and indicates areas of treatment need.

**Psychological Testing (e.g., MMPI):** Reveals impairment in 1 or more areas. Note: Paranoid type usually shows little or no impairment.

## NURSING PRIORITIES

1. Promote appropriate interaction between client and environment.
2. Enhance physiologic stability/health maintenance.
3. Provide protection, ensure safety needs.
4. Encourage family/significant other(s) to become involved in activities to promote independent, satisfying lives.

## DISCHARGE CRITERIA

1. Physiologic well-being maintained with appropriate balance between rest and activity.
2. Demonstrates increasing/highest level of emotional responsiveness possible.
3. Interacts socially without decompensation.
4. Family displays effective coping skills and appropriate use of resources.

| NURSING DIAGNOSIS: | THOUGHT PROCESSES, ALTERED |
|---|---|
| May Be Related To: | Disintegration of thinking processes; impaired judgment. |
| | Psychologic conflicts; disintegrated ego boundaries (confusion with environment). |
| | Sleep disturbance. |
| | Ambivalence and concomitant dependence (part of need-fear dilemma interferes with ability to self-initiate fulfilling diversional activities). |
| Possibly Evidenced By: | Presence of delusional system (may be grandiose, persecutory, of reference, of control, somatic, accusatory); commands, obsessions. |
| | Symbolic and concrete associations; blocking; ideas of reference. |
| | Inaccurate interpretation of environment; cognitive dissonance; impaired ability to make decisions. |
| | Simple hyperactivity and constant motor activity (ritualistic acts, stereotyped behavior) to withdrawal and psychomotor retardation. |
| | Interrupted sleep patterns. |
| Desired Outcomes/Evaluation Criteria—Client Will: | Recognize changes in thinking/behavior. |
| | Identify delusions and increase capacity to cope effectively with them by elimination of pathologic thinking. |
| | Maintain reality orientation. |
| | Establish interpersonal relationships. |

## ACTIONS/INTERVENTIONS

### Independent

Assess the presence/severity of client's altered thought processes, noting form (dereistic, autistic, symbolic, loose and/or concrete associations, blocking); content (somatic delusions, delusions of grandeur/persecution, ideas of reference); and flow (flight of ideas, retardation).

Establish a therapeutic nurse-client relationship.

Use therapeutic communications (e.g., reflection, paraphrasing) to effectively intervene.

Structure communications to reflect consideration of client's socioeconomic, educational, and cultural history/values.

## RATIONALE

Identification of the symbolic/primitive nature of thinking/communications promotes understanding of the individual client's thought processes and enables planning of appropriate interventions.

Provides an emotionally safe milieu that enables interpersonal interaction and decreases autism.

Therapeutic communications are clear, concise, open, consistent, and require use of self. This reduces autistic thinking.

Lack of consideration of these factors can cause misdiagnoses/inaccurate interpretation (otherwise normal thinking viewed as pathologic).

217

| ACTIONS/INTERVENTIONS | RATIONALE |
|---|---|

### Independent

Express desire to understand client's thinking by clarifying what is unclear, focusing on the feeling rather than the content, endeavoring to understand (in spite of the client's unclearness), listening carefully, and regulating the flow of the thinking as needed.

Client is often unable to organize thoughts (easily distracted, cannot grasp concepts or wholeness but focuses on minutiae), and flow of thoughts is often characterized as racing, wandering, or retarded. Active-listening identifies patterns of client's thoughts and facilitates understanding. Expression of desire to understand conveys caring and increases client's feelings of self-worth.

Reinforce congruent thinking. Refuse to argue/agree with disintegrated thoughts. Present reality and demonstrate motivation to understand client (model patience). Share appropriate thinking and set limits if client tries to respond impulsively to altered thinking.

Decreases altered (disintegrated, delusional) thinking as client's thoughts compensate in response to presentation of reality. Provides opportunity for the client to control aggressive behavior. Enhances self-esteem and promotes safety for the client and others.

Assess rest/sleep pattern by observing capacity to fall asleep, quality of sleep. Graph sleep chart as indicated until acceptable pattern is established.

Delusions, hallucinations, etc., may interfere with client's sleep pattern. Fears may alter ability to fall asleep. Sleep deprivation can produce behaviors such as withdrawal, confusion, disturbance of perception. Sleep chart identifies abnormal patterns and is useful in evaluating effectiveness of interventions.

Structure appropriate times for rest and sleep; adjust work/rest activity patterns as needed.

Consistency in scheduling reduces fears/insecurities, which may be interfering with sleep. Sleep is enhanced by balancing activity (physical, occupational) with rest/sleep.

Help client identify/learn techniques that promote rest/sleep, e.g., quiet activities, soothing music before bedtime, regular hour for going to bed, drinking warm milk.

Enhances client's ability to optimize rest/sleep, enhancing ability to think clearly.

Assess presence/degree of factors affecting client's capacity for diversional activities.

Presence of hallucinations/delusions; situational factors such as long-term hospitalization (characterized by monotony, sensory deprivation); psychologic factors such as decreased volition; physical factors such as immobility contribute to deficits in diversional activity.

Monitor medication regimen, observing for therapeutic effect and side effects, e.g., anticholinergic (dry mouth, etc.), sedation, orthostatic hypotension, photosensitivity, hormonal effects, reduction of seizure threshold, agranulocytosis, and extrapyramidal symptoms. (Refer to ND: Knowledge Deficit [Learning Need].)

Enables identification of the minimal effective dose to reduce psychotic symptoms with the fewest adverse effects. Prevention of side effects/timely intervention may enhance cooperation with drug regimen. Identification of the onset of serious side effects, such as neuroleptic malignant syndrome, provides for appropriate interventions to avoid permanent damage.

### Collaborative

Administer medications as indicated, e.g.:
  antipsychotics (neuroleptics and psychotropics):
    phenothiazines, such as chlorpromazine (Thora-

Used for the reduction of psychotic symptoms. May be given orally or by injection. For long-term

| ACTIONS/INTERVENTIONS | RATIONALE |
|---|---|

### Collaborative

zine), thioridazine (Mellaril), fluphenazine (Prolixin), perphenazine (Trilafon); thioxanthenes, such as chlorprothixene (Taractan), thiothixene (Navane); butyrophenones, such as haloperidol (Haldol); dibenzoxazepines, such as loxapine (Loxitane);

maintenance therapy, depot neuroleptics may be the drugs of choice, when available, to maintain medication adherence and prevent relapse. When given at bedtime, the sedative effects of psychotropic medication can enhance quality of sleep and reduce hypotensive side effects.

clozapine (Clozaril),

Useful in treating clients resistant to other medications or in the presence of unacceptable side effects. Clozapine causes no muscular rigidity and a relatively low rate of akathisia. May not be used as first-line therapy because of a lowered seizure threshold or a 1%–2% potential for agranulocytosis, necessitating weekly blood testing for the duration of treatment. Note: Some sources use combination therapy, e.g., clozapine and a neuroleptic such as fluphenazine (Prolixin) or haloperidol.

risperidone (Risperdal);

Recently approved therapeutic agent proven effective that has been found to have few uncomfortable or serious side effects, especially agranulocytosis.

antiparkinsonism drugs, e.g.:

Used for relief of drug-induced extrapyramidal reactions and in treatment of all other forms of parkinsonism.

anticholinergics, such as trihexyphenidyl HCl (Artane), benztropine mesylate (Cogentin), procyclidine HCl (Kemadrin), biperiden HCl (Akineton);

Block action of acetylcholine, thereby reducing excitation of the basal ganglia.

antihistamines, such as diphenhydramine (Benadryl);

Suppresses cholinergic activity and prolongs action of dopamine by inhibiting its reuptake and storage.

miscellaneous, such as amantadine (Symmetrel).

Releases dopamine from presynaptic nerve endings in basal ganglia.

| NURSING DIAGNOSIS: | SENSORY/PERCEPTUAL ALTERATIONS (SPECIFY) |
|---|---|
| **May Be Related To:** | Panic levels of anxiety. |
| | Disturbance in thought, perception, affect, sense of self, volition, relationship to environment. |
| | Psychomotor behavior. |
| **Possibly Evidenced By:** | Illusions, delusions, and hallucinations. |
| | Disorientation. |
| | Changes in usual response to stimuli. |

| Desired Outcomes/Evaluation Criteria— Client Will: | Identify self in relationship to environment. |
| --- | --- |
| | Recognize reality and dismiss internal voices. |
| | Demonstrate improved cognitive, perceptual, affective, and psychomotor abilities. |

| ACTIONS/INTERVENTIONS | RATIONALE |
| --- | --- |

### Independent

| | |
| --- | --- |
| Assess the presence/severity of alterations in client's perceptions. Note possible causative/contributing factors, e.g., anxiety, substance abuse, fever, trauma, or other organic illnesses/conditions. | Provides information about client's behavior potentials regarding ADLs, sleep patterns, potential for violence (command hallucinations, homicide, suicide), nonverbal and verbal behaviors (content, form, style, flow). |
| Spend time with client, listening with regard and providing support for changes client is making. | Continued, consistent support/acceptance will reduce anxiety and fears and enable client to decrease altered perceptions. |
| Provide a safe environment by not arguing with or ridiculing the client. | Altered perceptions are frightening to the client and indicate loss of control. Because of lack of insight, client views altered perceptions as reality. Arguing only leads to defensiveness and a regressive struggle with the client. |
| Orient to reality by communicating effectively (clear, concise); reinforcing reality (of client's altered perceptions); and clarifying time, place, and person. | Client's distortion of reality is a defense against actual reality, which is more frightening. Reality orientation assists client to correctly interpret stimuli within the milieu. |
| Set limits on client's impulsive response to altered perceptions. Remain with the client and provide distraction when possible. | Client who is perceiving the environment incorrectly lacks internal controls to prevent impulsive response to misperceptions. Often client feels more in control if nurse remains in room. Distraction (music, TV, games) may also support client to regain capacity to control response to altered perceptions. |
| Be honest in expressing fears, especially if potential for violence is perceived. (Refer to ND: Violence, high risk for, directed at self/others.) | Informing client when behaviors are frightening and providing anticipatory guidance (by verbalizing actions) focuses attention on reality and assists in reducing anxiety. |

### Collaborative

| | |
| --- | --- |
| Provide external controls (quiet room, seclusion, restraints; inform client of intent to use touch) as indicated. | External limits and controls must be provided to protect client and others until client regains control internally and is able to ignore altered perceptions. |

| NURSING DIAGNOSIS: | COMMUNICATION, IMPAIRED, VERBAL |
| --- | --- |
| May Be Related To: | Psychologic barriers, psychosis. |
| | Autistic and delusional thinking. |
| | Alterations in perception. |

220

| **Possibly Evidenced By:** | Inability to verbalize rationally. |
| --- | --- |
| | Verbal expressions, such as neologisms, echo-lalia, associative/looseness, paralogic language. |
| | Nonverbal expressions, such as echopraxia-stereotypic behaviors (bizarre gesturing, facial expressions, and posturing). |
| **Desired Outcomes/Evaluation Criteria—Client Will:** | Verbalize or indicate an understanding of communication problems. |
| | Employ strategies to communicate effectively both verbally and nonverbally. |
| | Establish means of communication in which needs can be understood. |

| ACTIONS/INTERVENTIONS | RATIONALE |
| --- | --- |
| **Independent** | |
| Evaluate degree/type of communication impairment. | Degree of impairment of verbal/nonverbal communications (loose associations, neologisms, echolalia, and echopraxia) will affect client's ability to interact with staff and others and to participate in care. |
| Demonstrate a listening attitude within the nurse-client relationship. | A listening attitude enables the nurse to listen carefully, observe the client, and anticipate and watch certain patterns of client's communications that may emerge. |
| Acknowledge client's difficulty in communicating. | Recognition of client's difficulty in expressing ideas and feelings demonstrates empathy, lessening anxiety and enabling client to concentrate on communicating. |
| Provide a nonthreatening environment/safe forum for client's communications. | Atmosphere in which a person feels free to express self without fear of criticism helps to meet safety needs, increasing trust and providing assurance for tolerance and validation of appropriate negative communications. |
| Accept use of alternative communications, such as drawing, singing, dancing, mime. | Increases client's feelings of security, provides avenues for expressing needs. |
| Avoid arguing or agreeing with inaccurate communications; simply offer reality view in nonjudgmental style (communicate your lack of understanding to client). | Arguing is nontherapeutic and may cause the client to become defensive. Agreeing with the client's expression of inaccurate communication reinforces misinterpretation of reality. |
| Use therapeutic communications skills, such as paraphrasing, reflecting, clarification. | Client's flow of communications (too fast/too slow) may require regulation. These techniques assist with reality orientation, thereby minimizing misinterpretation and facilitating accurate communications. |

| ACTIONS/INTERVENTIONS | RATIONALE |
|---|---|
| **Independent** | |
| Be open and honest in therapeutic use of verbal and nonverbal communications. | Client has increased sensitivity to nonverbal messages. Honesty increases sense of trust, a loss of which is at the base of client's problem. Openness and genuineness in expression of feelings provide a role model for client. |
| Use a supportive approach to client by communicating desire to understand (ask client to help you do so). | Recognizes that client's past experiences have created distrust, which produces attempt to maintain distance by being vague and unclear in sending messages. |
| Identify the symbolic, primitive nature of the client's speech/communications. Note: Cultural beliefs (e.g., talking to dead relatives) may be accepted as normal within the client's culture. | Recognition of the symbolism of the client's primitive speech and thinking enables the nurse to better understand the client's feelings. Without this recognition, the actual communications may be vague and disorganized, indicating client's inability to focus and perceive clearly. Cultural attitudes need to be considered to avoid confusion with pathologic condition. |

| NURSING DIAGNOSIS: | COPING, INDIVIDUAL, INEFFECTIVE |
|---|---|
| **May Be Related To:** | Personal vulnerability; inadequate support system(s). |
| | Unrealistic perceptions. |
| | Inadequate coping methods. |
| | Disintegration of thought processes. |
| **Possibly Evidenced By:** | Impaired judgment, cognition, and perception. |
| | Diminished problem-solving/decision-making capacities. |
| | Poor self-esteem. |
| | Chronic anxiety and depression. |
| | Inability to perform role expectations. |
| | Alteration in social participation. |
| **Desired Outcomes/Evaluation Criteria— Client Will:** | Identify ineffective coping behaviors and consequences. |
| | Demonstrate understanding of and begin to use appropriate, constructive, effective methods for coping. |
| | Display behavior congruent with verbalization of feelings. |

| ACTIONS/INTERVENTIONS | RATIONALE |
|---|---|
| **Independent** | |
| Determine the presence/degree of impairment of client's coping abilities. | Provides information about perceived and actual coping ability, life change units, anxiety level, stresses (internal, external), developmental level of functioning, use of defense mechanisms, and problem-solving ability. |
| Assist client to identify/discuss thoughts, perceptions, and feelings. | Client is able to view how perceptions/thinking/affect is processed and to strengthen reality orientation and coping skills. |
| Encourage client to express areas of concern. Support formulation of realistic goals and learning of appropriate problem-solving techniques. | This disorder first manifests itself at an early age, before the client has had an opportunity to learn effective coping skills. In a trusting relationship (a climate of acceptance), the client can begin to learn these skills, without fear of judgment. |
| Encourage client to identify precipitants that led to ineffective coping, when possible. | Knowledge of stressors that have precipitated deteriorated coping ability enables client to recognize and deal with these factors before problems occur. |
| Explore how client's perceptions are validated prior to drawing conclusions. | With support, client has the opportunity to learn to validate perceptions before selecting ineffective/inappropriate coping methods (such as acting-out behavior). |
| Assist client to recognize/develop appropriate/effective coping skills. | Increased/more flexible problem-solving/coping behaviors prevent decompensation (distorted reality, delusional system). |

| | |
|---|---|
| **NURSING DIAGNOSIS:** | **SELF-ESTEEM, CHRONIC LOW/ROLE PERFORMANCE, ALTERED/PERSONAL IDENTITY DISTURBANCE** |
| **May Be Related To:** | Disintegrated thought processes (perception, cognition, affect). |
| | Loose/disintegration of ego boundaries. |
| | Perceived threats to the self. |
| | Disintegration of behavior, affect. |
| **Possibly Evidenced By:** | Expressions of worthlessness, negative feelings about self. |
| | Impaired judgment, cognition, and perception; protective delusional systems; disturbed sense of self (depersonalization and delusions of control). |
| | Role performance deterioration in family, social, and work areas. |

223

|  | Inadequate development of self-esteem and hopefulness. |
|---|---|
|  | Ambivalence and autism (interfering with acceptance of self and meaning of own existence). |
| **Desired Outcomes/Evaluation Criteria—Client Will:** | Demonstrate enhanced sense of self by decreasing episodes of depersonalization and delusions. |
|  | Verbalize feelings of value/worthwhileness and view self as competent and socially acceptable (by self and others). |
|  | Develop appropriate plans for improvement of role performance that promote highest possible level of adaptive functioning. |
|  | Demonstrate self-directedness by expressing own needs and desires and making effective decisions. |
|  | Participate in activities with others. |

| ACTIONS/INTERVENTIONS | RATIONALE |
|---|---|
| **Independent** | |
| Assess the degree of disturbance in client's self-concept. | Documents own and others' perceptions, client's goals, significant losses/changes. Provides basis for evaluation of progress/therapy needs. |
| Spend time with client; listen with positive regard and acceptance. | Conveys empathy, acceptance, support, which enhances client's self-esteem. Personal identity is strengthened as client identifies with the nurse and experiences therapeutic caring within the relationship. |
| Encourage client to verbalize areas of concern/feelings. | Self-esteem is improved by increased insight into feelings. Insight is gained as client verbalizes/identifies feelings, e.g., inadequacy, worthlessness, rejection, loneliness. |
| Assist client to identify how negative feelings decrease self-esteem. | Negative feelings can lead to severe anxiety and/or suspiciousness. Increased awareness/perception of factors that cause negative feelings can assist client to recognize how negative feelings cause deterioration. |
| Encourage client to recognize positive characteristics related to self. | Discussion of positive aspects of the self-system, such as social skills, work abilities, education, talents, and appearance, can reinforce client's feelings of being a worthwhile/competent person. |
| Review personal appearance and things client can do to enhance hygiene/grooming. (Refer to ND: Self-Care deficit [specify].) | Positive personal appearance enhances body image and respect for self. |
| Encourage client to participate in appropriate activities/exercise program. | Enhances capacity for interpersonal relationships (in 1:1 and small groups.) Activities that use the 5 senses increase the sense of self. Physical exercise promotes positive sense of well-being. |

| ACTIONS/INTERVENTIONS | RATIONALE |
|---|---|

### Independent

Assess client's capacity to tolerate use of touch carefully.

Use of touch can help client to reestablish body boundaries (if the experience can be tolerated).

Provide positive reinforcement for client's abilities/ efforts.

Positive feedback increases self-esteem, provides encouragement, and promotes a sense of self-direction.

Determine current level of role performance and note causative/contributing factors that affect it.

Factors such as inadequate knowledge, role conflict, alteration of self/others' perceptions of role, and change in usual patterns of responsibility can affect the client's physical and psychologic capacity for effective role performance.

Assist the client to adapt to changing role performance by working with client/significant other(s) to develop strategies for dealing with disturbances in role and enhancing expectations of coping effectively.

The client's eventual level of performance may be positively influenced by a support system that is responsive and caring.

Help client set realistic goals for managing life and performing own ADLs.

Client needs to be productive and benefits from being given the responsibility for own life and direction within limits of ability.

Assess the current sense of personal identity, considering if client acknowledges sense of self (observe how client addresses self, e.g., may refer to self in third person) or expresses feelings of unreadiness, merging with people/objects.

Identifies individual needs, appropriate interventions. Inability to identify self poses a major problem that can interfere with person's interactions with others.

Analyze the presence/severity of factors that alter personal identity, e.g., paranoia, blunted affect.

Disintegrated ego boundaries can cause a weakened sense of self. Clients often express fears of merging and losing personal identity.

Assess presence/severity of factors that affect client's religious/spiritual orientation. Note presence of religiosity.

Disintegrated behaviors create such factors as displaced anger toward God, expression of concern with meaning of life/death/values (may be expressed as delusions, hallucinations). These concerns may negatively affect the individual's sense of self-worth. Client may use religious beliefs as a defense against fears.

Use therapeutic communication skills to support client's verbalization of sense of self and to discover its relationship to meaning of existence.

Therapeutic communications, such as Active-listening, summarizing, reflection, can support client to find own solutions.

Facilitate early discharge for client when hospitalization has been required.

Clients can increase their sense of self by early return to own milieu surrounded by personal possessions.

### Collaborative

Administer appropriate tests, e.g., ask client to draw a stick figure of self, Body Image Aberration, Physical Anhedonia Scale.

These tests demonstrate client's view, concept of self, and its correlation to many variables.

| ACTIONS/INTERVENTIONS | RATIONALE |
|---|---|

### Collaborative

Refer to resources such as occupational therapist/movement therapy/Outdoor Education program; partial hospitalization program.

Provides activities that promote feelings of self-worth and accomplishment during involvement with others. Partial hospitalization may enhance return from hospital setting to community.

Initiate involvement in/refer to religious activities and resources as desired or appropriate. Note over-involvement in religious activity.

Spiritual resources such as a pattern of prayer, a sense of faith, or membership in an organized religious group may enhance the development of client's coping resources, sense of acceptance/self-worth. Strong attachment to an ideology (religiosity) may be used in an attempt to control feelings of anxiety.

| | |
|---|---|
| **NURSING DIAGNOSIS:** | **ANXIETY [specify level]/FEAR** |
| **May Be Related To:** | Disintegration of thought processes. |
| | Perception and affect occurring in response to overwhelming feelings of losing control; threat to self-concept. |
| | Change in environment, role functioning, interaction patterns. |
| | Extremes in psychomotor activity (occurring with chronicity or severity). |
| **Possibly Evidenced By:** | Inappropriate/regressed or absent responses; poor eye contact. |
| | Increased perception of danger; focus on self. |
| | Decreased problem-solving ability. |
| | Fear of perceived loss of control or approval from significant other(s); inappropriate response to such feelings; hurting self or others. |
| | Psychomotor disturbances varying from excited motor behavior to immobility. |
| **Desired Outcomes/Evaluation Criteria— Client Will:** | Respond appropriately to feelings of overwhelming anxiety (fears, loss of control, feelings of rejection) by decreasing regressive behaviors (disintegrated thinking/perception/affect). |
| | Communicate anxious feelings openly in an acceptable manner. |
| | Orient to reality as evidenced by interpreting milieu correctly. |
| | Verbalize no perceived danger in interactions with others. |

| ACTIONS/INTERVENTIONS | RATIONALE |
|---|---|
| **Independent** | |
| Note the level of the client's anxiety, considering severity, unfulfilled needs, misperceptions, present use of defense mechanisms, and coping skills. | The weakened ego of schizophrenia causes a decreased capacity to distinguish reality and a diminished capacity to problem-solve. This can result in a heightened sense of helplessness and anxiety. |
| Assess the degree and reality of the fears currently perceived by the client. | The client's experience of fear may contribute to decreased coping capacity and increased anxiety/fear. |
| Establish trust, through a patient, supportive, caring, and accepting relationship. | Trust, which is difficult for schizophrenic clients, is the basis of a therapeutic nurse-client relationship. The mutuality of the 1:1 experience enables clients to work through their fears and to identify appropriate methods for problem-solving by role-modeling within the 1:1. |
| Encourage the client to verbalize fears. | Verbalization of frightening perceptions (fears) reduces withdrawal and/or potential for violence (projection of aggressive impulses). |
| Assist client to identify/communicate sources of anxiety and areas of concern. Monitor for drug effectiveness/side effects. | Anxiety can arise from misperceived threats to self, unfulfilled needs, and perceived losses (of control/approval). Disintegration of thinking/perception/affect may be reduced as client verbalizes frightening feelings. Alertness for prevention of medication side effects can reduce frightening physiologic experiences that can escalate anxiety. |
| Demonstrate/encourage use of effective, constructive strategies for coping with anxiety, e.g., relaxation and thought-stopping techniques, meditation, and physical exercise. Use role-modeling, positive reinforcement. (Refer to NDs: Communication, impaired: verbal; Sensory/Perceptual alterations.) | Maladaptive coping needs to be examined with emphasis on ineffectiveness of outcomes. Reduces secondary gain and enables client to learn more adaptive/effective decision-making, problem-solving, coping skills. |
| Remain with the client and clarify reality. | Assists the client to achieve effective coping. The presence of a trusted individual can help client feel protected from external dangers and maintain contact with reality. |
| Involve client in planning treatment. | Participation in treatment increases client's sense of control and provides opportunity to practice problem-solving skills. |

| NURSING DIAGNOSIS: | SOCIAL ISOLATION |
|---|---|
| **May Be Related To:** | Disturbed thought processes that result in mistrust of others/delusional thinking. |
| | Environmental deprivation, institutionalization (as a result of long-term hospitalization). |

| Possibly Evidenced By: | Difficulty in establishing relationships with others; social withdrawal/isolation of self. |
| | Expressions of feelings of rejection. |
| | Dealing with problems using anger/hostility and violence. |
| Desired Outcomes/Evaluation Criteria— Client Will: | Verbalize willingness to be involved with othe |
| | Participate in activities/programs with others. |
| | Develop 1 : 1 trust-based relationship. |

| ACTIONS/INTERVENTIONS | RATIONALE |
| --- | --- |
| **Independent** | |
| Assess presence/degree of isolation by listening to client's comments about loneliness. | Mistrust can lead to difficulty in establishing r latationships, and client may have withdrawn fr close contacts with others. |
| Spend time with client. Make brief, short interactions that communicate interest, concern, and caring. | Establishes a trusting relationship. Consistent, brief, honest contact with the nurse can help the c begin to reestablish trusting interactions with othe |
| Plan appropriate times for activities (by limiting withdrawal, varying daily routine only as tolerated). | Consistency in 1 : 1 relationship and sameness milieu are required initially to enable client to crease withdrawn behavior. Motivation is stim lated by the humanistic sharing of a 1 : 1 experi ence. |
| Assist client to participate in diversional activities and limited/planned interaction situations with others in group meeting/unit party, etc. | With toleration of 1 : 1 relationship and strengt ened ego boundaries, client will be able to incr socialization and enter small-group situations. Brief encounters can help the client to become |
| more | comfortable in the company of others and prov an opportunity to try out new social skills. |
| Identify support systems available to the client, e.g., family, friends, coworkers, etc. | Support is an important part of the client's re-habilitation, providing a network to assist in so recovery. |
| Assess family relationships, communication patterns, knowledge of client condition. | Problems within family (poor social/relationsl skills, high expressed emotion) may interfere v client's progress and indicate need for family therapy. |
| Note client's sense of self-worth and belief about individual identity/role within milieu and family setting. (Refer to NDs: Self-Esteem, chronic low; Role Performance, altered; Personal Identity dis- | When client feels good about self and own valu interactions with others are enhanced. |

| NURSING DIAGNOSIS: | PHYSICAL MOBILITY, IMPAIRED, high risk for |
|---|---|
| Risk Factors May Include: | Disintegration of thought and behavior. |
| | Perceptual impairment; sensory overload/deprivation. |
| | Psychomotor retardation; diminished muscle strength; impaired coordination and limited range of motion/total immobility. |
| | Psychomotor activity (occurring with chronicity or severity) varying from excited motor behavior to immobility. |
| Possibly Evidenced By: | [Not applicable; presence of signs and symptoms establishes an **actual** diagnosis]. |
| Desired Outcomes/Evaluation Criteria— Client Will: | Maintain optimal mobility and muscle strength. |
| | Demonstrate awareness of the environment (psychomotor behavior) and capacity to regulate psychomotor activity. |
| | Engage in physical activities. |

| ACTIONS/INTERVENTIONS | RATIONALE |
|---|---|
| **Independent** | |
| Determine the level of impairment (rate from complete independence to dependence with social withdrawal) in relation to preillness capacity, considering age, meaning (motivation, desire, tolerance), onset, duration, coordination, range of motion, muscle strength, and control. Measure capacity for activity by observing endurance (attention span, psychomotor response, appropriateness of participation). | Provides information to determine the amount of nursing assistance required and client potentials. |
| Note the presence/severity of factors that affect the client's level of mobility, such as psychotic functioning, control needs, sensory overload/deprivation. | These factors need to be considered in planning nursing care, as they can affect client's ability to perform at appropriate activity level. |
| Encourage client to identify need for/plan resumption of activities/exercise. | As psychotic functioning decreases, the capacity to relate to milieu/others and to self-initiate increases. Involving client in scheduling activities provides client with sense of independence (control over environment). |
| Determine current activity level appropriate for client by assessing attention span, capacity to tolerate others in milieu. | Presence of psychotic features can cause mental/emotional withdrawal or agitation. |
| Structure appropriate times for exercise/activity (turning/moving unaffected body parts); monitor environmental stimulations such as radio, TV, visitors. | Movement reduces physiologic deterioration. Environmental stimulation can be used to maintain/promote sensory-perceptual capacity. |

229

| ACTIONS/INTERVENTIONS | RATIONALE |
|---|---|

**Independent**

| | |
|---|---|
| Schedule adequate periods of rest/sleep. Monitor client's response and set limits as needed. | Establishing a regular sleep pattern helps client to become rested, reducing fatigue, and may improve ability to think. When client is able to think more clearly, participation in treatment program may be enhanced. |

| NURSING DIAGNOSIS: | VIOLENCE, HIGH RISK FOR, DIRECTED AT SELF/OTHERS |
|---|---|
| Risk Factors May Include: | Disintegrated thought processes stemming from ambivalence and autistic thinking; hallucinations, delusions. |
| | Lack of development of trust and appropriate interpersonal relationships. |
| Possible Indicators: | Disintegrated behaviors. |
| | Perception of environmental and other stimuli/cues as threatening. |
| | Physical aggression to self; irrational, threatening, or assaultive behavior. |
| | Religiosity. |
| Desired Outcomes/Evaluation Criteria—Client Will: | Resolve conflicts and/or cope with anxiety without the use of threats or assaultive behavior (to self or others). |
| | Participate in care and meet own needs in an assertive manner. |
| | Demonstrate self-control, as evidenced by relaxed posture, nonviolent behavior. |

| ACTIONS/INTERVENTIONS | RATIONALE |
|---|---|

**Independent**

| | |
|---|---|
| Assess the presence/degree of client's potential for violence (toward self or others) on a 1–10 scale. Determine suicidal/homicidal intent, indications of loss of control over behavior (actual or perceived), hostile verbal/nonverbal behaviors, risk factors, and prior/present coping skills. | Information essential for planning nursing care and documents degree of intent. (May be no. 1 nursing priority if score is high.) Prior history of violent behavior increases risk for violence, as would factors such as command hallucinations. |
| Provide safe, quiet environment; tell client "you are safe." | Keeping environmental stimuli to a minimum and providing reassurance will help prevent agitation. |
| Be careful in offering a pat on the shoulder/hug, etc. | Touch may be misinterpreted as an aggressive gesture. |
| Encourage verbalizations of feelings and promote acceptable verbal outlet(s) for expression, e.g., yelling in room. | Ventilation of feelings may reduce need for inappropriate physical action. |

| ACTIONS/INTERVENTIONS | RATIONALE |
|---|---|

### Independent

| | |
|---|---|
| Assist client to identify situations that trigger anxiety/aggressive behaviors. | Promotes understanding of relationship between severe anxiety and situations that result in destructive feelings leading to aggressive actions. |
| Explore implications and consequences of handling these situations with aggression. | Helps client to realize the possibility and importance of thinking through a situation before acting. |
| Assist client to define alternatives to aggressive behaviors. Initially engage in solitary physical activities, instead of group. Monitor competitive activities; use with caution. | Enables client to learn to handle situations in a socially acceptable manner. Appropriate outlets will allow for release of hostility. Anxiety and fear may escalate during activities in which the client perceives self in competition with others and can trigger violent behavior. |
| Set limits, stating in a clear, specific, firm manner what is acceptable/unacceptable. Use demands only when situation requires. | Being clear and remaining calm increase chance that client will cooperate, lessening potential for violence. Having few but important limits enhances chances of having them observed. |
| Be alert to signs of impending violent behavior: increase in psychomotor activity; intensity of affect; verbalization of delusional thinking, especially threatening expressions; frightening hallucinations. | Therapeutic interventions are more effective before behavior becomes violent. |
| Accept verbal hostility without retaliation or defense. Nurse (caregiver) needs to be aware of own response to client behavior, e.g., anger/fear. | Behavior is not usually directed at nurse personally, and responding defensively will tend to exacerbate situations. Looking at meaning behind the words will be more productive. Awareness of own response allows nurse to express/deal with those feelings. |
| Isolate promptly in nonpunitive manner, using adequate help if violent behavior occurs. Hold client if necessary. Tell client to STOP behavior. | Removal to quiet environment can help calm client. Usually the individual is being self-critical and afraid of own hostility and does not need external criticism. Sufficient help will prevent injury to client/staff. Often holding client and/or saying "Stop" is enough to help client regain control. |

### Collaborative

| | |
|---|---|
| Apply restraints or put in seclusion as indicated, documenting reasons for action. | May be needed for short-term control until client regains control over self. |
| Administer medications as indicated. (Refer to ND: Thought Processes, altered.) | Used to reduce psychotic symptoms, decrease delusional thinking, and assist client to regain control of self. |

---

**NURSING DIAGNOSIS:**

**May Be Related To:**

**SELF-CARE DEFICIT (specify)**

Perceptual and cognitive impairment.

Immobility resulting from social withdrawal, isolation, and decreased psychomotor activity.

| | |
|---|---|
| | Autonomic nervous system side effects of psychotropic medications. |
| **Possibly Evidenced By:** | Inability/difficulty feeding self, keeping body clean, dressing appropriately, and/or toileting self. |
| | Bladder stasis/paralysis; urinary calculi formation. |
| | Decreased bowel activity with constipation, fecal impaction, and/or paralytic ileus. |
| **Desired Outcomes/Evaluation Criteria— Client Will:** | Perform self-care and ADLs at highest level of adaptive functioning possible. |
| | Recognize cues/maintain elimination patterns, preventing complications. |
| | Identify/use resources available for assistance. |

| ACTIONS/INTERVENTIONS | RATIONALE |
|---|---|
| **Independent** | |
| Determine current vs. preillness level of self-care (specify levels 0–4) re: feeding, bathing/hygiene, dressing/grooming, toileting. | Identifies potentials and determines degree of nursing care to be provided. |
| Assess presence/severity of factors that affect client's capacity for self-care, e.g., disintegrative perceptual/cognitive abilities, mobility status. | Impairment in these areas can alter client's ability/readiness for self-care. |
| Discuss personal appearance/grooming and encourage dressing in bright colors, attractive clothes. Give positive feedback for efforts. | Appearance affects how the client sees self. A rundown, disheveled appearance conveys a sense of low self-worth, while an attractive, well-put-together appearance conveys a positive sense of self to the client as well as to others. |
| Determine client's regular elimination patterns and compare with current pattern. Note contributing factors, e.g., anxiety, decreased attention span, disorientation, reduced psychomotor activity, as well as use of psychotropic medications. | Identifies appropriate interventions, as patterns of elimination are individually influenced by physiologic, cultural, and psychologic factors. These factors can affect toileting, e.g., client does not pay attention to cues; dehydration from inadequate intake results in lessened urinary output and contributes to constipation; anticholinergic effect of medication may result in urinary retention. |
| Encourage/provide diet high in fiber and at least 2 liters of fluid each day. (Refer to NDs: Fluid Volume deficit, high risk for; Nutrition, altered, less/more than body requirements.) | A diet high in fiber and residue promotes bulk formation and at least 2 liters of fluid daily regulates stool consistency (facilitating bowel elimination) and renal function. |
| Observe/record urinary output. Note changes in color, odor, clarity. Encourage client to observe/report changes. | Bladder paralysis/retention can occur from psychotropic medications, increasing risk of infection. |

232

| ACTIONS/INTERVENTIONS | RATIONALE |
|---|---|

### Independent

Establish increasing daily activity level as client progresses. Include regular intervals for toileting.

Adequate exercise increases muscle tone; consistency in daily routine stimulates bowel elimination. A schedule prevents accidents that can occur due to polyuria from psychotropic medication or decreased attentiveness to cues and psychomotor activity.

### Collaborative

Plan with client for effective use of community resources, such as nutritional programs, sheltered workshops, group/transitional/apartment homes, home care services.

Assists client to develop an effective plan for hygienic/self-care needs.

Administer laxatives/stool softeners, as indicated.

Used cautiously for brief period or as needed to enhance bowel function. Overuse promotes dependency.

| NURSING DIAGNOSIS: | FLUID VOLUME DEFICIT, HIGH RISK FOR |
|---|---|
| **Risk Factors May Include:** | Disintegrated patterns of thinking and behavior. |
| | Altered eating/drinking patterns. |
| | Excessive renal losses (side effects of some psychotropic medications). |
| **Possibly Evidenced By:** | [Not applicable; presence of signs and symptoms establishes an **actual** diagnosis.] |
| **Desired Outcomes/Evaluation Criteria— Client Will:** | Verbalize understanding of need for fluid. |
| | Recognize physical cues of thirst. |
| | Ingest indivdually appropriate amount of fluid. |
| | Demonstrate adequate fluid balance with appropriate urinary output, stable vital signs, moist mucous membranes, good skin turgor. |

| ACTIONS/INTERVENTIONS | RATIONALE |
|---|---|

### Independent

Assess presence/severity of factors that affect client's fluid intake.

Factors such as physical immobility, psychotropic medications, mental status, can cause fluid volume imbalance.

Record intake/output; monitor mental status, vital signs, weight, skin turgor. Note medication interactions/side effects.

Careful monitoring and early recognition of symptoms can prevent complications. If oral intake is not adequate, orthostatic hypotension may develop. Dehydration/reduced circulating volume directly affects cerebral perfusion/mentation. Dry mucous membranes, decreased skin turgor can oc-

## Independent

cur, increasing risk of tissue breakdown. Polyuria is a frequent side effect of psychotropics, further affecting fluid balance.

| ACTIONS/INTERVENTIONS | RATIONALE |
|---|---|
| Structure/encourage appropriate times for fluid intake. | Scheduling of intake provides for an accurate record and helps to ensure that adequate amounts are ingested. |
| Encourage measures such as frequent mouth care, chewing sugarless gum or sucking on hard (sugarless) candy, and drinking lemonade. | Reduces oral cavity discomfort associated with dehydration/effects of medication. Note: Omit gum/hard candy for aged client when danger of choking is present (e.g, phenothiazines alter the swallowing reflex.) |

| NURSING DIAGNOSIS: | NUTRITION, ALTERED, LESS/MORE THAN BODY REQUIREMENTS |
|---|---|
| May Be Related To: | Imbalance between energy needs and intake. |
| | Disintegration of thought and perception. |
| | Inability/refusal to eat. |
| Possibly Evidenced By: | Delusions or hallucinations related to food intake. |
| | Reported dysfunctional eating patterns, e.g., eating in response to internal cues other than hunger; increased appetite (side effect of some psychotropic medications). |
| | Weight loss/gain. |
| | Sore, inflamed buccal cavity. |
| Desired Outcomes/Evaluation Criteria—Client Will: | Maintain adequate/appropriate nutritional intake. |
| | Demonstrate progressive weight gain/loss toward expected goal. |
| | Identify behaviors/lifestyle changes to maintain appropriate weight. |

ACTIONS/INTERVENTIONS                      RATIONALE

## Independent

| | |
|---|---|
| Assess presence/severity of factors that create altered nutritional intake. | Factors such as psychotic thinking or excessive activity to prevent frightening thoughts may cause inability/refusal to eat. |
| Review dietary intake via 24-hour recall/diary noting eating pattern and activity level. | Provides accurate information for assessment of client's nutritional status and needs. Alterations in dietary intake (decreased/increased calories, salt, fats, sugars) can aid in correcting faulty eating patterns. Lack of knowledge of appropriate dietary |

| ACTIONS/INTERVENTIONS | RATIONALE |
|---|---|
| **Independent** | |
| | needs, perception of food, and activity/exercise (immobility) results in improper caloric intake. |
| Encourage client to regulate caloric intake with activity/exercise program. | A balance of activity/exercise with appropriate caloric intake maintains weight loss/gain, improves nutritional status, and can improve mental functioning. |
| Structure consistent times for eating and limit use of food for other than nutritional needs. | Positively reinforces client's appropriate eating behaviors. Limits behaviors (rituals, acting out) that allow client to withdraw/refuse meals or overeat. Secondary gains that may occur can be reduced by setting appropriate expectations. |
| Provide small, frequent feedings as indicated. | May enhance intake when psychotic thought/behavior interferes with eating. |
| Encourage client to choose own food, when possible. | Individual is more likely to eat chosen food than what has been arbitrarily given to him or her, especially when paranoid thoughts of poisoning are present. |
| Assess presence/severity of factors that affect client's oral mucous membranes. Identify strategies to relieve or minimize altered/irritated oral mucous membranes, such as: rinsing with water, chewing sugarless gum/candy or glycerin-based cough drops, drinking lemonade, and mouth care before and after meals. | Altered nutrition can cause dehydration, edema, oral lesions, or altered salivation, which can adversely affect/restrict intake. With relief of dry mouth, client's anxiety is reduced, medication compliance may be increased, and nutritional intake enhanced. |
| **Collaborative** | |
| Arrange consultation with dietitian/nutritional team, as indicated. | May be necessary to establish/meet individual dietary needs. |

| | |
|---|---|
| **NURSING DIAGNOSIS:** | **FAMILY COPING, ineffective: disabling** |
| **May Be Related To:** | Ambivalent family system/relationships. |
| | Difficulty family members have in coping effectively with client's maladaptive behaviors. |
| **Possibly Evidenced By:** | Client's expressions of despair at family's lack of reaction/involvement. |
| | Neglectful relationships with client; impaired restructuring of a meaningful life for individual family members. |
| | Extreme distortion regarding client's health problem, including extreme denial about its existence/severity or prolonged overconcern. |
| **Desired Outcomes/Evaluation Criteria— Family Will:** | Verbalize realistic perception of roles within limits of individual situation. |

Express feelings appropriately, honestly, and openly.

Demonstrate improvement in communications (clear), problem-solving, behavior control, and affective spheres of family functioning.

| ACTIONS/INTERVENTIONS | RATIONALE |
| --- | --- |

### Independent

Compare current and preillness level of family functioning.

Provides information about client and family to assist in developing plan of care and choosing interventions. Note: Some family members may demonstrate psychopathologies that may make their influence detrimental to the client.

Determine whether family is high in expressed emotion, e.g., criticism, disappointment, hostility, solicitude, extreme worry, overprotectiveness, or emotional overinvolvement.

The emotional climate of the client's family has been shown to significantly affect the client's recovery. Relapse is associated with the expression of certain feelings in specific ways rather than emotional openness itself. Relapse occurs significantly more often in families high in expressed emotion (EE), especially criticism and hostility. Note: Some studies suggest EE may be more a response to the client's bizarre behavior, rather than a family trait, and may lessen as the condition persists and the family becomes used to the symptoms.

Provide opportunity for family members to discuss feelings, impact of disorder on family, and individual concerns.

Feelings of guilt, shame, isolation; loss of hopes/expectations regarding client; and concerns for personal and client safety impact family's ability to manage crisis and support client. Chronic nature of condition, with a wide range of socially, emotionally, and intellectually disabling symptoms that come and go unpredictably, can physically, emotionally, and financially exhaust family. The disproportionate allocation of resources can create deep feelings of resentment and family conflict as time and energy are focused on the client to the possible exclusion of the needs of other family members, and monetary expenses may restrict the family's ability to take vacations, go to college, or even consider retirement.

Assess readiness of family members/significant other(s) to participate in client's treatment.

Family theorists believe that identified client also represents disintegrated/enmeshed schizophrenogenic family system. Aftercare of client must include family/SO(s) to raise level of interpersonal functioning.

Provide honest information about the nature and seriousness of the disorder and enlist cooperation of family members to help client to remain in the community.

The family that already has maladaptive coping skills may have difficulty dealing with diagnosis and implications of a long-term illness. Client's behavior may be difficult and embarrassing for some families who have problematic coping skills or have a high profile in the community.

| ACTIONS/INTERVENTIONS | RATIONALE |
|---|---|
| **Independent** | |
| Promote family involvement with nurses/others to plan care and activities. | Involvement with others provides a role model for individuals to learn new behaviors/ways of handling stress. |
| Encourage client/family/SO(s) to identify and change maladaptive behaviors. | Client's success in treatment is dependent on effective change of whole systems rather than treatment of client's behaviors as a separate entity. |
| Establish/encourage ongoing open communication within the family. | Promotes healthy interaction, allows for timely problem-solving, and maintains effective relationships. |
| **Collaborative** | |
| Promote family involvement in behavioral management programs. | Helps family members to realize that while they can have a positive or negative influence on the course of the illness, they are doing the best they can in a difficult situation, blame is to be avoided, and communication/problem-solving skills can be learned to reduce stress. |
| Encourage family to participate in family education, therapy, community support groups. | Multiple stressors, labile nature of disorder, lack of definitive treatment options or resolution of condition increases likelihood of family conflict, disorganization, and even dissolution. Providing information about the disorder and showing family how to help the client without neglecting needs of family members and better ways to communicate with one another and with the client, as well as training families to identify and solve problems as they arise, enhance family coping and may lessen the rate of relapse. |
| Promote involvement with mental health treatment team (e.g., mental health center, family physician/psychiatrist, psychiatric/public health nurse, social/vocational services, occupational/physical therapist), and respite care, when necessary. | When bizarre behavior is difficult for family to manage, assistance/support may enhance coping, improve the situation, and provide opportunity for individual growth, strengthening the family unit. |
| Provide client/family/SO(s) with assistance to deal with current life situation, e.g., therapy (family/couples/1:1); aftercare services (day care centers, night hospitals, halfway houses, sheltered workshops, rehabilitation services). | Aftercare may include efforts to enlarge social spheres and increase client's/family's level of functioning, enhancing ability to manage long-term illness and enabling the client to remain in the community. |

| NURSING DIAGNOSIS: | FAMILY PROCESSES, ALTERED |
|---|---|
| **May Be Related To:** | Stiuational crisis (schizophrenic disorder present in family which normally functions effectively).<br><br>Change of roles. |

237

| Possibly Evidenced By: | Deterioration in family functioning. |
| --- | --- |
| | Failure to adapt to change/deal with crisis in a constructive manner and meet needs of its members. |
| | Difficulty in relating to each other for mutual growth/development; failure to send/receive clear messages. |
| | Ineffective family decision-making process. |
| **Desired Outcomes/Evaluation Criteria—Family Will:** | Express feelings regarding illness and altered coping openly and appropriately. |
| | Verbalize understanding of illness, treatment regimen, and prognosis. |
| | Encourage and allow member who is ill to handle situation in own way. |
| | Engage in problem-solving for resumption of highest possible adaptive level of functioning. |

| ACTIONS/INTERVENTIONS | RATIONALE |
| --- | --- |
| **Independent** | |
| Determine current and preillness level of family functioning. Note factors such as problem-solving skills, level of interpersonal relationships, outside support systems, roles, boundaries, rules, and communications. | These factors affect the family's capacity for returning to precrisis level of adaptive functioning as well as set the tone/expectations for a favorable prognosis. |
| Assess readiness of the family/SO(s) to reintegrate client into system, such as family's ability to use assistance or to cope with crisis appropriately by adaptation or change. | Ability to tolerate and assist with management of client behavior affects client's reentry into the family system. |
| Assist family to identify potential for growth of family system and individual members. Role-model positive behaviors during this process. | Family that has previously functioned well has skills to build on and can learn new ways of dealing with changed family structure and challenges of marginally functioning family member. The nurse can provide an example for learning new skills. |
| **Collaborative** | |
| Provide information about/referrals to therapy (family, couples, group) and supportive community resources (halfway houses, vocational counseling, day care centers, sheltered workshops, night hospitals). | Can provide assistance to help the family cope effectively with client's disintegrative behaviors. Having opportunity to take time away from situation enhances ability to manage long-term illness. |

| NURSING DIAGNOSIS: | HEALTH MAINTENANCE ALTERED/HOME MAINTENANCE MANAGEMENT, IMPAIRED |
|---|---|
| May Be Related To: | Impaired perception, cognition, communication skills, and individual coping skills. |
| | Inadequate developmental task accomplishment; lack of knowledge. |
| | Inability or lack of cooperation. |
| | Lower socioeconomic group with limited resources. |
| | Impaired or diminished family functioning. |
| Possibly Evidenced By: | Mistrust, lack of autonomy, and disturbed capacity for relationship formation. |
| | Impairment of personal support system (e.g., family conflict/disorganization). |
| | Decreased capacity to identify and mobilize adequate support systems and maintain a safe, growth-promoting immediate environment. |
| Desired Outcomes/Evaluation Criteria— Client Will: | Maintain optimal health and family functioning through improved communications and coping skills. |
| | Return home and maintain optimal wellness with minimal complications. |
| | Identify and use resources effectively. |

| ACTIONS/INTERVENTIONS | RATIONALE |
|---|---|
| **Independent** | |
| Assess present and preillness level of home/health maintenance. Consider deficits in communication, knowledge, decision-making, developmental tasks, support systems and their effect on client's basic health practices. | Dysfunction in family (diminished problem-solving, poor financial management/inadequate resources, and ineffective support system; emotional impoverishment), and lack of motivation to participate in treatment can impair functioning. |
| Identify readiness of client/SO(s) to maintain safe, growth-promoting environment that meets individual's needs. | Assisting client/SO(s) to develop a plan for a safe, well-ordered household can enable nurse to assess capacity for/compliance with home/health management needs. |
| Assist client/family to identify appropriate health-care needs/practices, e.g., dental, physician/clinic, regular hygiene practices, as well as some social contacts. | Poor organizational capacity for ADLs and socialization as well as personal involvement can lead to neglect of these areas. |
| Involve client/SO(s) in the development of a long-term plan for optimal home health management, encouraging identification/use of resources. | Involvement increases the potential for cooperation with the plan. |

239

| ACTIONS/INTERVENTIONS | RATIONALE |
|---|---|

### Collaborative

Provide referrals to resources, e.g., appropriate support, health teams (mental health center group/day care; family, community, and other support systems).

Ineffective coping requires support/teaching, which often necessitates referrals. Legal assistance may be required to provide conservatorships and client advocacy.

| NURSING DIAGNOSIS: | **KNOWLEDGE DEFICIT, [LEARNING NEED] regarding condition, prognosis, and treatment needs** |
|---|---|
| **May Be Related To:** | Cognitive limitation (altered thought process/psychosis). |
| | Misinterpretation/inaccurate information; unfamiliarity with information resources. |
| | Chronic nature of the disorder. |
| **Possibly Evidenced By:** | Ambivalence and dependency strivings. |
| | Inappropriate or exaggerated behaviors; need-fear dilemma and withdrawal (can lead to abrupt termination of therapy, medication). |
| | Inaccurate follow-through of instructions; appearance of side effects of psychotropic medications. |
| | Recidivism. |
| **Desired Outcomes/Evaluation Criteria— Client Will:** | Verbalize understanding of disorder and treatment. |
| | Participate in learning process/treatment regimen. |
| | Assume responsibility for own learning within individual abilities. |

| ACTIONS/INTERVENTIONS | RATIONALE |
|---|---|

### Independent

Determine the current level of knowledge about the disorder and its management.

Identifies areas of need and misperceptions. Communication skills such as validation of perceptions can assist in assessment of accuracy of client's knowledge base and readiness to learn.

Assess the presence/severity of factors that affect client's cognitive framework for decision-making about disorder and management, noting lack of recall, ignorance of resources and their use.

Factors such as disintegrated thinking, cognitive deficits, ambivalence, denial, and dependency needs can limit learning/block use of knowledge for management of disorder.

Instruct client/family about disorder, its signs and symptoms, management (medication, ADLs, vocational rehabilitation, socialization needs).

Provides information and can promote independent behaviors within client's ability.

| ACTIONS/INTERVENTIONS | RATIONALE |
|---|---|
| **Independent** | |
| Identify/review risk factors of medications client is taking, e.g., sedation, postural hypotension, photosensitivity, hormonal effects, agranulocytosis, and extrapyramidal symptoms (tremors, akinesia/akathisia, dystonia, oculogyric crisis, and tardive dyskinesia). | The anticholinergic effects of psychotropics (and antiparkinsonian drugs that may be given concomitantly to decrease the incidence of extrapyramidal effects of neuroleptics) alter autonomic nervous system functioning and may cause dry mouth (xerostomia), oral lesions, or hemorrhagic gingivitis. Most side effects occur within the first few weeks of treatment and subside with time. However, signs indicative of agranulocytosis (sore throat, malaise), extrapyramidal symptoms, and tardive dyskinesia need immediate attention. |
| Emphasize importance of immediate medical attention for onset of high fever and severe muscle stiffness and discontinuation of the medication until seen by the doctor. | Severe muscle stiffness and high fever are the hallmarks of neuroleptic malignant syndrome, which can usually be effectively treated before it becomes life-threatening if it is detected early. |
| Have client verbalize/paraphrase knowledge gained. | Evaluates comprehension of information regarding disorder's characteristics and management needs and may reduce recidivism. |
| Assist the client to develop strategies for continuing treatment. Make contract with client to provide for actions to take when problems arise. | Instructing the client/SO(s) that feeling better is no indication for discontinuing medication and that no addiction can develop with continued treatment and providing for self-administration often enhances cooperation, reducing medication discontinuation. |
| Establish schedule for follow-up/postdischarge care. Assess client's verbalizations, refusal of medications, or other treatment strategies (socialization, vocation, exercise, and diet). | Monitoring of client's behavior may reveal indications of willingness/ability to continue treatment. |
| Identify group, family, and individual therapies and community support systems. | Promotes trusting relationships and encourages further cooperation with treatment plan. Adequate management plans and organizing social supports for the family enable these clients to remain in the community. |

| NURSING DIAGNOSIS: | SEXUAL DYSFUNCTION |
|---|---|
| **May Be Related To:** | Ego boundary disintegration; inability to distinguish between self and environment. |
| | Weakened sexual identification; gender identity confusion, which interferes with normal sexual orientation formation. |
| | Development of delusions around the primitive sexual orientation. |
| | Lack of drive and energy, normal social inhibitions, and passivity. |

| | |
|---|---|
| **Possibly Evidenced By:** | Uninhibited sexual behavior; involvement in multiple sexual liaisons. |
| | Preoccupation with sex or gender identity. |
| | Inability to find sexual partner. |
| | Endocrine changes associated with antipsychotic drugs, e.g., ejaculatory inhibitions, impotence in men/amenorrhea in women, decreased libido. |
| **Desired Outcomes/Evaluation Criteria— Client Will:** | Strengthen ego boundaries to enable identification and acceptance of sexual orientation. |
| | Verbalize understanding of, identify, and report changes in body functions (if they occur) while taking antipsychotics. |
| | Demonstrate behavioral restraint in public. |
| | Identify and use individually effective birth control method. |
| | Practice safer sex. |

| ACTIONS/INTERVENTIONS | RATIONALE |
|---|---|
| **Independent** | |
| Have client describe own perceptions of sexuality/sexual functioning. | When sexual/sexuality concerns/perceptions are shared, it provides an opportunity to understand the client's point of view and help the client to learn what is needed. |
| Assess presence/degree of factors that alter sexuality/sexual functioning. | Ego boundary disintegration can cause regressive behavior (withdrawal, preoccupation with self), which interferes with the formation of attachments and creates gender identity confusion. Antipsychotic medications can cause endocrine changes (amenorrhea, lactation in women; and impotence, ejaculatory inhibition, gynecomastia in men). |
| Provide information regarding medications, their effects and regulation, and counseling/teaching about problem-solving (expressing feelings of loss and seeking alternate solutions). | Lack of sufficient knowledge may be a contributing factor to the dysfunction. Information can provide assistance in the resolution of the problem(s). |
| Encourage client to identify/report any alterations in sexuality/sexual functioning. | Timely intervention may prevent future disintegration of ego boundaries and further side effects of medications. |
| Counsel client about birth control, genetic implications of having children. | Severely ill clients have difficulty with relationships and do not make good partners or parents. Although higher-functioning clients may find marriage supportive, they need to be aware that each child has a 12%–15% chance of becoming schizophrenic. Premarital expert eugenic counseling is extremely important. |

| ACTIONS/INTERVENTIONS | RATIONALE |
| --- | --- |

### Independent

Identify "safer sex" practices and discuss risk of contracting sexually transmitted diseases (STDs).

The lack of social inhibitions (multiple partners, unprotected sex) places these clients at risk for the possibility of contracting a sexually transmitted disease, and a poor level of function may result in neglect of treatment.

# SCHIZOAFFECTIVE DISORDER

## DSM IV
295.70  Schizoaffective Disorder

## DSM III-R
295.70  Schizoaffective Disorder (Specify)

Term that emphasizes the temporal relationship of schizophrenic and mood symptoms and is used for conditions that do not meet the criteria for either schizophrenia or a mood disorder.

## ETIOLOGIC THEORIES

### Psychodynamics

Refer to CP: Schizophrenia.

### Biologic

Refer to CP: Schizophrenia.

### Family Dynamics

Refer to CP: Schizophrenia.

## CLIENT ASSESSMENT DATABASE

### Neurosensory

Mood is depressed.
Pronounced manic and depressive features are intermingled with schizophrenic features.
Delusions and hallucinations may be noted.

### Teaching/Learning

May report previous episode(s) and remission with no permanent defect.

## DIAGNOSTIC STUDIES

Refer to CP: Schizophrenia.

## NURSING PRIORITIES

1. Provide protective environment; prevent injury.
2. Assist with self-care.
3. Promote interaction with others.
4. Identify resources available for assistance.
5. Support family involvement in therapy.

## DISCHARGE GOALS

1. Signs of physical agitation are abating and no physical injury occurs.
2. Improved sense of self-esteem, lessened depression, and elevated mood are noted.
3. Approaches and socializes appropriately with others, individually and in group activities.
4. Adequate nutritional intake is achieved/maintained.
5. Client/family displays effective coping skills and appropriate use of resources.

244

(Refer to CP: Schizophrenia for other NDs that apply, in addition to the following.)

| | |
|---|---|
| **NURSING DIAGNOSIS:** | **VIOLENCE, HIGH RISK FOR, DIRECTED AT SELF/OTHERS** |
| **Risk Factors May Include:** | Depressed mood; feelings of worthlessness; hopelessness. |
| | Unsatisfactory parent/child relationship; feelings of abandonment by significant other(s). |
| | Anger turned inward/directed at the environment. |
| | Punitive superego and irrational feelings of guilt. |
| | Numerous failures (learned helplessness). |
| | Misinterpretation of reality. |
| | Extreme hyperactivity. |
| **Possible Indicators:** | History of previous suicide attempts; making direct/indirect statements indicating a desire to kill self/having a plan. |
| | Hallucinations; delusional thinking. |
| | Self-destructive behavior (hitting body parts against wall/furniture); destruction of inanimate objects. |
| | Temper tantrums/aggressive behavior; increased agitation and lack of control over purposeless movements. |
| | Vulnerable self-esteem. |
| **Desired Outcomes/Evaluation Criteria— Client Will:** | Express improved sense of well-being/self-esteem. |
| | Manage behavior and deal with anger appropriately. |
| | Demonstrate self-control without harm to self or others. |

## ACTIONS/INTERVENTIONS

### Independent

Note direct statements of a desire to kill self; indi-. rect actions, e.g., putting affairs in order, writing a will, giving away prized possessions; presence of hallucinations and delusional thinking; history of previous suicidal behavior/acts; statements of hopelessness regarding life situation.

Ask client directly if suicide has been considered/ planned and if the means are available to carry out the plan.

Provide a safe environment for the client by removing potentially harmful objects from access (e.g., sharp objects; straps, belts, ties; glass items; smoking materials).

## RATIONALE

Direct and indirect indicators of suicidal intent need to be attended to and addressed as being potentially acted on.

The risk of suicide is greatly increased if the client has developed a plan and particularly if means exist for the execution of the plan.

Provides protection while treatment is being undertaken to deal with existing situation. Client's rationality is impaired and may harm self inadvertently.

245

| ACTIONS/INTERVENTIONS | RATIONALE |
|---|---|

### Independent

Assign to quiet unit, if possible.

Milieu unit may be too distracting, increasing agitation and potential for loss of control.

Reduce environmental stimuli, e.g., private room, soft lighting, low noise level, and simple room decor.

In hyperactive state, client is extremely distractible, and responses to even the slightest stimuli are exaggerated.

Stay with the client/request client remain in staff view. Provide supervision as necessary.

Provides support and feelings of security as agitation grows and hyperactivity increases.

Formulate a short-term verbal contract with the client that she or he will not harm self during specified period of time. Renegotiate the contract as necessary.

An attitude of acceptance of the client as a worthwhile individual is conveyed. Discussion of suicidal feelings with a trusted individual provides a degree of relief to the client. A contract gets the subject out in the open and places some of the responsibility for own safety with the client.

Ask client to agree to seek out staff member/friend if thoughts of suicide emerge.

The suicidal client is often very ambivalent about own feelings. Discussion of these feelings with a trusted individual may provide assistance before the client experiences a crisis situation.

Encourage verbalizations of honest feelings. Explore and discuss symbols of hope client can identify in own life.

Because of elevated anxiety, client may need assistance to recognize presence of hope in life situations.

Promote expression of angry feelings within appropriate limits. Provide safe method(s) of hostility release. Help client to identify true source of anger, and work on adaptive coping skills for continued use.

Depression and suicidal behaviors may be viewed as anger turned inward on the self, or anger may be expressed as hostile acting out toward others. If this anger can be verbalized and/or released in a nonthreatening environment, the client may be able to resolve these feelings, regardless of the discomfort involved.

Orient client to reality, as required. Point out sensory/environmental misperceptions, taking care not to belittle client's fears or indicate disapproval of verbal expressions.

Elevated level of anxiety may contribute to distortions in reality. Client may require assistance to distinguish between reality and misperceptions of the environment.

Spend time with the client on a regular schedule and provide frequent intermittent checks as indicated in response to client needs.

Provides a feeling of safety and security, while also conveying the message, "I want to spend time with you because I think you are a worthwhile person."

Provide structured schedule of activities that includes established rest periods throughout the day.

Structured schedule provides feeling of security for the client. Additional rest promotes relaxation for the agitated client.

Provide physical activities as a substitute for purposeless hyperactivity, e.g., brisk walks, housekeeping chores, dance therapy, aerobics.

Physical exercise provides a safe and effective means of relieving pent-up tension.

Observe for effectiveness and evidence of adverse side effects of drug therapy, e.g., anticholinergic (dry mouth, blurred vision), extrapyramidal (tremors, rigidity, restlessness, weakness, facial spasms).

Individual reactions to medications may vary, and early identification can assist with changes in dosage and/or drug choice, possibly preventing client from discontinuing drug therapy prematurely with potential loss of control.

| ACTIONS/INTERVENTIONS | RATIONALE |
|---|---|
| **Collaborative** | |
| Administer medication, as indicated, e.g.:<br>neuroleptics, e.g., chlorpromazine (Thorazine); | Pharmacologic interventions need to be directed at the presenting symptoms and used on a short-term basis. Antipsychotics may be effective in reducing the hyperactivity associated with mania. |
| antidepressants, e.g., imipramine (Tofranil); | Allows the accumulation of the neurotransmitters norepinephrine and serotonin, potentiating their antidepressant effect. |
| antimanics, e.g., lithium (Eskalith, Lithobid). | The exact mechanism of action is not known; however, it is thought to alter chemical transmitters in the CNS, reducing manic behavior. |
| Assist with electroconvulsive therapy (ECT). | May be indicated to alter mood until neuroleptics or antidepressants become effective. |
| Identify community resources that client may use as support system and from whom help may be sought if suicidal thoughts/feelings occur. | Having a concrete plan for seeking assistance during a crisis may discourage or prevent self-destructive behaviors. |

| NURSING DIAGNOSIS: | SOCIAL ISOLATION |
|---|---|
| **May Be Related To:** | Developmental regression. |
| | Depressed mood; feelings of worthlessness. |
| | Egocentric behaviors (which offend others and discourage relationships). |
| | Delusional thinking. |
| | Fear of failure. |
| | Impaired cognition fostering negative view of self. |
| | Unresolved grief. |
| **Possibly Evidenced By:** | Sad, dull affect. |
| | Absence of supportive significant other(s): family, friends, group. |
| | Uncommunicative/withdrawn behavior; absence of eye contact; seeking to be alone. |
| | Preoccupation with own thoughts; repetitive, meaningless actions. |
| | Assuming fetal position; catatonic behaviors. |
| **Desired Outcomes/Evaluation Criteria— Client Will:** | Verbalize willingness to be with others. |
| | Spend time voluntarily with others, seek out group activities. |
| | Develop 1:1 trust-based relationship. |

| ACTIONS/INTERVENTIONS | RATIONALE |
|---|---|

### Independent

| | |
|---|---|
| Spend time with client. (This may mean sitting in silence for a while.) | Nurse's presence helps improve client's perception of self as a worthwhile person. |
| Develop a therapeutic nurse-client relationship through frequent, brief contacts and an accepting attitude. Show unconditional positive regard. | The nurse's presence, acceptance, and conveyance of positive regard enhance the client's feeling of self-worth and facilitate trust and interaction with others. |
| Encourage attendance in group activities, after client feels comfortable in the 1:1 relationship. May need to attend with client the first few times to offer support. Accept client's decision to remove self from group situation if anxiety becomes too great. | The presence of a trusted individual provides emotional security for the client. Moving slowly into a more threatening activity and accepting client's decision to leave promote self-trust and sense of control. |
| Provide positive reinforcement for client's voluntary interactions with others. | Positive reinforcement enhances self-esteem and encourages repetition of desirable behaviors. |
| Verbally acknowledge client's absence from any group activities. | Knowledge that absence was noticed may reinforce the client's feelings of self-worth. |
| Assist client to learn assertiveness techniques. | Knowledge of the use of assertive techniques could improve client's relationships with others. |
| Devise a plan of therapeutic activities and provide client with a written time schedule. | The depressed client needs structure because of the impairment in decision-making/problem-solving ability. A structured schedule provides security until the client is able to function independently. |
| Help client to learn skills that may be used to approach others in a socially acceptable manner. Practice these skills through role-play, beginning with simple assignments, e.g., introduce self in safe environment. | With practice, these skills become easier in real-life situations, and client feels more comfortable performing them. |
| Limit group activities, when agitated. Help client to establish 1 or 2 close relationships. | Client's ability to interact with others is impaired. More security is felt in a 1:1 relationship that is consistent over time. |

| | |
|---|---|
| **NURSING DIAGNOSIS:** | **NUTRITION, ALTERED, LESS THAN BODY REQUIREMENTS** |
| **May Be Related To:** | Energy expenditure in excess of calorie intake. |
| | Refusal/inability to sit still long enough to eat meals. |
| | Lack of attention to/recognition of hunger cues. |
| **Possibly Evidenced By:** | Lack of interest in food; weight loss. |
| | Pale conjunctiva and mucous membranes. |
| | Poor muscle tone/skin turgor. |

**Desired Outcomes/Evaluation Criteria—Client Will:**

Amenorrhea.

Abnormal laboratory findings, e.g., anemias, electrolyte imbalances.

Identify and formulate plan to meet individual dietary needs.

Demonstrate adequate intake to maintain individual nutritional balance/provide desired weight gain.

Exhibit no signs of malnutrition.

| ACTIONS/INTERVENTIONS | RATIONALE |
|---|---|
| **Independent** | |
| Determine individual daily caloric requirement, considering body structure, height, and activity level. | Important for the provision of adequate nutrition and realistic weight gain. |
| Have juice and snacks available at all times. | Nutritious intake is required on a regular basis to compensate for increased caloric requirements due to hyperactivity. |
| Maintain accurate record of intake, output, and calorie count. | Necessary to make an accurate nutritional assessment, identify individual needs, and maintain client safety. |
| Weigh daily. | Helpful in evaluating therapeutic needs and effectiveness of treatment plan. |
| Determine client's dietary likes and dislikes. | Client is more likely to eat foods that are particularly enjoyed. |
| Pace or walk with client as finger foods are taken. As agitation subsides, sit with client during meals. Offer support and encouragement. | Presence of a trusted individual may provide feeling of security and decrease agitation. Encouragement and positive reinforcement increase self-esteem and foster repetition of desired behaviors. |
| Assist client to learn the importance of adequate nutrition and fluid intake. | Client may have inadequate or inaccurate knowledge regarding the contribution of good nutrition to overall wellness. |
| **Collaborative** | |
| Consult with dietitian as indicated. | Helpful in establishing individual needs/program and provides educational opportunity. |
| Provide high-protein, high-calorie, nutritious finger foods and drinks that can be consumed on the run. | The client may have difficulty sitting still long enough to eat a meal because of hyperactive state. The likelihood is greater that food and drinks that can be carried around and eaten with little effort will be consumed. |
| Administer vitamin and mineral supplements, as indicated. | To improve and/or restore nutritional well-being. |
| Monitor laboratory values, and report significant changes. | Provides an objective assessment of nutritional status, therapeutic needs/effectiveness. |

# DELUSIONAL (PARANOID) DISORDER

## DSM IV
297.1 Delusional Disorder

**Erotomanic:** Delusions that another person of higher status is in love with the individual.
**Grandiose:** Delusions of inflated worth, power, knowledge, identity, or special relationship to a deity or famous person.
**Jealous:** Delusions that one's sexual partner is unfaithful.
**Persecutory:** Delusions that one (or someone to whom one is close) is being malevolently treated in some way.
**Somatic:** Delusions that one has some physical defect or general medical condition.
**Mixed:** Delusions characteristic of more than one of the above types, but no one theme predominates.

## DSM III-R
297.10 Delusional (Paranoid) Disorder/Specify Type

Delusional disorders are defined as the presence of persistent, nonbizarre delusions that are not related to a known toxic state or underlying metabolic condition.

## ETIOLOGIC THEORIES

### Psychodynamics

Emotional development is delayed because of a lack of maternal stimulation/attention. The infant is deprived of a sense of security and fails to establish basic trust. A fragile ego results in severely impaired self-esteem, a sense of loss of control, fear, and severe anxiety. A suspicious attitude toward others is manifested and may continue throughout life. Projection is the most common mechanism used as a defense against feelings.

### Biologic

There appears to be a relatively strong familial pattern of involvement with these disorders. Individuals whose family members manifest symptoms of these disorders are at greater risk for development than the general population. Twin studies have also suggested genetic involvement.

### Family Dynamics

Some theorists believe that paranoid persons had parents who were distant, rigid, demanding, and perfectionistic, engendering rage, a sense of exaggerated self-importance, and mistrust in the individual. The clients become vulnerable as adults because of this early experience.

## CLIENT ASSESSMENT DATABASE

Refer to CP: Schizophrenia for physical symptoms.

### Ego Integrity

May present with severe anxiety; inability to relax, exaggeration of difficulties, being easily agitated.
Expresses feelings of inadequacy, worthlessness, lack of acceptance, and trust of others.
Demonstrates difficulty in coping with stress, uses maladjusted coping mechanisms, e.g., excessive use of projection and aggressive behavior, takes unnecessary precautions, avoids accepting blame.

### Neurosensory

Nonbizarre delusional system of at least 1 month's duration.

Experiencing emotions and behavior congruent with the content of belief system/fears that either self or significant others are in danger, are being followed/conspired against, poisoned, infected; having a disease; being deceived by one's spouse, cheated by others; loving; loved at a distance.

Exhibits controlled, cold, unemotional affect; guarded/evasive/distrustful behavior.

Vigilant, looks for hidden motives, every person/event is under suspicion.

Perception is keen; will demonstrate impaired judgment about the perception.

Delusions of reference or control that may incorporate the FBI, CIA, radio/TV.

(Prominent auditory or visual hallucinations not usually present.)

### Safety

May display assaultive/violent behavior.

### Social Interactions

Significant impairment in social/marital functioning may be noted; usually behavior in all other areas of life appears normal.

Litigiousness common.

### Teaching/Learning

Onset most often occurs in middle or late adult life.

May have history of substance abuse/physical illness.

## DIAGNOSTIC STUDIES

Refer to CP: Schizophrenia.

## NURSING PRIORITIES

1. Promote safe environment, safety of client/others.
2. Provide open, honest atmosphere in which client can begin to trust self/others.
3. Encourage client/family to focus on defining methods for copng with anxieties and life stressors.
4. Promote a sense of self-worth and increased self-esteem.

## DISCHARGE GOALS

1. Coping with anxiety without the use of threats or assaultive behavior.
2. Reality is recognized, and client agrees to give up or live with the delusional system.
3. Client/family/SOs participating in therapy, e.g., behavioral, group.
4. Family/SO(s) are providing emotional support for the client.

| NURSING DIAGNOSIS: | VIOLENCE, HIGH RISK FOR, DIRECTED AT SELF/OTHERS |
|---|---|
| Risk Factors May Include: | Perceived threats of danger. |
| | Increased feelings of anxiety. |

| Possible Indicators: | Acting out in an irrational manner. |
| --- | --- |
| | Becoming threatening or assaultive in the face of perceived threat. |
| **Desired Outcomes/Evaluation Criteria— Client Will:** | Verbalize awareness of delusional system. |
| | Resolve conflicts, coping with anxiety without the use of threats or assaultive behavior. |

| ACTIONS/INTERVENTIONS | RATIONALE |
| --- | --- |

### Independent

| | |
| --- | --- |
| Note prior history of violent behavior when under stress. | Indicator of increased risk for recurrence of aggression/violent behavior. |
| Assess client to identify situations that trigger anxiety and aggressive behaviors. | Understanding relationship between severe anxiety and aggressive feelings can help client to identify options to avoid violent behavior. |
| Explore implications and consequences of handling these situations with aggression. | Emphasizes importance of thinking through situations before acting. |
| Encourage to engage in solitary activity instead of group activities to begin with. | Anxiety, fear, suspiciousness may escalate if involved in competitive/group activities. |
| Be careful in offering a pat on the shoulder/hug, etc. | Gestures involving touch may be misinterpreted as aggressive by the suspicious person. |
| Assist client to define alternatives to aggressive behaviors. Engage in physical activities such as Ping-Pong, foosball. (Monitor competitive activities; use with caution.) | Enables client to learn to handle situations in a socially acceptable manner. Appropriate outlets will allow for release of hostility. Note: Competition can trigger violent behavior. |
| Encourage verbalizations of feelings and promote outlet for expression. | Ventilation of feelings reduces need for physical action. |
| Be alert to signs of impending violent behavior, e.g., increase in psychomotor activity, intensity of affect, verbalization of delusional thinking, especially threatening expressions. | Therapeutic interventions are more effective before behavior becomes violent. |
| Accept verbal hostility without retaliation or defense. Nurse (caregiver) needs to be aware of own response to client behavior, e.g., anger/fear. | Behavior is not usually directed at nurse personally, and responding defensively will tend to exacerbate situation. Looking at meaning behind the words will be more productive. Awareness of own response allows nurse to confront/deal with those feelings. |
| Provide safe, quiet environment; tell client he or she is "safe." | Keeping environmental stimuli to a minimum will help reassure client and assist with prevention of agitation. |
| Isolate promptly in nonpunitive manner, using adequate help, if violent behavior occurs. Hold client if necessary. Tell client to STOP behavior. | Removal to a quiet environment can help calm client. Sufficient help will prevent injury to client/staff. Usually the individual is being self-critical and afraid of hostility and does not need external criticism. Saying "Stop" may be enough to allow client to regain control. |

| ACTIONS/INTERVENTIONS | RATIONALE |
|---|---|

### Collaborative

| ACTIONS/INTERVENTIONS | RATIONALE |
|---|---|
| Administer medications, as indicated. (Refer to ND: Anxiety, severe). | Antipsychotic/antianxiety drugs may decrease anxiety and delusional thinking, decreasing suspicious thoughts/aggressive behaviors and aiding client in maintaining control. |

| NURSING DIAGNOSIS: | ANXIETY [severe] |
|---|---|
| May Be Related To: | Inability to trust (has not mastered tasks of trust vs. mistrust). |
| Possibly Evidenced By: | Rigid delusional system (provides relief from stress that justifies the delusion). |
| | Frightened of other people and own hostility. |
| Desired Outcomes/Evaluation Criteria— Client Will: | Acknowledge delusion and deal with it appropriately. |
| | Define methods to decrease own anxiety level. |
| | Report anxiety is reduced to a manageable level. |
| | Demonstrate a relaxed manner. |

| ACTIONS/INTERVENTIONS | RATIONALE |
|---|---|

### Independent

| ACTIONS/INTERVENTIONS | RATIONALE |
|---|---|
| Develop primary nurse/client relationship. | The continuity of a primary care relationship can provide the time necessary to form an alliance with the suspicious person. |
| Assist client to identify sources of anxiety and concerns. | Increases awareness of problems/contributing factors. Client needs to become aware of how behavior affects others and take responsibility for it. |
| Explore present patterns of coping with anxiety and how effective they have been (e.g., threatening harm and/or shouting at others, believing "they are out to get me/my family"). | Increases awareness that aggressive acts may have destructive outcome. |
| Discuss alternatives to current ineffective behaviors. | Client has been using maladjusted coping; identifying effective, constructive strategies to handle fearful situations can be an impetus to change. |
| Encourage implementation of new strategies, giving feedback on effectiveness. | Reinforces acceptable behaviors. |
| Avoid confrontation of delusion. | Logic does not work, and forcing the client to give up the delusion increases anxiety. |
| Observe for side effects of medications: note changes in behavior/response to environment, level of consciousness, intellectual responses/thought control; reports of dry mouth, blurred vision. Monitor vital signs, intake/output, weight. | Adverse reactions such as extrapyramidal symptoms, tardive dyskinesia, orthostatic hypotension, decreased sensation of thirst, constipation, urinary retention, weight gain may occur; paradoxical exacerbations of psychotic symptoms may develop and may actually heighten anxiety, suspiciousness. |

## ACTIONS/INTERVENTIONS

## RATIONALE

### Collaborative

Develop behavioral therapy program with input and agreement of client, family/SO, and therapeutic team.

Administer medications as indicated, e.g., fluphenazine (Prolixin), haloperidol (Haldol).

Hypersensitivity to the actions of others has been learned and can be unlearned. Breaking this cycle assists in reducing sensitivity to criticism and improving client's social skills.

Decreases anxiety and delusional thinking, which can increase ability to problem-solve. Note: Decreased sensation of thirst and sensitivity to sun/photophobia are side effects of antipsychotic drugs that require increased fluid intake and avoidance of prolonged exposure to sun.

| NURSING DIAGNOSIS: | POWERLESSNESS |
|---|---|
| May Be Related To: | Lifestyle of helplessness: Feelings of inadequacies, sense of severely impaired self-esteem. |
| | Interpersonal interaction. |
| Possibly Evidenced By: | Verbal expressions of having no control/influence over situation(s). |
| | Use of paranoid delusions, aggressive behavior to compensate. |
| | Expressions of recognition of damage paranoia has caused self and others. |
| Desired Outcomes/Evaluation Criteria—Client Will: | State belief that outcome of situations causing concern can be significantly affected by own actions. |
| | Identify individual actions to effect control. |
| | Demonstrate necessary behaviors/lifestyle changes to maintain control without use of aggression. |

## ACTIONS/INTERVENTIONS

## RATIONALE

### Independent

Encourage client to do as much for self as able, providing choices when possible.

Assist client to identify when feelings of loss of control began and events/situations that led to feelings of powerlessness and aggressive acts.

Review previous relationships/social contacts. If no longer involved in these relationships, have client describe what happened.

Permits/enables control of situation so suspicion can be reduced.

Increases understanding of sources of stressful events and that aggression is an attempt to compensate for feeling powerless.

Knowledge can be gained of how the client establishes relationships and why they deteriorated or remained intact, providing insight to change own behavior and enhancing future relationships.

| ACTIONS/INTERVENTIONS | RATIONALE |
|---|---|

### Independent

| | |
|---|---|
| Discuss predelusional period and how events might precede panic state. | Helps client discern how much of delusion is real and how much relates to anxiety state. |
| Explore alternate ways to regain control without resorting to aggression. (Refer to ND: Violence, high risk for, directed at self/others.) | Provides knowledge of constructive coping mechanisms. |
| Give positive feedback when client demonstrates use of constructive alternatives. | Enhances self-esteem and reinforces acceptable behaviors. |

| | |
|---|---|
| **NURSING DIAGNOSIS:** | **THOUGHT PROCESSES, ALTERED** |
| **May Be Related To:** | Psychologic conflicts. |
| | Increasing anxiety and fear (characteristic of the suspicious person). |
| **Possibly Evidenced By:** | Interference with the ability to think clearly and logically, difficulties in the process and character of thought, fragmentation and autistic thinking, delusions. |
| **Desired Outcomes/Evaluation Criteria—Client Will:** | Recognize changes in thinking and behavior. |
| | Identify the meaning of the delusion. |
| | Deal with anxieties/fears as evidenced by more logical/reality-based thinking. |

| ACTIONS/INTERVENTIONS | RATIONALE |
|---|---|

### Independent

| | |
|---|---|
| State reality matter-of-factly. Communicate in clear, concise terms with clearly stated rules about what client can/cannot do. | The very suspicious/delusional client needs to have straight information that differentiates him or her from the seemingly dangerous surroundings. Knowledge of the rules can provide this person with a sense of control. |
| Note impulsive behaviors and request client to stop. If client does not stop, evaluate basis of behavior and whether it is potentially harmful. (Refer to ND: Violence, high risk for, directed at self/others.) | These behaviors are often the result of psychotic thought/perceptual distortions and not willful actions. |
| Gradually involve in learning activities, occupational/recreational/activity therapies. (Refer to ND: Self-Esteem disturbance). | As thought processes improve, task mastery opportunities can enhance self-esteem and enable the client to feel good about accomplishments. |

| NURSING DIAGNOSIS: | COPING, INDIVIDUAL, INEFFECTIVE |
|---|---|
| **May Be Related To:** | Maladjusted method of coping with stress. |
| | Delusional system. |
| **Possibly Evidenced By:** | Beliefs and behaviors of suspicion/violence. |
| | Inappropriate ways of dealing with others. |
| **Desired Outcomes/Evaluation Criteria— Client Will:** | Recognize relationship of paranoid ideation to current situation. |
| | Verbalize awareness of own coping abilities. |
| | Demonstrate appropriate, constructive, effective coping skills. |

| ACTIONS/INTERVENTIONS | RATIONALE |
|---|---|

### Independent

| | |
|---|---|
| Provide outlet(s) for expression of fears/anxieties in 1:1 or group settings. | In a trusting relationship, feelings can be freely expressed without fear of judgment. |
| Assist in identifying/discussing thoughts, perceptions, and own conclusions of reality. | Increases comprehension of what client sees as problems and gives insight into how information is being processed. |
| Encourage client to identify when fears/suspicions began and events that led to these feelings. | Gaining knowledge of stressors that have precipitated deterioration in coping ability may help prevent recurrence of these behaviors. |
| Explore how perceptions are validated prior to drawing conclusions. Discuss successes and failures of these attempts. | Validation of perceptions may prevent drawing the wrong conclusion and acting-out behaviors. |
| Guide in defining methods to decrease anxiety and fears without distortion of reality or using delusional system. Encourage development of exercise programs/relaxation techniques. | Increases repertoire of coping behaviors, may prevent decompensation. Note: Use of guided imagery may exacerbate delusional thinking. |

| NURSING DIAGNOSIS: | SELF-ESTEEM DISTURBANCE |
|---|---|
| **May Be Related To:** | Underdeveloped ego, fixation in earlier level of development, inability to trust. |
| | Lack of positive feedback. |
| **Possibly Evidenced By:** | Delusional system (attempt to hurt or strike out at someone else in order to protect the self); self-destructive behavior. |
| | Inability to accept positive reinforcement. |
| | Not taking responsibility for self-care; nonparticipation in therapy. |

| **Desired Outcomes/Evaluation Criteria— Client Will:** | Verbalize feelings of increased self-value/worth. |
|---|---|
| | Identify self as a person capable of problem-solving and functioning in society in a manner acceptable to self and others. |
| | Demonstrate adaptation to changes by active participation in treatment program. |

| ACTIONS/INTERVENTIONS | RATIONALE |
|---|---|

### Independent

| | |
|---|---|
| Provide clear, consistent verbal/nonverbal communication. Be truthful and honest; follow through on commitments. | Helpful in establishing trust and reaffirming that the individual has value and worth. |
| Encourage client to verbalize feelings of inadequacies, worthlessness, fear of rejection/need for acceptance by others. | Must have insight into feelings in order to begin to improve self-esteem. |
| Explore how these negative feelings could lead to severe anxiety and suspiciousness. | Increases awareness of internal factors that cause feelings of inadequacy and how these feelings lead to decompensation. |
| Encourage client to identify positive aspects about self related to social skills, work abilities, education, talents, and appearance. | Reinforces own feelings of being a worthwhile person capable of adaptive functioning. |
| Give positive feedback regarding abilities and how they can be used to increase self-esteem. | Provides encouragement and promotes a sense of self-direction. |
| Engage in activities, increasing socialization and interaction with others as tolerated. | Opportunity to interact with others reduces isolation, enhances feelings of self-worth, and promotes social skills. |

| **NURSING DIAGNOSIS:** | **SOCIAL INTERACTION, IMPAIRED** |
|---|---|
| **May Be Related To:** | Disturbed thought processes, mistrust of others/delusional thinking. |
| | Knowledge/skill deficit about ways to enhance mutuality. |
| **Possibly Evidenced By:** | Discomfort in social situations, difficulty in establishing relationships with others. |
| | Expressions of feelings of rejection, no sense of belonging; isolation of self/withdrawal. |
| | Dealing with problems with anger/hostility and violence. |
| **Desired Outcomes/Evaluation Criteria— Client Will:** | Verbalize willingness to be involved with others. |
| | Participate in activities/programs with others with lessened discomfort. |

| ACTIONS/INTERVENTIONS | RATIONALE |
|---|---|

### Independent

Establish 1:1 relationship, use Active-listening, and provide safe environment for self-disclosure.

Consistent, brief, honest contact can help the client initiate and master tasks associated with learning to trust others.

Determine degree of impairment, listening to client's comments about loneliness. Note sense of self-esteem. (Refer to ND, Self-Esteem disturbance.)

Mistrust can lead to difficulty establishing relationships, and client may have withdrawn from close contacts with others.

Encourage client to verbalize feelings of discomfort about social situations and perceptions of reasons for problems.

Acknowledgment helps client to become aware of feelings and begin to deal with them.

Observe and describe social/interpersonal behaviors in objective terms.

Provides insight into how others view them and may serve as a beginning for change.

Identify support systems available to the client: family, friends, coworkers, etc.

Can be an important part in the client's rehabilitation by improving socialization and diminishing sense of isolation.

Assess family relationships, communication patterns, knowledge of client condition.

Problems within the family may preclude members providing adequate support/continuing relationship and may interfere with client's progress. (Refer to ND: Family Coping, ineffective: compromised/Family Processes, altered).

Explore and role-play means of changing social interactions/behaviors. Provide positive feedback for efforts.

Provides safe environment to try out new behaviors. Encouragement enhances repetition and risk taking.

---

| **NURSING DIAGNOSIS:** | **FAMILY COPING, ineffective: compromised/FAMILY PROCESSES, ALTERED** |
|---|---|
| **May Be Related To:** | Temporary family disorganization/role changes. |
| | Inadequate or incorrect information or understanding by a primary person. |
| | Prolonged progression of condition that exhausts the supportive capacity of significant other(s). |
| **Possibly Evidenced By:** | Family system does not meet physical/emotional/spiritual needs of its members. |
| | Inability to express/accept wide range of feelings/feelings of members. |
| | Inappropriate or poorly communicated family rules, rituals, symbols. |
| | Inappropriate boundary maintenance. |
| | Significant person describes preoccupation with personal reactions, withdraws or enters into limited or temporary personal communication with client at time of need. |

| **Desired Outcomes/Evaluation Criteria— Family Will:** | Express feelings freely and appropriately. |
| --- | --- |
| | Identify/verbalize resources within itself to deal with the situation. |
| | Interact appropriately with the client. |
| | Provide opportunity for client to deal with situation in own way. |
| | Identify need for outside support and use appropriately. |

| ACTIONS/INTERVENTIONS | RATIONALE |
| --- | --- |
| **Independent** | |
| Identify individual factors that may contribute to difficulty of family in providing needed assistance to the client. | Each member of a family system has an effect on other members, and members of this family may be in constant conflict with other members. |
| Determine information available to and understood by family/significant other(s). | Lack of understanding of illness can lead to angry responses in family members, resulting in continuing conflict. |
| Discuss underlying reasons for client's behaviors, e.g., fear of loss of control, extreme sensitivity, use of projection and blame to avoid looking at own responsibility. | Promotes understanding of client and provides opportunity for changing ineffective responses to positive, growth-promoting behaviors. |
| Encourage and assist client/family to develop problem-solving skills. | This client's behavior creates conflict among family members, and learning to resolve issues in an open, nonjudgmental manner lessens angry responses, allowing for resolution of the conflict. |
| Help individuals to look at own behavior in relation to the client's. | Interaction among family members often enables the client to maintain suspicions and paranoid ideation, and when this behavior is acknowledged and dealt with, behavior can begin to change. |
| **Collaborative** | |
| Refer to appropriate resources such as marital/family therapy, psychotherapy, support groups. | Since conflict is so prevalent in this family, and divorce is common, long-term assistance may be needed to maintain relationships or achieve amicable parting. |

## CHAPTER 8

# MOOD DISORDERS

## DEPRESSIVE DISORDERS: Major Depression/ Dysthymic Disorder

**DSM IV**
**DEPRESSIVE DISORDERS**
296.xx  Major Depressive Disorder
296.2x  Single Episode
296.3x  Recurrent
300.4   Dysthymic Disorder
311     Depressive Disorder NOS

**DSM III-R**
293.2x  Major Depression, Single Episode
296.3x  Major Depression, Recurrent
300.40  Dysthymia

A disturbance of mood, characterized by a full or partial depressive syndrome, or loss of interest or pleasure in usual activities and pastimes with evidence of interference in social/occupational functioning.

## ETIOLOGIC THEORIES

### Psychodynamics

Psychoanalytic theory focuses on an early unsatisfactory parent/child relationship, with an unresolved grieving process. This results in the individual remaining fixed in the anger stage of the grieving process and turning it inward on the self. The ego remains weak, while the superego expands and becomes punitive.

Cognitive theory projects a belief that depression occurs as a result of impaired cognition, fostering a negative evaluation of self through disturbed thought processes. The individual is pessimistic and views self as inadequate and worthless and life as hopeless.

Learning theorists propose that depressive illness arises out of the individual's having experienced numerous failures (either real or perceived). A feeling of inability to succeed at any endeavor ensues. This "learned helplessness" is viewed as a predisposition to depressive illness.

The behavioral model states that the cause of depression is in the person-behavior-environment interaction. Although people are seen as capable of exercising control over their behavior, they are not totally free of environmental influence.

## Biologic

There may be a family history of major affective disorders, and recently the disease has been found to have a genetic marker as shown by numerous studies that support the involvement of heredity in depressive illness.

Biochemical factors, e.g., electrolyte imbalances, appear to play a role in depressive illness. An error in metabolism results in the transposition of sodium and potassium within the neuron. Another theory implicates the biogenic amines norepinephrine, dopamine, and serotonin. The levels of these chemicals are deficient in individuals with this illness. Controversy remains as to whether these changes cause the illness or if the biochemical changes occur because of the depression. In recent years, a common form of major depression called seasonal affective disorder (SAD) has been identified. Recurring each year, starting in fall or winter and ending in spring, the symptoms are largely typical of depression, with some atypical symptoms (excessive sleep, increased appetite, and weight gain). It is believed that this disorder is caused by the decreased availability of sunlight and is related to circadian cycles, which are set by individual internal biological clock. They are more precisely adjusted and coordinated by the alternation of darkness and light.

## Family Dynamics

Object loss theory suggests that depressive illness occurs if the person is separated from or abandoned by a significant other during the first 6 months of life. The bonding process is interrupted, and the child withdraws from people and the environment.

## CLIENT ASSESSMENT DATABASE

### Activity/Rest

Fatigue, malaise, decreased energy level, lethargy.

Sleep disturbances, e.g., insomnia, occur in 90% of cases, either anxiety insomnia (falling asleep is difficult) or depressive insomnia (early morning awakening occurs, accompanied by painful ruminations); may experience hypersomnia (restless and unrefreshing, particularly in SAD).

May report feeling best early in the morning, then continually worsen as the day progresses (dysthymia); or the opposite may be true (severe depression).

### Ego Integrity

Feelings of worthlessness: self-derogatory statements, expressions of guilt, or exaggeration of minor inadequacies; may assume delusional proportions with presentations of unrealistic evidence of self-worth/intense focus on self, e.g., feeling oneself responsible for major tragedies and catastrophes or persecuted for a failure.

Actual loss or life stressor perceived as a loss (e.g., retirement, job loss, divorce, illness, aging, etc.), may or may not see a connection between perceived losses and the onset of the depression. Symptoms must persist for at least 2 months after the loss/death of a loved one.

Feelings of helplessness, hopelessness, powerlessness, pessimism, irritability, excessive anger.

### Elimination

Constipation, urinary retention may be present.

### Food/Fluid

Decreased/increased appetite accompanied by significant change in weight (average gain of 10 pounds in SAD).

## Neurosensory

Dejected or sad mood with loss of interest/enjoyment in usual activities. Depressed mood for most of day, for more days than not, for at least 2 years (dysthmia).

Expressed sadness, dejection, not caring about anything, not seeing any future for self; sighing and tearful.

Irritability, headache.

Psychotic features with prominent delusions and/or hallucinations (major depression).

**Psychomotor Retardation:** May present a "slow motion" picture with slowed speech and latencies (long pauses before responding), decreased amount of speech, and slowed body movements; or agitation: constant, rapid, purposeless movements (severe depression).

Thinking characterized by poor concentration and decreased memory, indecision, ideas of suicide.

Posture may be bent/slouched (defeated-looking).

## Safety

Thoughts of suicide/wanting to die may be frequent, occurring at variable times in course of illness; may range in severity from indifference about the consequences of behavior, e.g., lack of cooperation with medical treatment or dangerous driving, to wishing it were "over" or for death, to specific suicide plans and attempts.

## Sexuality

Disinterest in sexual activities and/or impotence.

## Social Interactions

Participation diminished, difficulty starting activities, withdrawn (e.g., housebound or remains in a single room/bed).

## Teaching/Learning

Family history of depression, high rates of alcoholism/other drug abuse.

## DIAGNOSTIC STUDIES

(The several biochemical alterations in depression are not, by themselves, indicative of depression but, combined with clinical observation, may indicate best pharmacologic response.)

**Thyroid-Stimulating Hormone Response to Thyrotropin-Releasing Hormone:** Decreased level suggests depression.

**Dexamethasone-Suppression Test (DST)** (an indirect marker of melancholia): Post-dexamethasone cortisol levels exceeding 5 g/dl, indicate abnormal/positive result.

**EEG Sleep Profile:** Shows reduced latency of rapid eye movement (REM) sleep.

Other medical tests that may be included:

**Platelet Monoamine Oxidase Activity (MAO):** Increased.

**Biogenic Amines** (especially norepinephrine and serotonin levels): Decreased (clients with low serotonin levels are 10 times more likely to commit suicide within a year).

**α-Acid Glycoprotein** (inhibitor of serotonin transporter): Elevated.

**Urinary 3-methoxy-4-hydroxyphenylglycol (MHPG):** Low levels indicate decreased norepinephrine output.

**Cerebrospinal fluid level of 5-hydroxytryptamine (5HIAA):** Reduced.

**Minnesota Multiphasic Personality Inventory (MMPI):** Scale 2 consistently elevated.

**Wechsler Adult Intelligence Scale—Revised (WAIS-R):** Overall performance score significantly lower than verbal score.

**Rorschach Test:** Long reaction times, chromatic color responses diminished.

**Thematic Apperception Test (TAT):** Short, stereotyped responses/simple descriptions of cards.

**Zung** (or similar) **Depressive Scale (ADS):** Self-report reflecting affective, psychic, somatic characteristics of depression.

## NURSING PRIORITIES

1. Promote physical safety with special focus on suicide prevention.
2. Provide for client's basic needs, promoting highest possible level of independent functioning.
3. Provide experience/interactions that enhance self-esteem, sense of personal power.
4. Support client/family participation in follow-up care/community treatment.

## DISCHARGE GOALS

1. Absence of suicidal ideation/self-violent behaviors.
2. Physiologic stability achieved with responsibility for self demonstrated.
3. Client expressing feelings appropriately with some optimism and hope for the future.
4. Client/family participating in follow-up care/community treatment.

| NURSING DIAGNOSIS: | VIOLENCE, HIGH RISK FOR, SELF-DIRECTED |
| --- | --- |
| **Risk Factors May Include:** | Depressed mood. |
| | Feelings of worthlessness and hopelessness. |
| **Possible Indicators:** | Verbalization of suicidal ideation/plan or futility of trying ("What's the use?"). |
| | Giving possessions away/making a will. |
| | Sudden mood elevation/appears more energized or displays calmer, more peaceful manner. |
| | Refusal/reluctance to sign a "no harm" contract. |
| **Desired Outcomes/Evaluation Criteria— Client Will:** | Voluntarily comply with suicide precautions, sign "no harm" contract. |
| | Verbalize a decrease/absence of suicidal ideas. |
| | State 2 reasons for not harming self. |
| | Commit no acts of self-violence. |

| ACTIONS/INTERVENTIONS | RATIONALE |
| --- | --- |

### Independent

Identify degree of risk/potential for suicide through direct questions, e.g., "Have you thought about killing yourself?" Assess seriousness of suicidal tendency, noting behaviors, e.g., gestures, threats, giving away possessions, previous attempts, presence of hallucinations or delusions. (Use scale of 1–10 and prioritize care according to severity of threat, availability of means.)

The degree of hopelessness expressed by the client is an important indicator of the severity of the depression and suicide risk. Eight of 10 clients who state an intention to commit suicide, do. The more thought-out the plan, the higher the chances of completing it. The chances of suicide increase if there was a previous attempt or if a family history of suicide and depression is present. Impulsive clients are more likely to attempt suicide without giving clues, including those with psychotic thinking who are especially at risk when hallucinations or delusions encourage self-harm.

263

| ACTIONS/INTERVENTIONS | RATIONALE |
|---|---|

### Independent

Reevaluate potential for suicide periodically at key times (e.g., mood changes, initiation of/changes in medication regimen, increasing withdrawal; when discharge planning becomes active; before sending out on pass, before discharge from program).

Suicide risk is the greatest during the first few weeks following admission to treatment. Over half of suicides by hospitalized patients occur out of the hospital, on leave or unauthorized absence. (The highest risk is when the client has both suicidal ideation and sufficient energy with which to act, e.g., at the point when the client begins to feel better.)

Implement suicide precautions, such as:

Explain to client that you are concerned for client safety and that you will be helping client to stay "safe."

Communicates caring and provides sense of protection.

Create a time-specific contract with client on what client and nurse will do to provide for client's safety. Renew contract as appropriate. Place a copy of the "contract," signed by client and staff, in the chart/file and give a copy to the client to keep.

Documents actions taken to prevent suicide and client response. Also promotes communication and can be helpful to the client to realize others care what happens. Short-term contracts encourage client to deal with the here and now and provide opportunity to reassess situation.

(When hospitalized:)

Provide close observation (1:1 or 15-minute checks for most acute risk). Place in room close to nurse's station; do not assign to a single room. Accompany to off-ward activities if attendance is indicated. Ask client to stay in view of staff member at all times.

Being alert for suicidal and escape attempts facilitates being able to prevent or interrupt harmful behavior.

Be alert to use of hazardous equipment; remove hazardous personal items (e.g., scarves, belts, razor blades, scissors).

Provides environmental safety; removes objects that may prompt suicidal thoughts/attempts.

Check all items brought in to or by the client as indicated. Ask family, visitors to avoid bringing hazardous items.

Suicidal clients may bring harmful items back from pass or may ask family for items with a plan in mind.

Maintain special care in administration of medications.

Prevents saving up to overdose or discarding and not taking.

Be alert when client is using bathroom.

While decreasing the client's privacy may seem awkward, it is essential that the suicidal client be within easy reach at all times to prevent self-harm, e.g., hanging.

Make rounds at frequent, irregular intervals (especially at night, toward early morning, at change of shift, or other predictably busy times for staff).

Prevents staff surveillance from becoming predictable. To be aware of client's location is important, especially when staff is busy and least available/observant.

Routinely check environment for hazards. Provide for environmental safety, e.g., lock doors/windows when not supervised, block access to stairways/roof, and construction areas, monitor cleaning chemicals/repair supplies.

Minimizing opportunities for self-harm is an ongoing issue requiring constant attention and consideration of the unusual.

| ACTIONS/INTERVENTIONS | RATIONALE |
|---|---|

## Independent

Review medical regimen, including electroconvulsive therapy (ECT), allowing client/family to ask questions and express feelings freely.

Antidepressant drugs may take 3 or more weeks to lift mood. In the meantime, other forms of therapy may be required to provide protection for suicidal client. ECT is generally a second line of treatment, used if depression has not responded to pharmacologic treatment and/or client continues to display suicidal ideation, sleeplessness, refusal to eat and drink. Client may fear ECT, and nurse needs to empathize with client's fears while being supportive of ECT as a positive treatment alternative.

Be aware of staff attitudes toward the use of ECT and avoid influencing client negatively.

When nurses/others have negative/ambivalent feelings toward this treatment, these feelings can be communicated to the client, causing confusion/reluctance to accept appropriate therapy.

## Collaborative

Administer medications as indicated, e.g.:
 cyclic antidepressants:
  unicyclic, e.g., bupropion (Wellbutrin);
  bicyclic, e.g., fluoxetine (Prozac);
  tricyclic, e.g., amitriptyline (Elavil), amoxapine (Asundin), doxepin (Sinequan), nortriptyline (Pamelar);
  tetracyclic, e.g., maprotiline (Ludiomil);
 other, e.g., trazodone (Desyrel);
 monoamine oxidase inhibitors (MAOIs), e.g. phenelzine (Nardil), isocarboxazid (Marplan), tranylcypromine (Parnate).

Cyclic antidepressants are generally considered safer and easier to manage and so are started first. If response is not noted in 4 to 6 weeks, an MAOI may be the drug of choice. These drugs act by blocking enzyme degradation of neurotransmitters (norepinephrine, serotonin). Note: Medications inhibiting reuptake of serotonin, or unicyclic drugs (e.g., bupropion), are usually preferred for treating depression in bipolar disorders, whereas imipramine and MAOIs may increase possibility of switch to manic behavior.

Assist with ECT as indicated.

ECT becomes essential and in some cases lifesaving when depression does not respond to other treatments and suicide is a major risk. (Eighty to 90% of clients with major depression show marked improvement after ECT.)

| NURSING DIAGNOSIS: | GRIEVING, DYSFUNCTIONAL |
|---|---|
| May Be Related To: | Multiple life changes, actual/perceived loss including loss of physiopsychosocial well-being (poor nutrition, little or no exercise). |
| | Thwarted grieving response to a loss, lack of resolution of previous grieving response. |
| | Absence of anticipatory grieving. |
| Possibly Evidenced By: | Perception of areas in life as unfulfilled or as losses; denial of loss; expression of unresolved issues, guilt. |

|  | Crying/labile affect. |
|---|---|
| | Interference with life functioning, alterations in concentration/pursuit of tasks, changes in eating habits, sleep/dream patterns, activity level, libido. |
| **Desired Outcomes/Evaluation Criteria— Client Will:** | Demonstrate progress in dealing with stages of grief at own pace. |
| | Participate in work/self-care activities at level of ability. |
| | Verbalize a sense of progress toward resolution of the grief and hope for the future. |

| ACTIONS/INTERVENTIONS | RATIONALE |
|---|---|

### Independent

| | |
|---|---|
| Assess losses that have occurred in the client's life. Discuss meaning these have had for the client. | Denial of the impact/importance of a loss may be contributing to severity of depression. |
| Determine cultural factors and ways individual has dealt with previous loss(es). | Cultural beliefs affect how people express and accept grieving processes. |
| Encourage verbalization of and assist in identification of feelings and relationship between feelings and event/stressor, when the event is known. | Verbalization of feelings in a nonthreatening environment can help client begin to deal with unrecognized/unresolved issues that may be contributing to depression. Helps client in realizing response (feeling) is connected to the stressor or precipitating event. |
| Discuss ways to identify and cope with underlying feelings, e.g., hurt, rejection, anger. Set limits regarding destructive behavior. | Begins to increase the client's repertoire of coping strategies. Learning that choices are available for behaving differently can often decrease the feeling of being stuck. "Storytelling" of how others have handled situations may be helpful, not only in providing potential solutions but also in giving the idea that the problem is manageable. |
| Identify normal stages of grief and acknowledge reality of associated feelings, e.g., guilt, anger, powerlessness. | Helps client understand normalcy of feelings and may alleviate some of the guilt generated by these feelings. |
| Assist client to identify need to address problem differently. Describe all aspects of the problem through the use of therapeutic communication skills. | Contracting for change begins with agreeing on "the problem." Helps the client to consider all aspects of the problem in order to clearly define what the client is dealing with. |
| Assist the client to recognize early symptoms of depression and plan ways to alleviate them. Help client to formulate steps to take for outside support if symptoms continue. | Involves the client actively, reducing sense of powerlessness. Rehearsal promotes generalization of recently learned coping strategies to new situations. May help to minimize recurrence of depressive feelings. |

| ACTIONS/INTERVENTIONS | RATIONALE |
|---|---|
| **Independent** | |
| Reinforce the positive aspects of being able to reach out for help. | Encourages the client to learn how to manage/take care of self. It is important that the client has support available should help be needed and that the client experience needing to reach out as positive, reflecting sense of empowerment and own self-worth. |
| Encourage participation in regular exercise program, sporting activities, occupational/recreational therapy including brisk walks, jogging, punching bag, volleyball. | Participation in individually prescribed activities and large motor exercises provides safe, effective methods for discharging pent-up tensions, learning to trust self, and enhancing self-esteem. |

| | |
|---|---|
| **NURSING DIAGNOSIS:** | **ANXIETY [moderate to severe]/THOUGHT PROCESSES, ALTERED** |
| **May Be Related To:** | Psychologic conflicts; unconscious conflict about essential values/goals of life. |
| | Unmet needs. |
| | Threat to self-concept. |
| | Sleep deprivation. |
| | Interpersonal transmission/contagion. |
| **Possibly Evidenced By:** | Reports of nervousness or fearfulness, feelings of inadequacy. |
| | Agitation, angry or tearful outbursts, rambling and discoordinated speech. |
| | Restlessness, hand rubbing or wringing, tremulousness. |
| | Poor memory and concentration, decreased ability to grasp ideas, inability to follow, impaired ability to make decisions, circumstantiality (unable to get to the point). |
| | Numerous, repetitious physical complaints without organic cause. |
| | Ideas of reference, hallucinations/delusions. |
| **Desired Outcomes/Evaluation Criteria— Client Will:** | Verbalize awareness of feelings of anxiety, changes in thinking/behavior. |
| | Identify ways to deal effectively with decision-making. |
| | Converse appropriately with staff or in groups. |
| | Attend to and complete tasks (ADL, occupational therapy projects, etc.) of increasing length and difficulty. |
| | Report anxiety is reduced to manageable level. |

| ACTIONS/INTERVENTIONS | RATIONALE |
|---|---|
| **Independent** | |
| Evaluate/reevaluate level of anxiety. | Approaches are different dependent on level of anxiety. (Refer to CP: Generalized Anxiety Disorder.) |
| Recognize and deal with own feelings in response to client's anxiety. | Anxiety is highly communicable. If the nurse becomes anxious (or impatient, irritable, etc.), this will be communicated and feed client's anxiety. |
| Listen nonjudgmentally to client's expressions; convey empathy; acknowledge or label feelings for client. | Helps client identify basis for anxious feelings, communicates acceptance, and assists in reducing current level of anxiety. |
| Use short, concrete communication. Assume calmed, "in-control-of-things" manner. Let client know about safety and supportive attentions of the staff/facility. | Attention, concentration, and problem-solving are compromised by anxiety. Benign attentions/monitoring by staff may be interpreted in a paranoid manner by the client. |
| Decrease environmental stimulation; remove to quiet area away from other clients. Suggest activity that may be relaxing, e.g., warm bath, back rub. Involve in a quiet activity when calmer. | Reduces anxiety-provoking stimuli and distractions. Helps client refocus away from anxiety. |
| Maintain a calm attitude and use physical touch, if acceptable to client. | May prove helpful if anxiety stems from delusions/hallucinations; touch can restore client to reality. Caution is required with suspicious clients who may interpret touch as aggression. |
| Defer problem-solving, assessment of precipitating factors until anxiety is reduced to a more manageable level. | Ability to problem-solve is compromised, and such requests may increase anxiety. |
| Analyze incident with client and staff to identify precipitating factors, early signs of building anxiety, previously helpful interventions. | Develops an individualized plan that will help decrease anxiety; establishes/reestablishes previous coping skill. Client needs to learn how to manage own anxiety by recognizing the signs and then acting to lower the anxiety. |
| Decrease decision-making for client by offering only a choice between 2 options, for example, whether to have cereal or eggs rather than a full menu. | Decreasing options lessens the amount of information to process and enhances decision-making. As ability to think through incoming information increases, more options can be added. |
| Choose for the client when necessary, based on knowledge of the client's interest and activity level, telling client how the choice was decided. | Judicious choosing for the client may decrease sense of inadequacy when client feels overwhelmed and provide role-modeling of decision-making process. |
| Discourage use of caffeine. | Can produce anxietylike symptoms, compounding clinical picture and client's perception of situation. |
| Assist client to learn relaxation/imagery exercises. Use tapes of relaxation exercises and calm music. Reinforce practice of these, and prompt client to use them when becoming anxious. (Note: It may be necessary to stay with anxious client.) | Develops skills for coping with anxiety responses. Staying with the client can keep client focused on the relaxation exercises and provide sense of worth and confidence. |
| Encourage practice sessions when not feeling anxious. | Enables client to use skill more effectively (automatically) as needed. |

| ACTIONS/INTERVENTIONS | RATIONALE |
|---|---|

### Independent

Encourage creative activities and development of greater leisure skills.

Helps expand positive energy and attention. Enhances self-esteem.

Involve in group settings, encouraging and reinforcing appropriate participation. Redirect into activities, e.g., interaction with others, as indicated.

Increases opportunities for/reinforcement of desired, productive interaction style. Sharing with others decreases sense of being the only one. Client may learn new coping styles from stress of participation as well as from peers who have experienced similar stressors.

Deal with physical complaints in matter-of-fact style. Investigate appropriately if new; redirect if not new or validated. Do not ask how client is or feels. Help client recognize physical symptoms as anxiety signals when appropriate. Note history of mitral valve prolapse.

Detection of physical problems and prevention of discounting client's discomfort are important. Reduces reinforcement for focusing on self and symptoms while providing opportunity and reinforcement for other-directed, more appropriate interaction style. Note: Focus on physical complaints occurs in depressed persons in about 25% of cases. Palpitations resulting from MVP may increase anxiety to panic state and require medical evaluation/treatment.

### Collaborative

Provide phototherapy as indicated.

Light therapy using white fluorescent lights (2500 to 10,000 lux) at a distance of 3 feet from the client for several hours a day has been found to improve mood within 2 to 4 days in presence of SAD. Treatment has few disadvantages, although relapse is common if therapy is discontinued. For this reason, light therapy may be combined with medication.

| | |
|---|---|
| **NURSING DIAGNOSIS:** | **PHYSICAL MOBILITY, IMPAIRED/SELF-CARE deficit (SPECIFY)** |
| **May Be Related To:** | Disinterest or unconcern; lack of energy/inertia; psychomotor retardation. |
| | Impaired self-concept; depression; severe anxiety. |
| **Possibly Evidenced By:** | Impaired ability to make decisions, such as whether to get out of bed, what to wear/eat; disheveled appearance. |
| | Reports of "I can't/don't want to" or "Wait until later" to perform self-care activities. |
| | Requests for help in the absence of physical incapacity. |
| | Inactivity. |

| ACTIONS/INTERVENTIONS | RATIONALE |
| --- | --- |

### Independent

| | |
| --- | --- |
| Speak directly to client; respect individuality and personal space as appropriate. | Promotes sense of worthwhileness of the person. |
| Provide structured opportunities for client to make choices of care, e.g., what to wear today, what activity to participate in. | Begins to establish own ability to make decisions and accept/deal with consequences. |
| Be aware of the amount of time client actually spends in bed/chair, especially clients who appear in a poor nutritional state. | Immobility places client at increased risk for skin lesions/decubitus, circulatory stasis, constipation, and infection. |
| Examine skin over bony prominences for redness (include heels) after client has been in bed/chair a while. | Identifies compromised tissues receiving decreased circulation (because of prolonged pressure) and requiring intervention. |
| Provide skin care with attention to cleanliness, massage and lotion every 2–3 hours. Change position every 2 hours, including bed to chair or to stroll "once around the day room." Progress to regular exercise program. | Until etiologic factors are remedied (immobility and nutritional status) these actions are helpful in preventing skin breakdown by alleviating pressure and promoting circulation. Also stimulates peristalsis, enhancing elimination. |
| Set progressive activity goals with client. | Reduces risks of complications related to sedentary lifestyle/immobility. Activity can also release natural endorphins, which aid in elevating mood. |
| Monitor intake and output. Note color/concentration of urine. Observe for complications of reduced fluid intake, e.g., dry mucous membranes and lips, poor skin turgor, constipation, and treat accordingly. | Direct indicators of individual needs/presence of problems. Poor hydration directly affects tissues (increasing risk of damage/breakdown in face of decreased mobility) and elimination. |
| Offer fluids frequently/leave small amounts of fluid within easy reach. Encourage intake of at least 1500–2000 ml/day. | Improves overall intake in depressed person to whom everything seems too difficult. Client may drink because it is available. Small amounts prevent guilt over things being "wasted" if all not consumed. Prevents options for negative self-reinforcement, e.g., "nothing available," "can't drink that much." |
| Note dietary intake/deficits. Implement individual dietary changes, e.g., increase roughage; provide fruit juices, stimulant beverages (hot or caffeine-containing, if tolerated). | Promotes general well-being, helps increase energy level, and promotes improved pattern of elimination. Fiber improves stool consistency and bowel function. Caffeine has a cholinergic effect, and some juices, such as prune, have a by-product that stimulates intestinal mobility. |

| ACTIONS/INTERVENTIONS | RATIONALE |
|---|---|
| **Independent** | |
| Perform/assist with needed self-care activities for client, as necessary. Note frequency of elimination pattern. | Ensures that needed activities are accomplished if client is unable/unwilling to perform alone. |
| Provide/obtain needed equipment, client's own supplies, clothing. | Availability may prompt performance; having one's own things enhances self-esteem, autonomy. |
| Choose one self-care activity and plan with client how to implement in a simple, concrete fashion. | Assisting client toward self-care in a slow and achievable manner is important. Depressed clients feel overwhelmed, and it is important that success is experienced 1 task at a time. |
| Provide low-key reinforcement for improved functioning in this area. | Enhances self-esteem; low-key style avoids provoking discounting, self-derogation. |
| Give low-key reminder regarding need to perform a self-care activity. | Gentle prodding can be helpful to the client; however, reminders may be perceived as criticism and can feed into self-derogatory thinking. |
| **Collaborative** | |
| Refer to occupational/recreational therapy involving motor activities, e.g., walking, working with clay, aerobic exercise, crafts, activities of daily living. | These activities help to discharge anger and aggression and relieve guilt, as well as build self-confidence and prepare client for return to previous occupation/leisure time activities. |
| Encourage beautician/barber appointments, if available. | Can enhance self-image, stimulate participation in self-care activities. |
| Administer stool softener/bulk preparation. | May be used to supplement dietary inadequacies/soften stool until normal stool is established. |
| Provide glycerine suppository or laxative product according to protocol if no bowel movement occurs. | Prevents impaction and helps to restore regular pattern. |

| NURSING DIAGNOSIS: | NUTRITION, ALTERED, LESS/MORE THAN BODY REQUIREMENTS |
|---|---|
| **May Be Related To:** | Inappropriate nutritional intake to meet metabolic needs. |
| **Possibly Evidenced By:** | Lack of interest in eating/food or choosing nutritional foods; aversion to eating. |
| | Dysfunctional eating patterns, e.g., eating in response to internal cues other than hunger. |
| | Recent weight loss; poor muscle tone; decreased subcutaneous fat/muscle mass; pale conjunctiva and mucous membranes; or weight gain. |
| | Sedentary activity level. |

271

| Desired Outcomes/Evaluation Criteria—Client Will: | Demonstrate progressive weight gain/loss toward goal with normalization of laboratory values. |
| --- | --- |
| | Be free of signs of malnutrition. |
| | Identify actions/lifestyle changes to regain and/or to maintain appropriate weight. |

| ACTIONS/INTERVENTIONS | RATIONALE |
| --- | --- |
| **Independent** | |
| Monitor/record amount and type of food eaten, calculate total calorie intake. Note how client perceives food and the act of eating. | Provides database and documents change/progress toward goal. |
| Explain to client that malnutrition itself decreases energy levels and ability to think cohesively (e.g., decreased protein and vitamin B affect and may deepen depression). | May provide incentive to eat, increasing cooperation with regimen and intake of nutritious foods. |
| Determine calorie requirements based on physical factors and activity. Increase calorie intake as activity level increases. | Caloric requirements need to be adapted to provide sufficient energy to meet expenditures/maintain appropriate weight. |
| Monitor body weight, depending on the seriousness of the problem and the client's response to being weighed. | Provides information about therapeutic needs/effectiveness. Note: Increased appetite is one of the earliest responses to antidepressants. |
| Avoid getting into a "power struggle" about these issues. | Focuses attention on food and weight, overemphasizing them (possibly providing secondary gain) rather than underlying dynamics. |
| Provide small meals and interval feedings, emphasizing nutritious choices (e.g., high protein-carbohydrates, high fiber). | A full meal may look like an insurmountable challenge, especially for client who is depressed. |
| Identify and obtain foods client thinks would be interesting/appealing. Use family/friends as resources as indicated. | May enhance desire to eat and promote increased/balanced intake. Family can provide information about client's likes and dislikes, other helpful ideas to increase food intake. |
| Feed client if indicated by physical condition and refusal/inability to eat. | Assisting client to eat can help to meet nutritional needs. |
| **Collaborative** | |
| Consult with dietitian as necessary. | Helpful in determining individual needs, alternate dietary therapy, reinforcing proper eating habits. |
| Monitor laboratory studies, e.g., serum albumin, glucose, electrolytes, nitrogen balance. | Detects deficiencies/imbalances, identifies therapeutic needs/effectiveness. |
| Administer vitamin/mineral supplements. | Aids in correcting deficiencies until needs are met by balanced diet. |
| Provide tube feeding, as indicated. | May be necessary when client refuses or is unable to eat and client safety/condition requires. |

| NURSING DIAGNOSIS: | SLEEP PATTERN DISTURBANCE |
|---|---|
| **May Be Related To:** | Biochemical alterations (decreased serotonin). |
| | Unresolved fears and anxieties. |
| | Inactivity. |
| **Possibly Evidenced By:** | Difficulty in falling/remaining asleep; early morning awakening/awakening later than desired. |
| | Reports of not feeling rested. |
| | Physical signs, e.g., dark circles under eyes, excessive yawning. |
| | Hypersomnia, using sleep as an escape. |
| **Desired Outcomes/Evaluation Criteria—Client Will:** | Identify interventions to promote/enhance sleep. |
| | Report falling asleep within 30 minutes of retiring and sleeping 4–6 hours before awakening. |
| | Verbalize having had a satisfactory night's sleep/feeling well rested. |
| | Refrain from using sleep as a means of escaping real feelings and fears. |

| ACTIONS/INTERVENTIONS | RATIONALE |
|---|---|
| **Independent** | |
| Identify nature of sleep disturbance and variation from usual pattern, e.g., insomnia (difficulty falling asleep or may awaken early and be unable to return to sleep) or hypersomnia. | Patterns provide clues to help client and nurse to work together to solve the problem. |
| Assess what client does when awake and plan with client to change pattern as indicated. | Clients often awaken and ruminate about themselves in a hopeless/helpless manner. Having client set aside a period during the day to ruminate may extinguish this behavior at night. |
| Establish a realistic goal with client. | Some individuals have unrealistic ideas of a "normal" night's sleep. |
| Identify previous bedtime rituals that may have been interrupted by illness/hospitalization, and reestablish when possible. | Restoring familiar, successful rituals may allow the client to reestablish usual pattern. |
| Decrease afternoon and evening caffeine intake (coffee, tea, chocolate, colas). | Avoids stimulants, which may affect ability to fall/stay asleep. |
| Restrict evening fluids and have client void before retiring. | Reduces need to rise at night to void. |
| Provide light bedtime nourishment, such as milk, if client likes it and it is not otherwise contraindicated. | Milk (with L-tryptophan) is thought to be helpful in promoting sleep. Snack may prevent awakening during night due to hunger. |
| Encourage relaxation exercises to soft music prior to sleep. | Aids in release of tension and promotes falling asleep. |

273

| ACTIONS/INTERVENTIONS | RATIONALE |
|---|---|
| **Independent** | |
| Reduce environmental stimuli, e.g., lights, noises, loudspeakers, etc. | Decreases distracting stimuli that may interfere with sleep. |
| Provide night lights, environmental control (room adequately warm or cool); appropriate nightwear/bedding, including special blanket/pillow, which can be brought from home. | May prevent confusion upon awakening. Ensures personal comfort, promotes sleep, sense of security. |
| Schedule treatments, procedures, assessments, and medications during the daytime. | Prevents unnecessary interruption during sleep. |
| Increase daytime activity, including stimulating diversionary activities in daily schedule. Set limits on time spent in room, discourage returning to bed during the day. | Increased activity without overexertion promotes sleep. Note: If client must nap, morning napping disrupts sleep less than afternoon naps. |
| Explore fears and feelings that sleep is helping to suppress. | Identifies these factors so they can be dealt with to enable client to progress with therapy. |
| **Collaborative** | |
| Give hypnotic or sedative only if other methods fail. | Products may suppress REM sleep, resulting in not feeling rested upon awakening. |
| Administer/recommend that antidepressants or other medication with sedative side effects be taken at bedtime when possible. | Decreases daytime drowsiness and aids sleeping at night. |

| NURSING DIAGNOSIS: | **SOCIAL ISOLATION/SOCIAL INTERACTION, IMPAIRED** |
|---|---|
| **May Be Related To:** | Alterations in mental status/thought processes (depressed mood). |
| | Inadequate personal resources; decreased energy/inertia. |
| | Difficulty engaging in satisfying personal relationships. |
| | Feelings of worthlessness/low self-concept; inadequacy in or absence of significant purpose in life. |
| | Knowledge/skill deficit about social interactions. |
| **Possibly Evidenced By:** | Verbalization/demonstration of awareness that interpersonal or social interactions do not have desired, satisfactory, or reinforcing outcomes. |
| | Changes in patterns of interacting/communication (e.g., slowed speech, latencies, decreased amount of speech, muteness). |

**Desired Outcomes/Evaluation Criteria— Client Will:**

Decreased involvement with others; expressed feelings of difference from others; dysfunctional interaction with peers, family, and/or others.

Refusing invitations/suggestions of social involvement; remaining in home/room/bed.

Attend/then participate in a specific number of activities per day/week.

Participate in 1 : 1 interaction for specified number of minutes.

Complete errands, initiate socialization activities a specific number of times per week.

Reinstate 2 previously enjoyed activities involving others or develop new ones.

Verbalize increased satisfaction with outcomes of social interactions.

| ACTIONS/INTERVENTIONS | RATIONALE |
|---|---|
| **Independent** | |
| Be consistent and on time in planned meetings with client. | Client will experience lateness as further evidence of decreased self-worth. In building trust, client needs to know that the nurse will follow through on previously agreed meetings/commitments. |
| Greet routinely, beginning with client's name and personal comment (e.g., appearance, clothing); share pertinent information from shift report, observations, etc., without concern for response by client. | Reinforces individuality, gets attention. Provides a "no-demand" acceptance, opportunity to interact if client chooses. Matter-of-fact manner prevents demand for client to provide a response when depressed feelings interfere. |
| Use touch, unless contraindicated. | Touch is a basic form of communication and can help client in interactions, demonstrate caring, and reinforce sense of self-worth. |
| Start conversation and "give" client a topic, e.g., unit or world event, OT project, etc. | Initiating activity is often very difficult for client, and having an assignment helps get the activity started. |
| Keep input fairly short and concrete. Ask only 1 question (about 1 thing) at a time. Avoid asking "yes-no" and "why" questions. | Requires less effort for client to attend to and retain. Promotes focus and requires that client put thinking into response. "Why" questions are often perceived as threatening. |
| Take adequate time; wait patiently for responses. Observe and give feedback regarding the feeling tone conveyed and interaction style observed. | Indicates interest, enhances self-esteem. Recognition of these feelings demonstrates empathy, sensitivity. Promotes understanding of how client is perceived by others, where discomfort and feelings of inadequacy have been experienced and provides opportunity for insight/change. |

| ACTIONS/INTERVENTIONS | RATIONALE |
|---|---|

### Independent

Emphasize attendance at routine unit activities as well as nondemanding activities (e.g., movies). Initially emphasize attendance rather than participation or enjoyment to be gained.

Starting with achievable goals gives client the ability to succeed and enhance self-esteem. Attendance precedes participation.

Contract with client (e.g., for nonsuicidal client, 1 hour of attendance at an activity is rewarded by 1 hour in room without being "pestered").

Involving client in decision-making increases sense of control over situation and may promote cooperation.

Gradually increase activity schedule. Involve with one other person or in quiet activity in day area.

Enhances chances of cooperation, diminishes threat, promotes progression of interaction.

Avoid taking client's difficulty in responding or negative/hostile responses personally.

Client will try to reinforce feeling of "worthlessness" by trying to create negative responses from others. Working with depressed client requires much patience and ability to recognize small goals as improvement.

Encourage visits by friends, relatives, other social contacts identified/located by family member.

Helps reestablish neglected, previously rewarding relationships.

Determine what the client's interests/activities were, and ask client to share those. Let client teach others about past skills by asking questions, indicating desire to learn about client's contributions to job and family. Obtain hobby equipment from home, if indicated.

Revitalizes memories from a time when client felt better, promoting client's individuality and sense of offering self to others. Encourages resumption of previously enjoyed activities, reduces sense of isolation, and increases sense of purpose.

Involve family and friends to escort/transport on outings and functional (shopping, business, obtaining belongings at home) or social activities (a brief meal, church or temple service, etc.).

Events such as these require little of client but increase social involvement and yield social reinforcement. Decreases sense of isolation from outside world.

Assist individual to assess own satisfaction with outcome(s) of interpersonal interactions. Avoid asking client if activities are "enjoyable" or "fun."

Helps client plan what is to be expected from interacting and how client can behave to realize those expectations. Involves the client in problem identification and helps to evaluate whether goals are realistic. Note: Avoid cheerfulness, as it may be interpreted as false.

Request feedback on outings and activities from both client and others involved (therapists, companions).

The goal is to increase involvement, and because client will likely report a less successful event than a more objective observer, input is important from both. The client can also hear others' perception of an event, which can serve to validate/add to the client's perception.

Use social skills training model to assist client to identify alternative strategies; role-play/rehearse new (more effective) behavior; obtain feedback and reinforcement; try new behavior in a "real situation."

Client may need to learn social skills and practice new behaviors. Improved social skills are more likely to have results that satisfy/reinforce interactions.

Use group situations for maximum impact/reinforcement, e.g., group therapy, OT, RT, etc.

The group provides more opportunity for interaction, feedback, reinforcement.

| ACTIONS/INTERVENTIONS | RATIONALE |
|---|---|

### Independent

Give positive reinforcement regarding attendance, performance (e.g., increased involvement in groups, demonstration of more effective social skills) matter-of-factly and low key.

Assist in identifying the natural reinforcers that occur with more effective interactions.

Client is unable to discount reinforcement and is thus reinforced for participation. Positive reinforcement increases the reward for trying the new tactics, encourages repetition of desired behaviors.

These reinforcers will increase the client's confidence and strengthen the behavior.

| NURSING DIAGNOSIS: | SEXUAL DYSFUNCTION/SEXUALITY PATTERNS, ALTERED |
|---|---|
| **May Be Related To:** | Decreased energy and concern, apathy; loss of sexual desire. |
| | Decreased self-esteem; values conflict. |
| | Misinformation/misconceptions about sexual functioning/behavior. |
| | Impaired relationship with SO; psychosocial abuse, e.g., harmful relationships. |
| **Possibly Evidenced By:** | Reported difficulties, limitations, or changes in sexual behaviors/activities (e.g., inability to achieve desired satisfaction, women may express a loss of interest; men may experience impotence and loss of libido). |
| | Actual/perceived limitation imposed by condition/therapy. |
| | Alteration in relationship with partner. |
| **Desired Outcomes/Evaluation Criteria— Client Will:** | Verbalize understanding of effect of depression on sexual functioning. |
| | Identify stressors that contribute to dysfunction. |
| | Resume sexual functioning at level desired/as agreed on by client and partner. |

| ACTIONS/INTERVENTIONS | RATIONALE |
|---|---|

### Independent

Assess client's sexual history and degree of satisfaction prior to depression.

Assist client to define expectations for sexual satisfaction and decide what can be done to attain these.

Establishes a baseline and elicits client's feelings about previous sexual satisfaction. Note: May need to discuss this when client is well into recovery, as feelings of self-worth are intertwined with feelings about sexual satisfaction.

Planning can help the client identify more clearly what own desires are and whether they are reasonable/attainable.

277

| ACTIONS/INTERVENTIONS | RATIONALE |
|---|---|

### Independent

| | |
|---|---|
| Provide sex education as necessary. Include significant other/partner as appropriate. | Often sexual problems are partly ignorance and misconceptions about sexual facts, and knowledge can assist with problem resolution. Note: Client may need support to terminate abusive relationships/initiate involvement with others. |
| Review medication regimen; observe for side effects of drugs prescribed. | Many medications can affect libido and/or cause impotence. Evaluation of drug and individual response is important to ascertain whether drug is responsible for the problem. |

### Collaborative

| | |
|---|---|
| Refer for further counseling/sex therapy as indicated. | May need additional and/or in-depth assistance if problems are severe/unresolved as depression lifts. |

| NURSING DIAGNOSIS: | FAMILY PROCESSES, ALTERED |
|---|---|
| **May Be Related To:** | Situational crises of illness of family member. |
| | Developmental crisis (e.g., loss of family member/relationship). |
| **Possibly Evidenced By:** | Expressions of confusion; statements of difficulty coping with situation. |
| | Family system not meeting needs of its members; difficulty accepting or receiving help appropriately. |
| | Ineffective family decision-making process; failure to send and to receive clear messages. |
| **Desired Outcomes/Evaluation Criteria— Family Will:** | Express feelings freely and appropriately. |
| | Demonstrate individual involvement in problem-solving processes directed at appropriate solutions for the situation/crisis. |
| | Encourage and allow member who is ill to handle situation in own way, progressing toward independence. |
| | Identify/use community resources appropriately. |

| ACTIONS/INTERVENTIONS | RATIONALE |
|---|---|

### Independent

| | |
|---|---|
| Assess degree of family dysfunction and current coping methods of individual members. | Identifies problems of individual family members, provides direction for intervention. |
| Identify family developmental stage (e.g., newly married couple/divorced, children leaving home); components of family and client's role in the family constellation. | Developmental stage may be a factor in current situation and client's depression. Disruption of client's role may contribute to family disorganization/strain on other family members who have to step in and assume duties client usually takes care of. |

## ACTIONS/INTERVENTIONS

## RATIONALE

### Independent

Identify patterns of communication within the family. Are feelings freely expressed? Is blame or fault assigned? What is the process of decision-making in the family and who makes the decisions? What is the interaction between family members?

Dysfunctional communication contributes to feelings of inadequacy, rejection, and inability to cope on the part of the members of the family.

Acknowledge difficulties observed while giving permission to express feelings and discussing more effective methods of communication.

Reassures family that feelings are acceptable and can be dealt with appropriately.

Provide information as necessary in verbal, written, and/or tape format as appropriate.

Provides opportunity for family members to review and incorporate new knowledge to assist in resolution of current situation.

Establish/discuss goals and expectations of family members/client following discharge. Let individuals know the importance of taking it slow and not pressuring each other to change.

Realistic expectations of abilities of client to assume place in the family are crucial to continued recuperation. Family needs to understand that members need to continue to work on new style of communication and changing ways of dealing with conflict issues.

### Collaborative

Involve in group/family therapy, as indicated.

Opportunity to hear others discuss shared problems and ways of handling can encourage family members to look at new ways of interacting.

Provide information about resources available as needed, e.g., social services, homemaker assistance, counseling, visiting nurse services.

Assistance may be needed for family members to assimilate new skills and begin to make necessary lifestyle changes to promote wellness.

| | |
|---|---|
| **NURSING DIAGNOSIS:** | **KNOWLEDGE DEFICIT [LEARNING NEED] regarding diagnosis, treatment needs, and prognosis** |
| **May Be Related To:** | Lack of information about pathophysiology and treatment of depression. |
| | Misconceptions about mental illness. |
| **Possibly Evidenced By:** | Inaccurate statements about own situation and potential for recovery. |
| | Lack of follow-through with treatment regimen. |
| | Inappropriate behavior, apathy. |
| **Desired Outcomes/Evaluation Criteria— Client Will:** | Exhibit increased interest, participating in learning process. |
| | Verbalize understanding of condition, prognosis, and therapeutic regimen. |
| | Assume responsibility for following through on treatment options. |
| | Identify/use resources appropriately. |

279

| ACTIONS/INTERVENTIONS | RATIONALE |
|---|---|

**Independent**

| | |
|---|---|
| Determine level of knowledge, mental/emotional readiness for learning. | May be first experience with illness/mental health system. Previous experience may or may not have provided accurate information. May be too depressed to access information accurately. |
| Provide information about depression/treatment as indicated. Give written information as well as verbal. | Provides opportunity for client to learn about own situation and enhances recall. |
| Provide information about drug therapy and potential side effects, e.g., anticholinergic effects, sedation, orthostatic hypotension of antidepressants; possibility of hypertensive crisis if individual consumes foods containing tyramine while taking MAOIs; dysrhythmias; photosensitivity; reduction of seizure threshold. | Client needs to know what to expect from drug trial. Knowledge can increase cooperation with drug regimen. Particularly, clients need to be aware that improvement may not occur until 4–6 weeks and that side effects will generally improve/disappear within 2 weeks. |
| Encourage frequent fluids, lip salve, ice chips, as indicated. | Provides relief of dry mouth caused by anticholinergic effect of drug therapy. |
| Suggest medication dosage be taken at bedtime, when appropriate. | Sedative effect may be helpful in promoting and maintaining sleep. |
| Discuss importance of monitoring blood pressure as indicated. Suggest client rise slowly from sitting/lying position. | Most common side effect of antidepressants is orthostatic hypotension, which can result in dizziness, injury following sudden position change. |
| Review diet restrictions, e.g., tyramine-free diet (avoid aged cheeses, fermented foods, wine/beer, liver, sour cream/yogurt, soy sauce, yeast products), limitation of caffeine. | Necessary to avoid interaction (hypertensive crisis) when MAOIs are used and for 2 weeks following discontinuation. |
| Stress necessity to avoid driving or operating dangerous machinery during initiation/changes in medication regimen. | Side effects of drowsiness or dizziness are usually self-limiting but require adjustment in activities until resolved. |
| Encourage client to stop smoking, avoid alcohol intake. | Smoking increases metabolism of tricyclic medications, necessitating adjustment in dosage to achieve therapeutic effect. Alcohol potentiates CNS effects of antidepressants. |
| Instruct client to contact provider before taking other prescription or OTC medications. | Many medications contain substances that, in combination with antidepressants, could precipitate a life-threatening hypertensive crisis. |
| Discuss use of identification bracelet/card, notification of other health caregivers. | Provides information, if needed, in emergency situation to prevent sudden termination of medication, which could be detrimental. |
| Reinforce importance of not stopping drugs abruptly. | Sudden cessation of drugs can result in untoward effects, e.g., may aggravate condition, deepening depression, and cause withdrawal with nausea/vomiting and diarrhea. |
| Refer to resources/agencies, e.g., social services, homemaker/baby-sitting, support groups. | May be helpful to client for long-range planning for regaining/maintaining wellness. |

| NURSING DIAGNOSIS: | INJURY, HIGH RISK FOR [effects of therapy] |
|---|---|
| Risk Factors May Include: | Electroconvulsive effects on the cardiovascular, respiratory, musculoskeletal, and nervous systems. |
| | Pharmacologic effects of anesthesia. |
| Possibly Evidenced By: | [Not applicable; presence of signs and symptoms establishes an **actual** diagnosis.] |
| Desired Outcomes/Evaluation Criteria— Client Will: | Maintain physiologic stability, free of injury/complications. |

## ACTIONS/INTERVENTIONS

### Independent

Review medical testing, e.g., CBC, electrocardiograph, chest x-ray, urinalysis, and x-rays of lateral aspects of the spine.

Discuss what will be done, e.g., anesthesia, muscle relaxants, oxygenation, drugs used, who will be with the client, and how the client is likely to feel after ECT.

Verify informed consent/signed permission form has been obtained.

Have client empty bladder, remove jewelry/hair decorations, eyeglasses/contacts, and dentures before treatment.

Orient client upon awakening after the treatment, and support client until immediate confusion clears.

Monitor vital signs every 15 minutes until stable.

Have emergency equipment, suction, ambu bag, etc., available.

### Collaborative

Restrict oral intake as indicated.

Provide supplemental oxygen as necessary.

Administer preprocedural medications as indicated, e.g., atropine sulfate.

## RATIONALE

A complete medical workup can identify preexisting problems and the potential for problems, which should be reported to personnel involved with procedure.

Knowledge can reduce anxiety and decrease fear response and is necessary for informed consent to procedure. Client will feel more secure knowing nurse will be there upon awakening. Awareness that confusion/memory loss are temporary helps alleviate associated fears.

Indicates that client agrees to procedure and should have been given information.

Reduces risk of injury/aspiration.

Short-term memory may be affected, and client awakens confused. May be frightened by amnesia. Confusion increases with each treatment, and knowledge that aftereffects disappear will be reassuring.

Premedication, muscle relaxants, and anesthesia may produce dysrhythmias and respiratory depression, which need immediate intervention.

Prompt treatment of respiratory depression/airway obstruction can prevent/correct life-threatening complications.

Reduces risk of vomiting/aspiration.

Provides for optimum oxygenation during period of reduced ventilation.

Decreases secretions to prevent aspiration and increases heart rate to offset response to vagal stimulation caused by ECT.

# BIPOLAR DISORDERS

## DSM IV
Bipolar I Disorders
    296.0x  Single Manic Episode
    296.40  Most Recent Episode Hypomanic
    296.4x  Most Recent Episode Manic
    296.6x  Most Recent Episode Mixed
    296.7    Most Recent Episode Unspecified
    296.5x  Most Recent Episode Depressed (Refer to CP: Depressive Disorders)
296.89  Bipolar II Disorder (Recurrent Major Depressive Episodes with Hypomania)
301.13  Cyclothymic Disorder
296.80  Bipolar Disorder NOS

## DSM III-R
296.6x  Bipolar Disorder, Mixed
296.4x  Bipolar Disorder, Manic
296.5x  Bipolar Disorder, Depressed
301.13  Cyclothymia

Recurrent moods swings of varying degree from depression to elation with intervening periods of normalcy. Milder mood swings such as cyclothymia may be manifested or viewed as everyday creativity rather than an illness requiring treatment. Hypomania can actually enhance artistic creativity and creative thinking/problem-solving. This plan of care focuses on treatment of the manic phase. (Note: Bipolar II is characterized by periods of depression and hypomania, but without manic episodes.) Refer to CP: Depressive Disorders for care of depressive episode.

## ETIOLOGIC THEORIES

### Psychodynamics

Psychoanalytic theory explains the cyclic behaviors of mania and depression as a response to conditional love from the primary caregiver. The child is maintained in a dependent position, and ego development is disrupted. This gives way to the development of a punitive superego (anger turned inward or depression) or a strong id (uncontrollable impulsive behavior or mania). In the psychoanalytic model, mania is viewed as the mirror image of depression, a "denial of depression."

### Biologic

There is increasing evidence to indicate that genetics plays a strong role in the predisposition to bipolar disorder. Incidence among relatives of affected individuals is higher than in the general population. Biochemically there appear to be increased levels of the biogenic amine, norepinephrine, in the brain, which may account for the increased activity of the manic individual.

### Family Dynamics

Object loss theory suggests that depressive illness occurs if the person is separated from or abandoned by a significant other during the first 6 months of life. The bonding process is interrupted, and the child withdraws from people and the environment. Rejection by parents in childhood or spending formative years with a family that sees life as hopeless and has a chronic expectation of failure makes it difficult for the individual to be optimistic. The mother may be distant and unloving, the father a less powerful person, and the child expected to achieve high social and academic success.

### CLIENT ASSESSMENT DATABASE (MANIC EPISODE)

#### Activity/Rest

Reports disrupted sleep pattern or extended periods without sleep/decreased need for sleep, e.g., feels well rested with 3 hours of sleep.

Physically hyperactive.

#### Ego Integrity

Inflated self-esteem typical, with unrealistic self-confidence.

Grandiosity may be expressed in a range from unrealistic planning and persistent offering of unsolicited advice (where no expertise exists) to grandiose delusions of a special relationship to important persons, including God, or persecution because of "specialness."

Humor attitude may be caustic/hostile.

#### Food/Fluid

Weight loss often occurs.

#### Hygiene

Grooming and clothing choices may be inappropriate, flamboyant, and bizarre.

Inattention to ADLs common.

#### Neurosensory

Prevailing mood is remarkably expansive, "high," or irritable.

Reports of activities that are disorganized and flamboyant or bizarre, denial of probable outcome, perception of mood as desirable and potential as limitless.

Mood is labile: predominantly euphoric, but easily changed to anger or dispair with slightest provocation. Mood swings may be profound with intervening periods of normalcy.

**Mental Status:** Concentration/attention poor (responds to multiple irrelevant stimuli in the environment), leading to rapid changes in topics (flight of ideas) in conversation and inability to complete activities.

Delusions and psychotic phenomena may be noted.

Poor judgment and irritability usual.

Speech rapid and pressured.

Psychomotor agitation.

#### Safety

May demonstrate a degree of dangerousness to self and others; acting on misperceptions.

#### Sexuality

Sexual interest increased; behavior may be uninhibited.

#### Social Interactions

History of overinvolvement with other people and with activities; ambitious, unrealistic planning; acts of poor judgment regarding social consequences (uncontrolled spending, reckless driving, problematic or unusual sexual behavior).

Marked impairment in social activities, relationship with others, school/occupational functioning, periodic changes in employment/frequent moves.

#### Teaching/Learning

First full episode usually occurs between ages 15 and 24 years, with symptoms lasting at least 1 week.

May have been hospitalized for previous episodes of manic behavior.
Periodic alcohol or other drug abuse.

## DIAGNOSTIC STUDIES

**Drug Screen:** Rule out possibility that symptoms are drug-induced.
**Electrolytes:** Excess of sodium within the nerve cells may be noted.
**Lithium Level:** Done when client is receiving this medication to assure therapeutic range between 0.5 and 1.5 mEq/liter.

## NURSING PRIORITIES

1. Protect client/others from the consequences of hyperactive behavior.
2. Provide for client's basic needs.
3. Promote reality orientation and realistic problem-solving and foster autonomy.
4. Support client/family participation in follow-up care/community treatment.

## DISCHARGE GOALS

1. Remains free of injury with decreased occurrence of manic behavior(s).
2. Balance between activity and rest is restored.
3. Meeting basic self-care needs.
4. Communicating logically and clearly.
5. Client/family participating in ongoing treatment and understands importance of drug therapy/monitoring.

| NURSING DIAGNOSIS: | TRAUMA, HIGH RISK FOR/VIOLENCE, HIGH RISK FOR, DIRECTED AT OTHERS |
|---|---|
| **Risk Factors May Include:** | Emotional difficulties; irritability and impulsive behavior; delusional thinking; angry response when ideas are refuted/wishes denied. |
| | Manic excitement. |
| | History of assaultive behavior. |
| **Possible Indicators:** | Body language, increased motor activity. |
| | Difficulty evaluating the consequences of own actions. |
| | Overt and aggressive acts; hostile, threatening verbalizations. |
| **Desired Outcomes/Evaluation Criteria—Client Will:** | Demonstrate self-control with decreased hyperactivity. |
| | Acknowledge why behavior occurs. |
| | Verbalize feelings (anger, etc.) in an appropriate manner. |
| | Use problem-solving techniques instead of violent behavior/threats or intimidation. |

| ACTIONS/INTERVENTIONS | RATIONALE |
|---|---|

### Independent

Decrease environmental stimuli, avoiding exposure to areas or situations of predictable high stimulation and removing stimulation from area if client becomes agitated.

Client may be unable to focus attention on only relevant stimuli and will be reacting/responding to *all* environmental stimuli.

Continually reevaluate the client's ability to tolerate frustration and/or individual situations.

Facilitates early intervention and assists client to manage situation independently, if possible.

Provide safe environment, removing objects and rearranging room to prevent accidental/purposeful injury to self or others.

Grandiose thinking, e.g., "I am Superman," and hyperactive behavior can lead to destructive actions such as trying to run through the wall/into others.

Intervene when agitation begins to develop, with strategies such as being verbally direct, prompting more effective behavior, redirecting or removing from the provoking situation, voluntary "Time out" in room or a quiet place, physical control (e.g., holding).

Intervention at earliest sign of agitation can assist client in regaining control, preventing escalation to violence and allowing treatment in least restrictive manner.

Defer problem-solving regarding prevention of violence and information collection about precipitating or provoking stimuli until agitation/irritability is diminished (e.g., no "why," analytical questions).

Questions regarding prevention increase frustration because agitation decreases ability to analyze situation.

Concretely communicate rationale for staff action.

Agitated persons are unable to process complicated communication.

Allow client to enter areas of increased stimuli gradually when he or she is ready to leave "Time out" seclusion area.

Tolerance of environmental stimuli is reduced, and gradual reentry fosters coping ability.

Avoid arguing when client verbalizes unrealistic or grandiose ideas or "put-downs."

Prevents triggering agitation in predictably touchy areas.

Ignore/minimize attention given to undesired behaviors (e.g., bizarre dress, use of profanity), while setting limits on destructive actions.

Avoids giving reinforcement to these behaviors, while providing control for potentially dangerous activities.

Avoid unnecessary delay of gratification. Give concrete and nonjudgmental rationale if refusal is necessary.

In hyperactive state, client does not tolerate waiting or deal well with abstractions, and unnecessary delay can trigger aggressive behavior.

Offer alternatives when available ("I don't have any coffee. Would you like a glass of juice?").

Uses client's distractibility to help decrease the frustration of being refused.

Provide information regarding more independent and alternative problem-solving strategies when client is not labile or irritable.

Improves retention, as agitated person will not be able to recall or use strategies discussed.

Encourage client, during calm moments, to recognize antecedents/precipitants to agitation.

Promotes early recognition of developing problem, allowing client to plan for alternative responses and intervene in a timely fashion.

Assist client in identifying alternative behaviors that are acceptable to both client and staff. Roleplay, if indicated. Intervene as necessary to protect client when behavior is provocative or offensive. (Refer to ND: Social Interaction, impaired.)

Client will be more apt to follow through on alternatives if they are mutually acceptable. Practice in a nonagitated time helps client learn new behavior. Client may become physically violent with others when behavior is socially unacceptable/rejected.

| ACTIONS/INTERVENTIONS | RATIONALE |
|---|---|

### Independent

| | |
|---|---|
| Provide reinforcement/positive feedback when client attempts to handle frustrating incidents without violence. | Increases feeling of success and the likelihood of client repeating that behavior again. |

### Collaborative

| | |
|---|---|
| Analyze any violent incidents with involved staff/observers, identifying antecedents or provoking situations, client indicators of increasing agitation, client response(s) to intervention attempted, etc. | Information is used to develop individualized and proactive interventions based on experience. |
| Administer medications, as indicated:<br>Antimanic drugs, e.g., lithium carbonate (Lithobid, Eskalith); | Lithium is the drug of choice for mania. It is indicated for alleviation of hyperactive symptoms. |
| Antipsychotic drugs, e.g., chlorpromazine (Thorazine), haloperidol (Haldol); or some benzodiazepines, e.g., clonazepam (Klonipin). | Useful in decreasing the level of extreme hyperactivity and ameliorating accompanying thought disorder until therapeutic level of lithium can be achieved, or when lithium is ineffective. |
| Provide seclusion and/or restraint (according to agency policy). | May be required for brief period when other measures fail to protect client, staff, or others. |
| Prepare for electroconvulsive therapy as indicated. | ECT may be required in presence of severely manic decompensation. (Refer to CP: Depressive Disorders, ND: Injury, high risk for.) |

| | |
|---|---|
| **NURSING DIAGNOSIS:** | **NUTRITION, ALTERED, LESS THAN BODY REQUIREMENTS** |
| **May Be Related To:** | Inadequate intake in relation to metabolic expenditures. |
| **Possibly Evidenced By:** | Body weight 20% or more below ideal weight. |
| | Observed inadequate intake. |
| | Inattention to mealtimes. |
| | Distraction from task of eating. |
| | Laboratory evidence of nutritional deficits/imbalances. |
| **Desired Outcomes/Evaluation Criteria—Client Will:** | Verbalize importance of adequate intake. |
| | Display increased attention to eating behaviors. |
| | Demonstrate weight gain toward goal. |
| | Display normalization of laboratory values. |

| ACTIONS/INTERVENTIONS | RATIONALE |
|---|---|
| **Independent** | |
| Monitor/record nutritional and fluid intake (including calorie count) and activity level on an ongoing basis. | Helps determine deficits/needs and progress toward goal. |
| Weigh routinely. | Provides information about therapeutic needs/effectiveness. |
| Offer meals in area with minimal distracting stimuli. | Promotes focus on task of eating and prevents distractions from interfering with food intake. |
| Walk or sit with client during meals/snack times. | Provides support and encouragement to eat adequate amounts of nutritious foods even if client is unable to sit through meal time. |
| Have snack foods, juices available at all times. | Nutritious intake is required on a regular basis to compensate for increased caloric requirements due to hyperactivity. |
| Provide opportunity to select foods when client is ready to deal with choices. | If alternatives do not add confusion, can provide favored foods, sense of control. |
| **Collaborative** | |
| Refer to dietitian. | Helpful in determining client's individual needs and most appropriate options to meet needs. |
| Offer high-protein/carbohydrate diet. Provide interval feedings, using finger foods. | Maximizes nutritional intake and allows additional opportunity to "boost" dietary intake as client may eat foods that are easily picked up and/or carried around. Note: As mania subsides, caloric requirements decline, necessitating adjustment of diet based on client's weight, health status, and activity level. |
| Review laboratory studies as indicated, e.g., chemistry profile (including electrolytes) and urinalysis. | Indicates nutritional status, identifies therapeutic needs/effectiveness. |
| Administer supplemental vitamins and minerals. | Corrects dietary deficiencies, improving nutritional status. |

| | |
|---|---|
| **NURSING DIAGNOSIS:** | **SLEEP PATTERN DISTURBANCE** |
| **May Be Related To:** | Psychologic stress, lack of recognition of fatigue/need to sleep, hyperactivity. |
| **Possibly Evidenced By:** | Denial of need to sleep. |
| | Interrupted nighttime sleep, one or more nights without sleep. |
| | Changes in behavior and performance, increasing irritability/restlessness. |
| | Dark circles under eyes. |

| Desired Outcomes/Evaluation Criteria—Client Will: | Recognize cues indicating fatigue/need for sleep. |
|---|---|
| | Reestablish sleep pattern as individually appropriate. |
| | Report feeling well rested and appear relaxed. |

## ACTIONS/INTERVENTIONS / RATIONALE

### Independent

| ACTIONS/INTERVENTIONS | RATIONALE |
|---|---|
| Decrease environmental stimuli in room and from common areas. | Manic client is unable to relax and decrease attention to stimuli, affecting ability to fall asleep. Note: May need private room, seclusion. |
| Restrict intake of caffeine, e.g., coffee, tea, cocoa, cola drinks. | May stimulate CNS, interfering with relaxation, ability to sleep. |
| Offer small snack/warm milk at bedtime or when awake during the night. | Inattention to personal needs may have led to a less than adequate intake, and hunger at night may distract from sleep. |
| Encourage engaging in physical activities/exercise during morning/afternoon. Restrict activity in the evening prior to bedtime. | Enhances sense of fatigue and promotes sleep/rest. Evening activity may actually stimulate client and interfer with/delay sleep. |
| Encourage routine bedtime activities, relaxation techniques. | Reinforces need for rest, "setting stage" for client to quiet mind and prepare for sleep. |
| Reroute to bed matter-of-factly, without providing the distraction of other activities. | Avoids providing distracting stimuli or provoking irritability. |

### Collaborative

| ACTIONS/INTERVENTIONS | RATIONALE |
|---|---|
| Administer medications as indicated, e.g.:<br>    sedatives; | Careful use may assist in reestablishing sleep pattern. |
|     antipsychotics. | Produces a calming effect, reducing hyperactivity and promoting rest/sleep. |

| NURSING DIAGNOSIS: | SELF-CARE DEFICITS: grooming/hygiene, management of personal belongings |
|---|---|
| May Be Related To: | Lack of concern; impulsivity; poor judgment. |
| | Hyperactivity. |
| Possibly Evidenced By: | Unkempt appearance, dirty, wearing inadequate and/or inappropriate clothing. |
| | Giving away clothing, money, etc., spending or "charging" extravagantly. |
| Desired Outcomes/Evaluation Criteria—Client Will: | Perform self-care activities within level of own ability. |
| | Use resources/assistance as needed. |
| | Take responsibility for/manage personal belongings. |

| ACTIONS/INTERVENTIONS | RATIONALE |
|---|---|
| **Independent** | |
| Assess current level of functioning; reevaluate daily. | Provides information about changes in individual abilities necessary for planning/altering care. |
| Provide physical assistance, supervision and simple directions/reminders, encouragement and support, as needed. | Helps focus attention on task. Providing only required assistance fosters autonomous functioning. |
| Acquire needed supplies, including clothing, if not immediately available. Obtain client's own toiletries/clothing as soon as possible. | May not have own necessities if disorganized prior to hospitalization or hospitalized as an emergency measure. Having own supplies/clothing supports autonomy, self-esteem. |
| Limit the selection of clothing available, as indicated. | May be necessary during time of extreme hyperactivity and distractibility until client is able to refrain from bizarre dress and/or care for personal belongings. |
| Monitor ability to manage money and valuables as well as other personal effects. | May give possessions away, spend money extravagantly, or become involved in grandiose plans, necessitating intervention. |
| Intervene to protect client from own impulsivity and from exploitation, if indicated, decreasing restrictions as soon as possible. | Provides protection from deleterious consequences of impulsivity without compromising or undue restriction of civil/personal liberties or autonomous functioning. |
| Set goals to establish minimum standards for self-care as condition improves, e.g., take a bath every other day, brush teeth twice a day. | Promotes idea that client can begin to assume responsibility for self, enhances sense of self-worth. |

| | |
|---|---|
| **NURSING DIAGNOSIS:** | **SENSORY/PERCEPTUAL ALTERATIONS (SPECIFY)[overload]** |
| **May Be Related To:** | Decrease in sensory threshold; psychologic stress (narrowed perceptual fields). |
| | Chemical alteration: endogenous. |
| | Sleep deprivation. |
| **Possibly Evidenced By:** | Increased distractibility and agitation (in areas/times of increased environmental stimuli); anxiety. |
| | Disorientation; poor concentration; bizarre thinking; auditory/visual hallucinations. |
| | Motor incoordination. |
| **Desired Outcomes/Evaluation Criteria— Client Will:** | Verbalize awareness/causes of sensory overload. |
| | Demonstrate behaviors to reduce/manage sensory input, e.g., sits quietly, attends to simple tasks and completes them. |

Initiate and/or take "Time out" in quieter area when prompted.

Attend and be appropriately involved in activities (e.g., unit meeting, groups).

| ACTIONS/INTERVENTIONS | RATIONALE |
|---|---|
| **Independent** | |
| Orient to reality, e.g., identify primary caregiver, where room is. Keep communications simple. | May be disoriented/confused as a result of change of surroundings, multiple distractions. |
| Assist client in focusing on input or task, e.g., address by name; use short, 1-stage directions; provide a low-stimulus area for interview, meals, tasks. | Decreases distractions/choices that are available, helping to gain client's attention in presence of multiple distractions. |
| Avoid looking at watch, taking notes, talking to others when focusing on client. | Causes distracting stimuli, adding to stimulation, which can increase hyperactivity. |
| Remove to area of lower environmental stimulus level if client shows increasing agitation or distractibility. | Reduces distractions, thereby reducing stimulation and diminishing hyperactive behavior. |
| Explain upcoming events, necessary treatments in advance, giving reasons and using simple terms. | Stimuli may be less overwhelming when client is prepared. |
| Limit invasion of personal space, e.g., touching clothing, items in room. Use physical touch judiciously. | Reduces stimuli, shows respect for client, who may view touch as threatening. |
| Observe/monitor for indicators of improved tolerance for multiple sensory stimuli; and increase exposure toward environment, people, activities accordingly. | Allows greatest possible participation in treatment milieu, personal freedom. |

| NURSING DIAGNOSIS: | SOCIAL INTERACTION, IMPAIRED |
|---|---|
| **May Be Related To:** | Poor judgment; impulsivity; self focus/egocentricity. |
| | Hyperactivity. |
| **Possibly Evidenced By:** | Inappropriate behavior, e.g., interrupts, is intrusive, demanding, hypercritical and verbally caustic/hostile, provocative and/or teasing, does not respect others' personal space. |
| | Inappropriate and/or flamboyant social behavior with bizarre dress. |
| | Problematic sexual behavior. |
| **Desired Outcomes/Evaluation Criteria— Client Will:** | Listen/converse without consistent interruptions. |
| | Participate appropriately or constructively in 1:1, group, OT. |

Demonstrate social behavior and dress individually consistent with social norms of the client's peer group.

Respect the privacy and personal property of others.

| ACTIONS/INTERVENTIONS | RATIONALE |
|---|---|
| **Independent** | |
| Be aware, gently confront manipulative behaviors (e.g., not taking responsibility for own actions, getting others to do things they normally would not do). | Grandiose behavior may be inappropriately used with client becoming demanding and overbearing, interfering with relationships with others. Clients who are manic are attuned to sources of conflict and may consciously or unconsciously escalate the conflict to refocus attention from self, thus putting others on the defensive. |
| Discuss consequences of client's behavior and ways in which client attempts to attribute them to others. | Client needs to accept responsibility for own behavior before adaptive change can occur. |
| Redirect or suggest more appropriate behavior using low-key, matter-of-fact, nonjudgmental style. | Avoids triggering agitated/angry response. Helps reduce and control exaggerated/unrealistic thinking and behaviors. |
| Ask client to wait until a specified time and give rationale if gratification of a request is not possible. | When the client believes staff responses have reasons, refusals will provoke less agitation. |
| Maintain a nondefensive response to criticisms or suggestions regarding better ways to run things such as the unit. Use suggestions when appropriate. | A low-key response can reduce the volatility of the situation. (This may be frustrating when the client is either outrageous or partly correct.) |
| Act, as needed, to protect the client from harmful responses when behavior is provocative or offensive. | When the client is not taking this responsibility, the nurse needs to/is responsible for protecting the client's safety. |
| Offer feedback (positive as well as negative) regarding the impact of social behavior, in 1:1, OT, group therapy. | The manic client is "outward oriented" and responsive to reinforcement. |
| Help client identify positive aspects about self, recognize accomplishments, and feel good about them. | As self-esteem is increased, client will feel less need to manipulate others for own gratification. |
| Problem-solve with client (when able) regarding more effective ways to achieve goals. | When lability and poor concentration have improved, client will be able to focus and to control behavior enough to learn/"try out" new behaviors. |

| NURSING DIAGNOSIS: | SELF-ESTEEM DISTURBANCE [specify] |
|---|---|
| **May Be Related To:** | Retarded ego development; unmet dependency needs; lack of positive feedback. |
| | Unrealistic self-expectations; personal vulnerability. |
| | Perceived lack of control in some aspect of life; experience of real or perceived failures. |

| **Possibly Evidenced By:** | Demonstration of exaggerated expectations or sense of own abilities; grandiosity. |
| --- | --- |
| | Unsatisfactory interpersonal relationships; imperious, demanding behavior; criticism of others. |
| | Hypersensitivity to slights or criticism; excessively seeking reassurance. |
| **Desired Outcomes/Evaluation Criteria— Client Will:** | Verbalize appropriate/realistic evaluation of own abilities. |
| | Identify feelings and methods for coping with underlying negative perception of self. |
| | Formulate realistic plans for recovery. |
| | Describe strategies for minimizing future impact of personal actions, which can contribute to control of illness. |

| ACTIONS/INTERVENTIONS | RATIONALE |
| --- | --- |

### Independent

| | |
| --- | --- |
| Ask how client would like to be addressed. Avoid approaches that imply a different perception of the client's importance. | Grandiosity is thought actually to reflect low self-esteem. |
| Explain rationale for requests by staff, unit routine, etc. Maintain a nondefensive stance; strictly adhere to respectful/courteous approaches, matter-of-fact style, passive, friendly attitude. | Nursing approaches should reinforce patient dignity, worth. Understanding reasons enhances cooperation with regimen. Nondefensive stance promotes reasoned response, may reduce conflict. |
| Encourage verbalization and identification of feelings related to issues of chronicity, lack of control impacting self-concept. | Problem-solving begins with agreeing on "the problem." |
| Assist client to identify aspects where control is possible in the hospital and encourage appropriate assertion of personal control/autonomy. | Allows client to "practice," provides experience of assuming control. |
| Provide choices of activities (e.g., when to bathe, food desired, participation in social interactions), when possible. | This strategy reduces the client's sense of powerlessness. |
| Assist client, as reasonable, to maintain personal privacy. | Provides sense of appreciation for the client's dignity. |
| Offer matter-of-fact feedback regarding unrealistic plans, self-evaluation; use 1:1, group, OT, etc. | Provides an opportunity to cast doubt on unrealistic self-evaluation in the context of accepting relationships. |
| Identify and reinforce successes and gains made in 1:1, group, and OT settings. | Addressing issues of self-esteem allows the client to be positively reinforced for realistic successes. |
| Encourage client to view life after discharge and identify aspects over which control is possible. Identify how the client will demonstrate that control. | Role rehearsal is helpful in returning client to level of independent functioning. When individual is functioning well, sense of self-esteem is enhanced. |

292

| ACTIONS/INTERVENTIONS | RATIONALE |
|---|---|

### Independent

Frame relationship with health care provider after discharge as one of collaboration. Emphasize choices, decisions, personal control that will be possible.

Enhances the client's self-perception and sense of control in relation to "experts" promoting feelings of self-worth.

Assist client to identify a plan that will prevent/ minimize severe recurrence of illness. Encourage identification of signs of recurrence and concete response to symptoms, e.g., "If I go 2 nights with- out sleep, I will call my doctor."

Establishes some concrete guidelines and a plan that will allow community-based care providers to intervene, perhaps preventing an acute episode.

---

| NURSING DIAGNOSIS: | POISONING [lithium toxicity], HIGH RISK FOR |
|---|---|
| Risk Factors May Include: | Narrow therapeutic range of drug. |
| | Client's ability (or lack of) to follow through with medication regimen. |
| | Denial of need for information. |
| Possibly Evidenced By: | [Not applicable; presence of signs and symp- toms establishes an **actual** diagnosis.] |
| Desired Outcomes/Evaluation Criteria— Client Will: | List the symptoms of lithium toxicity and appro- priate actions to take. |
| | Identify factors that can cause lithium level to change and ways of avoiding this. |

---

| ACTIONS/INTERVENTIONS | RATIONALE |
|---|---|

### Independent

Observe for/review signs of impending drug tox- icity, e.g., blurred vision, ataxia, tinnitus, persistent nausea/vomiting, and severe diarrhea. Differenti- ate from common side effects, e.g., mild nausea, loose stools, thirst/polyuria, metallic taste, head- ache, tremor.

As there is a very narrow margin between thera- peutic and toxic levels, toxicity can occur quickly and requires immediate intervention. The common side effect of tremor may be lessened by use of low doses of propranolol (Inderal) or atenolol (Tenor- min).

Assess current understanding, perceptions about medications. Evaluate ability to self-administer medication correctly.

Identifies misinformation/misconceptions about drug therapy and establishes learning needs and likelihood of successful medication routine.

Provide information regarding lithium with a structured format and informational handout.

Structured client education is more effective. Hand- out provides a memory prompt.

Frame adherence to medication and follow-up treatment, attention to lifestyle as ways of assum- ing personal control.

Linking follow-up treatment to the client's goals for self-control may enhance feelings of self-esteem and continued participation in care.

293

| ACTIONS/INTERVENTIONS | RATIONALE |
|---|---|
| **Independent** | |
| Draw parallel to other kinds of chronic illness, e.g., diabetes, epilepsy. | Supports the need for ongoing care and normalcy of lifelong medication. |
| Stress importance of adequate sodium and fluid in diet. | Sodium and fluid are required for appropriate lithium excretion, which is necessary to the prevention of toxicity. |
| Discuss use of nonsteroidal, anti-inflammatory drugs, e.g., ibuprofen (Motrin, Advil, Nuprin) or thiazide diuretics. | Use of NSAIDs and some diuretics can alter renal clearance of lithium, increasing blood levels and risk of toxicity. Note: Potassium-sparing diuretics, e.g., amiloride (Midamor) or triamterene (Dyrenium), appear to have a higher level of safety in combination with lithium therapy. |
| Encourage involvement of family in regimen/monitoring. | Enhances understanding of reason for/importance of drug therapy. |
| Provide opportunity for client to demonstrate learning after initial class and at least once again before discharge. Clarify misconceptions, confusion about drug use/follow-up care. | Determines success of client education/additional needs, and helps to plan appropriate follow-up |
| Document information that has been given and how client/family demonstrate learning. | Provides continuity, communicates to other providers the level of client's/family's knowledge. |
| **Collaborative** | |
| Monitor serum lithium levels at least twice a week upon initiation of drug therapy until serum levels are stable, then weekly to bimonthly, as indicated. | Narrow therapeutic range increases risk of developing toxicity. Early detection and prompt intervention may prevent serious complications. |
| Provide a schedule for regular laboratory testing and follow-up appointments at discharge. | Assists client to stay on medication and maintain improved state. |

| NURSING DIAGNOSIS: | **FAMILY PROCESSES, ALTERED** |
|---|---|
| **May Be Related To:** | Situational crises (illness, economic, change in roles). |
| | Euphoric mood and grandiose ideas/actions of client. |
| | Manipulative behavior and limit-testing; client's refusal to accept responsibility for own actions. |
| **Possibly Evidenced By:** | Statements of difficulty coping with situation. |
| | Lack of adaptation to change or not dealing constructively with illness; ineffective family decision-making process. |

**Desired Outcomes/Evaluation Criteria—Family Will:**

Failure to send and to receive clear messages; inappropriate boundary maintenance.

Express feelings freely and appropriately.

Demonstrate individual involvement in problem-solving processes directed at appropriate solutions.

Verbalize understanding of illness, treatment regimen, and prognosis.

Encourage and allow member who is ill to handle situation in own way, progressing toward independence.

| ACTIONS/INTERVENTIONS | RATIONALE |
|---|---|
| **Independent** | |
| Determine individual situation and feelings of individual family members, e.g., guilt, anger, powerlessness, despair, and alienation. | Living with a family member with bipolar illness engenders a multitude of feelings and problems that can affect interpersonal relationships/functioning and may result in dysfunctional responses/family disintegration. |
| Assess patterns of communication, e.g., are feelings expressed freely? Who makes decisions? What is the interaction between family members? | Provides clues to degree of problem being experienced by individual family members and coping skills being used to handle crisis of illness. |
| Assess boundaries of family members, e.g., Do members share family identity and have little sense of individuality, or do they seem emotionally distant? | Degree of symbiotic involvement/distancing of family members affects ability to resolve problems related to behavior of identified patient. |
| Determine patterns of behavior displayed by client in relationships with others, e.g., manipulation of self-esteem of others, perceptiveness to vulnerability and conflict, projection of responsibility, progressive limit-testing, and alienation of family members. | These behaviors are typically used by the manic individual to manipulate others. These clients are sensitive to others' vulnerability and can intentionally escalate conflict, shifting responsibility from self to others and putting the other person on the defensive. Family members assume blame and continually try to keep peace at any cost. The client will test limits, constantly getting concessions from others and creating feelings of guilt and ambivalence. The result of these behaviors is alienation, and high rates of divorce occur. |
| Assess role of client in family, e.g., nurturer, provider, and how illness affects the roles of other members. | When the role of the ill person is not filled, dissonance and family disintegration can occur. The spouse and children of the manic individual may not understand what is happening and react in an adversarial manner, escalating the conflicts that exist. |
| Acknowledge difficulties observed while reinforcing that some degree of conflict is to be expected and can be used to promote growth. | Provides support for family members who may feel helpless to change the client and/or what is happening in their lives. |

| ACTIONS/INTERVENTIONS | RATIONALE |
|---|---|
| **Independent** | |
| Provide information about behavior patterns and expected course of the illness. Encourage discussion of the acute episode with the client. | Assist families to understand normal aspects of bipolar illness. This knowledge may relieve guilt and promote family discussion of the problems and solutions. Family members tend to hide the illness of the client and excuse the manic's behavior with a variety of rationalizations. |
| Encourage the family members to confront the client's behavior. | Family may be afraid to discuss the behavior because of the client's volatile temper. Confrontation can promote insight into the dynamics of the illness and bring about a positive resolution of the family situation. |
| Encourage use of stress management techniques, e.g., appropriate expression of feelings, use of relaxation exercises, imagery (when appropriate). | Assists individuals to develop coping skills to deal with the client and difficult situations. Imagery may be counterproductive when patient is not in touch with reality. |
| **Collaborative** | |
| Involve client and family members with support groups, clergy, psychologic counseling/family therapy. | Use of these support systems can assist individuals to cope with illness, which creates problems of relationships and daily living. |

# CHAPTER 9

# ANXIETY DISORDERS

## GENERALIZED ANXIETY DISORDER

### DSM IV
300.02  Generalized Anxiety Disorder
### DSM III-R
300.02  Generalized Anxiety Disorder

Although some degree of anxiety is normal in life's stresses, it can be adaptive or maladaptive. Problems arise when coping mechanisms are inadequate to deal with the danger, which may be recognized or unrecognized. The essential feature is unrealistic or excessive anxiety and worry about life circumstances.

### ETIOLOGIC THEORIES
#### Psychodynamics

Freudian view is that of conflict between demands of the id and superego, with the ego serving as mediator. Anxiety occurs when the ego is not strong enough to resolve the conflict.

Sullivanian theory states that fear of disapproval from the mothering figure is the basis for anxiety. Conditional love results in fragile ego and lack of self-confidence. The individual has low self-esteem, fears failure, and is easily threatened.

Dollar and Miller believe anxiety is a learned response based on an innate drive to avoid pain. Anxiety results from being faced with two competing drives or goals.

Cognitive theory suggests that there is a disturbance in the central mechanism of cognition or information processing with the consequent disturbance in feeling and behavior. Anxiety is maintained by this distorted thinking with mistaken or dysfunctional appraisal of a situation. The individual feels vulnerable, and the distorted thinking results in a negative outcome.

#### Biologic

Although biologic and neurophysiologic influences in the etiology of anxiety disorders have been investigated, no relationship has yet been established. However, there does seem to be a genetic influence with a high family incidence.

The autonomic nervous system discharge that occurs in response to a frightening impulse and/or emotion is mediated by the limbic system, resulting in the peripheral effects of the autonomic nervous system seen in the presence of anxiety.

Some medical conditions have been associated with anxiety and panic disorders, such as abnormalities in the hypothalamic-pituitary-adrenal and hypothalamic-pituitary-thyroid axes, acute myocardial infarction, pheochromocytomas, substance intoxication and withdrawal, hypoglycemia, caffeine intoxication, mitral valve prolapse, and complex partial seizures.

### Family Dynamics

The individual exhibiting dysfunctional behavior is seen as the representation of family system problems. The "identified patient" is carrying the problems of the other members of the family, which are seen as the result of the interrelationships (disequilibrium) between family members rather than as isolated individual problems.

It is recognized that multiple factors contribute to anxiety disorders.

## CLIENT ASSESSMENT DATABASE

### Activity/Rest

Restlessness, pacing anxiously, or, if seated, restlessly moving extremities.
Feels keyed up/on edge, unable to relax.
Easily fatigued.
Difficulty falling or staying asleep; restless, unsatisfying sleep.

### Circulation

Heart pounding or racing/palpitations; cold and clammy hands; hot or cold spells, sweating; flushing, pallor.
High resting pulse, increased blood pressure.

### Ego Integrity

Excessive worry about a number of events/activities, occurring more days than not for at least 6 months.
Complains vociferously about inner turmoil, difficulty in controlling worry.
May demand help.
Facial expression in keeping with level of anxiety felt (e.g., furrowed brow, strained face, eyelid twitch).
May report history of threat to either physical integrity (illness, inadequate food and housing, etc.) or self-concept (loss of significant other; assumption of new role).

### Elimination

Frequent urination; diarrhea.

### Food/Fluid

Lack of interest in food, dysfunctional eating pattern (e.g., responding to internal cues other than hunger).
Dry mouth, upset stomach, discomfort in the pit of the stomach, lump in the throat.

### Neurosensory

Absence of other mental disorder, such as depressive disorder or schizophrenia.
Motor tension: shakiness, jitteriness, jumpiness, trembling, muscle tension, easily startled.
Dizziness, lightheadedness, tingling hands or feet.
Apprehensive expectation: anxiety, worry, fear, rumination, anticipation of misfortune to self or others, inability to act differently (feeling stuck).
Excessive vigilance/hyperattentiveness resulting in distractibility, difficulty in concentrating or mind going blank, irritability, impatience.
Free-floating anxiety usually chronic or persisting over weeks/months.

### Pain/Discomfort

Muscle aches, headaches.

### Respiratory

Increased respiratory rate, shortness of breath, smothering sensation.

### Sexuality

Women twice as likely to be affected as men.

### Social Interactions

Significant impairment in social/occupational functioning.

### Teaching/Learning

Age of onset usually 20s and 30s.

## DIAGNOSTIC STUDIES

**Drug Screen:** Rule out drugs as contribution to cause of symptoms.

Other diagnostic studies may be conducted to rule out physical disease as basis for individual symptoms, e.g., ECG for severe chest pain, echocardiogram for mitral valve prolapse, EEG to identify seizure activity, thyroid studies.

## NURSING PRIORITIES

1. Assist client to recognize own anxiety.
2. Promote insight into anxiety and related factors.
3. Provide opportunity for learning new, adaptive coping responses.
4. Involve client/family in educational/support activities.

## DISCHARGE GOALS

1. Feelings of anxiety are recognized and handled appropriately.
2. Coping skills are developed to manage anxiety-provoking situations.
3. Resources are identified and used effectively.
4. Client/family participating in ongoing therapy program.

| **NURSING DIAGNOSIS:** | **ANXIETY [severe]/POWERLESSNESS** |
| --- | --- |
| **May Be Related To:** | Real or perceived threat to physical integrity or self-concept (may or may not be able to identify the threat). |
| | Unconscious conflict about essential values (beliefs) and goals of life; unmet needs. |
| | Negative self-talk. |
| **Possibly Evidenced By:** | Persistent feelings of apprehension and uneasiness (related to unidentified stressor or stimulus) that client has difficulty alleviating. |
| | Sympathetic stimulation; restlessness; extraneous movements (foot shuffling, hand/arm fidgeting, rocking movements). |

|  | Poor eye contact; focus on self. |
|---|---|
|  | Impaired functioning; verbal expressions of having no control or influence over situation, outcome, or self-care. |
|  | Free-floating anxiety. |
|  | Nonparticipation in care or decision-making when opportunities are provided. |
| **Desired Outcomes/Evaluation Criteria— Client Will:** | Verbalize awareness of feelings of anxiety. |
|  | Identify effective coping mechanisms to successfully deal with stress. |
|  | Report anxiety is reduced to a manageable level. |
|  | Demonstrate problem-solving skills/lifestyle changes as indicated for individual situation. |

| ACTIONS/INTERVENTIONS | RATIONALE |
|---|---|
| **Independent** | |
| Establish and maintain a trusting relationship through the use of warmth, empathy, and respect. Provide adequate time for response. Communicate support of the client's self-expression. | The client may perceive the nurse as a threat, increasing the client's anxiety. Attending behaviors can increase the degree of comfort the client experiences with the nurse. |
| Be aware of any negative or anxious feelings nurse may have because of client's conscious or unconscious resistance of nurse's helpful efforts. | Negative reactions to the client will block future progress. Anxiety is "contagious," and nurse needs to recognize and control own anxiety. |
| Identify behaviors of the client that produce anxiety in the nurse. Explore these behaviors with the client when relationship is established. | Promotes growth and change and helps client realize how own behavior affects others. |
| Have client identify and describe the sensations of emotional and physical feelings. Assist the client to link behavior and feelings. Validate all inferences and assumptions with the client. | In order to adopt new coping responses, the "5 R's" of anxiety reduction are used. The client first needs to **RECOGNIZE** anxiety and be aware of feelings, how they link to certain maladaptive coping responses, and own responsibility in learning to control behavior. |
| Help to explore conflictual issues by beginning with nonthreatening topics and progressing to more conflict-laden ones. | Anxious client does not think clearly, and beginning with simple topics promotes comfort level, increasing sense of success and progress. |
| Monitor the anxiety level of the nurse/client interction on an ongoing basis. | Moderate anxiety may be productive for/motivate client, but too high a level can interfere with the interaction and ability to attend to information. |
| Use supportive confrontation as indicated. | Confrontation can be useful when client progress is blocked but may heighten anxiety to a level that is detrimental to the therapy process; therefore, it should be used with caution. |

| ACTIONS/INTERVENTIONS | RATIONALE |
|---|---|

### Independent

Assist the client to identify the situations and interactions that immediately precede the anxiety. Suggest the client keep an anxiety notebook that focuses on feelings and what is going on in the environment when anxious feelings begin.

After the client recognizes feelings of anxiety, examination of the development of the anxiety (e.g., what precipitates it, the strength of the stressor[s], and what resources are available) can help the client develop new coping skills. Writing serves to decrease the anxiety while the client is learning about it, making it more tangible/controllable.

Help client to correlate cause-and-effect relationships between stressor and anxiety.

Gives more control over situation. Increases sense of power if client can identify cause of anxiety.

Note when reports of anxiety move from one area to another (e.g., money, health, relationship), and help client recognize what is happening.

Feelings of anxiety can become "free-floating," becoming attached to one concern after another, and the client needs to recognize this so it can be dealt with.

Link the present experience with relevant ones from the past. Ask questions like, "Does that seem familiar to you? What does it remind you of from the past?"

Provides opportunity for client to make connections between these events and development of current anxiety, promoting insight and learning experience.

Assist the client to learn new, adaptive coping mechanisms by exploring how the client dealt with anxiety in the past and what methods produced relief. Help to identify the maladaptive effects of present coping responses.

The client is capable of learning new, adaptive coping responses by analyzing coping mechanisms used previously, identifying available resources, and accepting personal responsibility for change, effectively **REMOVING** the threat or stressors underlying the anxiety. (Refer to ND: Coping, individual, ineffective.)

Encourage use of adaptive coping responses that have worked in the past.

Increases confidence in own ability to deal with stress.

Keep the focus of responsibility for change on the client.

Increases feelings of self-control and self-esteem.

Include significant others as resources and social supports in helping client learn new coping responses.

Enhances ability to cope when one does not feel alone. In addition, since anxiety may have an interpersonal basis, involvement of SO(s) can enhance the client's relationship skills. **RELATIONSHIPS** can provide support, help, and reassurance, enabling the use of others as resources rather than withdrawal.

Expose client slowly to anxiety-provoking situations, use role-playing as appropriate.

**RE-ENGAGEMENT** allows the client time to identify/implement and practice new, adaptive coping responses and to become comfortable in using them.

Assist to reevaluate goals, modify behavior, use resources, and test out new coping responses.

Goals may have been too rigid and may have set up client for anxiety that could be avoided by change in behavior/responses.

Develop regular physical activity program.

Excess energy is discharged in a healthful manner through physical exercise. Biochemical effects of exercise decrease feelings of anxiety.

301

| ACTIONS/INTERVENTIONS | RATIONALE |
|---|---|

### Independent

Encourage client to use relaxation techniques, e.g., meditation, massage, breathing techniques, exercises, guided imagery, and biofeedback.

**RELAXATION** is the ultimate stress management technique because it brings about a decreased heart rate, lowers metabolism, and decreases respiration. The relaxation response is the physiologic opposite of the anxiety response.

### Collaborative

Administer medication as indicated, e.g., buspirone (BuSpar), alprazolam (Xanex), clonazepam (Klonopin), clorazepate (Tranxene), chlordiazepoxide (Librium), diazepam (Valium), oxazepam (Serax).

Antianxiety medication provides relief from the immobilizing effects of anxiety.

| NURSING DIAGNOSIS: | COPING, INDIVIDUAL, INEFFECTIVE |
|---|---|
| **May Be Related To:** | Level of anxiety being experienced by the client. |
| | Inadequate coping methods. |
| | Personal vulnerability; unmet expectations; inadequate support systems. |
| | Little or no exercise. |
| | Multiple stressors, repeated over period of time. |
| **Possibly Evidenced By:** | Maladaptive coping skills; verbalization of inability to cope. |
| | Chronic worry, emotional tension; muscular tension/headaches; chronic fatigue, insomnia. |
| | Inability to problem-solve. |
| | Alteration in societal participation. |
| | High rate of accidents; overeating/excessive smoking, and/or drinking/drug use. |
| **Desired Outcomes/Evaluation Criteria— Client Will:** | Identify ineffective coping behaviors and consequences. |
| | Express feelings appropriately. |
| | Identify options and use resources effectively. |
| | Use effective problem-solving techniques. |

| ACTIONS/INTERVENTIONS | RATIONALE |
|---|---|

### Independent

Assess current functional capacity, developmental level of functioning, and level of coping. Determine defense mechanisms used, e.g., denial, repression, conversion, dissociation, reaction formation, undoing, displacement, or projection.

Knowing how the individual's coping ability is being affected by current events determines need for/kind of intervention. People tend to regress during illness/crisis and need acceptance and support to regain/improve coping ability.

| ACTIONS/INTERVENTIONS | RATIONALE |
|---|---|
| **Independent** | |
| Identify previous methods of coping with life problems. | How client has handled previous life problems is a reliable predictor of how current problems will be handled. |
| Determine use of substances (e.g., alcohol, other drugs; smoking habits; eating patterns). | Substances are often used as coping mechanism to control anxiety and can interfere with client's ability to deal with current situation. |
| Observe and describe behavior in objective terms. Validate observations with client as possible. Note physical complaints. | Provides accurate picture of client situation and avoids judgmental evaluations. Anxious people may have increased somatic concerns. (Refer to CP: Somatoform Disorders.) |
| Assess for premenstrual tension syndrome when indicated. | Increased progesterone may cause increased anxiety for women during the luteal phase of the menstrual cycle. |
| Active-listen client concerns and identify perceptions of what is happening. | Promotes sense of self-worth and value for beliefs and clarifies client view of situation. |
| Confront client behaviors in context of trusting relationship, pointing out differences between words and actions, when appropriate. | Helps client to become aware of distortions of reality resulting from anxiety state. |
| Provide information about different ways to deal with situations that promote anxious feelings, e.g., identification and appropriate expression of feelings and problem-solving skills. | Provides opportunity for client to learn new coping skills and incorporate these into own lifestyle. |
| Use role-play and rehearsal techniques as indicated. | Promotes practice of new skills in a nonthreatening environment. |
| Encourage and support client in evaluating lifestyle, noting activities and stresses of family, work, and social situations. | Helps client to look at difficult areas that may contribute to anxiety and to make changes gradually without undue/debilitating anxiety. |
| Have client identify short- and long-term goals that are attainable, prioritized according to individual client needs and realistic time requirements. | Helps provide direction, enables evaluation of progress, promotes feelings of success as goals are attained. Unrealistic goals set client up for failure and reinforce feelings of powerlessness. |
| Recommend dividing tasks into manageable units. Let client know it is OK to say "No" to requests for additional work/other commitments. | Provides focus to achieve goals by small steps. Giving permission not to take on more than individual can handle frees client from added stressors, increasing likelihood of success. |
| Suggest simplifying work environment; interrupting stressful periods with breaks for relaxation. | Enhances coping skills by reducing distractions, promoting sense of control, and allowing individual to return to task refreshed. |
| Stress importance of structuring life to provide adequate exercise/sleep, diversional activities, and nutrition. | Structure provides feeling of security for the anxious client. Promotes a less stressful lifestyle, enhances feelings of general well-being and ability to cope. |
| **Collaborative** | |
| Refer to outside resources, e.g., groups, psychotherapy, counselor, religious resources, sexual counseling, as indicated. | May need additional assistance or support to maintain improvement/control. |

303

| NURSING DIAGNOSIS: | SOCIAL INTERACTION, IMPAIRED/ SOCIAL ISOLATION |
|---|---|
| May Be Related To: | Use of unsuccessful social interaction behaviors.<br><br>Inadequate personal resources; absence of available significant others or peers.<br><br>Self-concept disturbance.<br><br>Altered mental status, hypervigilance. |
| Possibly Evidenced By: | Verbalized/observed discomfort in social situations; dysfunctional interactions.<br><br>Expression of feelings of difference from others; preoccupation with own thoughts, irritability, impatience, difficulty in concentrating.<br><br>Sad, dull affect; uncommunicative, withdrawn behavior; absence of eye contact. |
| Desired Outcomes/Evaluation Criteria— Client Will: | Recognize anxiety and identify factors involved with feelings of isolation/impaired social interactions.<br><br>Participate in activities to enhance interactions with others.<br><br>Give self positive reinforcement for changes that are achieved. |

| ACTIONS/INTERVENTIONS | RATIONALE |
|---|---|
| **Independent** | |
| Listen to client comments regarding sense of isolation. Differentiate isolation from solitude and loneliness. | Provides information about individual concerns/ problems of feelings of aloneness. Client may not be aware of difference between being alone by choice and feeling of being alone even when others are around. |
| Spend time with client, discussing areas of concern, e.g., reasons anxious feelings interfere with ability to be involved with others. Express positive regard for the client; Active-listen concerns. | Provides opportunity for learning ways to deal with feelings of anxiety in social situations. Communicates belief in client's self-worth and provides safe environment for self-disclosure. |
| Develop plan of action with client; look at available resources, risk-taking behaviors, appropriate self-care. | Involvement of client communicates sense of competence and ability to change behavior, even in presence of anxious feelings. |
| Assess client's use of coping skills and defense mechanisms. | Awareness of defenses individual is using provides for choice of changing behavior. Helps to develop skills that can be used to manage anxiety and promote social interaction. |
| Assist client to learn social skills and use role-playing for practice. | Provides for new ways to handle anxiety in interaction with others. |

## ACTIONS/INTERVENTIONS

## RATIONALE

### Independent

Encourage journal-keeping and recording social interactions of each day for review.

Noting the comfort/discomfort that is experienced and possible causes can provide insight, may reduce anxiety, and is useful in evaluating individual responses/coping behaviors. (Refer to ND: Coping, individual, ineffective.)

Recommend client share/discuss situation with peers/coworkers.

Helps others understand condition, reducing risk of misinterpretation and decreasing individual anxiety. Provides opportunity for client to hear own words, gain new perspective, and begin to problem-solve new ways of handling stressors.

### Collaborative

Involve in classes/programs directed at resolution of problems, e.g., assertiveness training, group therapy, outdoor education program.

Developing positive social skills/behaviors provides opportunity for diminishing anxiety and promoting involvement with others.

| NURSING DIAGNOSIS: | SLEEP PATTERN DISTURBANCE |
|---|---|
| May Be Related To: | Psychologic stress. |
| | Repetitive thoughts. |
| Possibly Evidenced By: | Reports of difficulty in falling asleep/awakening earlier or later than desired; not feeling rested. |
| | Dark circles under eyes; frequent yawning. |
| Desired Outcomes/Evaluation Criteria— Client Will: | Verbalize understanding of relationship of anxiety and sleep disturbance. |
| | Identify appropriate interventions to promote sleep. |
| | Report improvement in sleep pattern, increased sense of well-being, and feeling well-rested. |

## ACTIONS/INTERVENTIONS

## RATIONALE

### Independent

Determine type of sleep pattern disturbance present, including usual bedtime, rituals/routines, number of hours of sleep, time of arising, environmental needs, and how much of a problem it is to client.

Identification of individual situation and degree of interference with functioning determines need for/ appropriate interventions.

Provide quiet environment, comfort measures (e.g., back rub, wash hands/face, bath), and sleep aids, such as warm milk. Restrict use of caffeine and alcohol before bedtime.

Promotes relaxation and cues for falling asleep. Stimulating effects of caffeine/alcohol interfere with ability to fall asleep.

Discuss use of relaxation techniques/thoughts, visualization.

Promotes reduction of anxious feelings, resulting in improved sleep/rest.

305

| ACTIONS/INTERVENTIONS | RATIONALE |
|---|---|

### Independent

| | |
|---|---|
| Suggest ways to handle waking/not sleeping, e.g., do not lie in bed and think, get up and remain inactive, or do something boring. | Having a plan can reduce anxiety about not sleeping. |
| Involve in exercise program, avoiding exercise within 2 hours of going to bed. | Increases fatigue, promotes sleep but avoids excessive stimulation from activity before bedtime. |
| Avoid use of sedatives, when possible. | Sedative drugs interfere with REM sleep and affect quality of rest. A rebound effect may lead to intense dreaming, nightmares, and more disturbed sleep. |

| NURSING DIAGNOSIS: | FAMILY COPING, ineffective: compromised, high risk for |
|---|---|
| Risk Factors May Include: | Inadequate or incorrect information or understanding by a primary person. |
| | Temporary family disorganization and role changes. |
| | Prolonged disability that exhausts the supportive capacity of significant other(s). |
| Possibly Evidenced By: | [Not applicable, presence of signs and symptoms establishes an **actual** diagnosis.] |
| Desired Outcomes/Evaluation Criteria— Family Will: | Identify resources within themselves to deal with situation. |
| | Interact appropriately with the client, providing support and assistance as needed. |
| | Recognize own needs for support, seek assistance, and use resources effectively. |

| ACTIONS/INTERVENTIONS | RATIONALE |
|---|---|

### Independent

| | |
|---|---|
| Assess information available to and understood by family/significant others. | Lack of understanding of client's behavior can lead to dysfunctional interactional patterns, which contribute to anxiety in family members. |
| Identify role of the client in family and how the illness has changed the family organization, e.g., mother who does not maintain household, father who does not go to work. | Degree of disability suffered by the client that interferes with performance of usual family role can contribute to family stress/disorganization. |
| Note other factors besides illness that affect the ability of family members to provide needed support, e.g., anxiety, personality disorders. | Systems theory maintains that other members of the family also exhibit dysfunctional behavior, but the client is the "identified patient." |
| Discuss underlying reasons for client's behaviors. | Helps family understand and accept behaviors that may be difficult to handle. |

| ACTIONS/INTERVENTIONS | RATIONALE |
|---|---|

### Independent

Assist family and client to understand "who owns the problem" and who is responsible for resolution.

Promotes responsibility of knowing that whoever has the problem has to solve it. The individual can ask for help, but others do not rescue or try to solve it for the person.

Encourage development of problem-solving skills.

Assists family in learning new ways to deal with conflicts and reduce anxiety-provoking situations.

### Collaborative

Refer to appropriate resources as indicated, e.g., counseling, psychotherapy; financial, spiritual advisors.

May need additional assistance to maintain family integrity.

# PANIC DISORDERS/PHOBIAS

## DSM IV
### Panic Disorder

300.01 Without Agoraphobia
300.21 With Agoraphobia
300.22 Agoraphobia without History of Panic Disorder
300.23 Social Phobia (Social Anxiety Disorder)
300.29 Specific Phobia (Simple Phobia)

## DSM III-R

300.21 Panic Disorder with Agoraphobia
300.01 Panic Disorder without Agoraphobia
300.22 Agoraphobia without History of Panic Disorder
300.23 Social Phobia, Specify
300.29 Simple Phobia

A discrete period of intense fear or discomfort with onset spontaneous/unpredictable or situationally bound, usually lasting 5–30 minutes.

## ETIOLOGIC THEORIES

### Psychodynamics

Phobic object may symbolize the underlying conflict, although there is not always a clear connection. Personal perceptions, life experiences, and cultural values color the meaning of the symbol for the client.

Freudian view is that anxiety feelings stem from loss of love and support from mothering figure, which increases the client's dependency needs. The client combats the diffuse intolerable anxiety by an exaggerated use of displacement on a particular object or situation, which makes the anxiety more manageable.

Phobic partners may develop in the family; these are "helpers" who stand by and participate in maintaining phobic behavior, protecting phobic client from acute panic and anxiety. Participation of partner furthers the unconscious wish of phobic client to be taken care of and to be in control.

### Biologic Theories

Refer to CP: Generalized Anxiety Disorder.

It has been suggested that temperament is a factor in that some fears are innate. These fears represent a part of the overall characteristics with which one is born that influence how the individual responds to specific situations throughout his or her life.

### Family Dynamics

Refer to CP: Generalized Anxiety Disorder.

## CLIENT ASSESSMENT DATABASE

### Circulation

Palpitations or tachycardia.
Chest pain or discomfort.
Sweating, hot flashes, or chills.

### Ego Integrity

Reports a persistent fear of some object/situation that poses no actual danger or in which the danger is magnified out of proportion to its seriousness; tries to avoid or escape contact with the feared object or situation.

Degree of discomfort may vary from mild anxiety to incapacitation; may be unable to move, speak, or identify ways of decreasing anxiety or may begin running about aimlessly and shouting.

May express a sensation of dread and a certain knowledge that death is at hand or may fear dying, going crazy, or doing something uncontrolled.

### Food/Fluid

Nausea/abdominal distress.

### Neurosensory

May exhibit one of three types of phobias:

**Agoraphobia:** Fears any situation where may feel helpless or humiliated by frequent panic attacks, not only open places but also any place where client cannot readily escape from public view.

**Specific/Simple Phobia:** Involves a specific object such as spiders or snakes or situations such as heights, darkness, or closed spaces.

**Social Phobia:** Fears talking or writing in public and/or eating, blushing, or urinating; fears that these behaviors will result in public scorn. May avoid sexual involvement because of fear of arousal, particular sexual acts, and/or relationships.

Preoccupied with bodily symptoms and feelings of terror.

May experience brief periods of delusional thinking, hallucinations, inability to test reality.

Feelings of faintness, dizziness, or lightheadedness; trembling/shaking.

Depersonalization or derealization.

Paresthesias (numbness or tingling sensations).

May occur in conjunction with other disorders such as major depression, somatization disorder, schizophrenia.

### Respiratory

Shortness of breath (dyspnea), smothering sensations, choking, hyperventilation.

### Sexuality

Occurs more frequently in women than in men.

### Social Interactions

More common among people who have experienced an early traumatic loss, such as the death of a parent.

Manipulates environment and depends on others to avoid confrontation with the object or situation.

Some constriction of life activities present.

### Teaching/Learning

Usually begins in late teens or early adulthood.

No history of a physical disorder (e.g., hyperthyroidism, hypoglycemia); mitral valve prolapse may be present.

## DIAGNOSTIC STUDIES

**Drug Screen:** Identifies drugs that may be used by client to reduce anxiety, rule out drugs that may produce symptoms.

Other diagnostic studies may be conducted to rule out physical disease as basis for individual symptoms, e.g.:

**EKG:** In the prsence of severe chest pain to rule out cardiac conditions.

**Thyroid Studies:** Rule out hyperthyroidism.

## NURSING PRIORITIES

1. Provide for physical safety.
2. Assist client to recognize onset of anxiety.
3. Help client learn alternative responses.
4. Assist with desensitization to phobic object/situation, if present.
5. Promote involvement of client/family in group or community support activities.

## DISCHARGE GOALS

1. Stays in feared situation even when discomfort is experienced.
2. Identifies techniques to lower/keep fear at manageable level.
3. Confronts the phobia and is desensitized to the stimulus.
4. Demonstrates greater independence and an increasingly freer lifestyle.

(Refer to CP: Generalized Anxiety Disorder for needs/concerns in addition to the following NDs).

| NURSING DIAGNOSIS: | FEAR |
| --- | --- |
| **May Be Related To:** | Unfounded morbid dread of a seemingly harmless object/situation, e.g., fear of being alone in public places, snakes, spiders, dark, heights, stormy weather (virtually any object/situation). |
| **Possibly Evidenced By:** | Physiologic symptoms, mental/cognitive behaviors indicative of panic. |
| | Withdrawal from or total avoidance of situations that place client in contact with feared object. |
| **Desired Outcomes/Evaluation Criteria— Client Will:** | Acknowledge and discuss fears. |
| | Demonstrate understanding through use of effective coping behaviors and active participation in treatment regimen. |
| | Resume normal life activities. |

| ACTIONS/INTERVENTIONS | RATIONALE |
| --- | --- |

### Independent

| | |
| --- | --- |
| Encourage discussion of the phobia. Investigate sexual concerns, noting problems expressed, e.g., sex is a duty/obligation that is not enjoyed by the client. | Only when a difficulty is acknowledged can it be dealt with. Note: Phobic reaction to sex may indicate a problem of incest/sexual abuse. |
| Provide for client's safety, e.g., a secure environment, staying with the client, letting the client know the nurse will provide for safety. | In severe anxiety, client fears total disintegration and loss of control. |

| ACTIONS/INTERVENTIONS | RATIONALE |
| --- | --- |

**Independent**

| | |
| --- | --- |
| Suggest that the client substitute positive thoughts for negative ones. | Emotion is hooked to thought, and changing to a more positive one can decrease the level of anxiety experienced. This also gives the client an alternative way of looking at the problem. |
| Discuss the process of thinking about the feared object/situation before it occurs. | Anticipation of a future phobic reaction allows client to deal with the physical manifestations of fear. |
| Encourage client to share the seemingly unnatural fears and feelings with others, especially nurse therapist. | Clients are often reluctant to share feelings for fear of ridicule and may have repeatedly been told to ignore feelings. Once the client begins to acknowledge and talk about these fears, it becomes apparent that the feelings are manageable. |
| Share own experience with client as indicated when relationship has been established. | If nurse therapist has successfully dealt with a phobia in own life, the client may be encouraged by the fact that someone has overcome a similar problem. Use judiciously to avoid meeting own needs rather than focusing on the client's needs. |
| Encourage to stop, wait, and not rush out of feared situation as soon as experienced. Support use of relaxation exercises. | Phobics fear "fear" itself. If client waits out the beginnings of anxiety and decreases it with relaxation exercises, then client may be ready to continue confronting the fear. |
| Explore things that may lower fear level and keep it manageable, e.g., use of singing while dressing, practicing positive self-talk while in a fearful situation. | Provides the client with a sense of control over the fear. Distracts the client so that fear is not totally focused on and allowed to escalate. |
| Use desensitization approach, e.g.: | Client fears disorganization and loss of control of body and mind when exposed to the fear-producing stimulus. This fear leads to an avoidance response, and reality is never tested. Gradual systematic exposure of the client to the feared situation under controlled conditions allows the client to begin to overcome the fear. |
| Expose client to a predetermined list of anxiety-provoking stimuli rated in hierarchy from the least frightening to the most frightening; | Experiencing fear in progressively more challenging but attainable steps allows client to realize that dangerous consequences will not occur. |
| Pair each anxiety-producing stimulus with arousal of another affect of an opposite quality, strong enough to suppress anxiety, e.g., relaxation, exercise, biofeedback; | Helps client to achieve physical and mental relaxation as the anxiety becomes less uncomfortable. |
| Help client to learn how to use these techniques when confronting an actual anxiety-provoking situation. Provide for practice sessions (e.g., role-play), deal with phobic reactions in real-life situations. | Client needs continued confrontation to gain control over fear. Practice helps the body become accustomed to the feeling of relaxation, enabling the individual to handle feared object/situation. |
| Encourage client to set increasingly more difficult goals. | Develops confidence and movement toward improved functioning and independence. |

311

| ACTIONS/INTERVENTIONS | RATIONALE |
|---|---|

## Collaborative

Administer antianxiety medications as indicated: benzodiazepines, e.g., alprazolam (Xanax), clonazepam (Klonopin), diazepam (Valium), lorazepam (Ativan), chlordiazepoxide (Librium), oxazepam (Serax); or antidepressants, e.g., imipramine (Tofranil), fluoxetine (Prozac), sertraline (Zoloft).

Biologic factors are thought to be involved in phobic/panic reactions, and these medications (particularly alprazolam) produce a rapid calming effect and may assist client to change behavior by keeping anxiety low during learning and desensitization sessions. Addictive tendencies of CNS depressants need to be weighed against benefit from the medication.

| NURSING DIAGNOSIS: | ANXIETY [severe to panic] |
|---|---|
| May Be Related To: | Unidentified stressor(s). |
| | Contact with feared object/situation. |
| | Limitations placed on ritualistic behavior. |
| Possibly Evidenced By: | Attacks of immobilizing apprehension. |
| | Physical, mental, and cognitive behaviors indicative of panic. |
| | Expressed feelings of terror and inability to cope. |
| Desired Outcomes/Evaluation Criteria—Client Will: | Verbalize a reduction in anxiety to a manageable level. |
| | Use individually appropriate techniques to interrupt progression of anxiety to panic level. |
| | Demonstrate increasing tolerance to phobic object/situation. |
| | Identify and use resources effectively. |

| ACTIONS/INTERVENTIONS | RATIONALE |
|---|---|

## Independent

Establish and maintain a trusting relationship by listening to the client; displaying warmth, answering questions directly, offering unconditional acceptance; being available and respecting the client's use of personal space.

Therapeutic skills need to be directed toward putting the client at ease, because the nurse who is a stranger may pose a threat to the highly anxious client.

Be aware and in control of own feelings; explore the cause and use this understanding therapeutically.

The nurse's anxiety can be communicated to the client, which only adds to the client's sense of terror. Discussion of these feelings can provide a role model for the client and show a different way of dealing with them.

Provide simple, clear explanations and instructions.

During period of increased anxiety, client may have difficulty focusing on/comprehending communications.

| ACTIONS/INTERVENTIONS | RATIONALE |
|---|---|

### Independent

| | |
|---|---|
| Support the client's defenses initially. | The client is using the defense in an attempt to deal with an unconscious conflict, and giving up the defense prematurely results in increased anxiety. |
| Verbally acknowledge the reality of the pain of the client's present coping mechanism (panic) without focusing on the symptoms that are being expressed. | The symptoms that the client is using relieve some of the intolerable anxiety felt by the client. If client is unable to release this tension, the anxiety will only increase, and client may lose control. |
| Provide feedback about behavior, stressors, and coping responses. Validate what you observe with the client. | Sets groundwork for dealing with anxiety when client is calmer. Includes client in plan of care, providing sense of control/self-worth. |
| Stress the relationship between physical and emotional health and reinforce that this is an area to be explored when client feels better. | Client needs to be aware of mind-body relationship and the physiologic changes that cause discomfort. |
| Observe for increasing anxiety. Assume a calm manner, decrease environmental stimulation, and provide temporary isolation, as indicated. | Early detection and intervention facilitate modifying client's behavior by changing the environment and the client's interaction with it to minimize the spread of anxiety. |
| Assist client/family to recognize and modify situations that cause anxiety when precipitating factor can be identified. (Note: Simple phobias are usually specific and object centered; this is not so with all phobic disorders.) | Recognition of causes/relationships provides opportunity to intervene before anxiety escalates/loss of control occurs. |
| Determine/discuss use of alcohol and other drugs. | May be used to reduce anxiety/avoid panic attacks and can lead to abuse. (Refer to Ch. 5, Substance-Related Disorders.) |
| Note diagnosis of mitral valve prolapse. | This cardiac abnormality affects between 1/4 and 1/2 of panic disorder clients. Heart palpitations resulting from the failure of the valve to close properly can increase anxiety and trigger panic attacks. |
| Determine use of caffeine-containing beverages. | These clients may be more sensitive to the anxiety-producing effects of caffeine, which may precipitate panic/anxiety attacks. |
| Administer supportive physical measures, such as warm baths/whirlpool, massage. | Provides physical relaxation and helps client manage anxiety/maintain control. |
| Encourage interest in outside activity through the following actions: | Increases participation in life while decreasing the amount of time and energy available for maladaptive coping mechanisms. |
| Share an activity with the client; | This is emotionally supportive and reinforces socially acceptable behavior. |
| Provide for physical exercise/activity of some type within client toleration; | Uses energy in constructive ways. Endorphins (the body's naturally produced "narcotics") induce feelings of wellness/euphoria and are thought to be released during exercise. Note: 1/2 of clients have increased anxiety with exercise. |

| ACTIONS/INTERVENTIONS | RATIONALE |
|---|---|

### Independent

Structure the client's day with a list of planned activities realistic to client's capabilities. Include others in client's care to provide support.

Provides opportunity to experience success, which enhances self-esteem and increases self-confidence.

Identify signs/symptoms of escalating anxiety and appropriate responses, e.g., relaxation, stopping negative self-talk.

Helps client become proactive in interrupting progression of anxiety to panic. Enhances sense of control.

Discuss side effects of medications, noting reactions that may occur, e.g., drowsiness, ataxia, confusion, headache, slurred speech, lethargy, giddiness, dizziness, vertigo, and impaired visual accommodation.

Side effects of antianxiety medications may cause concern and heighten anxiety and may require evaluation/treatment.

### Collaborative

Administer medication as indicated:
antianxiety agents, e.g., alprazolam (Xanax), clonazepam (Klonipin);

Provides relief from the immobilizing effects of anxiety and promotes participation in ADLs and therapy program.

monoamine-oxidase inhibitors (MAOIs), e.g., phenelzine sulfate (Nardil);

These drugs have been found to be effective in treating panic attacks. Side effects may be temporary, and caution needs to be exercised about food that should not be consumed while on these drugs.

propranolol (Inderal).

Several antihypertensive agents such as this beta blocker have potent effects on the somatic manifestations of anxiety (e.g., palpitations, tremors, etc.), although they have less dramatic effects on the psychologic component of anxiety.

Refer client/family to counseling, psychotherapy, or groups, as indicated.

May need additional assistance/long-term support to make lifestyle changes necessary to achieve maximum recovery.

# OBSESSIVE-COMPULSIVE DISORDER

**DSM IV**

300.3 Obsessive-Compulsive Disorder

**DSM III-R**

300.30 Obsessive-Compulsive Disorder

An obsession is an intrusive/inappropriate repetitive thought, impulse, or image that the individual recognizes as a product of his or her own mind but is unable to control. A compulsion is a repetitive urge that the individual feels driven to perform and cannot resist without great difficulty (severe anxiety).

## ETIOLOGIC THEORIES

### Psychodynamics

Freud placed origin for obsessive-compulsive characteristics in the anal stage of development. The child is mastering bowel and bladder control at this developmental stage and derives pleasure from controlling own body and indirectly the actions of others.

Erikson's comparable stage is autonomy vs. shame and doubt. The child learns that to be neat and tidy and to handle bodily wastes properly gains parental approval and to be messy brings criticism and rejection.

The obsessional character develops the art of the need to obtain approval by being excessively tidy and controlled. Frequently the parents' standards are too high for the child to meet, and the child continually is frustrated in attempts to please parents.

The defensive mechanisms used in obsessive-compulsive behaviors are unconscious attempts by the client to protect the self from internal anxiety. The greater the anxiety, the more time and energy will be tied up in the completion of the client's rituals. First, the client uses regression, a return to earlier methods of handling anxiety. Second, the obsessive thoughts are either devoid of feeling or are attached to anxiety. Thus isolation is utilized. Third, the client's overt attitude toward others is usually the opposite of the unconscious feelings. Thus reaction formation is being used. Last, compulsive rituals are a symbolic way of undoing or resolving the underlying conflict.

### Biologic

Although biologic and neurophysiologic influences in the etiology of anxiety disorders have been investigated, no relationship has yet been established. The mind-body connection is well accepted; however, it is difficult to establish whether the biologic changes cause anxiety or whether the emotional state causes physiologic manifestations. However, recent findings suggest neurobiologic disturbances may play a role in obsessive-compulsive disorder, with physiologic and biochemical factors playing significant roles.

### Family Dynamics

The individual exhibiting dysfunctional behavior is seen as the representation of family system problems. The "identified patient" is carrying the problems of the other members of the family, which are seen as the result of the interrelationships (disequilibrium) between family members rather than as isolated individual problems.

It is recognized that multiple factors contribute to anxiety disorders.

## CLIENT ASSESSMENT DATABASE

(Also refer to CPs: Generalized Anxiety Disorder; Panic Disorders/Phobias.)

315

### Activity/Rest

Difficulty relaxing.
Pleasurable activities cause anxiety.

### Ego Integrity

May be very controlled from within.
Preonset stressors (e.g., family death, pregnancy/childbirth, sexual failures) may be present.

### Hygiene

Characteristic rituals may impact/include repetitive hand washing, intensive cleanliness, activities of daily living, e.g., dressing and undressing a number of times, placing articles in a specific order.

### Neurosensory

Obsessive thoughts may be destructive or delusional, with most frequent themes including contamination/dirt, health/illness, orderliness or need for symmetry, aggression, morality/religion, sex (e.g., shameful/degrading acts).
Thinking processes are rigid, intellectual, and sharply focused toward tasks; may express belief that nonpurposeful and nondirected activity is unsafe and bad.
Repetitive mental acts, e.g., praying, counting, repeating words silently.
Impaired problem-solving ability.
Ritualistic speech often noted.

### Social Interactions

More frequent occurrence in upper-middle class, with higher levels of intellectual functioning.
Interference with normal routines, occupational functioning, social activities/relationships.
May focus on details but be unproductive in work situations because of narrow scope and rigidity of ideas.

### Teaching/Learning

Most often seen in adolescence and early adulthood (average age of onset is 20).

## DIAGNOSTIC STUDIES

Refer to CPs: Generalized Anxiety Disorder; Panic Disorder/Phobias.

## NURSING PRIORITIES

1. Assist client to recognize onset of anxiety.
2. Explore the meaning and purpose of the behavior with the client.
3. Assist client to limit ritualistic behaviors.
4. Help client learn alternative responses to stress.
5. Encourage family participation in therapy program.

## DISCHARGE GOALS

1. Anxiety is decreased to a manageable level.
2. Ritualistic behaviors are managed/minimized.
3. Environmental and interpersonal stress is decreased.

4. Client/family are involved in support group/community programs.

(Refer to CP: Generalized Anxiety Disorder for needs/concerns in addition to the following NDs.)

| | |
|---|---|
| **NURSING DIAGNOSIS:** | **ANXIETY [severe]** |
| **May Be Related To:** | Earlier life conflicts (may be reflected in the nature of the repetitive actions and recurring thoughts). |
| **Possibly Evidenced By:** | Repetitive action (e.g., hand washing). |
| | Recurring thoughts (e.g., dirt and germs). |
| | Decreased social and role functioning. |
| **Desired Outcomes/Evaluation Criteria— Client Will:** | Verbalize understanding of significance of ritualistic behaviors and relationship to anxiety. |
| | Demonstrate ability to cope effectively with stressful situations without resorting to obsessive thoughts or compulsive behaviors. |

## ACTIONS/INTERVENTIONS

## RATIONALE

### Independent

Establish relationship through use of empathy, warmth, and respect. Demonstrate interest in client as a person through use of attending behaviors.

Anything about which the client feels anxious will serve to increase the ritualistic behaviors. Establishing trust provides support and communicates that the nurse accepts the client as a person with the right to self-determination.

Acknowledge behavior without focusing attention on it. Verbalize empathy toward client's experience rather than disapproval or criticism. Better to say: "I see you undress 3 times every morning. That must be tiring for you" rather than "Try to dress only 1 time today."

Ignoring ritualistic behaviors can result in diminishing them. As anxiety is reduced, the need for the behaviors is reduced. Reflecting the client's feelings may reduce the intensity of the ritualistic behavior.

Use a relaxed manner with the client; keep the environment calm.

Any attempts to decrease stress will help the client to feel less anxious, thus reducing the intensity of the ritualistic behaviors.

Assist client to learn stress management, e.g., thought stopping, relaxation exercises, imagery. Identify what the client perceives as relaxing, e.g., warm bath, music.

Stress management techniques can be used, instead of ritualistic behaviors, to break habitual pattern.

Engage in constructive activities such as quiet games that require concentration, as well as arts and crafts such as needlework, woodwork, ceramics, and painting.

Planned activities allow the client less time for compulsive behavior and distract the client in a manner that allows creativity and positive feedback.

Give positive reinforcement for noncompulsive behavior. Avoid reinforcing compulsive behavior. Help significant other(s) learn the value of not focusing on the ritualistic behaviors.

This approach will prevent the client from obtaining secondary gains from the maladaptive behaviors.

317

| ACTIONS/INTERVENTIONS | RATIONALE |
|---|---|

### Independent

Assist the client to find ways to set limits on own behaviors. At the same time allow adequate time during the daily routine for the ritual(s).

Encourages the client to problem-solve limiting own behaviors while also recognizing that behaviors cannot be stopped by others or anxiety will be increased. If the time required for performing the rituals is not considered in planning care, then the client feels rushed and anxious in performing behaviors. A mistake is more likely to be made, and the whole ritual will have to be started again, resulting in increased anxiety, possibly to an unmanageable level.

Limit the amount of time allotted for the performance of rituals. Encourage client to gradually decrease this time.

Provides initial control of maladaptive behaviors until client is able to enforce own limits and substitute more adaptive responses(s) to stress.

Encourage client to explore the meaning and purpose of behaviors; to describe the feelings when the behaviors occur, intensify, or are interrelated; and to examine the precipitating factors to the performance of the rituals.

This exploration provides an opportunity to begin to understand the process and gain control over the obsessive-compulsive sequence. When opportunity for ritualistic behavior does not occur, the client fears that something bad will happen. Recognizing precipitating factors allows client to interrupt escalating anxiety.

### Collaborative

Administer medications as indicated, e.g.:
   clomiprimine (Anafranil), fluoxetine (Prozac);

The most commonly used agents to decrease feelings of anxiety, reduce need for ritualistic behavior(s), and allow for learning of other methods of stress reduction.

   buspirone (Buspar) and lithium (Eskalith);

Refractory clients may require combination therapy, e.g., buspirone and fluoxetine or lithium and clomiprimine.

   sertraline (Zoloft), venlafaxine (Effexor).

These drugs are being used investigationally with some success for the treatment of obsessive-compulsive behaviors.

| NURSING DIAGNOSIS: | SKIN/TISSUE INTEGRITY, IMPAIRED/HIGH RISK FOR |
|---|---|
| May Be Related To: | Repetitive behaviors related to cleansing, such as hand washing, brushing teeth, showering. |
| Possibly Evidenced By (Actual): | Disruption of skin surfaces; destruction of skin layers/tissues (e.g., mucous membranes). |
| Desired Outcomes/Evaluation Criteria— Client Will: | Identify risk factors. |
| | Verbalize understanding of treatment/therapy regimen. |
| | Engage in behaviors/techniques to prevent skin/tissue breakdown. |

| ACTIONS/INTERVENTIONS | RATIONALE |
|---|---|
| **Independent** | |
| Assess changes in skin/tissue, e.g., alterations in skin turgor, edema, dryness, altered circulation, and presence of infections. | Repetitive behaviors, such as hand washing with detergents or cleaning with caustic substances, can damage the skin and underlying tissues. |
| Encourage use of mild soap and hand creams while using methods previously described in ND: Anxiety (severe) to decrease repetitive behaviors. | Helps to minimize tissue trauma until other forms of therapy reduce damaging behaviors. |
| Discuss measures client can take during/after cleaning behaviors, e.g., use of rubber gloves and application of antiseptic cream. | Protects skin and tissues in the presence of constant hand washing, use of caustic substances. |

| NURSING DIAGNOSIS: risk | ROLE PERFORMANCE, ALTERED, high for |
|---|---|
| Risk Factors May Include: | Psychologic stress. Health-illness problems. |
| Possibly Evidenced By: | [Not applicable; presence of signs and symptoms establishes an **actual** diagnosis.] |
| Desired Outcomes/Evaluation Criteria— Client Will: | Identify conflicts within work/family situations. Talk with family/SO(s) about situation and changes that have occurred. |

| ACTIONS/INTERVENTIONS | RATIONALE |
|---|---|
| **Independent** | |
| Determine client's role within family and extent to which illness-related thoughts and actions affect role relationships. | Identifies areas of concern and provides accurate information to formulate plan of care. |
| Discuss client's perceptions of role, how obsessive-compulsive behaviors affect role, and whether perceptions are realistic. | Client may deny extent of effect that behaviors have on daily activities. |
| Identify conflicts that exist within the family system and specific relationships that are affected. Encourage family members to begin to discuss identified problem areas. | Knowing what stressors as well as what adaptive and maladaptive responses are occurring helps individuals begin the process of positive change. |
| Explore options for changes or adjustments in role and practice using role-play. | Planning and rehearsal of potential role transitions can reduce anxiety. |
| Encourage participation by all family members in problem-solving process and plans for change. | Likelihood of positive change increases when family system is involved in resolution of situations arising from client's ritualistic behaviors. |
| Provide positive reinforcement for movement toward resuming role responsibilities and decreasing ritualistic behaviors. | Enhances self-esteem and promotes repetition of desired behaviors. |

319

# POSTTRAUMATIC STRESS DISORDERS

## DSM IV

309.81  Posttraumatic Stress Disorder (specify acute, chronic, or delayed onset)
308.3    Acute Stress Disorder

## DSM III-R

309.89  Posttraumatic Stress Disorder (specify if delayed onset [onset of symptoms at least 6
         months after the trauma])

An anxiety disorder resulting from exposure to a traumatic event in which the individual has experienced, witnessed, or been confronted with an event or events that involve actual or threatened death/serious injury or a threat to the physical integrity of the self or others. The individual's response involved intense fear, helplessness, or horror. Note: A thorough physical examination should be done to rule out neurologic/organic problems.

## ETIOLOGIC THEORIES

### Psychodynamics

The client's ego has experienced a severe trauma often perceived as a threat to physical integrity or self-concept. This results in severe anxiety, which is not controlled adequately by the ego and manifests in symptomatic behavior. Because the ego is vulnerable, the superego may become punitive and cause individual to assume guilt for traumatic occurrence; the id may assume dominance, resulting in impulsive, uncontrollable behavior.

### Biologic

Refer to CP: Generalized Anxiety Disorder.

### Family Dynamics

Refer to CP: Generalized Anxiety Disorder

## CLIENT ASSESSMENT DATABASE

### Activity/Rest

Sleep disturbances, recurrent intrusive dreams of the event, nightmares, difficulty in falling
    or staying asleep; hypersomnia. (Note: Intrusive thoughts, flashbacks, and/or night-
    mares are the triad symptomatic of PTSD.)
Easy fatigability, chronic fatigue.

### Circulation

Increased heart rate, palpitations; increased blood pressure.
Hot/cold spells, excessive perspiration.

### Ego Integrity

Various degrees of anxiety with symptoms lasting days, weeks, or months (2 days to maxi-
    mum of 4 weeks occurring within 4 weeks of traumatic event [acute stress disorder];
    duration of symptoms less than 3 months [acute PTSD], more than 3 months [chronic
    PTSD], or onset at least 6 months after traumatic event [delayed]).
Difficulty seeking assistance (e.g., medical, legal) or mobilizing personal resources (e.g.,
    telling family members/friends of experience).
Feelings of guilt, helplessness, powerlessness.
Sense of a bleak or foreshortened future (e.g., expects failing relationships, early death).

## Neurosensory

Cognitive disruptions, difficulty concentrating and/or completing usual life tasks; hypervigilence.

Excessive fearfulness of objects and/or situations in the environment triggered by reminders or internal cues that resemble or symbolize the events; e.g., startle response to loud noises (someone who experienced combat trauma), breaking out in a sweat when riding an elevator (for someone who was raped in an elevator).

Persistent recollection (illusions, dissociative flashbacks, hallucinations) or talk of the event, despite attempts to forget; impaired/no recall of an important aspect of the trauma.

Poor impulse control with unpredictable explosions of aggressive behavior or acting out of feelings such as anger, resentment, malice, ill will (dudgeon).

Mental status examination may reveal: change in usual behavior (moody, pessimistic, brooding, irritable); loss of self-confidence, depressed affect.

Muscular tension, tremulousness, motor restlessness.

## Pain/Discomfort

Pain/physical discomfort of the injury may be exaggerated beyond expectation in relation to severity of injury.

## Respiratory

Increased respiratory rate, dyspnea.

## Safety

Angry outbursts, suicidal ideation, previous attempts.

## Sexuality

Loss of desire; avoidance of/dissatisfaction with relationships.
Inability to achieve sexual satisfaction/orgasm; impotence.

## Social Interactions

Avoidance of people/places/activities that arouse recollections of the trauma, decreased responsiveness, psychic numbing, emotional detachment/estrangement from others.

Markedly diminished interest/participation in significant activities, including work.

Restricted range of affect, absence of emotional responsiveness (e.g., absence of loving feelings).

## Teaching/Learning

Occurrence of PTSD is often preceded or accompanied by physical illness/harm.
Use/abuse of alcohol or other drugs.

## DIAGNOSTIC STUDIES

Refer to CPs: Generalized Anxiety Disorder; Panic Disorders/Phobias.

## NURSING PRIORITIES

1. Provide safety for client/others.
2. Assist client to enhance self-esteem and regain sense of control over feelings/actions.
3. Encourage development of assertive, not aggressive behaviors.
4. Promote understanding that the outcome of the present situation can be significantly affected by own actions.
5. Assist client/family to learn healthy ways to deal with/realistically adapt to changes and events that have occurred.

## DISCHARGE GOALS

1. Self-image is improved/enhanced.
2. Individual's feelings/reactions are acknowledged, expressed, and dealt with appropriately.
3. Physical complications are treated/minimized.
4. Appropriate changes in lifestyle are planned/made.

| NURSING DIAGNOSIS: | ANXIETY [severe to panic]/FEAR |
|---|---|
| **May Be Related To:** | Current memory of past traumatic life event, such as natural disasters, accidental/deliberate man-made disasters, and events such as rape, assault, or combat. |
| | Threat to self-concept/death, change in environment. |
| | Negative self-talk (preoccupation with trauma). |
| **Possibly Evidenced By:** | Increased tension/wariness; restlessness. |
| | Sense of helplessness; apprehension, fearfulness, uncertainty/confusion. |
| | Somatic complaints; sympathetic stimulation, e.g., palpitations, shortness of breath, diaphoresis, pupil dilation. |
| | Sense of impending doom: fright, terror, panic, and/or withdrawal. |
| **Desired Outcomes/Evaluation Criteria— Client Will:** | Verbalize awareness of feelings of anxiety/sense of control over fearful stimuli. |
| | Identify healthy ways to manage feelings. |
| | Demonstrate ability to confront situation using problem-solving skills. |
| | Report/display reduction of physiologic symptoms. |

| ACTIONS/INTERVENTIONS | RATIONALE |
|---|---|
| **Independent** | |
| Assess degree of anxiety/fear present, associated behaviors, and reality of threat perceived by client. | Identifies needs for developing plan of care/interventions. Clearly understanding client's perception is pivotal to providing appropriate assistance in overcoming the fear. |
| Develop trusting relationship with the client. | Trust is the basis of a therapeutic nurse/client relationship and enables them to work effectively together. Note: Some clients may need to participate ingroup situations and hear others relate their own experiences before they can speak about their own experiences or begin to trust others. |

| ACTIONS/INTERVENTIONS | RATIONALE |
|---|---|

### Independent

Identify whether incident has reactivated preexisting or coexisting situations (physical/psychologic).

Observe for and elicit information about physical injury, and assess symptoms such as numbness, headache, tightness in chest, nausea, and pounding heart.

Note presence of chronic pain or pain symptoms in excess of degree of physical injury.

Evaluate social aspects of trauma/incident, e.g., disfigurement, chronic conditions, permanent disabilities.

Identify psychologic responses, e.g., anger, shock, acute anxiety (panic), confusion, denial. Note laughter, crying, calm or agitation, excited (hysterical) behavior, expressions of disbelief and/or self-blame. Record emotional changes.

Determine degree of disorganization.

Note signs of increasing anxiety, e.g., silence, stuttering, inability to sit still/pacing.

Identify development of phobic reactions to ordinary articles (e.g., knives), situations (e.g., strangers ringing doorbell, walking in crowds of people), occurrences (e.g., car backfires).

Stay with client, maintaining a calm, confident manner. Speak in brief statements, using simple words.

Provide for nonthreatening, consistent environment/atmosphere.

Gradually increase activities/involvement with others.

Discuss with client perception of what is causing anxiety.

Assist client to correct any distortions being experienced. Share perceptions with client.

---

Concerns/psychologic issues will be recycled every time trauma is reexperienced and affect how the client views current situation.

Physical injuries may have occurred during incident/panic of recurrence, which may be masked by anxiety of current situation. These need to be identified and differentiated from anxiety symptoms so appropriate treatment can be given.

Psychologic responses may enhance/exacerbate physical symptoms.

Problems that occurred in the original trauma may have left visible reminders that have to be dealt with on a daily basis.

Although these are normal responses at the time of the trauma, they will recycle again and again until they are adequately dealt with.

Indicator of level of intervention that is required, e.g., may need to be hospitalized when disorganization is severe.

May be indicative of inability to handle current happenings, e.g., feelings or therapy, suggesting need of more intensive evaluation/intervention.

These may trigger feelings from original trauma and need to be dealt with sensitively, accepting reality of feelings and stressing ability of client to handle them. (Refer to CP: Panic Disorders/Phobias.)

Can help client to maintain control when anxiety is at a panic level.

Minimizes stimuli, reducing anxiety and calming the individual, and is helpful in breaking the cycle of anxiety/fear.

As anxiety (panic) level is decreased, client can begin to tolerate interaction with others. Activity further releases tension in an acceptable manner. (Refer to ND: Violence, high risk for, directed at self/others.)

Increases ability to connect symptoms to subjective feeling of anxiety, providing opportunity for client to gain insight/control and make desired changes.

Perceptions based on reality will assist to decrease fearfulness. How the nurse views the situation may help client to see it differently.

323

| ACTIONS/INTERVENTIONS | RATIONALE |
|---|---|

### Independent

Help client to identify feelings being experienced and focus on ways to cope with them.

Increases awareness of affective component of anxiety and ways to control and manage it.

Explore with client the manner in which the client has coped with anxious events before the trauma.

Helps client regain sense of control and recognize significance of trauma.

Engage client in learning new coping behaviors, e.g., progressive muscle relaxation, thought-stopping.

Replacing maladaptive behaviors can enhance ability to manage anxiety and deal with stress. Interrupting obsessive thinking allows client to use energy to address underlying anxiety, while continued rumination about the incident can actually retard recovery.

Give positive feedback when client demonstrates better ways to manage anxiety and is able to calmly and/or realistically appraise own situation.

Provides acknowledgment and reinforcement, encouraging use of new coping strategies. Enhances ability to deal with fearful feelings and gain control over situation, promoting future successes.

### Collaborative

Administer medications as indicated, e.g.:
    antidepressants: fluoxetine (Prozac), amoxapine (Asendin), doxepin (Sinequan), imipramine (Trofranil), MAO inhibitor-phenelzine (Nardil);

Used to decrease anxiety, lift mood, aid in management of behavior, and ensure rest until client regains control of own self.

    valporic acid (Depakene), carbamazepine (Tegretol), or clonidine (Catapres);

May be used in combination with tricyclic antidepressants or beta-adrenergic receptor antagonists.

    benzodiazepines: alprazolam (Xanax), clonazepam (Klonopin);

May be used in combination with phenelzine or fluoxetine. Note: Use with caution as some degree of unpredictable disinhibition may occur.

    phenothiazines: chlorpromazine (Thorazine).

May be used for the reduction of psychotic symptoms when loss of contact with reality occurs.

Use Eye Movement Desensitization/Reprocessing (EMD/R) as appropriate.

When used by a trained therapist, this short-term method of therapy is particularly effective with individuals who have been traumatized or who have problems with anxiety and depression.

---

| NURSING DIAGNOSIS: | POWERLESSNESS |
|---|---|
| **May Be Related To:** | Interpersonal interaction (lack of control of traumatic event). |
| | Being overwhelmed by symptoms of anxiety (e.g., intrusive thoughts, flashbacks; physical manifestations). |
| | Lifestyle of helplessness/poor coping skills. |
| **Possibly Evidenced By:** | Verbal expression of lack of control over present situation/future outcome; passivity and/or anger. |

| | |
|---|---|
| **Desired Outcomes/Evaluation Criteria— Client Will:** | Reluctance to express true feelings. |
| | Dependence on others. |
| | Nonparticipation in care or decision-making when opportunities are provided. |
| | Identify areas over which individual has control. |
| | Express sense of control over present situation/future outcome. |
| | Demonstrate involvement in care and planning for the future. |

| ACTIONS/INTERVENTIONS | RATIONALE |
|---|---|
| **Independent** | |
| Identify present/past effective coping behaviors and reinforce use. | Awareness of past successes enhances self-confidence and increases options for current use, promoting a sense of control. |
| Note ethnic background, cultural/religious perceptions and beliefs about the occurrence, e.g., retribution from God. | Sense of own responsibility (blame) and guilt about not having done something to prevent incident or not having been good enough to deserve surviving are strong beliefs in individuals who are influenced by background and cultural factors. |
| Formulate plan of care with client, setting realistic goals for achievement. | Actively involves client, providing a measure of control over life situation. |
| Encourage client to identify factors under own control as well as those not within own ability to control. | Recognition of areas of control decreases sense of helplessness. Confronting issues outside of client's control may encourage acceptance of that which cannot be changed. |
| Assist client to identify precipitating factors when feelings of powerlessness and loss of control began. | Increases understanding of sources of stressful events that trigger these feelings. |
| Explore actions client can use during periods of stress, e.g., deep breathing, counting to 10, reviewing the situation, reframing. | Provides information to assist client with learning constructive ways to cope with feeling of powerlessness and to regain control. Reframing stressors/situation in other words/positive ideas can help client look at alternatives. |
| Give positive feedback when client uses constructive methods to regain control. | Acknowledgment and reinforcement encourage repetition of desirable behaviors. |
| Promote involvement in group therapy. | Provides an opportunity for client to learn new coping behaviors from peers who have experienced similar traumatic events/reactions in the past. |

| | |
|---|---|
| **NURSING DIAGNOSIS:** | **VIOLENCE, [actual]/HIGH RISK FOR, DIRECTED AT SELF/OTHERS** |
| **Related/Risk Factors May Include:** | Intrusive memory of event causing a sudden acting out of a feeling as if the event were occurring; startle reaction. |

| | |
|---|---|
| | Rage reactions: breaking through of rage that has been walled off; rage at the sense of helplessness/dependency or at those who were exempted from the trauma. |
| **May Be Evidenced By/Possible Indicators:** | Increased motor activity (pacing, excitement, irritability, agitation). |
| | Argumentative, dissatisfied, overreactive, hypersensitive, provocative behaviors; hostile, threatening verbalizations. |
| | Overt and aggressive acts; goal-directed destruction of objects in environment. |
| | Self-destructive behavior (including substance abuse) and/or active, aggressive suicidal/homicidal acts. |
| **Desired Outcomes/Evaluation Criteria— Client Will:** | Acknowledge realities of the situation and precipitating factors. |
| | Verbalize awareness of positive ways to cope with feelings. |
| | Demonstrate self-control as evidenced by relaxed posture/manner, use of problem-solving rather than threats or assaultive behavior to resolve conflicts and/or cope with anxiety. |

| ACTIONS/INTERVENTIONS | RATIONALE |
|---|---|
| **Independent** | |
| Evaluate for presence of self-destructive and/or suicidal/homicidal behaviors, e.g., mood/behavior changes, increasing withdrawal. Assess seriousness of threat, e.g., gestures, previous attempts. (Use scale of 1–10 and prioritize according to severity of threat, availability of means.) | Client may be in such despair or self-esteem may be so low that behaviors may be engaged in that are violent toward self/others with conscious or unconscious wish for suicide. (Note: If scale is high, this may be no. 1 nursing diagnosis.) |
| Encourage client to identify and verbalize triggering stimuli, causative/contributing factors that lead to potential or actual violence by client. | Client needs to learn to recognize what precipitates anger and tension. Early recognition and prompt intervention may prevent occurrence of violence. |
| Negotiate contract with client regarding actions to be taken when feeling out of control. | Contracting to let nurse/significant person know when feeling overwhelmed helps the client obtain assistance as needed and maintain a sense of control. |
| Assist client to understand that feelings of anger may be appropriate in the situation but need to be expressed verbally or in an acceptable manner rather than acted on in a destructive way. | Learning to discharge anxiety and affect in a socially acceptable manner reduces likelihood of violent outbursts. |
| Tell the client to STOP violent behaviors. Use environmental controls (such as providing a quiet place for client to go, holding the client) if behavior continues to escalate. Talk to client in gentle, quiet manner while holding him or her. | Saying "Stop" may be sufficient to assist client to regain control, but external controls may be required if client is unable to call up internal controls. Note: Physical holding can provide a sense of contact and caring to help the client to regain control. |

| ACTIONS/INTERVENTIONS | RATIONALE |
|---|---|
| **Independent** | |
| Give client as much control as possible in other areas of life, helping to identify more appropriate solutions and responses to tension and anxiety. | Learning new ways of responding to impulsive tendencies increases capacity for controlling impulses. |
| Involve in exercise program, in outdoor activity program (hiking, wall/rock climbing, etc.); encourage sporting activities (group or individual). | Relieves tension and increases sense of well-being, promotes self-esteem. When activity is geared to individual interests, participation and therapeutic benefits are enhanced. |
| **Collaborative** | |
| Use seclusion or restraints until control is regained, as indicated. | Provides external control to prevent injury to client/staff/others. |
| Administer medications, as indicated, e.g., lithium carbonate (Eskalith). | Low-dose therapy may be used to reduce explosive behavior. |

| NURSING DIAGNOSIS: | COPING, INDIVIDUAL, INEFFECTIVE |
|---|---|
| **May Be Related To:** | Personal vulnerability; unmet expectations; unrealistic perceptions. |
| | Inadequate support systems/coping method(s). |
| | Multiple stressors, repeated over period of time; overwhelming threat to self. |
| **Possibly Evidenced By:** | Verbalization of inability to cope or difficulty asking for help. |
| | Muscular tension/headaches. |
| | Emotional tension; chronic worry. |
| **Desired Outcomes/Evaluation Criteria— Client Will:** | Identify ineffective coping behaviors and consequences. |
| | Verbalize awareness of own coping abilities. |
| | Express feelings appropriately. |
| | Identify options and use resources effectively. |

| ACTIONS/INTERVENTIONS | RATIONALE |
|---|---|
| **Independent** | |
| Identify and discuss degree of dysfunctional coping (e.g., denial, rationalization), including use/abuse of chemical substances. | Identifies needs/depth of interventions required. Individuals display different levels of dysfunctional behavior in response to stress, and often the choice of alcohol and/or other drugs is a way of deadening the psychic pain. |

327

| ACTIONS/INTERVENTIONS | RATIONALE |
|---|---|
| **Independent** | |
| Review consequences of behaviors, how relationships/functioning are affected. | Helps client recognize negative impact on life and provides focus to begin addressing problems. |
| Be aware of and assist client to use ego strengths in a positive way and acknowledge ability to handle what is happening. | Often the firm statement of the nurse's conviction that the client can handle what is happening connects with the inner belief in self that is inherent in people. |
| Permit free expression of feelings at client's own pace. Do not rush client through expressions of feelings too quickly; avoid reassuring inappropriately. | Nonjudgmental listening to all feelings conveys acceptance of the worth of the client. Taking own time to talk about what has happened and allowing feelings to be fully expressed aids in the healing process. If rushed, client may believe pain and/or anguish is misunderstood. Statements such as "You don't understand" or "You weren't there" are a defense, a way of pushing others away. |
| Encourage client to become aware and accepting of own feelings and reactions when identified. | There are no bad feelings, and accepting them as signals that need to be attended to and dealt with can help the client move toward resolution. |
| Give "permission" to express/deal with anger at the assailant/situation in acceptable ways. | Being free to express anger appropriately allows it to be dissipated so that underlying feelings can be identified and dealt with, strengthening coping skills. |
| Keep discussion on practical and emotional level, rather than intellectualizing the experience. | When feelings (the experience) are intellectualized, uncomfortable insights and/or awareness are avoided by the use of rationalization, blocking resolution of feelings and impairing coping abilities. |
| Identify supportive persons available for the client. | Having unconditional support from loving/caring others can assist the client to confront situation, cope with it, and move on to live more fully. |
| **Collaborative** | |
| Provide for sensitive counselors/therapists who are especially trained in crisis management and use therapies such as psychotherapy (in conjunction with medications), implosive therapy, flooding, hypnosis, relaxation, Rolfing, memory work, or cognitive restructuring. | While it is not necessary for the helping person to have experienced the same kind of trauma, sensitivity and listening skills are important to helping the client confront fears and learn new ways to cope with what has happened. Therapeutic use of desensitization techniques (flooding, implosive therapy) provides for extinction through exposure to the fear. Body work can alleviate muscle tension. Some techniques (Rolfing) help to bring blocked emotions to awareness as sensations of the traumatic event are reexperienced. |

| ACTIONS/INTERVENTIONS | RATIONALE |
|---|---|
| **Collaborative** | |
| Refer to occupational therapy, vocational rehabilitation. | Assistance with new activities and learning new skills may be needed to help the client develop coping skills to reintegrate into the work setting. New activities/work skills, while generating some anxiety, will help with the process of desensitization and reduction/elimination of anxiety. |

| | |
|---|---|
| **NURSING DIAGNOSIS:** | **GRIEVING, DYSFUNCTIONAL** |
| **May Be Related To:** | Actual/perceived object loss (loss of self as seen before the traumatic incident occurred, as well as other losses incurred in/after the incident). |
| | Loss of physiopsychosocial well-being. |
| | Thwarted grieving response to a loss; absence of anticipatory grieving; lack of resolution of previous grieving response. |
| **Possibly Evidenced By:** | Verbal expression of distress at loss; difficulty in expressing loss; expression of guilt. |
| | Expression of unresolved issues; reliving of past experiences. |
| | Denial of loss; anger, sadness, crying; labile affect. |
| | Alterations in eating habits, sleep and dream patterns, activity level, libido. |
| | Alterations in concentration and/or pursuit of tasks. |
| **Desired Outcomes/Evaluation Criteria— Client Will:** | Demonstrate progress in dealing with/movement through stages of grief. |
| | Participate in work and self-care/activities of daily living as able. |
| | Verbalize a sense of progress toward resolution of the grief and hope for the future. |

| ACTIONS/INTERVENTIONS | RATIONALE |
|---|---|
| **Independent** | |
| Note verbal/nonverbal expressions of guilt or self-blame. | "Survivor's guilt" affects most people who have survived trauma in which others have died, and client questions, "Why was I spared?" or perhaps believes, "I am not worthy, and others may have been." |
| Acknowledge reality of feelings of guilt, and assist client to take steps toward resolution. | Acceptance of feelings and support of new coping skills allow for taking risk of new behaviors. |

329

| ACTIONS/INTERVENTIONS | RATIONALE |
|---|---|

### Independent

| | |
|---|---|
| Reinforce that client made the best decision he or she could have made at the time. | Regardless of the choices made, the client survived the event(s). The client needs unconditional positive acceptance and validation of decisions in order to resolve feelings of guilt and begin to deal with grief. |
| Note signs and stage of greiving for self and/or others, e.g., denial, anger, bargaining, depression, acceptance. | Identification and understanding of stages of grief assist with choice of interventions, plan of care, and movement toward resolution. |
| Be aware of avoidance behaviors, e.g., anger, withdrawal. | Client has avoided dealing with the feelings, leading to current situation. Recognition at this time can help with beginning new approach to solving the problem(s). |
| Provide information about normalcy of feelings/ actions in relation to stages of grief. | Individual may believe it is unacceptable to have these feelings, and knowing they are normal can provide sense of relief. |
| Give "permission," when the client is depressed, to be at this point. | Provides opportunity for the client to accept self and feel satisfied with current progress. |
| Encourage verbalization without confrontation about realities. | Helps client to begin resolution and acceptance. Confrontation may convey lack of acceptance and actually impede progress. |
| Identify cultural factors and ways individual has dealt with previous loss(es). Point out individual strengths/positive coping skills. | Different cultures deal with loss in different ways, and it is important to allow client to deal with situation in own way. How the client has dealt with losses in the past can be a reliable predictor of how current losses are being dealt with and how they may be dealt with in the future, effectively or ineffectively. Client may discount own capabilities. |
| Reinforce use of previously effective coping skills. | Identification of helpful ways client is already dealing with problems allows client to feel positive about self. |
| Assist significant other(s) to cope with client response. | Support and understanding of reasons for client's behavior provide opportunity for family to work with client in development of new coping skills to resolve grief. |

### Collaborative

| | |
|---|---|
| Refer to other resources, e.g., peer/support group, counseling, psychotherapy, spiritual advisor. | May need additional help to resolve situation/ concomitant problems. |

| | |
|---|---|
| **NURSING DIAGNOSIS:** | **SLEEP PATTERN DISTURBANCE** |
| **May Be Related To:** | Psychologic stress (anxiety, depression with recurring disruptive dreams). |
| **Possibly Evidenced By:** | Verbal reports of difficulty in falling asleep/not feeling well rested. |

| **Desired Outcomes/Evaluation Criteria— Client Will:** | Insomnia that causes awakening. |
| | Reports of sleep disturbances, e.g., nightmares, dreams of personal death, disaster-related dreams, flashbacks, intrusive/trauma images, fear of re-experiencing the event. |
| | Hypersomnia (as a way of avoiding behaviors, events, or situations that arouse recollections). |
| | Verbalize understanding of sleep disorder/problem. |
| | Identify behaviors to promote sleep. |
| | Sleep adequate/appropriate number of hours for individual needs. |
| | Report increased sense of well-being and feeling rested. |

## ACTIONS/INTERVENTIONS

## RATIONALE

### Independent

| Assess sleep pattern disturbance by observation and reports from client and/or significant others. | Subjective and objective information provides assessment of individual problems and direction for interventions. |
| Identify causative and contributing factors, e.g., intrusive/repetitive thoughts, nightmares, severe anxiety level. Note use of caffeine and/or alcohol, other drugs. | These factors interfere with ability to fall asleep and with the REM cycle of sleep, affecting quality of rest. |
| Provide a quiet environment; arrange to have uninterrupted sleep as much as possible. | Assists in establishing optimal sleep/rest routine. |
| Encourage client to develop behavior routine when insomnia is present, e.g., no napping after noon, having warm bath/milk before bed, relaxing thoughts, getting out of bed 10 minutes after awakening if unable to fall asleep again, limiting sleep to 7 hours each night. | Rituals assist in decreasing anxiety and fear of facing a sleepless night. Note: Tryptophan in milk is believed to induce sleep. |

### Collaborative

| Administer sedative, hypnotic, or antianxiety drugs as indicated. (Refer to ND: Anxiety [severe to panic]/Fear.) | May require short-term drug therapy to decrease sense of exhaustion/fear and promote relaxation to enhance sleep. (These drugs should be used sparingly to avoid dependence and addiction.) |

| **NURSING DIAGNOSIS:** | **SOCIAL ISOLATION/SOCIAL INTERACTION, IMPAIRED** |
| **May Be Related To:** | Reduced involvement with the external world; numbing of responsiveness to the environment/affective numbing; difficulty in establishing and/or maintaining relationships with others. |

331

|                                                    |                                                                                                                                                                                                                                                                                           |
| -------------------------------------------------- | ------------------------------------------------------------------------------------------------------------------------------------------------------------------------------------------------------------------------------------------------------------------------------------------- |
| **Possibly Evidenced By:**                         | Feelings of guilt and shame/survivor's guilt.                                                                                                                                                                                                                                             |
|                                                    | Unacceptable social behaviors/values.                                                                                                                                                                                                                                                     |
|                                                    | Conflicts with family, significant others; withdrawal and avoidance of others/absence of supportive others; expressed feelings of rejection/alienation; observed discomfort in social situations/use of unsuccessful social interaction behaviors.                                          |
|                                                    | Chronic loss of interest and energy for work and relationships.                                                                                                                                                                                                                           |
|                                                    | Sense of vulnerability over fear of loss of control of aggressive impulses.                                                                                                                                                                                                               |
|                                                    | Sense of responsibility (guilt) for inciting event or failing to control it; rage at those exempted from loss or injury.                                                                                                                                                                  |
|                                                    | Drug (alcohol) abuse.                                                                                                                                                                                                                                                                     |
| **Desired Outcomes/Evaluation Criteria—Client Will:** | Verbalize recognition of causes of impaired interactions/isolation.                                                                                                                                                                                                                     |
|                                                    | Acknowledge willingness to be more involved with others.                                                                                                                                                                                                                                  |
|                                                    | Demonstrate involvement/participation in appropriate activities and programs.                                                                                                                                                                                                             |

## ACTIONS/INTERVENTIONS

### Independent

Assess degree of isolation. Note withdrawn behavior and use of denial. Ascertain client's perceptions of reasons for problems.

Help client differentiate between isolation and loneliness/aloneness.
ated

Identify support systems available to client (e.g., family, friends, coworkers).

Explore with client and role-play ways of making changes in social interactions/behaviors.

Acknowledge any positive efforts client makes in establishing contact with others.

### Collaborative

Encourage client to continue and/or seek outside or outpatient therapy/peer group activities.

## RATIONALE

Indicates need for/choice of interventions. Withdrawing and denial can inhibit/sabotage participation in therapy.

Time for the client to be alone is important to the maintenance of mental health, but the sadness cre-

by isolation and loneliness need different interventions.

Involvement of significant others can help to build and/or reestablish support system and reintegrate client into a social network.

Developing and practicing strategies promotes and enhances possibility of change.

Positive reinforcement of movement toward others can decrease sense of isolation and encourage repetition of behaviors, enhancing socialization.

Will need ongoing support and encouragement to reestablish social connections and develop/strengthen relationships.

| ACTIONS/INTERVENTIONS | RATIONALE |
| --- | --- |

### Collaborative

| | |
| --- | --- |
| Refer for employment counseling, if indicated. (Refer to ND: Coping, individual, ineffective.) | Interpersonal difficulties may have affected work relationships and performance, and client may need help to reintegrate into current job or relocate. |

| | |
| --- | --- |
| **NURSING DIAGNOSIS:** | **FAMILY PROCESSES, ALTERED** |
| **May Be Related To:** | Situational crises. |
| **Possibly Evidenced By:** | Expressions of confusion about what to do and that family is having difficulty coping with situation; difficulty accepting/receiving help appropriately. |
| | Not adapting to change or dealing with traumatic experience constructively; ineffective family decision-making process. |
| | Difficulty expressing individual and/or wide range of feelings. |
| | Family system does not meet physical/emotional/spiritual needs of its members. |
| **Desired Outcomes/Evaluation Criteria— Family Will:** | Express feelings freely and appropriately. |
| | Verbalize understanding of trauma, treatment regimen, and prognosis. |
| | Demonstrate individual involvement in problem-solving processes directed at appropriate solutions for the situation. |

| ACTIONS/INTERVENTIONS | RATIONALE |
| --- | --- |

### Independent

| | |
| --- | --- |
| Determine family members' understanding of client's illness/PSTD. | Family members and SO often do not recognize that client's present behavior is the result of trauma that has occurred. |
| Identify patterns of communications in the family, e.g.: Are feelings expressed clearly and freely? Do family members talk to one another? Are problems resolved equitably? What are interactions among/ between members? | How family members communicate provides information about their ability to problem-solve, understand one another, cooperate in making decisions, and resolve problems resulting from trauma. |
| Encourage family members to verbalize feelings (including anger) about client's behavior. | SO/spouse may feel angry/unloved and believe client is rejecting, rather than recognizing behaviors as a sign of client's pain. |

333

| ACTIONS/INTERVENTIONS | RATIONALE |
|---|---|

### Independent

Acknowledge difficulties each member is experiencing while reinforcing that conflict is to be expected and can be used to promote growth.

Recognition of what the person is feeling/going through provides a sense of acceptance. Most people have the fantasy that once the conflict has been resolved, everything will be fine. Discussing conflict as an ongoing problem that can be resolved so all parties win can help family members begin to believe a new method of handling it can be learned.

Identify and encourage use of previous successful coping behaviors.

In the stress of current situation, family members tend to focus on negative behaviors, feel hopeless, and neglect looking at positive behaviors used in the past.

Encourage use of stress-management techniques, e.g., appropriate expression of feelings, relaxation exercises, guided imagery.

Reduction of stress enables individuals to begin to think more clearly/develop new behaviors to cope with client.

Present information about PSTD and provide opportunity to ask questions/discuss concerns.

These materials can help family members learn more about client's condition and assist in resolution of current crisis.

### Collaborative

Refer to other resources as indicated, e.g., support groups, clergy, psychologic counseling/family therapy.

Additional/ongoing support and/or therapy may be needed to help family resolve family crisis and look at potential for growth.

| NURSING DIAGNOSIS: | SEXUAL DYSFUNCTION/SEXUALITY PATTERNS, ALTERED |
|---|---|
| **May Be Related To:** | Biopsychosocial alteration of sexuality (stress of posttrauma response). |
| | Loss of sexual desire. |
| | Impaired relationship with a significant other. |
| **Possibly Evidenced By:** | Alterations in achieving sexual satisfaction/relationship with significant other. |
| | Change of interest in self and others; preoccupation with self. |
| | Irritation, lack of affection. |
| **Desired Outcomes/Evaluation Criteria— Client Will:** | Verbalize understanding of reasons for sexual problems/changes that have occurred. |
| | Identify stresses involved in lifestyle that contribute to the dysfunction. |
| | Demonstrate improved communication and relationship skills. |
| | Participate in program designed to resume desired sexual activity. |

| ACTIONS/INTERVENTIONS | RATIONALE |
|---|---|

### Independent

| | |
|---|---|
| Inquire in a direct manner if there has been a change in sexual functioning/if problems exist, preferably in a conjoint session. | Client may prefer to dwell on reliving details of trauma and may not complain about this area of life. SO may not recognize relation of trauma to marital discord/sexual problems, and being with the client provides an opportunity for them to begin to talk realistically about what is happening. Note: Men typically have loss of sexual desire and occasional impotence; women experience lack of sexual pleasure and anorgasmia. |
| Determine intimate behavior/closeness between couple recently and in comparison to quality of sexual relationship before the trauma, when appropriate. | May reveal problems that have not been acknowledged previously by the couple. Client may deny existence of difficulties, excusing self as being "sick" or "needing time to recover from trauma." |
| Provide information about the effect anxiety and anger have on sexual desire/ability to perform. | When SO does not know this, it is easy to feel unloved and not cared about or believe mate is having an affair. With understanding/insight into cause(s), SO's anxiety may be relieved, and support and affection can be extended to the client. |
| Encourage expression of feelings and emotions (e.g., crying) openly and appropriately. | Client/SO may believe they are helping by being stoic and not expressing feelings of powerlessness, helplessness, fear, etc., to each other. |
| Help client who has been the victim of sexual assault to understand relationship of reluctance to have mate touch/make sexual advances to the event that occurred. | Client may have difficulty recognizing and feel embarrassed by the fact that mate's advances are reminder(s) of the trauma. |
| Discuss substance use and relationship to sexual difficulties. | Some clients use alcohol and other drugs to dull the pain of PSTD. These substances interfere with sexual functioning, causing diminished desire and inability to achieve and maintain an erection. Note: It is not known what effect chronic use of alcohol has on female sexual functioning. |
| Review relaxation skills. (Refer to ND: Coping, individual, ineffective.) | Learning to relax assists with reduction of anxiety and allows client/SO to focus on learning skills to regain sexual functioning. |

### Collaborative

| | |
|---|---|
| Refer to other resources as indicated, e.g., sex therapist. | Specific techniques may be used to assist the couple in regaining comfort level/ability to engage in nongenital/genital activity and intimacy. |

| | |
|---|---|
| **NURSING DIAGNOSIS:** | **KNOWLEDGE DEFICIT [LEARNING NEED]** *regarding situation, prognosis, and treatment needs* |
| **May Be Related To:** | Lack of exposure to/misinterpretation of information.<br>Unfamiliarity with information resources. |

| | |
|---|---|
| **Possibly Evidenced By:** | Lack of recall. |
| | Verbalization of the problem; statement of misconception. |
| | Inaccurate follow-through of instruction. |
| | Inappropriate or exaggerated behaviors, e.g., hysterical, hostile, agitated, apathetic. |
| **Desired Outcomes/Evaluation Criteria— Client Will:** | Participate in learning process. |
| | Assume responsibility for own learning and begin to look for information/ask questions. |
| | Identify stress situations and specific action(s) to deal with them. |
| | Initiate necessary lifestyle changes and participate in treatment regimen. |

| ACTIONS/INTERVENTIONS | RATIONALE |
|---|---|
| **Independent** | |
| Provide information about what reactions client may expect and let client know these are common reactions. Phrase in neutral terms, e.g., "may or may not happen." | Knowing what to expect can reduce anxiety and help the client in learning new behaviors to handle stressful feelings/situations. Having information about the commonality of experiences helps the individual feel less alone/strange, aiding in acceptance of these feelings. |
| Assist client to identify factors that may have created a vulnerable situation and that she or he may have power to change to protect self in the future. Avoid making value judgments. | Separates issues of vulnerability from blame. Factors such as body stance, carelessness, and not paying attention to negative cues may provide opportunity for tragic consequences that could possibly have been avoided/minimized. However, any inference that client is responsible for the incident is not therapeutic. |
| Discuss contemplated changes in lifestyle and how they will contribute to recovery. | Client needs to be able to look at these changes, what will be accomplished and determine whether they are realistic/necessary. |
| Assist with learning stress-management techniques. | Relaxation is a useful coping skill for dealing with stress of recurrent fears/stress response. |
| Discuss recognition of and ways to manage "anniversary reactions," letting client know normalcy of thoughts and feelings at this time. | Planning ahead and knowing some skills to handle this time can help to avoid severe regression. |
| Identify available resources, e.g.: psychiatric consultation/group participation; | Assists with understanding of and ways to deal with/help client. |
| support group for significant other(s); | Additional assistance may be required if client is overly violent or inconsolable or does not seem to be making an adjustment. |
| family/marital counselors as indicated. | Client problems affect others in family/relationships, and further counseling may help resolve issues of enabling behavior/communication problems. |

# CHAPTER 10

# SOMATOFORM DISORDERS

## SOMATOFORM DISORDERS

### DSM IV
300.81  Somatization Disorder
300.11  Conversion Disorder
300.7  Hypochondriasis
300.7  Body Dysmorphic Disorder
**Pain Disorder**
   307.80  Associated with Psychological Factors
   307.89  Associated with Both Psychological Factors and a General Medical Condition
300.81  Undifferentiated Somatoform Disorder
300.81  Somatoform Disorder NOS

### DSM III-R
300.81  Somatization Disorder
300.11  Conversion Disorder
307.80  Somatoform Pain Disorder
300.70  Hypochondriasis
300.70  Body Dysmorphic Disorder

Somatization refers to all those mechanisms by which anxiety is translated into physical illness or bodily complaints. The expression of physical symptoms suggests the presence of physiologic disorder, but there are no demonstrable organic findings/known pathologic mechanisms, or the symptoms are not fully explained by any physical disorder. That is, the symptoms are in excess of what would be expected from the history, physical examination, or laboratory findings. There does exist, however, positive evidence, or a strong presumption, that the symptoms are linked to psychologic factors or conflicts. These disorders are more common in women than in men, with somatization disorder rare in men.

## ETIOLOGIC THEORIES

### Psychodynamics

It is thought that this disorder represents an unconscious transformation of internal conflicts into physical symptoms that can be explained in terms of the ego's ability to control the sensory and motor apparatus, which may have specific meaning for the client.

Dependency is common in individuals with somatoform disorders, and fixation in an earlier level of development may be evident.

Repression is the primary defense mechanism, as severe anxiety is repressed and manifested by the presence of physical symptoms.

### Biologic

Although biologic and neurophysiologic influences in the etiology of anxiety have been investigated, no relationship has yet been established. However, there does seem to be a genetic influence with a high family incidence.

The autonomic nervous system discharge that occurs in response to a frightening impulse and/or emotion is mediated by the limbic system, resulting in the peripheral effects of the autonomic nervous system seen in the presence of anxiety. These manifestations of anxiety may be related to physiologic abnormalities.

### Family Dynamics

The family contributes to these conditions by initiating, reinforcing, and perpetuating the behavior patterns. The children learn (overtly or covertly) that physical complaints are acceptable ways of coping with stress and obtaining attention, care, and gratification of dependency needs. The client may gain attention and meet these needs by overdramatization of the symptoms, with resultant overinvolvement of other family members in enmeshed patterns of behavior. In the beginning, client may exaggerate minor symptoms to prove he or she is really ill when others ignore reports of illness.

## CLIENT ASSESSMENT DATABASE

### Activity/Rest

Fatigue.
General weakness.

### Circulation

Heart rate may be elevated if symptoms mimic those of cardiopulmonary disease (similar to those experienced during panic attack).

### Ego Integrity

Preoccupation with imagined defect in appearance or markedly excessive concern with slight physical anomaly not better accounted for by another mental disorder, e.g., dissatisfaction with body shape/size in anorexia nervosa (body dysmorphic disorder).
Evidence of severe psychologic stress preceding onset/exacerbation of the physical symptoms, e.g., death of a loved one (conversion).
Preoccupation with fear of having a serious disease (hypochondriasis).
Use of denial, evidence that presence of the symptoms alleviates or promotes avoidance of the psychologic conflict.
Feelings of anger, helplessness, powerlessness.
Report of issues suggesting unconscious secondary gain, e.g., attention of others, financial reimbursement, change in role expectations/responsibilities.

### Elimination

Urinary retention.
Constipation, diarrhea.

### Food/Fluid

Two or more GI symptoms, e.g., nausea, vomiting, bloating, intolerance of several different foods, difficulty swallowing (somatization).
Changes in eating patterns (loss of appetite/excessive intake).
Weight loss/gain.

## Neurosensory

Mental Status Exam:
> Fearful; preoccupation with belief of having serious disease; anxious (symptoms associated with moderate to severe level) or *la belle indifference* (lack of concern over loss of physical functioning).
> Depressed.
> Amnesia.
> Communication patterns: ruminating about physical symptoms.

May display loss of consciousness other than fainting (somatization).

Apparent loss or alteration in voluntary motor or sensory functioning that suggests neurologic disease, e.g., blindness, double vision, deafness, paralysis, anosmia, aphonia, episodic seizure activity, and coordination disturbances (especially common in conversion disorder).

## Pain/Discomfort

Pain in 1 or more anatomic sites of at least 6 months' duration and of sufficient severity to warrant clinical attention (pain disorder); involving 4 different sites of function, e.g., head, abdomen, back, joints, chest, during urination/menstruation/sexual intercourse (somatization).

Excessive use of analgesics with minimal relief of pain.

## Respiration

Respiratory rate may be increased.
Shortness of breath without exertion.

## Safety

May report suicidal ideations, inability to continue in current situation.

## Social Interactions

Observed/reported impairment in social, occupational, or other areas of functioing.

## Sexuality

One or more sexual/reproductive symptoms other than pain, e.g., decreased libido/sexual indifference, irregular menses/excessive menstrual bleeding, erectile/ejaculatory difficulties, pseudocyesis [false pregnancy], somatization.

## Teaching/Learning

Reports of physical symptoms of several years' duration beginning before the age of 30 (somatization).

History of a past experience with true serious organic disease, in self or close family member (hypochondriasis).

History of frequent visits to physicians (doctor shopping) to obtain relief/requests for surgery despite medical reassurance of absence of organic pathology.

Failure to improve despite multiple approaches/therapies.

Expression of anger and frustration toward physicians for "inability to determine cause of physical symptoms."

## DIAGNOSTIC STUDIES

Virtually any diagnostic procedure (including exploratory surgery) may be performed as deemed appropriate to rule out organic pathology in light of the physical symptom(s) presented by the client.

Urine and/or serum toxicology screen: to determine evidence of substance use/abuse.

339

## NURSING PRIORITIES

1. Alleviate/minimize physical symptoms/chronic pain.
2. Promote client safety.
3. Resolve potentially dysfunctional areas of client/family dynamics.
4. Promote independence in self-care activities.
5. Provide information and support for lifestyle changes.

## DISCHARGE GOALS

1. Relief from admitting physical symptom(s) obtained.
2. Client/family recognizes relationship between psychologic stressors and onset/exacerbation of physical symptom(s).
3. Stress management techniques used appropriately to prevent the occurrence/exacerbation of the physical symptom(s).
4. Level of function/independence increased.

| NURSING DIAGNOSIS: | COPING, INDIVIDUAL, INEFFECTIVE |
|---|---|
| **May Be Related To:** | Severe level of anxiety, repressed; personal vulnerability. |
| | Unrealistic perceptions. |
| | History of self or loved one having experienced a serious illness. |
| | Retarded ego development; fixation in earlier level of development; unmet dependency needs. |
| | Inadequate coping skills. |
| **Possibly Evidenced By:** | Verbalized inability to cope/problem-solve. |
| | High illness rate, multiple physical complaints that are not fully explained by a known general medical condition. |
| | Decreased functioning in social/occupational settings. |
| | Narcissistic tendencies, with total focus on self and physical symptoms; demanding behaviors. |
| | History of "doctor shopping." |
| | Inappropriate use of defense mechanisms (e.g., denial of correlation between physical symptoms and psychologic problems); refusal to attend therapeutic activities. |
| **Desired Outcomes/Evaluation Criteria—Client Will:** | Verbalize need for change within dysfunctional system. |
| | Recognize correlation between physical symptoms and psychologic problems. |
| | Demonstrate adaptive coping strategies in the face of stressful situations, discontinuing use of physical symptoms as a response. |
| | Report reduction of/relief from physical complaints. |

| ACTIONS/INTERVENTIONS | RATIONALE |
|---|---|

### Independent

Review laboratory and diagnostic results with the client in simple, easy-to-understand terminology. Answer any questions that may have arisen from discussions with the physician.

Client has the right to knowledge about own care. Honest explanation may help client to understand psychologic implications. Anxiety is high, so learning is difficult, thus explanations need to be kept simple and concrete.

Show unconditional positive regard. Convey that you understand the symptom is real to the client, even though no organic pathology can be found.

Denial of the client's feelings is nontherapeutic and interferes with establishment of a trusting nurse/client relationship.

Discuss possibility of and client's perceptions of behavior(s) as self-destructive. Determine suicidal risk as appropriate.

Limitations imposed by chronic "illness/disabilities" prevent client from full participation in life activities. In conjunction, multiple conflicts (e.g., medical, financial, family, legal) increase the likelihood of feelings of depression, helplessness, hopelessness, which may lead to substance abuse, dependence on pharmacologic agents, and/or suicidal ideation necessitating additional therapeutic interventions.

Be available to assist the client with basic dependency needs in the initial stages of the relationship. Recognize, however, that the client may be using the physical condition to preserve the dependency role.

To deny client this need at this time would result in an increased anxiety level and intensification of maladaptive behaviors.

Gradually decrease response to time and assistance required by the client as the trusting relationship is established. Encourage independent behaviors and respond with positive reinforcement.

Positive reinforcement enhances self-esteem and encourages repetition of desirable behaviors. Doing things for oneself helps to develop independence and improves coping ability.

Encourage verbalizations of honest feelings, including feelings of anger within appropriate limits. Provide safe method of hostility release, e.g., pounding pillows. Help client to identify true source of anger and work on adaptive coping skills for use outside the therapeutic setting.

Verbalization of feelings in a nonthreatening environment may help the client come to terms with unresolved issues. Presence of depression and/or suicidal behaviors may be viewed as anger turned inward on the self. When this anger is verbalized in a nonthreatening environment, the client may resolve these feelings, regardless of the discomfort involved.

Withdraw attention if rumination about physical symptoms begins.

Lack of response to maladaptive behaviors may discourage their repetition.

Help client identify symbols of hope in own life through exploration and discussion.

Encourages client to focus on reasons for wanting to change life.

Explore past experiences with client and correlate appearance of physical symptoms with times of stress.

Until denial defense is eliminated, change required for improvement will not occur.

Discuss possible alternative coping behaviors client may use in response to stress (e.g., relaxation techniques, deep breathing, physical activities, such as jogging, aerobics, brisk walks, housekeeping chores, sex). Offer positive reinforcement for use of these alternatives.

Because of high level of anxiety, client may require assistance in problem-solving and the ability to recognize available alternatives. Positive reinforcement enhances self-esteem and encourages repetition of desirable coping behaviors. Note: Stimulating activities/discussions should be avoided in late evening hours to prevent increasing level of anxiety, which could interfere with sleep.

| ACTIONS/INTERVENTIONS | RATIONALE |
|---|---|

### Independent

Report/investigate any new physical complaint.

Although physical symptoms have been used as a way of coping by the client, the possibility of organic pathology must always be considered to prevent jeopardizing client safety.

### Collaborative

Administer medications, as indicated:

Psychopharmacologic treatment is generally not indicated unless anxiety/depression are prominent.

    antianxiety agents, e.g., diazepam (Valium), chlordiazepoxide (Librium), alprazolam (Xanax);

Antianxiety medications have a calming effect on the client, masking the feelings of anxiety, which may minimize physical response. Careful monitoring of use of antianxiety agents is important because of high addiction potential. Note: Sedative side effects may induce sleep during day, therefore interfering with client's sleep at night.

    antidepressants, e.g., amitriptyline (Elavil), imipramine (Tofranil).

Antidepressant medication may elevate the mood as it increases level of energy and decreases feelings of fatigue. Note: Potential for suicide increases as energy level improves.

Discourage excessive sleep during the day, and encourage establishment of a routine pattern of sleep and activity with inclusion of customary bedtime rituals, e.g., warm baths, massage, warm/nonstimulating drinks or reduction of fluid intake, light snacks.

Daytime sleep may be used as a defense to deal with pain/stressors. Ritualistic patterns and a realistic balance of activity and rest induce relaxation, promote inducement of sleep at appropriate times, and decrease interruptions of sleep. Obtaining quality sleep enhances client's ability to deal with pain and develop new coping strategies.

| NURSING DIAGNOSIS: | PAIN, CHRONIC |
|---|---|
| **May Be Related To:** | Severe level of anxiety, repressed. |
| | Low self-esteem; unmet dependency needs. |
| | History of self or loved one having experienced a serious illness. |
| **Possibly Evidenced By:** | Multiple reports of severe/prolonged pain. |
| | Guarded movement/protective behaviors; facial mask of pain; fear of reinjury. |
| | Altered ability to continue previous activities; social withdrawal. |
| | Changes in weight, sleep patterns. |
| | History of seeking assistance from numerous health-care professionals; demands for therapy/medication. |

| Desired Outcomes/Evaluation Criteria— Client Will: | Acknowledge relationship between psychologic problems and onset/exacerbation of pain.<br><br>Demonstrate techniques to interrupt escalating anxiety/pain.<br><br>Verbalize noticeable reduction/relief of pain. |
|---|---|

| ACTIONS/INTERVENTIONS | RATIONALE |
|---|---|

### Independent

Note and record the duration and intensity of the pain. Assess factors that precipitate the onset of pain. Observe and report any new or different pattern of pain behavior to physician.

The correlation of these factors provides client with information to become aware of cause/effect relationship and to gain control of outcome. Note: Changes in pain necessitate evaluation to rule out development of organic pathology.

Convey to client your belief that the pain is indeed real, even though no organic pathology can be found.

Denying or belittling the client's feelings is nontherapeutic and interferes in the development of a trusting relationship.

Provide nursing comfort measures with a matter-of-fact approach that does not provide added attention to the pain behavior (e.g., back rub, warm bath, heating pad).

May serve to provide some temporary relief of pain for the client. Secondary gains from solicitous behavior may provide positive reinforcement and can actually prolong use of maladaptive behaviors.

Assist client with activities that distract from focus on self and pain.

Helps the client to focus on adaptive behavior patterns and serves as a transition to higher levels of therapy.

Use these distractors to facilitate initiation of discussion of unresolved psychologic issues, e.g., open expression of feelings such as guilt, fear about life events.

Unresolved psychologic issues must be dealt with before maladaptive patterns can be eliminated.

Help client connect times of onset/exacerbation of pain to times of increased anxiety. Identify specific situations that cause anxiety to rise, and demonstrate techniques to interrupt the pain response, e.g., visual or auditory distractions, guided imagery, breathing exercises, massage, application of heat or cold, relaxation techniques.

Client's ability to connect pain to times of increased anxiety helps to decrease denial and is the first step in resolution of the problem. Use of techniques described may help to maintain anxiety at manageable level and prevent the pain from becoming disabling.

Provide positive reinforcement for times when client is not focusing on pain.

Positive reinforcement, in the form of the nurse's presence and attention, may encourage a continuation of these more adaptive behaviors by the client.

### Collaborative

Review ongoing assessments by physician and laboratory/other diagnostic results.

The possibility of organic pathology needs to be ruled out.

Administer medications as indicated, e.g.:
  aspirin, ibuprofen (Motrin, Advil);

ASA, nonsteroidal anti-inflammatory agents have minimal side effects and low addiction potential and are useful in treating episodic exacerbations of chronic pain.

343

| ACTIONS/INTERVENTIONS | RATIONALE |
|---|---|

## Collaborative

low-dose antidepressants, e.g., amitriptyline (Elavil), doxepin (Sinequan), phenelzine (Nardil);

Helps combat depression, may enhance sleep, reduce level of fatigue, and promote feelings of well-being.

anticonvulsants, e.g., phenytoin (Dilantin), carbamazepine (Tegretol), clonazepam (Klonopin);

Studies suggest short-term use may be of some benefit in treating neuropathic and neuralgic pain while other therapeutic interventions are initiated.

sedative medications at bedtime, e.g., triazolam (Halcion).

Level of repressed anxiety/physical symptoms may interfere with obtaining quality sleep, negatively impacting energy level and coping ability. Sedatives should not be used for longer than a 3-week period, as they eventually interfere with, rather than promote, sleep.

Refer to chronic pain clinic.

May be helpful to learn ways to manage residual pain on a long-term basis.

| NURSING DIAGNOSIS: | BODY IMAGE DISTURBANCE |
|---|---|
| May Be Related To: | Severe level of anxiety, repressed. |
| | Low self-esteem; unmet dependency needs. |
| Possibly Evidenced By: | Preoccupation with real or imagined change in bodily structure and/or function that is out of proportion to any actual abnormality that may exist. |
| | Negative feelings about body/self. |
| | Fear of negative reaction or rejection by others; change in social involvement. |
| Desired Outcomes/Evaluation Criteria— Client Will: | Verbalize realistic perception of bodily condition. |
| | Express positive feelings about body. |
| | Function independently and interact socially without experiencing discomfort. |

| ACTIONS/INTERVENTIONS | RATIONALE |
|---|---|

## Independent

Ascertain client's perception of own body image. Acknowledge that disability is real to the client, even in the absence of evidence of organic pathology.

Information about the way in which the individual views self aids in developing accurate plan of care. Denial of client's feelings is nontherapeutic and impedes the development of trust.

Help client to see that image is distorted and out of proportion to reality of actual change in structure and/or function. Correct inaccurate perceptions in a matter-of-fact, nonthreatening manner.

Recognition that a misperception/distortion exists is necessary before client can accept reality and reduce significance of impairment.

| ACTIONS/INTERVENTIONS | RATIONALE |
|---|---|

### Independent

Withdraw attention when preoccupation with distorted image persists.

Lack of attention may encourage elimination of undesirable behavior.

Assist client to recognize personal body boundaries.

Use of touch may help client recognize acceptance of self by others and reduce fear of rejection.

Assist client to recognize normal feelings associated with the grieving process and offer support as the client progresses toward acceptance of change in self.

May need to deal with actual loss/impairment as well as problematic behavior. Progress through the grieving process is facilitated by client's recognition of feelings as acceptable and own ability to acknowledge ownership of those feelings.

Explore with client stressful life situations that may have symbolic correlation to the loss when the loss of function has no organic etiology, e.g., blindness in response to witnessing a traumatic event; aphonia in response to inner conflict associated with verbal expression of rage.

Client needs to recognize and accept that there is a relationship between the loss of function and anxiety associated with stressful life situations if improvement is to occur. Denial of psychologic implications impedes positive change.

Encourage verbalization of fears and anxieties associated with identified stressful life situations. Discuss ways in which client may respond more adaptively in the future.

Verbalization of feelings with a trusted individual may help the client come to terms with unresolved issues. A plan of action formulated with assistance and at a time when anxiety is low may prevent later dysfunctional response by client.

Encourage and give positive feedback for independent self-care behaviors, while gradually withdrawing attention from dependent behaviors.

Lack of attention to maladaptive behaviors discourages their repetition. Positive reinforcement enhances self-esteem and promotes repetition of desirable behaviors.

| **NURSING DIAGNOSIS:** | **SELF-CARE DEFICIT (SPECIFY)** |
|---|---|
| **May Be Related To:** | Paralysis of body part. |
| | Inability to see, hear, speak. |
| | Pain, discomfort. |
| **Possibly Evidenced By:** | Inability to bring food from a receptacle to the mouth; obtain or get to water sources; wash body or body parts; regulate temperature or flow of water. |
| | Impaired ability to put on or take off necessary items of clothing, obtain or replace articles of clothing, fasten clothing, maintain appearance at a satisfactory level. |
| | Inability to get to toilet or commode (impaired mobility); manipulate clothing for toileting; flush toilet or empty commode; sit on or rise from toilet or commode; carry out proper toilet hygiene. |

| Desired Outcomes/Evaluation Criteria—Client Will: | Display willingness to participate in ADLs. |
| --- | --- |
| | Demonstrate techniques/lifestyle changes to meet self-care needs. |
| | Perform self-care activities independently within level of ability |

| ACTIONS/INTERVENTIONS | RATIONALE |
| --- | --- |

### Independent

| | |
| --- | --- |
| Assess degree of impairment; note level of disability as well as areas of strength. | Establishes client needs and identifies individual potentials. |
| Encourage client to perform ADLs to own level of ability. Intervene only when client is unable to perform. | Loss of function may be related to unfulfilled dependency needs. Intervening when client is capable of performing independently serves to foster dependency in the client. |
| Convey a nonjudgmental attitude as nursing assistance with self-care activities is provided. Remember that the physical symptom is real to the client and is not within the client's conscious control. | A judgmental attitude interferes with the nurse's ability to provide therapeutic care for the client, provoking defensiveness that blocks client's willingness to look at own behavior/dynamics. |
| Provide positive reinforcement for ADLs performed independently. | Positive reinforcement enhances self-esteem and encourages repetition of desirable behaviors. |
| Encourage client to discuss feelings regarding the disability and the need for dependency it creates. Help the client to see the purpose this disability is serving. | Self-disclosure and exploration of feelings with a trusted individual may help client fulfill unmet needs and come to terms with unresolved issues, thus eliminating the need for maladaptive physical responses. |
| Involve family members in care at level of their ability/willingness. | Feelings of anger toward the client may interfere with ability to provide care in a therapeutic/nonjudgmental manner. |

### Collaborative

| | |
| --- | --- |
| Refer to occupational/physical therapy, community resources/supports. | Involvement with these programs provides role models, enhances client's self-esteem, promoting ability to care for self. |

| NURSING DIAGNOSIS: | SENSORY/PERCEPTUAL ALTERATIONS (SPECIFY) |
| --- | --- |
| May Be Related To: | Psychologic stress (narrowed perceptual fields caused by anxiety, expression of stress as physical problems/deficits). |
| | Poor quality of sleep. |
| | Presence of chronic pain. |

| Possibly Evidenced By: | Reported change in voluntary motor or sensory function, e.g., paralysis, anosmia, aphonia, deafness, blindness, loss of touch or pain sensation. |
|---|---|
| | "La belle indifference " (lack of concern over functional loss). |
| Desired Outcomes/Evaluation Criteria— Client Will: | Verbalize understanding of emotional problems as a contributing factor to alteration in physical functioning. |
| | Identify adaptive ways of coping with stress and community support systems to whom she or he may go for help. |
| | Demonstrate recovery of lost function. |

## ACTIONS/INTERVENTIONS

### Independent

Identify gains that the physical symptom is providing for the client, e.g., increased dependency, attention, distraction from other problems.

Assist client with ADLs with which the physical symptom is interfering.

Allow client to be as independent as possible without focusing on the disability. Intervene only when client requires assistance.

Encourage client to participate in therapeutic activities to the best of ability. Do not allow client to use disability as an excuse for nonparticipation. Withdraw attention if client continues to focus on physical limitation. Reinforce reality as required while ensuring maintenance of a nonthreatening environment.

Encourage client to verbalize fears and anxieties. Help client recognize that physical symptom appears at time of extreme stress and is a way of coping with that stress.

Help client identify positive coping mechanisms that can be used when faced with stressful situations.

Explain/review assertiveness techniques and use role-play to practice use.

Identify SO(s), other support systems who can provide assistance to the client.

### Collaborative

Monitor ongoing assessments, laboratory findings, and other data.

## RATIONALE

Important assessment data to be used in helping the client with problem resolution.

Comfort and safety are priorities for nursing care.

Encourages client to begin to assume responsibility for self. Giving attention to the use of the maladaptive response reinforces secondary gain, such as dependency.

Gently confronting reality of client's abilities while minimizing attention to problem helps client begin to accept own responsibility.

May be unaware of relationship between physical symptom and emotional stress.

Client has been used to using maladaptive coping to retreat from reality and needs to begin to change to more realistic ways of dealing with problems.

Enhances self-esteem and minimizes anxiety in interpersonal relationships.

Satisfactory supports can help client cope with overwhelming stress.

Assures that possibility of organic pathology is clearly ruled out. Failure to do so may jeopardize client safety.

| NURSING DIAGNOSIS: | SOCIAL INTERACTION, IMPAIRED |
|---|---|
| **May Be Related To:** | Inability to engage in satisfying personal relationships. |
| | Preoccupation with self and physical symptoms; altered state of wellness, chronic pain. |
| | Rejection by others due to focus on self/physical symptoms. |
| **Possibly Evidenced By:** | Preoccupation with own thoughts; repetitive verbalization about self/physical symptoms. |
| | Seeking to be alone; uncommunicative, withdrawn; no eye contact; sad, dull affect. |
| | Absence of supportive significant other(s)— family, friends, social contacts. |
| **Desired Outcomes/Evaluation Criteria— Client Will:** | Spend time voluntarily with others in group activities. |
| | Interact with others without apparent discomfort. |
| | Demonstrate interest in others, while discontinuing use of statements that focus on self/physical symptoms. |

| ACTIONS/INTERVENTIONS | RATIONALE |
|---|---|
| **Independent** | |
| Spend time with client after setting limits on attention-seeking behaviors. Withdraw presence if ruminations about physical symptoms begin. | The nurse's presence conveys a sense of worthwhileness to the client. Lack of reinforcement of maladaptive behaviors may help to decrease their repetition. |
| Increase amount of time/attention given during times when client is not focusing on physical symptoms. | This separates the person from the behavior and increases feelings of self-worth as unconditional acceptance is experienced by the client without need for the physical symptoms. |
| Describe client's interpersonal behaviors objectively. Emphasize how the focus on self/physical symptoms discourages relationships with others. | Client may not realize how own behavior is perceived by others/results in alienation. |
| Assist client in learning assertiveness techniques, especially the ability to recognize the difference between passive, assertive, and aggressive behaviors and the importance of respecting the human rights of others while protecting one's own basic human rights. | Use of these techniques enhances self-esteem and facilitates communication and mutual acceptance in interpersonal relationships. |
| Encourage attendance in group activities after client is interacting appropriately in the 1:1 relationship. Accompany the client the first few times. | As a trusted individual, the nurse provides objective feedback about client's behavior in the group. Subsequent discussion and role-play on a 1:1 basis may help prepare client for future group encounters and may promote success with this endeavor. |
| Provide positive feedback for any attempts at social interaction in which the client's focus is on others rather than self/physical symptoms. | Positive feedback enhances self-esteem and encourages repetition of desirable behaviors. |

| NURSING DIAGNOSIS: | KNOWLEDGE DEFICIT [LEARNING NEED] regarding condition, prognosis, and treatment needs |
|---|---|
| **May Be Related To:** | Strong denial defense system. |
| | Severe level of anxiety, repressed. |
| | Preoccupation with self and pain. |
| | Lack of interest in learning. |
| **Possibly Evidenced By:** | Verbalization of denial statements, such as, "I don't know why the doctor put me on the psychiatric unit. I have a physical problem." |
| | History of "doctor shopping" for evidence of organic pathology to substantiate physical symptoms. |
| | Lack of follow-through with psychiatric treatment plan. |
| **Desired Outcomes/Evaluation Criteria— Client Will:** | Verbalize understanding of psychologic implications of physical symptoms. |
| | Report relief from physical symptoms. |
| | Demonstrate more appropriate coping mechanisms to employ in response to stress. |

| ACTIONS/INTERVENTIONS | RATIONALE |
|---|---|

### Independent

| | |
|---|---|
| Ascertain client's level of knowledge regarding effects of psychologic problems on the body. Be aware of degree to which denial defense controls client's behavior. | Knowing what information the individual already has provides a base that is necessary to develop an effective plan of care for the client. Strong denial system needs to be penetrated before learning can begin. |
| Assess client's level of anxiety and readiness to learn. | Learning does not take place when level of anxiety is moderate to severe. |
| Explain purpose and review results of laboratory and diagnostic testing, as well as aspects of the physical examination. | Client has basic right to knowledge about care. Objective knowledge about physical condition may help to break through the strong denial defense. |
| Have client keep 2 separate records: (1) a diary of the appearance, duration, and intensity of physical symptoms, and (2) documentation of situations that the client finds especially stressful. | Comparison of these records may provide objective data from which to observe the relationship between physical symptoms and stress. |
| Help client identify needs that are being met through the sick role (e.g., dependency needs, attention seeking, and cover-up for painful conflicts in life situation). Help client recognize and accept more adaptive means for fulfilling these needs. Practice through role-playing. | Client usually does not realize that the physical symptoms are fulfilling unmet needs. Recognition needs to be achieved before change can occur. Roleplay can relieve anxiety by helping client anticipate responses to stressful situations. |
| Demonstrate/encourage use of adaptive methods of stress management, e.g., relaxation techniques, physical exercises, meditation, breathing exercises, autogenics. | These techniques may be employed in an attempt to relieve anxiety and discourage the use of physical symptoms as a maladaptive response. |

349

| ACTIONS/INTERVENTIONS | RATIONALE |
|---|---|

### Independent

| | |
|---|---|
| Incorporate occupational/recreational therapy activities in treatment plan to help client learn adaptive coping mechanisms. | Daily activities can provide opportunities to learn/practice specialized techniques for coping with stress (e.g., decision-making, problem-solving, housekeeping, art therapy, plant therapy, bowling, volleyball, weight lifting). |
| Encourage participation in outdoor education program, e.g., wall/rock climbing, hiking, caving. | Involvement in activities that challenge physical and psychologic abilities can help the client learn to become more self-aware and confident and increase self-esteem. |
| Include family/SO(s) in learning opportunities, assisting them to understand underlying reasons for client's behavior. | Having understanding support from significant other(s) can help client to accept reality of situation and make required changes. |

| | |
|---|---|
| **NURSING DIAGNOSIS:** | **SEXUAL DYSFUNCTION, actual/high risk for** |
| **May Be Related To:** | Perceived or actual loss of bodily structure or function. |
| | Preoccupation with physical symptoms; total focus on self/chronic pain response. |
| | Fear of contracting a serious disease. |
| **Possibly Evidenced By (Actual):** | Alterations in relationship with SO. |
| | Actual/perceived limitation imposed by condition. |
| | Change of interest in self/others; sexual indifference. |
| | Lack of pleasure/pain [dyspareunia] during intercourse. |
| | Inability to achieve or maintain erection. |
| | Desire to achieve greater satisfaction in sexual role. |
| **Desired Outcomes/Evaluation Criteria—Client Will:** | Identify underlying stressors that contribute to the dysfunction. |
| | Discuss concerns/perceptions with partner. |
| | Demonstrate techniques to control stressors. |
| | Verbalize achievement of sexual functioning at a mutually desired level. |

| ACTIONS/INTERVENTIONS | RATIONALE |
|---|---|

### Independent

Obtain sexual history, including previous pattern of functioning and client's perception of current problem.

Identifies individual problem(s) in order to develop an appropriate plan of care.

Determine pattern of drug use, including type, amount, and frequency of use.

Certain types of drugs can interfere with sexual functioning, e.g., alcohol, tranquilizers, narcotics, antihypertensives, antidepressants.

Identify stressors in client's life. Explore correlation of stressful situations to onset of sexual dysfunction.

Recognition and acceptance of psychologic implications (progression beyond the denial defense) need to occur before positive change can be effected.

Be aware of pathophysiology that could negatively affect sexual functioning, e.g., hypertension, diabetes.

Organic pathology as an etiologic factor needs to be considered in problem-solving when setting goals and identifying appropriate interventions.

Provide education regarding sexual functioning and alternative methods of fulfillment, as client indicates need and desire for this type of information.

Client may have misinformation about normal bodily functioning that may interfere with sexual fulfillment. Alternative methods may help to meet a need until desired level of functioning is attained.

Include significant other in as many sessions as seems appropriate and is possible.

Input from client's sexual partner will have a significant influence on client's progress. The couple should be treated as a unit. An absence of mutual trust and unwillingness to discuss each other's needs interferes with the goals of remediation.

### Collaborative

Refer to appropriate resources, such as clinical specialist, professional sex therapist, or family counselor.

May require individuals with a greater degree of knowledge and expertise in this specialty area to achieve resolution of persistent problem(s).

# CHAPTER 11

# DISSOCIATIVE DISORDERS

## DISSOCIATIVE DISORDERS

### DSM IV
300.12 Dissociative Amnesia
300.13 Dissociative Fugue
300.14 Dissociative Identify Disorder (Multiple Personality Disorder)
300.6  Depersonalization Disorder

### DSM III-R
300.14 Multiple Personality Disorder
300.13 Psychogenic Fugue
300.12 Psychogenic Amnesia
300.60 Depersonalization Disorder
300.15 Dissociative Disorder NOS

A disturbance or alteration in the normally integrative functions of identity, memory, or consciousness. The individual blocks off part of his or her life from consciousness during periods of intolerable stress. The stressful emotion becomes a separate entity, as the individual "splits" from it and mentally drifts into a fantasy state.

## ETIOLOGIC THEORIES

### Psychodynamics

Selective repression of distressing mental contents from conscious awareness as a mechanism for protecting the individual from emotional pain or expressing self in dangerous ways. The stressor(s) may arise from external circumstances or internal sources with onset of symptoms sudden or gradual and of transient or chronic nature. Intrapsychic conflict thus uses denial and "ego splitting" to decrease anxiety.

Physical sensations, such as in hysteria and hypochondria, may represent forbidden wishes that have been somatized. The use of the defense mechanism of displacement allows the feeling(s) to be directed away from the ego-threatening object toward one less threatening. In psychoanalytic terms, dissociation is a form of denial in which the object denied is part of the self or ego.

### Biologic

Research on the basis of these disorders is increasing as more recognition of the mind-body connection is accepted. It is difficult to determine whether the biologic changes (fight-

or-flight mechanism) that accompany severe anxiety precede or precipitate the emotional state. Biochemical, physiologic, and endocrine systems have an intimate connection with actual physical changes occurring in all body systems via the autonomic nervous system. Some studies have shown EEG abnormalities that have been associated with cerebral mechanisms in the temporal and limbic regions of the brain, which mediate identity formation and a sense of personal boundaries and may affect development of gender and generation boundaries.

Some organic causes of pathologic dissociative experiences are known or suspected, such as temporal lobe epilepsy, sensory deprivation, sleep loss, strokes, encephalitis, and Alzheimer's disease. Drugs may also induce amnesia or depersonalization directly or indirectly in some incidences. However, most dissociative states are not associated with any obvious organic conditions and the diagnosis of dissociative disorder requires that the condition is not due to the direct effects of a substance or a general medical condition.

## Family Dynamics

Systems theory sees the family as a system in which the process (interaction between members of the family) is the prime determinant. Level of differentiation and level of anxiety determine the degree of pathology.

Psychosocial theory states that individuals who develop dissociative disorders have often experienced severe physical, sexual, and/or emotional abuse early in life—stress so severe that the only way to cope with the painful emotions is to detach from them. The child learns to respond to stressful situations in this manner. One parent may be abusive, with the other being a passive participant, not taking care of the child. Psychiatric diagnoses (especially alcoholism) in close relatives are common, although multiple personality diagnosis is not.

Certain behaviors observed in childhood, while considered normal, may be identified as dissociative, including construction of imaginary playmates, use of different names or ages for themselves, taking on the role of an animal, imagining self as having been adopted or coming from another family, separation from the past, gender confusion, and regressive behavior. Responding to stressful situations with dissociative behaviors then becomes a method of coping for some individuals into adulthood, when there is less control over the dissociative states. The response becomes maladaptive in that the individual escapes from the stressful situation rather than facing it.

## CLIENT ASSESSMENT DATABASE

### Activity/Rest

Insomnia.

### Ego Integrity

Confusion about personal identity, may have assumed a new identity either partial or complete (fugue).
Anxiety responses, report of phobias; fears of going crazy.

### Neurosensory

Memory lapses/amnesia; disorientation; inability to recall important personal information/specific incidents not due to direct effects of a substance, general medical condition, or ordinary forgetfulness.
May report hallucinations, delusions.
Mood swings; psychologic conflicts; family/peers may describe client's behavior as erratic, unpredictable, or unreliable.
Sudden, unexpected travel away from familiar surroundings of work, with inability to recall past (fugue).

353

Persistent/recurrent experiences of feeling detached from own mental processes or body, although reality testing remains intact (depersonalization).

Presence of 2 or more distinct identities or personality states (mean average of 13), with each a fully integrated, complex unit with unique memories, behaviors, and relationships (or may be a personality state that does not have as wide a range of patterns) recurrently taking control of client's behavior, with transition from one personality to another being sudden/associated with psychosocial stress. Alternate personalities vary in their awareness of others, may be of opposite gender, and are commonly children, although some may be stated to be older than the individual (multiple personalities).

Transient changes in facial expression, voice, and posture; tastes/habits that seem to change quickly or often.

## Safety

Suicidal feelings/behaviors.
Evidence of self-mutilation.

## Sexuality

History of severe childhood incest/sexual and/or physical abuse.
Sexually inhibited and/or promiscuous.

## Social Interactions

Significant distress or impairment in social, occupational, or other important areas of functioning.

## Teaching/Learning

More common in women than in men, in persons with some higher education, and in white-collar workers.

Age of onset is early childhood, although often not diagnosed until the third decade.

Seldom diagnosed upon initial clinical contact (accurate diagnosis may be delayed by a period of months to years).

Substance abuse may be reported (but is not cause of disorder).

Absence of organic brain disorders (e.g., temporal lobe epilepsy).

History of major depression greater than 90% (multiple personalities).

## DIAGNOSTIC STUDIES

Evaluations to rule out an underlying or concurrent disease process are based on individual symptoms.

Neurologic testing, for example, EEG, CT scan, and MRI, to rule out organic brain conditions related to trauma, tumor, congenital defects, and temporal lobe epilepsy, symptoms of which often parallel manifestations of multiple personality disorder.

Psychosocial assessment, such as Rorschach, Thematic Apperception Test (TAT), Minnesota Multiphasic Personality Inventory (MMPI), Weschler Adult Intelligence Scale (WAIS), Dissociative Experiences Scale (DES), Dissociative Disorders Interview Schedule (DDIS), and hypnosis or amobarbital interviews as indicated, as these clients are frequently misdiagnosed initially because of blurring of symptoms that parallel other psychiatric problems, commonly depression, neuroses, personality disorders, and schizophrenia. Behavioral observation and documentation describing the character, duration, frequency, and precipitation of behavioral changes and client comments or complaints are essential to the diagnostic process.

**Drug Screen:** Assess for concomitant substance use.

## NURSING PRIORITIES

1. Provide safe environment; protect client/others from injury.
2. Assist client to recognize anxiety.
3. Promote insight into relationship between anxiety and development of dissociative state/other personalities.
4. Support client/family in developing effective coping skills and participating in therapeutic activities.

## DISCHARGE GOALS

1. Recognizes potentially dangerous behaviors/personalities and contracts for safety.
2. Effective coping skills/understanding of underlying dynamics of condition are demonstrated.
3. Client/family are participating in therapeutic regimen.
4. Recovers deficits in memory.
5. Major/emerging personality has been chosen and accepted (multiple personalities) or managing stress without resorting to dissociation.

| NURSING DIAGNOSIS: | ANXIETY [severe/panic]/FEAR |
|---|---|
| May Be Related To: | Maladaptation of ineffective coping continuing from early life. |
| | Unconscious conflict(s); threat to self-concept, threat of death (perceived or actual). |
| | Unmet needs. |
| | Phobic stimulus. |
| Possibly Evidenced By: | Increased tension; apprehension, fright; restlessness. |
| | Feelings of inadequacy; focus on self or projection of personal perceptions onto the environment. |
| | Verbalized focus of fear, e.g., fear of "going crazy." |
| | Maladaptive response to stress (dissociating self/fragmentation of the personality). |
| | Sympathetic stimulation: cardiovascular excitation, superficial vasoconstriction, pupil dilation. |
| Desired Outcomes/Evaluation Criteria— Client Will: | Acknowledge and discuss feelings of anxiety and fear. |
| | Identify ways to manage anxiety/fear effectively. |
| | Demonstrate problem-solving skills. |
| | Use resources effectively. |

| ACTIONS/INTERVENTIONS | RATIONALE |
|---|---|

### Independent

| Develop rapport and trust; accept verbal expression of feelings/anxieties. | A trusting alliance facilitates early identification of the underlying sources of anxiety and development of an appropriate treatment approach. Learning to |

355

| ACTIONS/INTERVENTIONS | RATIONALE |
|---|---|
| **Independent** | |
| | turn to trusted others for support assists the client to develop healthy methods of dealing with anxiety. |
| Discuss with the client the availability of assistance in maintaining safety. (Refer to ND: Violence, high risk for, directed at self/others.) | Prevents a false assurance of safety, particularly when internal threats to safety may not be readily apparent, lack of awareness of need/failure to use resources increases the likelihood of isolation and destructive behaviors. Note: Expressions of anxiety may represent a very real threat to or from alternate personalities and/or others. |
| Identify stressor(s) that precipitate severe anxiety. (Refer to ND: Personal Identity disturbance.) | Helps in recognition of individual factors precipitating dissociative symptoms (e.g., splitting, fugue, amnesia), which interfere with development/use of adequate coping skills. |
| Maintain a neutral approach when confronted by an alternate personality or dissociative state. | Allows essential observation and documentation and promotes a trusting relationship. Also avoids the therapist/care provider consciously or unconsciously promoting fragmentation of the personality. Because multiple personality disorder has been sensationalized, personnel may be intrigued by manifestations and respond to the client in ways that reinforce the behaviors manifesting the disorder. |
| Provide support and encouragement during times of depersonalization. | Client experiences fear and anxiety at these times and may fear "going crazy." Acknowledging these feelings will help client deal appropriately with them. |
| Reduce alterable sources of stress. Provide calm environment; minimize external stimuli. Identify individual causes/precipitators of stress. | Manipulation of the environment to reduce extraneous sources of stress allows the client to recognize and develop skills in managing internal sources of conflict. |
| Discuss relationship between severe anxiety and depersonalization behaviors. | Awareness of this relationship provides opportunity to define problem, look at options for dealing with stressors in more effective ways. |
| Explore past experiences and painful situations (e.g., trauma, abuse) that may be repressed. | It is believed that traumatic experiences predispose individuals to dissociative disorders. |
| Provide positive reinforcement and expectations, and role-model desired behaviors. | This client is commonly very suggestible and responsive to the positive expectations and attention of trusted others. Development of healthy coping mechanisms helps in reducing anxiety. |
| Prepare client for any testing procedures; provide information about the reason for the test and what is to be expected from the results. | An explanation of the processes of each test can allay anxiety. Care needs to be taken that the physical assessment is presented as routine because the client may misperceive the test as indicative of the presence of a physical disorder and may be prone to a psychosomatic or conversion disorder. |

| ACTIONS/INTERVENTIONS | RATIONALE |
|---|---|
| **Independent** | |
| Review test results as indicated. | Receiving the results in a timely manner relieves anxiety. Once organic causes have been ruled out, it is unlikely that extensive examinations and/or testing will have to be repeated, reducing the likelihood that the client might adopt physical symptoms, providing secondary gain. |
| Observe for/review with client untoward effects/adverse reaction to medication regimen. Monitor level of alertness, vital signs; note urinary retention, dry mouth, blurred vision, Parkinson's-like symptoms, rigidity, or atypical response (excitability, restlessness, agitation). | Psychoactive medications (sedatives, minor tranquilizers, antipsychotic agents, and antidepressants) frequently produce hypotension and anticholinergic and extrapyramidal symptoms, in addition to the desired effect. Early intervention will alleviate prolonged difficulties and/or serious physical complications and may prevent/lessen anxiety about their presence. |
| **Collaborative** | |
| Coordinate and develop a combined treatment plan. Facilitate communication among team members. | It is essential that all members of the treatment team work together in the plan of care to ensure that goals and objectives are in agreement and continuity of care exists. A cohesive treatment plan prevents dissension between disciplines. These clients are prone to manipulative behaviors and may be resistant to therapy; they do better when dealing with one primary provider supported by a cohesive treatment team. |
| Administer antianxiety medications as indicated, e.g., alprazolam (Xanax), diazepam (Valium). | Antianxiety medications are given with caution for brief periods to allay panic states or disabling anxiety. Caution is essential as substance abuse is a common complication and also because of the potential for self-destructive behavior. |

| **NURSING DIAGNOSIS:** | **THOUGHT PROCESSES, ALTERED** |
|---|---|
| **May Be Related To:** | *Psychologic conflict; severe level of anxiety, repressed.* |
| | *Childhood trauma/abuse; threat to physical integrity/self-concept.* |
| **Possibly Evidenced By:** | *Memory loss/deficit—inability to recall selected events related to a stressful situation, inability to recall events associated with entire life, inability to recall own identity; disorientation.* |
| **Desired Outcomes/Evaluation Criteria— Client Will:** | *Verbalize understanding that loss of memory is related to stress.* |
| | *Begin discussing stressful situation(s).* |
| | *Recover deficits in memory.* |
| | *Develop more adaptive coping mechanisms to deal with life stressors.* |

| ACTIONS/INTERVENTIONS | RATIONALE |
|---|---|

### Independent

Determine degree/extent of memory deficits. Obtain information about client from family/SO, identifying likes, dislikes, important people, activities, music, pets, etc.

Helps to develop a realistic plan of care incorporating information about past to work with client on recovering memory.

Expose client to stimuli that represent pleasant experiences from the past, such as smells associated with enjoyable activities and music known to be pleasurable.

Providing pleasurable stimuli can lead client to remembering the past without risk of sudden trauma.

Avoid flooding client with data about past life.

May expose client to painful information from which the amnesia is providing protection. Client may decompensate even further into a psychotic state if recall is too rapid.

Engage in further activities that stimulate life experiences as memory returns.

Supports continued recall in a nonthreatening manner.

Encourage client to discuss situations that have been especially stressful and to explore the feelings associated with those times.

Verbalization of feelings in a nonthreatening environment may help client come to terms with unresolved issues that may be contributing to the dissociative process.

Discuss more adaptive ways to respond to anxiety.

Dissociative behaviors will no longer be needed when more effective responses are used.

### Collaborative

Administer medication as indicated, e.g.: methylphenidate (Ritalin), pemoline (Cylert), bupropion (Wellbutrin).

Anecdotal information suggests that use of agents that increase synaptic levels of dopamine may be beneficial in treating depersonalization disorder when the client is distressed by persistent symptoms.

Prepare for/assist with IV amobarbital (Amytal) therapy.

May help client regain memory in amnesic or fugue state.

| NURSING DIAGNOSIS: | COPING, INDIVIDUAL, INEFFECTIVE |
|---|---|
| **May Be Related To:** | Personal vulnerability; unmet expectations; inadequate support systems/coping methods. |
| | Multiple stressors/overwhelming trauma to the client as a small child, usually occurring in the family of origin. |
| **Possibly Evidenced By:** | Verbalization of inability to cope/problem-solve. |
| | Inappropriate use of defense mechanisms (dissociative states). |
| | Reports of chronic worry, anxiety, depression, poor self-esteem. |
| | Inability to meet role expectations; divorce and alienation. |

| **Desired Outcomes/Evaluation Criteria—Client Will:** | Identify ineffective coping behaviors and consequences that are creating problems for the client. |
|---|---|
| | Meet psychologic needs as evidenced by appropriate expression of feelings, identification of options, and use of resources. |
| | Demonstrate positive coping mechanisms. |

| **ACTIONS/INTERVENTIONS** | **RATIONALE** |
|---|---|
| **Independent** | |
| Discuss measures being taken to protect client. Stay with client as needed. | Reassures client of psychologic safety/security when dissociative behaviors and/or therapy are frightening to the client. Presence of a trusted person can provide sense of security. |
| Commit to long-term alliance. Contract with client to refrain from acting on destructive thoughts or ending therapy abruptly. (Refer to ND: Violence, high risk for, directed at self/others.) | These clients often have difficulty developing a therapeutic relationship. Because of high incidence of childhood abuse, client mistrusts authority and has a lifelong habit of "keeping secrets" from self and others. |
| Encourage discussion and verbalization of stressful situation and exploration of feelings associated with those times. Help client to understand that disequilibrium is to be expected, is understandable, and will resolve as integration occurs. | Ventilation in a nonthreatening environment may help the client to come to terms with issues that may be contributing to the dissociative process. Provides opportunity for client to relive traumatic experiences, purge associated feelings, and accept the memories. |
| Demonstrate acceptance during disclosure of painful experiences. | Fear of condemnation and criticism makes such disclosure difficult, even in a trusting relationship, and support provides reassurance that information will be treated tactfully. |
| Have client identify methods of coping with stress in the past, the purpose served, and consequences. Determine whether the response was adaptive or maladaptive. | As anxiety decreases, client can begin to develop insight into the appropriateness of the response and develop a plan of action for the future. It is important for client to understand and accept that the dissociative behavior was originally adaptive and allowed the individual to survive an intolerable situation. |
| Remain alert to possibility of substance use. | A significant percentage of these clients use substances, such as alcohol, as a means of coping. This can cloud symptomatology and interfere with progress. |
| Assist the client to explore alternative coping strategies, evaluating benefits and consequences of each. | Helps the client to learn new ways to problem-solve and make decisions, which will promote development of independence and use of adaptive coping skills. |
| Reinforce positive coping mechanisms. | Promotes repetition of adaptive behaviors. These clients are very responsive to positive attention. |

| ACTIONS/INTERVENTIONS | RATIONALE |
|---|---|

### Independent

Provide supportive, insight-oriented therapy: encourage expression of feelings; accept verbal expressions without judgment; encourage recognition of strengths, positive attributes, and progress toward wellness.

Dissociative symptoms arise from internal conflict. The behaviors protect the client from psychic pain. Subsequently, any stressor can precipitate a like reaction. Insight-oriented therapy in a supportive setting allows the client to confront and resolve past and present painful or fear-inducing events.

Discuss problems of discouragement with lengthy treatment.

Discouraged feelings are inevitable (in face of treatment that may last for years), and client may resort to old, maladaptive coping mechanisms and feel like giving up. (Refer to ND: Violence, high risk for, directed at self/others.)

Identify specific conflicts that remain unresolved and problem-solve possible solutions.

When these underlying conflicts are not resolved, any improvement in coping behaviors may be regarded as temporary.

### Collaborative

Encourage client to develop a network of support systems through family, friends, community resources, and school/work and church affiliations, as well as health and mental health care providers and internal resources.

The tendency to overdependency present in these individuals is antitherapeutic and draining to family, friends, and therapy providers. Development of a large support network and internal resources promotes autonomy.

| NURSING DIAGNOSIS: | VIOLENCE, HIGH RISK FOR, DIRECTED AT SELF/OTHERS |
|---|---|
| **Risk Factors May Include:** | Dissociative state/conflicting personalities. |
| | Depressed mood. |
| | Panic states. |
| | Suicidal behaviors. |
| **Possible Indicators:** | Increased motor activity, pacing, excitement, irritability, agitation. |
| | Self-destructive behaviors, active aggressive suicidal acts/threats; "internal homicide" (in which one personality attempts to kill another personality). |
| | Substance abuse. |
| **Desired Outcomes/Evaluation Criteria— Client Will:** | Verbalize understanding of why behavior occurs. |
| | Demonstrate self-control as evidenced by relaxed posture, nonviolent behavior. |
| | Express increased self-esteem and meet needs in an assertive manner. |
| | Use resources and support systems effectively. |

| ACTIONS/INTERVENTIONS | RATIONALE |
|---|---|

### Independent

Remain vigilant to behavioral changes that may signal destructive actions. Assess seriousness of suicidal tendency, gestures, threats, or previous attempts. (Use scale of 1–10 and prioritize according to severity of threat, availability of means.)

Client behavior may change abruptly and dramatically. Impulse control may be impaired. (May be # 1 nursing diagnosis if score is high.)

Minimize environmental stimuli, remove dangerous objects.

These measures may prevent escalation/occurrence of violence.

Help client identify/recognize precipitants to destructive behaviors.

Early detection permits timely intervention, allowing environmental manipulation to reduce the occurrence of injurious behaviors.

Structure the environment to reduce stressors that precipitate destructive behavior. Assist the client to reduce exposure to external stressors by avoidance when practical.

Calm surroundings permit the client to recognize personally distressing factors, thereby reducing externally disruptive behaviors.

Active-listen and encourage the client to seek restraint and/or support when self-destructive or violent impulses are present.

A therapeutic alliance promotes client responsibility for behavioral restraint while supplementing internal controls. Ventilation will reduce the need for action.

Arrange protection in presence of multiple personalities for "individual" that is prone to violent behavior. Another personality, usually the primary one, can be appointed to monitor/control the behavior of the suspect personality.

Usually one personality can be identified as having these behaviors, and use of another personality may keep the violence from occurring.

Assist the client to identify alternatives to aggression or self-destructive behaviors, e.g., verbal expression, physical activity, written expression.

Provides a substitute activity in response to overwhelming impulse to enable client to respond to impulses in a nondestructive manner.

Take immediate and decisive action when danger is imminent. Tell client to "STOP" and/or hold as necessary until client calms down.

The organized approach of a concerned response by caregivers allows for rapid resolution and minimizes potential for injury to the client/staff/others.

Encourage participation in exercise program/physical activities.

Promotes safe and effective way of relieving tension.

Note presence/degree of depression and reassess periodically, noting suicidal ideation.

Client may become discouraged and depressed, as treatment is a long-term process, possibly in excess of 10 years.

### Collaborative

Hospitalize as necessary.

Usually instituted for differential diagnosis, in response to self-destructive thoughts/behavior, violence or potential violence, and/or psychosomatic complaints or conversion reaction.

361

## Collaborative

| ACTIONS/INTERVENTIONS | RATIONALE |
| --- | --- |
| Place in isolation and provide physical restraint in a nonpunitive manner. Observe closely/stay with client. | Punishment has no therapeutic value, but external controls are necessary to ensure safety/provide reassurance to client when internal controls fail. Close observation following initial restraint will be necessary to assure the effectiveness of the restraints and that the client is not injured by the restraint, e.g., strangulation, impaired circulation, suffocation, aspiration. |
| Administer antianxiety/antidepressant medication as indicated. | May be required to reduce anxiety until internal controls are achieved and/or elevate mood to allow client to begin to deal with feelings/situation. |

| | |
| --- | --- |
| **NURSING DIAGNOSIS:** | **PERSONAL IDENTITY DISTURBANCE** |
| **May Be Related To:** | Psychologic conflicts (dissociative state[s]). |
| | Threat to physical integrity/self-concept; childhood trauma/abuse. |
| | Underdeveloped ego. |
| **Possibly Evidenced By:** | Memory loss (unable to recall selected events/own identity); presence of more than one personality within the individual. |
| | Confusion about sense of self, purpose or direction in life; alteration in perception or experience of the self. |
| | Loss of one's own sense of reality/the external world; poorly differentiated ego boundaries. |
| **Desired Outcomes/Evaluation Criteria—Client Will:** | **GENERAL** |
| | Acknowledge threat to personal identity. |
| | Engage in a therapeutic alliance. |
| | Integrate threat in a healthy, positive manner (e.g., make commitment to long-term therapy, state anxiety is manageable, make plans for future). |
| | **DISSOCIATIVE IDENTITY DISORDERS** |
| | Verbalize awareness of all personalities, their thoughts and behaviors (development of co-consciousness). |
| | Display cooperation among the personalities. |
| | Demonstrate more stable personalities with resolution of traumatic events, moving toward partial to full integration into one personality. |
| | Verbalize acceptance of positive feelings toward emerging personality. |

| ACTIONS/INTERVENTIONS | RATIONALE |
|---|---|

### Independent

Develop trusting relationship with individual (and "alters" or subpersonalities if present).

Trust is the basis of a therapeutic relationship, but it may be difficult to achieve as client is often demoralized and suspicious, believing life is unjust/hopeless, or even that she or he is evil. In Dissociative Identity Disorder, each of the personalities views itself as a separate entity and must initially be treated as such.

Determine client's perception of the extent of the threat to self-integrity and current response.

Degree of distress perceived by the client will assist in determining actions necessary for intervention.

Help client understand/accept reality of the disorder (e.g., other personalities) and meaning of lapses in memory.

May be unaware/lack understanding of condition, resulting in increased anxiety and confusion about self.

Ascertain what client does recall and compare with information obtained from family members/other personalities.

Helps in orienting to realities of past events and assists client toward memory integration.

Share information in small amounts over a period of time. Avoid giving too much information (flooding) at any one time.

Enables client to begin to deal with painful information for which the amnesia has provided protection in the past. Too much material at any one time can be difficult for client to handle, and decompensation could occur.

Facilitate identification of stressful situations that precipitate dissociative state/transition from one personality to another. (Refer to ND: Coping, individual, ineffective.)

Assists client to respond more adaptively and to eliminate the need for separation from self.

Encourage client to identify the need the behavior/each subpersonality serves in the overall identity of the individual.

Knowledge of these unfulfilled needs enables client to face unresolved issues without dissociation and is the first step toward integration of multiple personalities.

Provide psychotherapy with feedback relative to behavioral observations. Encourage journal-keeping and other methods designed to allow gradual insight.

Decreases denial and amnesia, providing an opportunity for the client to accept the presence of the disorder and begin to own behaviors/personality components. Acceptance and ownership assist the client toward cooperation within the individual and subsequent integration when multiple personalities are present.

Discuss integration of subpersonalities into a unified identity within the individual, and help client understand that all personalities will contribute to the whole.

The idea of total elimination generates fear and defensiveness within alters who function as separate entities.

### Collaborative

Plan use of confrontive methods with all team members. Use cautiously.

These methods need to be paced with the individual's ability to benefit therapeutically and planned within the team conference to avoid overstressing the individual and precipitating exacerbation or decompensation.

| ACTIONS/INTERVENTIONS | RATIONALE |
|---|---|

### Collaborative

| | |
|---|---|
| Use/assist with hypnosis as indicated. | Allows client to become familiar with dissociation and learn how to interrupt/control it. Provides opportunity for client to make traumatic memories/feelings conscious and realize this will not destroy them. May be used to gain access to multiple personalities, helping client to work through and accept realities of positive aspects of each personality and participate in rituals of joining/integration. |
| Engage in activities that reflect life experiences, using occupational/vocational/recreational/physical therapy. Begin with pleasurable stimuli (as identified by the client), e.g., events, smells, pets, or music associated with pleasurable activities. | Presents additional stimulation which may encourage recall of repressed material. Provides opportunity to experience positive feelings that have also been repressed and work toward beginning to deal with negative feelings/occurrences. |

| | |
|---|---|
| **NURSING DIAGNOSIS:** | **FAMILY COPING, ineffective: compromised/disabling** |
| **May Be Related To:** | Multiple stressors, repeated over period of time. |
| | Temporary family disorganization and role changes; prolonged progression of disorder that exhausts the supportive capacity of significant people. |
| | Significant person with chronically unexpressed feelings of guilt, anger, hostility, and so forth. |
| | High-risk family situation, e.g., recurrent episodes of neglect/abuse, substance abuse. |
| **Possibly Evidenced By:** | Significant person describes inadequate understanding or knowledge base that interferes with effective assistive or supportive behaviors. |
| | Expresses despair regarding family reactions/lack of involvement. |
| | Marital conflict (separation/divorce). |
| | Intolerance, abandonment, rejection, desertion. |
| | Neglectful care of client in regard to basic human needs. |
| | Distortion of reality regarding the client's health problem, including extreme denial about its existence or severity. |
| **Desired Outcomes/Evaluation Criteria— Family Will:** | Verbalize more realistic understanding and expectations of the client. |
| | Identify/verbalize resources within self to deal with the situation. |

Provide opportunity for client to deal with situation in own way.

Remain intact, or separate in healthy way, being supportive of the client and one another.

| ACTIONS/INTERVENTIONS | RATIONALE |
|---|---|

### Independent

Identify contributing factors within the family or environment.

Family and marital dysfunction are extremely likely to occur. These factors contribute to ongoing emotional stress for all family members.

Note family who are involved with client, e.g., by marriage (husband, children), family of origin (mother/father, siblings, extended family). Complete a genogram.

It is important for all family members who are interacting with the client to be involved in helping with the therapeutic regimen to allow for the best outcome possible for the client.

Provide client/family education relative to the disorder and treatment plan.

An understanding of the problem and the fact that the disorder can be treated reduces anxiety, frustration, and guilt and allows the client to progress within a supportive environment.

Explore family dynamics. Note enabling/sabotage behaviors, e.g., failure to attend therapy/keeping client from attending.

Other family members may be invested in keeping the "sick" member symptomatic in order to camouflage their own problems.

Provide for client safety within the family setting or arrange for alternative living arrangements if abuse or neglect is at issue. (Refer to CP: Parenting, regarding issues of current abuse/neglect).

If the client remains in the family of origin, a diagnosis of dissociative state/multiple personality disorder should alert personnel to the possibility of abuse/neglect. As the "responsible adult," client may be unable to meet needs of own child(ren)/family.

Assist the family to respond to the client in a manner that reinforces positive behaviors.

Without assistance, the family may provide secondary gain for continued illness versus wellness.

Encourage the family to ventilate negative feelings and continue as much as possible with usual daily activities. Discourage family from allowing client to escape responsibilities because of the illness.

Family members are less likely to abandon the affected member if they have an outlet for anger/frustration and are not overburdened in caretaking. Positive expectations from family members promote hope for recovery and self-esteem and decrease the likelihood of secondary gain.

### Collaborative

Refer for additional individual, family, or marriage counseling.

Concurrent psychiatric problems in other family members are common. If the client's symptoms are the most florid, that individual has likely been identified as the "sick" family member and others have not sought/received help.

365

# CHAPTER 12

# SEXUAL AND GENDER IDENTITY DISORDERS

## SEXUAL DISORDERS

**DSM IV**
**SEXUAL DYSFUNCTIONS**
**Sexual Desire Disorders**
302.71  Hypoactive Sexual Desire Disorder
302.79  Sexual Aversion Disorder
**Sexual Arousal Disorders**
302.72  Female Sexual Arousal Disorder
302.72  Male Erectile Disorder
**Orgasmic Disorders**
302.73  Female Orgasmic Disorder (Inhibited Female Orgasm)
302.74  Male Orgasmic Disorder (Inhibited Male Orgasm)
302.75  Premature Ejaculation
**Sexual Pain Disorders**
302.76  Dyspareunia (Not Due to a General Medical Condition)
306.51  Vaginismus (Not Due to a General Medical Condition)

(Refer to DSM IV Manual for Sexual Dysfunctions Due to a General Medical Condition.)

**PARAPHILIAS**
302.4   Exhibitionism
302.81  Fetishism
302.89  Frotteurism
302.2   Pedophilia
302.83  Sexual Masochism
302.84  Sexual Sadism
302.82  Voyeurism
302.3   Transvestic Fetishism

**DSM III-R**
**PARAPHILIAS**
302.40  Exhibitionism
302.81  Fetishism
302.89  Frotteurism

302.20  Pedophilia
302.83  Sexual Masochism
302.84  Sexual Sadism
302.30  Transvestic Fetishism
302.82  Voyeurism

**SEXUAL DYSFUNCTIONS (DESIRE DISORDERS)**

302.71  Hypoactive Sexual Desire Disorder
302.79  Sexual Aversion Disorder
302.72  Female Sexual Arousal Disorder
302.72  Male Erectile Disorder
302.73  Inhibited Female Orgasm
302.74  Inhibited Male Orgasm
302.75  Premature Ejaculation
302.76  Dyspareunia
302.51  Vaginismus
302.70  Sexual Disorder NOS

Sexual disorders include sexual dysfunctions and paraphilias. Sexual dysfunction is defined as a persistent impairment/disturbance of a normal or desired pattern in any phase of the sexual response cycle. Paraphilias are more specific disorders in which unusual or bizarre imagery or acts are necessary for realization of sexual excitement. Since many paraphiliac behaviors are illegal in most states, individuals generally come for psychiatric treatment because of pressure from others, partners, or the authorities.

## ETIOLOGIC FACTORS

### Psychodynamics

Individual causes of sexual desire disorders may include religious beliefs, obsessive-compulsive personality, conflicts with gender identity or sexual preference, sexual phobias, fear of losing control over sexual urges, secret sexual deviations, fear of pregnancy, inadequate grieving following the death of a spouse, depression, and aging-related concerns. Psychologic factors may also be involved in arousal disorders as well.

Psychoanalytic theories state that paraphilias are the product of childhood desires that survive into adulthood in their immature forms because emotional development has been inhibited, distorted, and diverted. These wishes are believed to be universal and are used to achieve arousal and release when ordinary forms of sexual activity are not available. Deviations arise when these immature forms of libido dominate adult sexual life. Fixation is thought to occur in Freud's oral, anal, and phallic phases when corresponding body parts provide sources of instinctual gratification. Conflict arises when an imperfect compromise occurs between these impulses and reality, resulting in fear, which the unconscious perceives as castration.

Behavioral theorists believe any paraphilia/sexual dysfunction can be acquired through conditioning, in which an initial pairing of an object is accidentally associated with/then becomes necessary for sexual release. This need may become generalized to other situations of tension/anxiety.

### Biologic

Sometimes the cause is clearly biologic, e.g., temporal lobe epilepsy that may cause changes in sexual behavior between seizures. It has also been suggested that the problem arises out of interference with brain pathways governing rage and sexual arousal. Sex hormones have been studied. Rat studies have demonstrated that small, properly timed doses of androgens (male hormones) or estrogens (female hormones) in the fetus or newborn can influence sexual behavior. Various organic reasons, medication and other drug use, physical illnesses (most notably diabetes mellitus), surgery (such as prostatectomy), and degenera-

367

tive neural disorders (e.g., multiple sclerosis) may be involved in sexual desire, arousal, and pain disorders.

It is generally accepted that abnormal hormonal activity and biologic (genetic) predisposition interacting with social and family factors influence the development of these fantasies/sexual acts, which may occur within normal sexual activity but when they become the primary source of sexual satisfaction result in problems for the individual/others.

### Family Dynamics

There appears to be some evidence that paraphilias run in families and may be the result of dysfunctional family interactions and social learning.

Sexual dysfunctions are believed to be influenced by what the individual has learned/not learned as a child within the family system and by values and beliefs that may be based on myths and misconceptions.

## CLIENT ASSESSMENT DATABASE (SEXUAL DYSFUNCTIONS)

### Neurosensory

Mental Status:
    Findings may be indicative of intense distress about situation/condition or coexisting psychiatric disorders.
    Mood and affect may reveal evidence of increased anxiety and depression.

### Sexuality

May be lifelong or acquired after a period of normal sexual functioning.
May report inhibition or interference with some part of the human response cycle, e.g., low sexual desire, aversion to genital sexual contact, arousal/erectile/orgasmic disturbances, premature ejaculation; genital pain during or after sexual intercourse, and involuntary spasm of the outer third of the vagina interfering with coitus.
May display negative attitude(s) toward sexuality.

### Social Interactions

Impairment may be noted in marital/conjugal relationships but rarely affects job performance.

### Teaching/Learning

Most commonly occur in early adulthood, although male erectile disorder may surface later in life.

## CLIENT ASSESSMENT DATABASE (PARAPHILIAS)

### Ego Integrity

May express shame or guilt about behavior.
May or may not act on fantasies.

### Neurosensory

Personality disturbances frequently accompany sexual disorder(s).

### Safety

Physical injury may be seen following episodes of sadomasochistic activity.

## Sexuality

Recurrent, intense sexual urges and fantasies involving the exposure of one's genitals to a stranger that have been acted on, cause severe distress, and may be accompanied by masturbation (exhibitionism).

Use of nonliving object(s) to stimulate recurrent intense sexual urges and sexually arousing fantasies, e.g., female undergarments (fetishism).

Rubbing and touching against a nonconsenting person to invoke recurrent, intense sexual urges and fantasies. It is the touching, not the coercive nature of the act, that is sexually exciting (frotteurism).

Sexual activity with a prepubescent child or children (pedophilia).

Participates in the act (real, not simulated) of being humiliated, beaten, bound, or otherwise made to suffer (sexual masochism).

Participates in acts (real, not simulated) in which the psychologic or physical suffering (including humiliation) of the victim is sexually exciting to the person (sexual sadism).

Cross-dressing activities (transvestic fetishism).

Observing unsuspecting person(s), usually a stranger, who is naked, in the process of disrobing or engaging in sexual activity (voyeurism).

## Social Interactions

May not view self as ill; however, behavior may cause distress for the individual or may bring suffering to others.

May be in conflict with partner or society because of behavior.

Interference with interpersonal/occupational functioning may be noted.

## Teaching/Learning

Occur mostly in males.

Some evidence of occurrence in families of paraphiliacs and of depressed individual; high correlation between pedophiles and family history of pedophilic activity.

## DIAGNOSTIC STUDIES

As indicated to rule out physical causes of sexual dysfunction.

Screen for sexually transmitted diseases (STDs) including HIV/AIDS.

## NURSING PRIORITIES

1. Assist client to understand the nature of the behavior (disorder/dysfunction).
2. Encourage use of acceptable methods for reduction of anxiety.
3. Help to recognize the legal/interpersonal consequences of paraphilic behaviors.
4. Explore options for change.
5. Encourage involvement of client/family (significant other) in treatment regimen.

## DISCHARGE GOALS

1. The nature of the problem and consequences for the individual/family are understood.
2. Options have been explored and appropriate one(s) chosen.
3. Anxiety is reduced/managed in acceptable ways.
4. Confidence in own capabilities/sense of self-worth is expressed.
5. Participating in treatment program and using community/treatment resources effectively.

| NURSING DIAGNOSIS: | SEXUAL DYSFUNCTION/SEXUALITY PATTERNS, ALTERED |
|---|---|
| **May Be Related To:** | Biophysical alteration of sexuality: ineffectual or absent role models; vulnerability; misinformation; physical/sexual abuse.<br><br>Lack of significant other.<br><br>Loss of sexual desire; disruption of sexual response pattern, e.g., premature ejaculation, dyspareunia.<br><br>Conflicts involving values; conflicts with variant preferences.<br><br>Knowledge/skill deficit about alternative responses. |
| **Possibly Evidenced By:** | Reported difficulties, limitations/changes in sexual behaviors or activities.<br><br>Alterations in achieving sexual satisfaction; difficulty achieving desired satisfaction in socially acceptable ways. |
| **Desired Outcomes/Evaluation Criteria— Client Will:** | Verbalize understanding of sexual anatomy/function and individual reasons for sexual problems.<br><br>Identify stressors involved in lifestyle that contribute to dysfunction; satisfying/acceptable sexual practices and some alternative ways of dealing with sexual expression.<br><br>Demonstrate improved communication/relationship skills. |

| ACTIONS/INTERVENTIONS | RATIONALE |
|---|---|
| **Independent** | |
| Take sexual history, noting when problem(s) began, degree of anxiety, presence of relationship, conflict between partners, displacement of pattern of arousal to other than the opposite sex, and client desire of/need for change. | Identification of individual situation promotes appropriate goal-setting and interventions. |
| Determine cultural/value conflicts, preexisting problems affecting current situation. | Stress in other areas of life will affect sexual functioning. Client may feel guilt and shame or feel depressed because of sexual difficulties/deviant behavior. |
| Explore possible drug use. | Substance/prescription use may affect sexual functioning/be used to relieve anxiety of sexually deviant behavior. |

| ACTIONS/INTERVENTIONS | RATIONALE |
| --- | --- |

### Independent

Avoid making value judgments.

Does not help client to deal with the situation or feel better about self.

Determine what client needs/wants to know and provide information accordingly. Review information regarding safety and/or consequences of actions.

Prevents unnecessary repetition of information/presenting information client is not willing to hear. Reviewing necessary information gives client message that it is important and serves as a reminder of own responsibility.

Encourage open discussion of concerns and expression of feelings and assist with problem-solving.

Promotes thinking about causes/results of behavior(s) and resolution of problem.

Provide sex information/education, as necessary.

Lack of knowledge may be significant to underlying problem(s).

Encourage completion of structured homework exercises dependent on behavior and individual needs, e.g., avoidance of coitus/orgasm, use of masturbation, planned progression of intimate activity, diary of feelings/perceptions.

Heightened sensory awareness and improved nonverbal communication with partner in an atmosphere free of demands for sexual performance may resolve sexual dysfunctions. Note: Clients without partners may benefit from assertiveness training, self-exploration, permission to fantasize, correction of misconceptions.

### Collaborative

Refer for assessment of physical conditions, e.g., presence of diabetes, vascular problems.

1/3–1/2 of clients with sexual dysfunction have a physical condition that interferes with sexual functioning.

Monitor penile tumescence during REM sleep, as indicated.

Impotence can be assessed by noting erectile ability occurring during sleep. Physical conditions are ruled out when erection occurs.

Refer to appropriate resources as necessary, e.g., clinical specialist psychiatric nurse, professional sex therapists, family counseling.

Additional/in-depth counseling, sex therapy may help client come to terms with underlying problems that interfere with recovery. Note: Use of sexual surrogates for clients without partners is no longer recommended because of questions of ethics, values, psychologic effects, and relevance to normal sexual relations.

| | |
| --- | --- |
| **NURSING DIAGNOSIS:** | **ANXIETY [moderate to severe]** |
| **May Be Related To:** | Unconscious conflict about sexual feelings. |
| | Threat to self-concept; threat to role-functioning. |
| | Unmet needs. |
| **Possibly Evidenced By:** | Increased tension (sexual). |
| | Feelings of inadequacy. |
| | Fear of unspecified consequences. |
| | Extraneous movements (foot shuffling, hand/arm movements). |

|  | Glancing about; poor eye contact; focus on self. |
| **Desired Outcomes/Evaluation Criteria— Client Will:** | Impaired functioning; immobility. |
|  | Verbalize awareness of feelings of anxiety and report reduction to a manageable level. |
|  | Demonstrate problem-solving skills and use resources effectively. |

| ACTIONS/INTERVENTIONS | RATIONALE |
| --- | --- |

### Independent

| Determine degree and precipitants of anxiety. | Sexual activity is usually undertaken to reduce a state of inner tension and pressure. Fear of "failure," of being found out and/or disapproved of also creates anxiety. Individual may have sought help because of these fears/coming to the attention of the legal system. |
| Identify client's perception of the threat represented by the situation. | The client may not perceive the behavior as a problem; however, it is the reaction of others and consequences that create anxiety. Circumstances that prevent the client from indulging in paraphilic behavior can lead to intense anxiety. |
| Assess withdrawn behavior and evaluate for substance use (alcohol, other drugs), sleep disturbances, limited/avoidance of interactions with others. | These behaviors may be used by the client to deal with anxiety/other feelings (e.g., guilt) instead of other, positive coping mechanisms. Substance use may be a factor in the occurrence of the dysfunction(s). |
| Note prodromal symptoms of irritability, restlessness, tension, and headache. | In the exhibitionist, these may be the response to abnormal discharges in the temporal lobes. |
| Encourage appropriate expression of feelings, e.g., crying (sadness), laughing (fear, denial), swearing (fear, anger). | Suppression of feelings has contributed to difficulties client has in dealing with anxiety and coping appropriately with sexual desires/dysfunction. |
| Provide calm, quiet environment. Display accepting attitude. | Promotes discussion of sensitive sexual issues/concerns. Sexual performance is closely tied to individual sense of self as male or female, making self-disclosure difficult. |
| Confront the client's illegal behavior without judgment. | Client needs to hear that behavior, not the individual, is not acceptable. |
| Assist the client to recognize a helpful degree of anxiety and ways to begin to use it. | Moderate degree of anxiety heightens awareness and permits the client to focus on dealing with the problems. |

### Collaborative

| Administer medication as indicated, e.g.: antiandrogen drugs: Depo-Provera; | These drugs have been useful for altering sexual behavior, but their use is limited because they suppress desired as well as unwanted sexual responses. |

| ACTIONS/INTERVENTIONS | RATIONALE |
|---|---|
| **Collaborative** | |
| antidepressants: fluoxetine (Prozac), imipramine (Tofranil), lithium. | Research suggests that some compulsive sexual activity viewed as excessive or out of control (e.g., compulsive masturbation, obsessional fantasies about sex with children, voyeurism) may be an atypical symptom of depression. Sexual desire may be reduced and sexual activity become more normal when antidepressants are used. |
| Refer to therapy as indicated, e.g.: psychotherapy; | Psychotherapy may be used to help the client recognize the problem of sadness and isolation caused by the dysfunction and deal with the emotional issues involved. May also be used to help client accept sexual nature when behavior is not damaging/dangerous, e.g., transvestism. |
| marital/family therapy; | May resolve problems of communication, which may be major factor in many sexual dysfunction problems. |
| behavioral therapy. | Aversion therapy, in which the unwanted sexual act/thought is linked to an unpleasant sensation such as an electric shock or nausea and/or imagining a frightening or disgusting event, is used as negative reinforcement and is designed to extinguish the desire. Desensitization to painful heterosexual coitus is used with limited long-lasting success. |

| NURSING DIAGNOSIS: | **SELF-ESTEEM DISTURBANCE [specify]** |
|---|---|
| **May Be Related To:** | Emotional insecurity; lack of self-confidence. |
| | Substance use. |
| | Biophysical/psychosocial factors, e.g., achievement of sexual satisfaction in deviant ways; failure to perform satisfactorily. |
| **Possibly Evidenced By:** | Verbalization of fear of rejection/reaction by others; negative feelings about body; feelings of helplessness, hopelessness, or powerlessness. |
| | Change in social involvement. |
| | Difficulty accepting positive reinforcement. |
| | Lack of follow-through. |
| | Self-destructive behaviors. |
| **Desired Outcomes/Evaluation Criteria— Client Will:** | Identify feelings and methods for coping with negative perception of self. |

373

Verbalize increased sense of self-esteem in relation to current situation, e.g., sees self as a worthwhile person.

Demonstrate adaptation to events that have occurred by setting realistic goals and active participation in treatment program.

Report satisfactory sexual experiences.

| ACTIONS/INTERVENTIONS | RATIONALE |
|---|---|
| **Independent** | |
| Determine individual situation that contributes to client's self-esteem, as well as client's perception of the threat to self and awareness of own responsibility for dealing with situation. | Failure to perform sexually can affect a person's sense of esteem and self-worth. When the problem is defined as paraphilic, the client may not recognize the sexual behavior as related to current problem(s). Identification of individual circumstances helps in choosing appropriate interventions. |
| Assess type of sexual dysfunction/problem by asking direct questions, e.g., describe the dysfunction client is experiencing, clarify relationship between partners, presence of power struggle, anger, concern regarding commitment or stability of relationship; preference for nonliving objects, dressing in clothes of the opposite sex, use of physical/mental pain as a source of sexual arousal. | Partners may have very different expectations of the relationship, and sexual disorder may serve to correct power imbalance or maintain emotional distance. Client may not see sexual deviance as a problem but may seek help for feelings of guilt and sadness. Asking directly can promote client recognition of these factors. |
| Provide information about sexual anatomy/physiology as needed. | Lack of information and myths/misconceptions are the basis of sexual functioning problems, and accurate knowledge may be crucial to resolution of the problems. |
| Ascertain if client has ever been arrested. | Pattern of involvement with the law can provide information about extent of the problem. |
| Determine client motivation for change. | When client accepts the fact that the sexual behavior is responsible for the problems that exist and makes the decision to change, therapy has more chance of being successful. If therapy is court-ordered, possibility for change is less likely but still possible. |
| Discuss what purpose (positive intention) the behavior serves for the client (e.g., sense of inadequacy as a male may be met by exhibitionistic behaviors) and what other options might be available to meet needs in more satisfying and socially acceptable ways. | Identification of the purpose allows opportunity for the client to examine whether the behavior meets the purpose in an adaptive or maladaptive manner. |
| Give positive reinforcement for progress noted. | Encouragement can support development of mature coping behaviors. |

| ACTIONS/INTERVENTIONS | RATIONALE |
|---|---|
| **Independent** | |
| Permit client to progress at own rate. | Immaturity is believed to be involved in the development of paraphilias, and adaptation to a change in self-concept depends on the significance the individual attaches to the change, how long this behavior has been used, and necessary changes in lifestyle. Learning to see oneself as a capable, competent adult who interacts in an adult sexual manner takes a long time. |
| Assist client to incorporate changes accurately into self-concept. | Helps client recognize and cope with events/alterations and sense of loss of control. |
| **Collaborative** | |
| Refer to classes, e.g., assertiveness training, positive self-image, communication. | Assists with learning skills to promote self-esteem. |

| | |
|---|---|
| **NURSING DIAGNOSIS:** | **FAMILY PROCESSES, ALTERED** |
| **May Be Related To:** | Situational crisis (e.g., change in roles/revelation of sexual deviance/dysfunction). |
| **Possibly Evidenced By:** | Expressions of confusion about what to do/difficulty coping with situation. |
| | Inappropriate boundary maintenance; family does not demonstrate respect for individuality and autonomy of its members. |
| | Family system does not meet emotional/security needs; does not adapt to change or deal with traumatic experience constructively. |
| | Difficulty accepting/receiving help appropriately. |
| **Desired Outcomes/Evaluation Criteria— Family Will:** | Express feelings freely and appropriately. |
| | Demonstrate individual involvement in problem-solving processes directed at appropriate solutions for the situation. |
| | Encourage and allow member who is involved to handle situation in own way, progressing toward independence. |

| ACTIONS/INTERVENTIONS | RATIONALE |
|---|---|
| **Independent** | |
| Determine crisis that has occurred and individual members' perceptions of the situation. | Dysfunction may be perceived as signaling the end of individual's sexual activity. Sexual behavior may have resulted in arrest and be new knowledge to family members. |

| ACTIONS/INTERVENTIONS | RATIONALE |
| --- | --- |

### Independent

| | |
| --- | --- |
| Identify patterns of communication in the family. | Interaction among family members provides information about family dynamics, boundaries, and role expectations and may be indicative of support client may receive. |
| Assess energy direction, whether efforts at resolution/problem-solving are purposeful or scattered. | Indicative of degree of disorganization family is experiencing. |
| Note cultural and/or religious factors. | Strong beliefs about sexual expression and deviance/dysfunction influence acceptance or rejection by individuals involved. |
| Assess support systems available outside the family. | May be needed to help client as well as family members if disorganization is severe. |
| Acknowledge difficulties observed while reinforcing that some degree of conflict is to be expected and can be used to promote growth. | Acceptance of the reality of what is going on helps client and family to feel comfortable/begin to deal with situation. |
| Stress importance of continuous open dialogue between family members. | Promotes understanding of each other's point of view and allows for resolution of misunderstandings/misconceptions. |
| Identify and encourage use of previously successful coping behaviors. | Family has used these in the past and may have neglected them during the stress of current situation. |
| Encourage use of stress-management techniques, e.g., appropriate expression of feelings, relaxation exercises/imagery. | Decreases anxiety and promotes opportunity to problem-solve in calm manner. |

### Collaborative

| | |
| --- | --- |
| Refer to additional resources as indicated, e.g., classes, psychologic counseling, family/multifamily group therapy. | Providing information, opportunity to share feelings/concerns with others can be helpful to positive resolution of problems. |
| (Also refer to CP: Gender Identity, NDs: Family Coping, ineffective: compromised and Family Coping, potential for growth.) | |

# GENDER IDENTITY DISORDERS

## DSM IV
### GENDER IDENTITY DISORDERS
302.6    In Children
302.85  In Adolescents and Adults (specify: attracted to males/females/both/neither)
302.6    Gender Identity Disorder Not Otherwise Specified (Intersex Conditions, Androgen Insensitivity Syndrome, or Congenital Adrenal Hyperplasia and Gender Dysphoria.)
313.82  Identity Problem (specific to sexual orientation and behavior)

## DSM III-R
302.60  Gender Identity Disorder of Childhood
302.50  Transsexualism (specify: asexual, homosexual, heterosexual, unspecified)
302.85  Gender Identity Disorder of Adolescence or Adulthood, Nontranssexual Type (specify asexual, homosexual, heterosexual, unspecified)
302.85  Gender Identity Disorder NOS
313.82  Identity Disorder

Severe distress regarding uncertainty about issues relating to personal identity, in this case sexual orientation and behavior. Consensual homosexuality in adults is not viewed as a mental disturbance and is only a concern when the individual experiences persistent and marked distress about his or her sexual orientation.

In Gender Identity Disorder, strong and persistent cross-gender identification and discomfort with one's sex or a sense of inappropriateness in the gender role of that sex exists, resulting in clinically significant distress/functional impairments, e.g., social, occupational.

## ETIOLOGIC THEORIES

### Psychodynamics

The libido is seen as the force that expresses sexual instinct and develops gradually during the oral stage, focusing on the mouth and lips. The central concern of the anal stage is the anus and the elimination/retention of feces. During the phallic stage, the male is concerned with love of mother, is jealous of father, and has castration anxiety (Oedipus complex). The female has penis envy, loves her father, and rejects her mother (Electra complex). This theory focuses on the biologic inferiority of women because they do not have penises, with subsequent envy of the male.

Developmental theories suggest that sexuality develops throughout life and especially during the formative years. Confusion in relation to one's individual personality and sexual identity affects the ability to be intimate, interfering with sexual development.

### Biologic

Androgen is necessary for masculinization in the fetal male, with the fetus developing as female without the addition of this hormone. When androgenic influences in the fetal hypothalamus are decreased in the male or increased in the female, homosexuality may occur.

Some research sources report that there is a neuroendocrine factor, for example, that the fetus was exposed to large amounts of androgenic hormones or that the mother may have received synthetic hormones at a crucial developmental period, preventing adequate stimulation for neural differentiation.

Current research allows monitoring of normal fetal exposure to testosterone in utero. When subsequent behavior is linked to this information, we will understand more than has been previously available from studies of abnormal exposure of the fetus to high levels of androgen, overdoses due to drugs, or adrenal malfunction. Research continues into the effect of prenatal brain-sexing on homosexual development. We know that lack of male hormone at a crucial state of male fetal development can lead to a feminine brain in a male body. It is clear that, as with other aspects of behavior, sexual orientation is crucially medi- **377** ated by hormonal influences on the developing brain in utero. It is believed that abnormal hormones interact with neurotransmitters, the chemicals that direct the construction of the brain, affecting the sex centers, mating centers, and the so-called gender-role centers, which assume their structure at different times of brain development (Moir & Jessel, 1991).

### Family Dynamics

Role-modeling is believed to play a part in the development of these disorders as well as in the context of a disturbed relationship with one or both parents. Imprinting and classic conditioning are thought by some to affect the development of gender identity.

In males, a symbiotic relationship appears to exist between mother and child. The father is usually absent, ineffectual, or hostile and is perceived as weak and distant, with the mother seen as strong and protective.

In females, the child may not be valued as a girl, or the mother may be absent, depressed, or suffer from other illness, resulting in inadequate mothering. The father may treat the daughter as his little boy, expecting "masculine" behavior.

## CLIENT ASSESSMENT DATABASE

### Ego Integrity

Believes feelings/reactions are typical of other sex.
May report considerable anxiety and depression, attributable to difficulty of living in role of assigned sex.

### Hygiene

Exhibits a persistent marked aversion to wearing sex-appropriate clothing.

### Neurosensory

Moderate to severe coexisting personality disturbance may be noted.
**Mental Status Exam:** Abnormal findings may be indicative of intense distress (e.g., ego-dystonic homosexuality) about general identity or coexisting psychiatric disorders.
Mood and affect may reveal evidence of increased anxiety and depression.

### Safety

History of suicide attempts.

### Sexuality

Higher occurrence in males than females (may be due to narrow study base).
Incongruence between assigned sex and the sense of knowing to which sex one belongs.
May report a persistent and intense distress about his or her assigned sex and the desire to be/insistence that he or she is of the other sex; belief that penis/testes are disgusting/will disappear, individual will not develop breasts/menstruate; or desire medical/surgical intervention to alter sexual characteristics to simulate the other sex.
A preoccupation with stereotypic activities/toys of the opposite sex and/or repudiation of anatomic structures may be noted/reported in childhood.
Sexual responsiveness.

### Social Interactions

May report impairment in social/occupational functioning.

### Teaching/Learning

May present at any age, can be identified in childhood, but most often in late adolescence or early adulthood, although may have a later onset.

## DIAGNOSTIC STUDIES

Psychologic testing to rule out concomitant psychiatric conditions.
Screens for sexually transmitted diseases (STDs) including HIV/AIDS.

## NURSING PRIORITIES

1. Assist client to reduce level of anxiety.
2. Promote sense of self-esteem.
3. Encourage development of social skills/comfort level with own sexual identity/preference.
4. Provide opportunities for client/family to participate in group therapy/other support systems.

## DISCHARGE GOALS

1. Anxiety is reduced/managed effectively.
2. Self-esteem/image is enhanced.
3. Client accepts and is comfortable with identity as established.
4. Client/family are participating in ongoing treatment/support programs.

| NURSING DIAGNOSIS: | ANXIETY [severe] |
|---|---|
| **May Be Related To:** | Ego-dystonic gender identification. |
| | Unconscious conflicts about essential values/beliefs. |
| | Threat to self-concept; unmet needs. |
| **Possibly Evidenced By:** | Increased tension/helplessness (hopelessness). |
| | Feelings of inadequacy, apprehension, uncertainty. |
| | Increased wariness; insomnia. |
| | Focus on self; impaired daily functioning. |
| **Desired Outcomes/Evaluation Criteria— Client Will:** | Verbalize awareness of feelings of anxiety and healthy ways to deal with them. |
| | Appear relaxed and report anxiety is reduced to a manageable level. |
| | Demonstrate problem-solving skills and use resources effectively. |

| ACTIONS/INTERVENTIONS | RATIONALE |
|---|---|
| **Independent** | |
| Assess level of anxiety and degree of interference with daily activities/life. | Necessary information to identify the extent of problem for the individual and plan appropriate interventions. |
| Review drug history (prescription/illicit), familial/physiologic factors, e.g., mental/physical illness, family disorganization. | Drugs may have been used to handle anxious feelings in the past. Other factors contribute to anxiety and may affect individual's ability to handle stress of dealing with own identity problems. |

379

| ACTIONS/INTERVENTIONS | RATIONALE |
|---|---|

### Independent

Assist client to identify feelings, conveying empathy and unconditional positive regard. Encourage free expression of feelings in appropriate ways.

Identification of feelings within a safe, therapeutic environment can help the client begin to explore causes of anxiety and begin to move toward acceptance of self as a worthwhile person.

Acknowledge reality of anxiety/fear. (Do not deny or reassure client that everything will be all right.)

Helps client accept own feeling(s) and learn trust in self. Denial of these feelings contributes to increased anxiety.

Provide accurate information to assist client to clarify reality base, reframe sexuality, and delineate boundaries.

Anxiety may be the result of misinterpretation or lack of knowledge about sexuality/gender identity, and client may fantasize unrealistic ideation.

Accept the client as he or she is.

Lack of acceptance of own self is the basis of much anxiety, and when others project an atmosphere of unacceptance also, anxiety is increased.

Identify things client has done previously when feeling nervous/anxious.

Assists the client to see which previous actions have been helpful and can be used in this situation, increasing sense of control/capability and allaying anxiety.

Assist with developing program of exercise, e.g., brisk walking, aerobic class.

Strenuous activity releases opiate-like endorphins, which create sense of well-being and decrease anxiety.

| NURSING DIAGNOSIS: | ROLE PERFORMANCE, ALTERED/ PERSONAL IDENTITY DISTURBANCE |
|---|---|
| **May Be Related To:** | Crisis in development in which person has difficulty knowing/accepting to which sex he or she belongs or is attracted. |
| | Sense of discomfort and inappropriateness about anatomic sex characteristics. |
| **Possibly Evidenced By:** | Confusion about sense of self, purpose or direction in life, sexual identification/preference. |
| | Verbalization of desire to be/insistence that person is the opposite sex. |
| | Change in self-perception of role. |
| | Conflict in roles. |
| **Desired Outcomes/Evaluation Criteria— Client Will:** | Talk with family/significant other(s) about situation and changes that are occurring/have occured. |
| | Develop realistic plans for adapting to new role/ role changes as appropriate. |
| | Verbalize realistic perception and acceptance of self. |

| ACTIONS/INTERVENTIONS | RATIONALE |
|---|---|
| **Independent** | |
| Identify type of role dysfunction/distress client is expressing, e.g., ego-dystonic heterosexual/homosexual feelings, gender dysphoria. | Lack of self-acceptance and conflicting feelings regarding sexual expression may require therapeutic intervention. Lack of public and religious acceptance, few legal protections for same-sex couples along with lack of role clarity/boundaries can create significant stressors for the client. Note: When the individual views sexual expression/feelings/behavior as adaptive, a healthy attitude exists, and intervention is unnecessary as long as behavior is within legal boundaries. |
| Identify degree of openness client feels about sexual orientation concerns. | Degree to which client previously shared individual situation impacts one's level of concern/comfort and degree of conflict present. The process of sharing or withholding one's situation requires much emotional energy. |
| Role-play sexual disclosure encounters. | Once the decision to disclose is made, open discussion and practice of responses is necessary to the success of disclosure. |
| Provide acceptance of the client as presented. | These clients are sensitive to others' beliefs and will pick up on prejudicial feelings. The client needs to be free to express any views/feelings in order to begin to solve the problems being faced. |
| Determine presence of support systems, e.g., family, social, work. | May feel "different" and isolate self from usual support systems. May be pressured by family/friends to be heterosexual, creating conflict within self. |
| Identify beliefs and values of the individual about hetero/homo/transsexuality. Discuss client's beliefs in detail, providing information as appropriate. | Client may be ignorant of the facts and base fears and ideas on hearsay, prejudice, and religious beliefs. Learning the facts and discussing them with an unbiased person provides an opportunity to make informed decisions. |
| Explore client's feelings about gender identity (transsexuality) and review options for change, e.g., hormonal therapy, psychotherapy, surgical reassignment. | The client who feels strongly that he or she is in the wrong body needs to have complete information about available choices to help him or her begin to accept self and feel comfortable with the decision. Note: Not all transsexuals decide to have surgery. |
| Assist client to develop strategies to cope with threat to identity. | Provides protection and gives client a sense of control to have thought about/decided on actions that can be taken when feeling threatened. |
| Assess response of family/SO. (Refer to NDs: Family Coping, ineffective: compromised; Family Coping, potential for growth.) | May be in shock when first learning of client's concerns and then may either reject or rally to support client. |
| Encourage client to deal with situation in small steps. | Helps client cope with the larger picture when in stress overload. |
| Provide accurate information about threat to and potential consequences for the individual. | Knowledge about gender identity issues helps client assess own situation and make decisions based on fact. |

381

| ACTIONS/INTERVENTIONS | RATIONALE |
|---|---|

### Independent

| | |
|---|---|
| Be aware of one's own biases. Seek assistance/ terminate therapeutic role as appropriate. | Personal values/beliefs and conflicts or biases can negatively impact the therapeutic relationship and effectiveness of interventions. |

### Collaborative

| | |
|---|---|
| Identify available resources/support groups. | Can provide positive role models, opportunity to discuss shared concerns, and facilitate problem-solving. |
| Refer to professionals who are expert in the field of human sexuality and sexual reassignment. | Client needs to be known to the therapist for a period of 3–6 months and demonstrate a sense of discomfort with self and a desire to live in the opposite sex role before a major life-changing decision is finalized. |
| Refer to a therapist expert in the field of sexual reassignment for a second opinion when surgery is contemplated. | Because these procedures are not reversible, the client needs to be sure the correct decision has been made and demonstrate success in living in the opposite role for a period of 1–2 years. |

| NURSING DIAGNOSIS: | SEXUALITY PATTERNS, ALTERED |
|---|---|
| **May Be Related To:** | Ineffective or absent role models. |
| | Conflicts with sexual orientation and/or preferences. |
| | Impaired relationship with a significant other. |
| **Possibly Evidenced By:** | Verbalizations of discomfort with sexual orientation and/or role. |
| | Lack of information about human sexuality. |
| **Desired Outcomes/Evaluation Criteria— Client Will:** | Verbalize understanding of sexuality and acceptance of self. |
| | Demonstrate behaviors directed at lifestyle changes necessary to achieve desired effects. |

| ACTIONS/INTERVENTIONS | RATIONALE |
|---|---|

### Independent

| | |
|---|---|
| Have client describe problem in own terms, noting comments of client/SO that may reveal discounting by overt/covert sexual expressions. | It may be difficult for client to talk about situation/ express feelings, and client may joke, make oblique remarks, or use sarcasm to convey/cover concerns. |
| Take sexual history, including perception of normal function, use of vocabulary, and concerns about sexual identity. | Provides information about level of knowledge about anatomy/physiology of human sexuality and identifies/clarifies concerns to be dealt with by the client/nurse. |

| ACTIONS/INTERVENTIONS | RATIONALE |
|---|---|
| **Independent** | |
| Note cultural and religious/value factors and conflicts that may exist. | Provides opportunity to give information/discuss resources available to client who may believe thoughts and feelings are sinful and feel guilty. |
| Explore knowledge of alternative sexual responses and expressions. | May only have knowledge gained in discussions with friends, from myths, and from misconceptions. |
| Inquire about drug use, including OTC/prescription, illicit, and alcohol. | Drug use can affect sexual functioning. Additionally, client may use substances to dull pain of indecision/anxiety of identity. |
| Provide atmosphere in which discussion of sexual problems is encouraged, promoting free expression of feelings. | Essential to identification and resolution of problems. Client may have concerns about sexual behavior and diseases, such as AIDS. |
| Encourage discussion of possibilities and alternatives for client situation. (Refer to ND: Role Performance, altered/Personal Identity disturbance.) | Full range of discussion can assist the client in reaching a decision about the identity that is comfortable and the course to pursue. |
| Review hormonal therapy as indicated. | Transsexuals who elect to undergo surgical reassignment, as well as others who for economic or other reasons choose to live in the transsexual role, usually receive long-term, high-dose estrogen or testosterone therapy. The client needs to understand the implications before making the decision to pursue this course of therapy. |
| **Collaborative** | |
| Refer to resources as indicated, e.g., homosexual/lesbian support group; Homosexuals Anonymous Fellowship; LAMBDA, AA, Gay and Lesbian; Common Bond; gender identity clinics. | Information from these groups can help client reach a decision about sexual preference and/or provide support once decision has been made. HAF is a Christian-based group that directs efforts to assisting the client toward a decision to become heterosexual. Other organizations are reference groups that provide information/support. |

| NURSING DIAGNOSIS: | FAMILY COPING, ineffective: compromised |
|---|---|
| **May Be Related To:** | Inadequate/incorrect information or understanding. |
| | Temporary preoccupation by a significant person who is trying to manage emotional conflicts and personal suffering and is unable to perceive or to act effectively in regard to client's needs. |
| | Temporary family disorganization and role changes. |
| | Client providing little support in turn for the primary person. |

383

| | |
|---|---|
| **Possibly Evidenced By:** | Client expresses/confirms a concern or complaint about family/SO(s) response to client's gender/sexual concerns. |
| | SO describes preoccupation with own personal reactions to client's situation. |
| | Family attempts supportive behaviors with less than satisfactory results/withdraw support when needed. |
| **Desired Outcomes/Evaluation Criteria—Family Will:** | Identify resources within itself to deal with situation. |
| | Interact appropriately with client and staff, providing support and assistance as indicated. |

| ACTIONS/INTERVENTIONS | RATIONALE |
|---|---|
| **Independent** | |
| Determine individual situation and identify factors that may contribute to difficulty family is having in providing needed assistance/support for the client. | Individuals may have problems of their own that interfere with ability to extend themselves to the client. Problems of prejudice, myth/misinformation, values may also cause separation between family members. |
| Note behaviors of family members, e.g., withdrawn, rejecting, supportive, willing to learn. (Refer to ND: Family Coping, potential for growth.) | Identifies individual needs and steps to be taken to resolve family disorganization/assist the family in moving toward growth. |
| Discuss underlying reasons/behaviors client is expressing/exhibiting. | Helps family understand and accept the person as having different values. |
| Encourage each individual to be responsible for own self, not taking on the problem(s) of others. | The concept of "who owns the problem" can help clarify issues of who has responsibility for solution of specific problems. |
| Encourage free expression of feelings and ideas about homosexuality/gender identity issues. | Promotes an atmosphere in which individual can reveal feelings of self-blame, revulsion, confusion, and anger, or blaming of other(s). Once these have been expressed, members can move on to resolution. |
| Provide information as appropriate. | Because much of the problem may center around lack of knowledge, information can help individuals make informed decisions/choices about what is happening. |
| Discuss options for individuals in regard to client's decision about sexual partner, gender identity/ surgical reassignment, e.g., separation/divorce for spouses, resolution of parent/child issues. | Family members may have difficulty accepting client's alternate sexual expression/sexual reassignment. Individual needs to make decision about willingness to accept other person in altered role. Children of transsexuals have questions such as "Who am I, as the daughter of a father who is now a woman?" |
| Provide time to talk with family to discuss views/ concerns about situation, feelings toward client's sexual partner. | Opportunity to ventilate feelings, ask questions, and express ideas helps resolve problems. |

384

| ACTIONS/INTERVENTIONS | RATIONALE |
|---|---|

### Independent

Assist members to develop effective communication skills, e.g., Active-listening, I-messages, problem-solving process. Provide role model with which the family may identify. Include SO as appropriate.

Helpful in dealing with current situation as well as providing skills that will assist with resolution of future problems. Role-modeling shows individuals that the skills can be helpful to them. Including partner provides opportunity for resolution of conflict, incorporation into family.

### Collaborative

Identify/refer to support groups/classes that deal with similar problems, e.g., Parents/Friends of Lesbians and Gays (PFLAG), gender identity clinics.

Talking with others who have been through similar experiences can provide opportunity for members to learn/accept client.

Refer for marriage counseling as appropriate.

May be needed to help couple decide whether separation or divorce is in the best interests of each person, or whether they want to work out their problems and stay together.

| NURSING DIAGNOSIS: | FAMILY COPING, POTENTIAL FOR GROWTH |
|---|---|
| **May Be Related To:** | Individual's basic needs are sufficiently gratified and adaptive tasks effectively addressed to enable goals of self-actualization to surface. |
| **Possibly Evidenced By:** | Family members attempt to describe growth impact of crisis on their own values, priorities, goals, or relationships. |
| | Family members are moving in direction of health-promoting and enriching lifestyle that supports client's search for self. |
| | Family members choosing experiences that optimize wellness. |
| **Desired Outcomes/Evaluation Criteria— Family Will:** | Express willingness to look at its own role in family's growth. |
| | Verbalize knowledge and understanding of client's gender choice. |
| | Express desire to undertake tasks leading to change. |

| ACTIONS/INTERVENTIONS | RATIONALE |
|---|---|

### Independent

Listen to family's expressions of hope, planning, and effect on relationships/life.

Provides clues to opportunities that exist to help family move toward growth and positive relationships. When family members are doing this, client is free to move toward a positive resolution of own life.

385

| ACTIONS/INTERVENTIONS | RATIONALE |
|---|---|

### Independent

Help the family in supporting the client in meeting own needs/making own decision.

Significant other(s) may not have skills/knowhow to give support even when desired, and giving information and providing support enables them to learn.

Note expressions of change of values, e.g., "He/she is still my son/daughter even though homosexual/lesbian or contemplating sex-change surgery."

Indicators of beginning of acceptance of the situation as it is and willingness to learn and support child.

Provide a role model with which the family may identify.

Modeling of accepting behaviors/communication skills enables family members to learn new ways of interacting with the client.

Discuss importance of open communication and harm secretive behavior produces.

Open communication allows all participants to have access to all information, enhancing resolution of problems/understanding of what is happening.

Encourage open discussions of concerns about lifestyle changes, fear of AIDS, and other sexually transmitted diseases.

Individuals may have unexpressed fears, and this provides the opportunity to ask questions and get accurate answers.

Provide experiences for the family, e.g., involvement with other families facing similar decisions.

Helps them learn ways of assisting/supporting client.

### Collaborative

Refer to community resources, e.g., same-gender, transsexual groups.

Provides ongoing support as client/family make necessary lifestyle changes, go on with their lives.

# CHAPTER 13

# EATING DISORDERS

## ANOREXIA NERVOSA/BULIMIA NERVOSA

### DSM IV
307.1   Anorexia Nervosa
307.51 Bulimia Nervosa
307.50 Eating Disorder NOS

### DSM III-R
307.10 Anorexia Nervosa
307.51 Bulimia Nervosa

Anorexia nervosa is an illness of starvation, brought on by severe disturbance of body image and a morbid fear of obesity. Presently, there is no strong evidence of heredity.

Bulimia (binge-purge syndrome) is characterized by extreme overeating, followed by self-induced vomiting; may include abuse of laxatives and diuretics.

### ETIOLOGIC THEORIES
### Psychodynamics

The individual reflects a developmental arrest in the very early childhood years. The tasks of trust, autonomy, and separation-individuation are unfulfilled, and the individual remains in the dependent position. Ego development is retarded. Symptoms are often associated with a perceived loss of control in some aspect of life.

### Biologic

It is suggested that the cause of these disorders may arise out of neuroendocrine abnormalities within the hypothalamus. Symptoms are linked to various chemical disturbances normally regulated by the hypothalamus.

### Family Dynamics

Issues of control become the overriding factors in the family of the patient with an eating disorder. These families often consist of a passive father, a domineering mother, and an overly dependent child. There is a high value placed on perfectionism in this family, and the child believes he or she must satisfy these standards.

### CLIENT ASSESSMENT DATABASE
### Activity/Rest

Disturbed sleep patterns, e.g., early morning insomnia; fatigue.

Feeling "hyper" and/or anxious; increased activity/avid exerciser, participation in high-energy sports.

## Circulation

Feels cold even when room is warm.
Low BP; tachycardia, bradycardia, dysrhythmias.

## Ego Integrity

Powerlessness/helplessness, lack of control over eating, e.g., cannot stop eating/control what or how much is eaten (Bulimia).
Distorted (unrealistic) body image—reports self as fat regardless of weight and sees thin body as fat; persistent overconcern with body shape and weight, fears gaining weight.
Stress factors, e.g., family move, onset of puberty.
High self-expectations.
Suppression of anger; emotional states of depression, withdrawal, anger, anxiety, pessimistic outlook.

## Elimination

Diarrhea/constipation.
Decreased frequency of voiding/urine output, urine dark amber (dehydration).
Vague abdominal pain and distress, bloating.
Laxative/diuretic use.

## Food/Fluid

Constant hunger or denial of hunger; normal or exaggerated appetite that rarely vanishes until late in the disorder (Anorexia).
Intense fear of gaining weight; may have prior history of being overweight.
Inordinate pleasure in weight loss, while denying self pleasure in other areas; refusal to maintain body weight over minimal norm for age/height (Anorexia).
Recurrent episodes of binge eating; minimum average of 2 binge eating episodes a week for at least 3 months (Bulimina).
Regularly engages in either self-induced vomiting (binge-purge syndrome [bulimia]) independently or as a complication of anorexia) or strict dieting or fasting; excessive gum chewing.
Weight loss/maintenance of body weight 15% or more below that expected (anorexia) or weight may be normal or slightly below (bulimia).
Cachectic appearance; skin may be dry, yellowish/pale, with poor turgor.
Preoccupation with food, e.g., calorie counting, gourmet cooking; hiding food, cutting food into small pieces, rearranging food on plate.
Peripheral edema.
Swollen salivary glands; sore, inflamed buccal cavity, erosion of tooth enamel; gums in poor condition; continuous sore throat (Bulimia).
Vomiting, bloody vomitus (may indicate esophageal tearing, Mallory-Weiss).

## Hygiene

Increased hair growth on body (lanugo); hair loss (axillary/pubic).
Hair dull/not shiny.
Brittle nails.

## Neurosensory

Appropriate affect, except in regard to body and eating, or depressive affect (depression).
Mental changes: apathy, confusion, memory impairment (brought on by malnutrition/starvation).

Hysterical or obsessive personality style; no other psychiatric illness or evidence of a psychiatric thought disorder present (although a significant number may show evidence of an affective disorder).

## Pain/Discomfort

Headaches, sore throat.

## Safety

Decreased body temperature.
Recurrent infectious processes (indicative of depressed immune system).
Eczema/other skin problems.

## Sexuality

History of sexual abuse, promiscuity.
Absence of at least 3 consecutive menstrual cycles.
Denial/loss of sexual interest.
Breast atrophy, amenorrhea.

## Social Interactions

Middle-class or upper-class family background.
Passive father/dominant mother, family members enmeshed, togetherness prized, personal boundaries not respected.
History of being a quiet, cooperative child.
Problems of control issues in relationships, engagement in power struggles; withdrawal from friends/social contacts.
Sense of helplessness.
May have history of legal difficulties, e.g., shoplifting.

## Teaching/Learning

Family history of higher than normal incidence of depression.
Onset of the illness usually between the ages of 10 and 22.
Health beliefs/practices, e.g., certain foods have "too many" calories, use of "health" foods.
High academic achievement.

## DIAGNOSTIC STUDIES

**CBC with Differential:** Determines presence of anemia, leukopenia, lymphocytosis. Blood platelets show significantly less than normal activity by the enzyme monoamine oxidase (thought to be a marker for depression).
**Electrolytes:** Imbalances may include decreased potassium, sodium, and chloride.
**Endocrine Studies:**
**Thyroid Function:** Thyroxine ($T_4$) levels usually normal; however, circulating triiodothyronine ($T_3$) levels may be low.
**Pituitary Function:** Thyroid stimulating hormone (TSH) response to thyrotropin releasing factor (TRF) is abnormal in anorexia nervosa. Propranolol-glucagon stimulation test (studies the response of human growth hormone) reveals depressed level of GH in anorexia nervosa. Gonadotropic hypofunction is noted.
**Cortisol:** Metabolism may be elevated.
**Dexamethasone Suppression Test (DST):** (Evaluates hypothalamic-pituitary function) dexamethasone resistance indicates cortisol suppression, suggesting malnutrition/depression.
**Luteinizing Hormone Secretions Test:** Pattern often resembles those of prepubertal girls.
**Estrogen:** Decreased.

**Blood Sugar and Basal Metabolism (BMR):** May be low.

**Other Chemistries:** AST (SGOT) elevated. Hypercarotenemia, hypoproteinemia, hypocholesterolemia.

**MHP 6 Levels:** Decreased, suggestive of malnutrition/depression.

**Urinalysis and Renal Function:** BUN may be elevated; ketones present reflecting starvation; decreased urinary 17-ketosteroids; increased specific gravity (dehydration).

**EKG:** Abnormal with low voltage, T-wave inversion, dysrhythmias.

**Magnesium Level:** Decreased, indicative of inadequate nutritional intake.

## NURSING PRIORITIES

1. Reestablish adequate/appropriate nutritional intake.
2. Correct fluid and electrolyte imbalance.
3. Assist client to develop realistic body image/improve self-esteem.
4. Provide support/involve SO, if available, in treatment program.
5. Coordinate total treatment program with other disciplines.
6. Provide information about disease, prognosis, and treatment.

## DISCHARGE GOALS

1. Adequate nutrition and fluid intake maintained.
2. Maladaptive coping behaviors and stressors that precipitate anxiety recognized.
3. Adaptive coping strategies and techniques for anxiety reduction and self-control implemented.
4. Self-esteem increased.
5. Disease process, prognosis, and treatment regimen understood.

| NURSING DIAGNOSIS: | NUTRITION, ALTERED, LESS THAN BODY REQUIREMENTS |
|---|---|
| **May Be Related To:** | Inadequate food intake; self-induced vomiting. |
| | Chronic/excessive laxative use. |
| **Possibly Evidenced By:** | Body weight 15% (or more) below expected (anorexia), or may be within normal range (bulimia). |
| | Pale conjunctiva and mucous membranes; poor skin turgor/muscle tone. |
| | Excessive loss of hair; increased growth of hair on body (lanugo). |
| | Amenorrhea. |
| | Bradycardia, cardiac irregularities, hypotension, edema, hypothermia. |
| | Electrolyte imbalances. |
| **Desired Outcomes/Evaluation Criteria—Client Will:** | Verbalize understanding of nutritional needs. |
| | Establish a dietary pattern with caloric intake adequate to regain/maintain appropriate weight. |
| | Demonstrate weight gain toward expected range. |

| ACTIONS/INTERVENTIONS | RATIONALE |
| --- | --- |

### Independent

Establish a minimum weight goal and daily nutritional requirements.

Malnutrition is a mood-altering condition leading to depression and agitation and affecting cognitive functioning/decision-making. Improved nutritional status enhances thinking ability, and psychologic work can begin.

Use a consistent approach. Sit with client while eating; present and remove food without persuasion and/or comment. Promote pleasant environment and record intake.

Client detects urgency and reacts to pressure. Any comment that might be seen as coercion provides focus on food. When the staff responds in a consistent manner, client can begin to trust their responses. The single area in which the client has exercised power and control is food/eating, and she or he may experience guilt or rebellion if forced to eat. Structuring meals and decreasing discussions about food will decrease power struggles with client and avoid manipulative games.

Provide smaller meals and supplemental snacks as appropriate.

Gastric dilation may occur if refeeding is too rapid following a period of starvation dieting. Note: Client may feel bloated for 3 to 6 weeks while body readjusts to food intake.

Make selective menu available and allow client to control choices, as much as possible.

Client who gains confidence in self and feels in control of environment is more likely to eat preferred foods.

Provide diet and snacks with substitutions of preferred foods when available.

Having a variety of foods available will enable the client to have a choice of potentially enjoyable foods.

Be alert to choices of low-calorie foods/beverages; hoarding food; disposing of food in various places such as pockets or wastebaskets.

Client will try to avoid taking in what is viewed as excessive calories and may go to great lengths to avoid eating.

Maintain a regular weighing schedule, such as M-W-F before breakfast in same attire, and graph results.

Provides accurate ongoing record of weight loss and/or gain. Also diminishes obsessing about gains and/or losses.

Weigh with back to scale (dependent on program protocols.)

Although some programs prefer client to see the results of weighing, this can force the issue of trust in client who usually does not trust others.

Avoid room checks and other control devices whenever possible.

External control reinforces feelings of powerlessness and are usually not helpful.

Provide 1:1 supervision and have the client with bulimia remain in the dayroom area with no bathroom privileges for a specified period (e.g., 2 hours) following eating, if contracting is unsuccessful.

Prevents vomiting during/after eating. Client may desire food and use a binge-purge syndrome to maintain weight. Note: Purging may occur for the first time in a client as a response to establishment of weight gain program.

Monitor exercise program and set limits on physical activities. Chart activity/level of work (pacing, etc.)

Moderate exercise helps in maintaining muscle tone/weight and combating depression. However, client may exercise excessively to burn calories.

| ACTIONS/INTERVENTIONS | RATIONALE |
|---|---|

### Independent

| | |
|---|---|
| Maintain matter-of-fact, nonjudgmental attitude if giving tube feedings, hyperalimentation, etc. | Perception of punishment is counterproductive to promoting self-confidence and faith in own ability to control destiny. |
| Be alert to possibility of client disconnecting tube and emptying hyperalimentation if used. Check fluid measurements and tape tubing snugly. | Sabotage behavior is common in attempt to prevent weight gain. |

### Collaborative

| | |
|---|---|
| Involve client with team in setting up/carrying out program of behavior modification. Provide reward for weight gain as individually determined; ignore loss. | Provides structured eating situation while allowing client some control in choices. Behavior modification may be effective only in mild cases or for short-term weight gain. |
| Administer liquid diet, tube feedings/hyperalimentation as appropriate. | When caloric intake is insufficient to sustain metabolic needs, nutritional support can be used to prevent malnutrition/death while therapy is continuing. High-caloric liquid feedings may be given as medication, at preset times separate from meals, as an alternate means of increasing caloric intake. |
| Blenderize and tube feed anything left on the tray after a given period of time if indicated. | May be used as part of behavior modification program to provide total intake of needed calories. |
| Avoid giving laxatives. | Use is counterproductive, as they may be used by client to rid body of food/calories. Note: Metamucil/bran may be used to treat constipation. |
| Monitor laboratory values, as appropriate. | Identifies therapeutic needs/effectiveness of treatment. |
| Administer medications as indicated, e.g.: cyproheptadine (Periactin); | A serotonin and histamine antagonist used in high doses to stimulate the appetite, decrease preoccupation with food, and combat depression. Does not appear to have serious side effects, although decreased mental alertness may occur. |
| tricyclic antidepressants, e.g., amitriptyline (Elavil, Endep); | Lifts depression and stimulates appetite. |
| antianxiety agents, e.g., alprazolam (Xanax); | Reduces tension, anxiety/nervousness and may help client to participate in treatment. |
| major tranquilizers, e.g., chlorpromazine (Thorazine). | Promotes weight gain and cooperation with psychotherapeutic program. Major tranquilizers are used only when absolutely necessary because of extrapyramidal side effects. |
| Prepare for/assist with electroconvulsive therapy (ECT) if indicated. Discuss reasons for use and help client understand this is not punishment. | In rare and difficult cases in which malnutrition is severe and may be life-threatening, a short-term ECT series may enable the client to begin eating and become accessible to psychotherapy. Client may not understand and may fear use of electricity, believing it will be painful. |

| ACTIONS/INTERVENTIONS | RATIONALE |
|---|---|
| **Collaborative** | |
| Transfer to medical setting for nutritional therapy, as indicated. | Cure of the underlying problem cannot happen without improved nutritional status. Hospitalization provides a controlled environment in which food intake, vomiting/elimination, medications, and activities can be monitored. It also separates the client from SO(s) (who may be contributing factor) and provides exposure to others with the same problem, creating an atmosphere for sharing. |

| NURSING DIAGNOSIS: | **FLUID VOLUME DEFICIT, HIGH RISK FOR OR ACTUAL** |
|---|---|
| **May Be Related To:** | Inadequate intake of food and liquids. |
| | Consistent self-induced vomiting. |
| | Chronic/excessive laxative/diuretic use. |
| **Possibly Evidenced By (Actual):** | Dry skin and mucous membranes, decreased skin turgor. |
| | Increased pulse rate, body temperature; hypotension. |
| | Output greater than input (diuretic use); concentrated urine/decreased urine output (dehydration). |
| | Weakness. |
| | Change in mental state. |
| | Hemoconcentration, altered electrolyte balance. |
| **Desired Outcomes/Evaluation Criteria— Client Will:** | Maintain/demonstrate improved fluid balance as evidenced by adequate urine output, stable vital signs, moist mucous membranes, good skin turgor. |
| | Verbalize understanding of causative factors and behaviors necessary to correct fluid deficit. |

| ACTIONS/INTERVENTIONS | RATIONALE |
|---|---|
| **Independent** | |
| Monitor vital signs, capillary refill, status of mucous membranes, skin turgor. | Indicators of adequacy of circulating volume. Orthostatic hypotension may occur with risk of falls/injury following sudden changes in position. |
| Monitor amount and types of fluid intake. Measure urine output accurately. | Client may abstain from all intake, resulting in dehydration, or may substitute fluids for caloric intake, impacting electrolyte balance. |
| Discuss strategies to stop vomiting and laxative/diuretic use. | Helping the client deal with the feelings that lead to vomiting and/or laxative/diuretic use may prevent continued fluid loss. Note: The client with bulimia has learned that vomiting provides a release of anxiety. |

393

| ACTIONS/INTERVENTIONS | RATIONALE |
|---|---|

### Independent

Identify actions necessary to regain/maintain optimal fluid balance, e.g., specific schedule of fluid intake.

Involving client in plan to correct fluid imbalances improves chances for success.

### Collaborative

Review results of electrolyte/renal function test results.

Fluid/electrolyte shifts/decreased renal function can adversely affect client's recovery/prognosis and may require additional intervention.

Administer/monitor IV, hyperalimentation;

Used as an emergency measure to correct fluid/electrolyte imbalance.

potassium supplements, oral or IV, as indicated.

May be required to prevent cardiac dysrhythmias.

---

| NURSING DIAGNOSIS: | THOUGHT PROCESSES, ALTERED |
|---|---|
| **May Be Related To:** | Severe malnutrition/electrolyte imbalance. |
| | Psychologic conflicts, e.g., sense of low self-worth, perceived lack of control. |
| **Possibly Evidenced By:** | Impaired ability to make decisions, problem-solve. |
| | Non–reality based verbalizations. |
| | Ideas of reference. |
| | Altered sleep patterns, e.g., may go to bed late (stay up to binge/purge) and get up early; fatigue. |
| | Altered attention span/distractibility. |
| | Perceptual disturbances with failure to recognize hunger; anxiety and depression. |
| **Desired Outcomes/Evaluation Criteria— Client Will:** | Verbalize understanding of causative factors and awareness of impairment. |
| | Demonstrate behaviors to change/prevent malnutrition. |
| | Display improved ability to make decisions, problem-solve |

---

| ACTIONS/INTERVENTIONS | RATIONALE |
|---|---|

### Independent

Be aware of client's distorted thinking ability.

Allows the caregiver to have more realistic expectations of the client and provide appropriate information and support.

Listen to and do not challenge irrational, illogical thinking. Present reality concisely and briefly.

It is not possible to respond logically when thinking ability is physiologically impaired. The client needs to hear reality, but challenging leads to distrust and frustration.

Adhere strictly to nutrition regimen.

Improved nutrition is essential to improved brain functioning. (Refer to ND: Nutrition, altered, less than body requirements.)

| ACTIONS/INTERVENTIONS | RATIONALE |
|---|---|

### Collaborative

Review electrolyte/renal function tests.

Imbalances negatively affect cerebral functioning and may require correction before therapeutic interventions can begin.

| **NURSING DIAGNOSIS:** | **BODY IMAGE DISTURBANCE/SELF-ESTEEM, CHRONIC LOW** |
|---|---|
| **May Be Related To:** | Morbid fear of obesity. |
| | Perceived loss of control in some aspect of life. |
| | Unmet dependency needs, personal vulnerability. |
| | Continued negative evaluation of self. |
| | Dysfunctional family system. |
| **Possibly Evidenced By:** | Distorted body image (views self as fat even in the presence of normal body weight or severe emaciation). |
| | Expresses little concern, uses denial as a defense mechanism, and feels powerless to prevent/make changes. |
| | Expresses shame/guilt. |
| | Overly conforming, dependent on others' opinions. |
| **Desired Outcomes/Evaluation Criteria— Client Will:** | Establish a more realistic body image. |
| | Acknowledge self as an individual. |
| | Accept responsibility for own actions. |

| ACTIONS/INTERVENTIONS | RATIONALE |
|---|---|

### Independent

Establish a therapeutic nurse/client relationship.

Within a helping relationship, client can begin to trust and try out new thinking and behaviors.

Promote self-concept without moral judgment.

Client sees self as weak-willed, even though part of person may feel a sense of power and control (e.g., dieting/weight loss).

Have client draw picture of self.

Provides opportunity to discuss client's perception of self/body image and realities of individual situation.

State rules clearly regarding weighing schedule, remaining in sight during medication and eating times, and consequences of not following the rules. Without undue comment, be consistent in carrying out rules.

Consistency is important in establishing trust. As part of the behavior-modification program, client knows risks involved in not following established rules (e.g., decrease in privileges). Failure to do so is viewed as the client's choice and accepted by the staff in matter-of-fact manner so as not to provide reinforcement for the undesirable behavior.

395

| ACTIONS/INTERVENTIONS | RATIONALE |
|---|---|

### Independent

Respond (confront) with reality when client makes unrealistic statements such as "I'm gaining weight, so there's nothing really wrong with me."

Client may be denying the psychologic aspects of own situation and is often expressing a sense of inadequacy and depression.

Be aware of own reaction to client's behavior. Avoid arguing.

Feelings of disgust, hostility, and infuriation are not uncommon when caring for these clients. Prognosis often remains poor even with a gain in weight, because other problems may remain. Many clients continue to see themselves as fat, and there is also a high incidence of affective disorders, social phobias, obsessive-compulsive symptoms, drug abuse, and psychosexual dysfunction. Nurse needs to deal with own response/feelings so they do not interfere with care of the client.

Assist the client to assume control in areas other than dieting/weight loss, e.g., management of own daily activities, work/leisure choices.

Feelings of personal ineffectiveness, low self-esteem, and perfectionism are often part of the problem. Client feels helpless to change and requires assistance to problem-solve methods of control in life situations.

Help client formulate goals for self (not related to eating) and create a manageable plan to reach those goals, a single goal at a time, progressing from simple to more complex.

Client needs to recognize ability to control other areas in life and may need to learn problem-solving skills in order to achieve this control. Setting realistic goals fosters success.

Assist client to confront sexual fears. Provide sex education as necessary.

Major physical/psychologic changes in adolescence can contribute to development of this problem. Feelings of powerlessness and loss of control of feelings (in particular sexual) and sensations lead to an unconscious desire to desexualize themselves. Clients often believe that these fears can be overcome by taking control of bodily appearance/development/function.

Determine history of sexual abuse and institute appropriate therapy.

Client may use eating as a means of gaining control in life when sexual abuse has been experienced.

Note client's withdrawal from and/or discomfort in social settings.

May indicate feelings of isolation and fear of rejection/judgment by others. Avoidance of social situations and contact with others can compound feelings of worthlessness.

Encourage client to take charge of own life in a more healthful way by making own decisions and accepting self as is at this moment (including inadequacies and strengths).

Client often does not know what she or he may want for self. Parents (mother) usually make decisions for client. Client may also believe she or he has to be the best in everything and hold self responsible for being perfect.

Let client know that it is acceptable to be different from family, particularly mother.

Developing a sense of identity as separate from family and maintaining sense of control in other ways, besides dieting and weight loss, is a desirable goal of therapy/program.

| ACTIONS/INTERVENTIONS | RATIONALE |
|---|---|

### Independent

Involve in personal development program, preferably in a group setting. Provide information about proper application of makeup and grooming.

Learning about methods of enhancing personal appearance may be helpful to long-range sense of self-esteem/image. Feedback from others can promote feelings of self-worth.

Suggest disposing of "thin" clothes as weight gain occurs. Recommend consultation with an image consultant.

Provides incentive to at least maintain and not lose weight. Removes visual reminder of thinner self. Positive image enhances sense of self-esteem.

Use interpersonal psychotherapy approach rather than interpretive therapy.

Interaction between persons is more helpful for the client to discover feelings/impulses/needs from within own self. Client has not learned this internal control as a child and may not be able to interpret/attach meaning to behavior.

Encourage client to express anger and acknowledge when it is verbalized.

Important to know that anger is part of self and as such is acceptable. Expressing anger may need to be taught to client, because anger is often considered unacceptable in the family, and therefore client does not express it.

Assist client to learn strategies other than eating for dealing with feelings. Have client keep a diary of feelings, particularly when thinking about food.

Feelings are the underlying issue, and clients often use food instead of dealing with feelings appropriately. Client needs to learn to recognize feelings and how to express them clearly and directly.

Assess feelings of helplessness/hopelessness.

Lack of control is a common/underlying problem for this client and may be accompanied by more serious emotional disorders. Note: 54% of clients with anorexia have a history of major affective disorder, and 33% have a history of minor affective disorder.

Be alert to suicidal ideation/behavior.

Intensity of anxiety/panic about weight gain, depression, hopeless feelings may lead to suicidal attempts, particularly if client is impulsive.

### Collaborative

Involve in group therapy.

Provides an opportunity to talk about feelings and try out new behaviors.

Refer to occupational/recreational therapy.

Can develop interests and skills to fill time that has been occupied by obsession with eating. Involvement in recreational activities encourages social interactions with others and promotes fun and relaxation.

Refer to therapist trained in dealing with sexuality.

May need professional assistance to accept self as a sexual adult.

---

**NURSING DIAGNOSIS:**

**May Be Related To:**

**FAMILY PROCESSES, ALTERED**

Issues of control in family.

Situational/maturational crises.

| | |
|---|---|
| **Possibly Evidenced By:** | History of inadequate coping methods. |
| | Dissonance among family members; family needs not being met. |
| | Family developmental tasks not being met; ill-defined family rules, functions, and roles. |
| | Focus on identified patient (IP); family member(s) acting as enablers for IP. |
| **Desired Outcomes/Evaluation Criteria— Family Will:** | Express feelings freely and appropriately. |
| | Demonstrate more autonomous coping behaviors with individual family boundaries more clearly defined. |
| | Demonstrate individual involvement in problem-solving processes directed at encouraging client toward independence. |
| | Recognize and resolve conflict appropriately with the individuals involved. |

| ACTIONS/INTERVENTIONS | RATIONALE |
|---|---|
| **Independent** | |
| Identify patterns of interaction. Encourage each family member to speak for self. Do not allow 2 members to discuss a third without that member's participation. | Helpful information for planning interventions. The enmeshed, overinvolved family members often speak for each other and need to learn to be responsible for their own words and actions. |
| Discourage members from asking for approval from each other. Be alert to verbal or nonverbal checking with others for approval. Acknowledge competent actions of client. | Each individual needs to develop own internal sense of self-esteem. Individual often is living up to others' (family's) expectations rather than making own choices. Acknowledgment provides recognition of self in positive ways. |
| Listen with regard when the client speaks. | Sets an example and provides a sense of competence and self-worth in that the client has been heard and attended to. |
| Encourage individuals not to answer to everything. Communicate message of separation, that it is acceptable for family members to be different from each other. | Reinforces individualization and return to privacy. Individuation needs reinforcement. Such a message confronts rigidity and opens options for different behaviors. |
| Encourage and allow expression of feelings (e.g., crying, anger) by individuals. | Often these families have not allowed free expression of feelings and will need help and permission to learn and accept this. |
| Prevent intrusion in dyads by other members of family. | Inappropriate interventions in family subsystems prevent individuals from working out problems successfully. |
| Reinforce importance of parents as a couple who have rights of their own. | The focus on the child with anorexia is very intense and often is the only area around which the couple interact. The couple needs to explore their own relationship and restore the balance within it in order to prevent its disintegration. |

| ACTIONS/INTERVENTIONS | RATIONALE |
|---|---|

### Independent

Prevent client from intervening in conflicts between parents. Assist parents in identifying and solving their marital differences.

Triangulation occurs in which a parent-child coalition exists. Sometimes the child is openly pressed to ally with 1 parent against the other. The symptom (anorexia) is the regulator in the family system, and the parents deny their own conflicts.

Be aware of and confront sabotage behavior on the part of family members.

Feelings of blame, shame, and helplessness may lead to unconscious behavior designed to maintain the status quo.

### Collaborative

Refer to community resources, such as family group therapy, parents' groups, as indicated; Parent Effectiveness classes.

May help reduce overprotectiveness, support/facilitate the process of dealing with unresolved conflicts and change.

| NURSING DIAGNOSIS: | SKIN INTEGRITY, IMPAIRED, HIGH RISK FOR OR ACTUAL |
|---|---|
| May Be Related To: | Altered nutritional state; edema. |
| | Dehydration/cachectic changes (skeletal prominence). |
| Possibly Evidenced By (Actual): | Dry/scaly skin with poor skin turgor; tissue fragility. |
| | Brittle/dry hair. |
| | Dry rash, reports of itching, dermal abrasions (from scratching). |
| Desired Outcomes/Evaluation Criteria— Client Will: | Verbalize understanding of causative factors and relief of itching. |
| | Identify and demonstrate behaviors to maintain soft, supple, intact skin. |

| ACTIONS/INTERVENTIONS | RATIONALE |
|---|---|

### Independent

Observe for reddened, blanched, excoriated areas.

Indicators of increased risk of breakdown requiring more intense treatment.

Encourage bathing every other day instead of daily.

Frequent baths contribute to dryness of the skin.

Use skin cream twice a day and after bathing.

Lubricates skin and decreases itching.

Massage skin, especially over bony prominences.

Improves circulation to the skin, enhances skin tone.

Discuss importance of frequent change of position, need for remaining active.

Enhances circulation and perfusion to skin by preventing prolonged pressure on tissues.

Stress importance of adequate nutrition/fluid intake. (Refer to ND: Nutrition, altered, less than body requirements.)

Improved nutrition and hydration will improve skin condition.

399

| NURSING DIAGNOSIS: | KNOWLEDGE DEFICIT (LEARNING NEED) regarding condition, prognosis, and treatment needs |
|---|---|
| May Be Related To: | Lack of exposure to/unfamiliarity with information resources; misinterpretation; lack of interest in learning. |
| Possibly Evidenced By: | Inappropriate behaviors, e.g., apathy. |
| | Inaccurate follow-through of instructions. |
| | Verbalization of misconception/need for information. |
| Desired Outcomes/Evaluation Criteria— Client Will: | Identify relationship of signs/symptoms (e.g., weight loss, tooth decay) to behaviors of not eating/binge-purging. |
| | Verbalize awareness of and plan for lifestyle changes to maintain individual goals for wellness. |
| | Seek out sources/resources to assist with making identified changes. |
| | Assume responsibility for own learning. |

| ACTIONS/INTERVENTIONS | RATIONALE |
|---|---|
| **Independent** | |
| Determine level of knowledge and readiness to learn. | Learning is easier when it begins where the learner is. |
| Note blocks to learning, e.g., physical/intellectual/ emotional. | Malnutrition, family problems, drug abuse, affective disorders, obsessive-compulsive symptoms can interfere with learning, requiring resolution before effective learning can occur. |
| Review dietary needs, answering questions as indicated. Encourage inclusion of high-fiber foods and adequate fluid intake. (Refer to ND: Nutrition, altered, less than body requirements.) | Client/family may need assistance with planning for new way of eating. As constipation may occur when laxative use is curtailed, dietary considerations may prevent need for more aggressive therapy. |
| Provide information and encourage the use of relaxation and other stress-management techniques, e.g., visualization, guided imagery, biofeedback. | New ways of coping with feelings of anxiety and fear will help client to manage these feelings in more effective ways, assisting in giving up maladaptive behaviors of not eating/binging-purging. |
| Assist with establishing a sensible exercise program. Caution regarding overexercise. | Exercise can assist with developing a positive body image and combats depression (release of endorphins in the brain enhances sense of well-being). Client may use excessive exercise as a way of controlling weight. |
| Provide written information for client/SO(s). | Helpful as reminder of and reinforcement for learning. |

| ACTIONS/INTERVENTIONS | RATIONALE |
| --- | --- |

**Independent**

Discuss need for information about sex and sexuality.

Because avoidance of own sexuality is an issue for this client, realistic information can be helpful in beginning to deal with self as a sexual being.

Refer to National Association of Anorexia Nervosa and Associated Disorders.

May be a helpful source of support and information for client and SO(s).

# OBESITY

**DSM IV**

316.00 Psychological Factors Affecting Medical Condition—Maladaptive Health Behaviors

**DSM III-R**

316.00 Psychological Factors Affecting Physical Condition

Although considered to be a type of eating disorder, obesity is a general medical condition coded on Axis III and has psychologic factors that adversely affect the course and treatment of the medical condition, creating additional health risk for the individual.

## ETIOLOGIC THEORIES

### Psychodynamics

Food is substituted by the parent for affection and love. The child harbors repressed feelings of hostility toward the parent, which may be expressed inward on the self. Because of a poor self-concept, the person has difficulty with other relationships. Eating is associated with a feeling of satisfaction and becomes the primary defense.

### Biologic

It is suggested that the cause of these disorders may arise out of neuroendocrine abnormalities within the hypothalamus, which result in various chemical disturbances. Familial tendencies have been identified, but obesity is not clearly identified as being hereditary. People who are overweight have more fat cells than thin people and are known to be less active. While overeating has long been believed to be the cause of obesity, research has not borne this out. Another popular theory has identified carbohydrates as the fattening substance. Currently, a high intake of fat in the diet is being identified as the reason for weight gain/inability to lose weight. The set-point theory proposes that people are programmed to maintain a certain level of weight to protect fat stores.

In recent research, genetics, metabolic changes placing some people at risk, and the way the body stores fat all play a part in the problems of obesity. Rather than a single, simple cause, obesity appears to be the result of a complex system reflecting all these factors.

### Family Dynamics

Parents act as role models for the child. Maladaptive coping patterns (overeating) are learned within the family system and are supported through positive reinforcement. Family systems may sabotage efforts at changing any part of the system in order to maintain the status quo.

## CLIENT ASSESSMENT DATABASE

### Activity/Rest

Fatigue, constant drowsiness.
Inability/lack of desire to be active or engage in regular exercise.
Increased heart rate/respirations with activity; dyspnea with exertion.

### Circulation

Hypertension, edema.

### Ego Integrity

Weight may/may not be perceived as a problem.
Perception of body image as undesirable.

Cultural/lifestyle factors affecting food choices; value for thinness/weight.
Eating relieves unpleasant feelings, e.g., loneliness, frustration, boredom.

## Food/Fluid

Normal/excessive ingestion of food.
History of recurrent weight loss and gain.
Experimentation with numerous types of diets (yo-yo dieting) with varied/short-lived results.
Weight disproportionate to height; endomorphic body type (soft/round).
Failure to adjust food intake to diminishing requirements (e.g., change in lifestyle from active to sedentary, aging).

## Pain/Discomfort

Pain/discomfort on weight-bearing joints or spine.

## Respiration

Dyspnea.
Cyanosis, respiratory distress (Pickwickian syndrome).

## Sexuality

Menstrual disturbances, amenorrhea.

## Social Interactions

Family/significant other(s) may be supportive or resistant to weight loss (sabotage client's efforts).

## Teaching/Learning

Problem may be lifetime or related to life event.
Family history of obesity.
Concomitant health problems may include hypertension, diabetes, gallbladder and cardiovascular disease, hypothyroidism.

## DIAGNOSTIC STUDIES

**Metabolic/Endocrine Studies:** May reveal abnormalities, e.g., hypothyroidism, hypopituitarism, hypogonadism, Cushing's syndrome (increased insulin levels), hyperglycemia, hyperlipidemia, hyperuricemia, hyperbilirubinemia. It is also suggested that the cause of these disorders may arise out of neuroendocrine abnormalities within the hypothalamus, which result in various chemical disturbances.

## NURSING PRIORITIES

1. Assist client to identify a workable method of weight control incorporating needed nutrients/healthful foods.
2. Promote improved self-concept, including body image, self-esteem.
3. Encourage health practices to provide for weight control throughout life.

## DISCHARGE GOALS

1. Healthy pattern for eating and weight control identified.
2. Weight loss toward desired goal established.
3. Positive perception of self verbalized.
4. Plans for future control of weight made.

| NURSING DIAGNOSIS: | NUTRITION, ALTERED, MORE THAN BODY REQUIREMENTS |
|---|---|
| **May Be Related To:** | Food intake that exceeds body needs. |
| | Psychosocial factors. |
| | Socioeconomic status. |
| **Possibly Evidenced By:** | Weight of 20% or more over optimum body weight; excess body fat by anthropometric measurements. |
| | Reported/observed dysfunctional eating patterns; intake more than body requirements. |
| | Denial of excessive food intake. |
| **Desired Outcomes/Evaluation Criteria— Client Will:** | Verbalize a more realistic self-concept/body image, mental and physical. |
| | Identify inappropriate behaviors and consequences associated with overeating or weight gain. |
| | Demonstrate change in eating patterns and involvement in individual exercise program. |
| | Display weight loss with optimal maintenance of health. |

| ACTIONS/INTERVENTIONS | RATIONALE |
|---|---|
| **Independent** | |
| Review individual factors for obesity, e.g., organic or nonorganic and associated stressors. | Identifies/influences choice of interventions. |
| Implement/review daily food diary, e.g., caloric intake, types of food, eating habits. | Provides the opportunity for the individual to focus on/internalize a realistic picture of the amount of food ingested and corresponding eating habits/feelings. Identifies patterns requiring changes and/or a base on which to tailor the dietary program. |
| Discuss emotions/events associated with eating. | Helps to identify when client is eating to satisfy an emotional need rather than physiologic hunger. |
| Formulate an eating plan with the client. | While there is no basis for recommending one diet over another, a good reducing diet should contain foods from the basic food groups with a focus on low-fat intake. It is helpful to keep the plan as similar to client's usual eating pattern as possible. Plan developed with and agreed to by the client is more apt to be successful. Note: It is important to maintain adequate protein intake to prevent loss of lean muscle mass. |

| ACTIONS/INTERVENTIONS | RATIONALE |
|---|---|
| **Independent** | |
| Use knowledge of individual's height, body build, age, gender, individual patterns of eating, and energy and nutrient requirements when developing plan. | Standard tables are subject to error when applied to individual situations, and circadian rhythms/lifestyle patterns need to be considered. |
| Stress the importance of a balanced diet. | Elimination of needed components can lead to metabolic imbalances, e.g., excessive reduction of carbohydrates can lead to fatigue, headache, instability and weakness, and metabolic acidosis (ketosis) interfering with effectiveness of weight loss program. |
| Discuss need to give self permission to include desired/craved food items in dietary plan. | Denying self by excluding desired/favorite foods results in a sense of deprivation and feelings of guilt/failure when individual succumbs to temptation. These feelings can sabotage weight loss. Knowing that it is important to include small portions of these foods can prevent negative feelings and promote cooperation with weight loss program. |
| Identify realistic increment goals for weekly weight loss. | Reasonable weight loss (1–2 pounds/wk) results in more lasting effects. Excessive/rapid loss may result in fatigue and irritability and ultimately lead to failure in meeting goals for weight loss. Motivation is more easily sustained by meeting "stair-step" goals. |
| Weigh periodically as individually indicated, and obtain appropriate body measurements. | Provides information about effectiveness of therapeutic regimen and visual evidence of success of client's efforts. During hospitalization for controlled fasting, daily weight may be required. Weekly weight is more appropriate after discharge. |
| Determine current activity levels and plan progressive exercise program (e.g., walking) tailored to individual goals and choice. | Exercise may enhance weight loss by burning calories and reducing appetite, increasing energy, toning muscles, and enhancing sense of well-being and accomplishment. Commitment on the part of the client enables the setting of more realistic goals and adherence to the plan. Note: No evidence exists that spot reducing or mechanical devices aid in weight loss in specific areas. Loss occurs on a generalized overall basis. |
| Develop an appetite reeducation plan with the client. | Signals of hunger and fullness often are not recognized, have become distorted, or are ignored. |

| ACTIONS/INTERVENTIONS | RATIONALE |
|---|---|
| **Independent** | |
| Stress the importance of avoiding tension at meal-times and not eating too quickly. | Reducing tension provides a more relaxed eating atmosphere and encourages more leisurely eating patterns. This is important because a period of time is required for the appestat mechanism to know the stomach is full. |
| Encourage client to eat only at a table or designated eating place and to avoid standing while eating. | Technqiues that modify behavior may be helpful in avoiding diet failure. |
| Discuss restriction of salt intake and diuretic drugs if used. | Water retention may be a problem because of increased fluid intake, as well as the result of fat metabolism. |
| Reassess caloric requirements every 2–4 weeks to determine need for adjustment. Be aware of plateaus when weight remains stable for periods of time. | Changes in weight and exercise will necessitate changes in diet. As weight is lost, changes in metabolism occur. Plateaus can create distrust and accusations of "cheating" on caloric intake, which are not helpful. Client may need additional support at this time. |
| **Collaborative** | |
| Consult with dietitian to determine caloric/nutrient requirements for individual weight loss. | Individual intake can be calculated by several different formulas, but weight reduction is based on the basal caloric requirement for 24 hours, depending on client's sex, age, current/desired weight, and length of time estimated to achieve desired weight. |
| Administer medications as indicated: appetite-suppressant drugs, e.g., diethylpropion (Tenuate), mazindol (Sanorex); | May be used with caution/supervision at the beginning of a weight loss program to support client during stress of behavioral/lifestyle changes. They are only effective for a few weeks and may cause problems of tolerance/dependence in some people. |
| hormonal therapy, e.g., thyroid (Euthroid); | May be necessary when hypothyroidism is present. When no deficiency is present, replacement therapy is not helpful and may actually be harmful. Note: Other hormonal treatments, such as human chorionic gonadotropin (HCG), although widely publicized, have no documented evidence of value. |
| vitamin, mineral supplementation. | Obese individuals have large fuel reserves, but are often deficient in vitamins and minerals. |
| Hospitalize for fasting regimen and/or stabilization of medical problems. | Aggressive therapy/support may be necessary to initiate weight loss, although fasting is not generally a treatment of choice. Client can be monitored more effecitvely in a controlled setting to minimize complications such as postural hypotension, anemia, cardiac irregularities, and decreased uric acid excretion with hyperuricemia. |
| Refer for evaluation of surgical options, e.g., gastric bypass, partitioning, as indicated. | May be necessary to assist the client lose weight when obesity is life-threatening. |

| NURSING DIAGNOSIS: | BODY IMAGE DISTURBANCE/SELF-ESTEEM, CHRONIC LOW |
|---|---|
| May Be Related To: | Biophysical/psychosocial factors, such as client's view of self (slimness is valued in this society, and negative messages may be received when thinness is stressed). |
| | Family/subculture encouragement of overeating. |
| | Control, sex, and love issues. |
| Possibly Evidenced By: | Verbalization of negative feelings about body (mental image often does not match physical reality); expressions of shame/guilt. |
| | Rejection of positive feedback and exaggeration of negative feedback about self. |
| | Feelings of hopelessness/powerlessness; fear of rejection/reaction by others. |
| | Lack of follow-through with diet plan; verbalization of powerlessness to change eating habits; hesitancy to try new things. |
| | Preoccupation with change (attempts to lose weight). |
| Desired Outcomes/Evaluation Criteria— Client Will: | Verbalize a more realistic self-image. |
| | Demonstrate beginning acceptance of self based on self-attributes, rather than an idealized image. |
| | Acknowledge self as an individual who has responsibility for own self. |
| | Seek information and actively pursue weight loss (as desired/if condition is life-threatening). |

| ACTIONS/INTERVENTIONS | RATIONALE |
|---|---|
| **Independent** | |
| Determine client's view of being fat and what it does for the individual. | Mental image includes our ideal and is usually not up to date. Fat and compulsive eating behaviors may have deep-rooted psychologic implications, e.g., compensating for lack of love and nurturing, or a defense against intimacy. |
| Provide privacy during care activities. | Individual usually is sensitive/self-conscious about body. |
| Have client recall coping patterns related to food in family of origin and explore how these may affect current situation. | Parents act as role models for the child. Maladaptive coping patterns (overeating) are learned within the family system and are supported through positive reinforcement. Food may be substitued by the parent for affection and love, and eating is associated with a feeling of satisfaction, becoming the primary defense. |

407

| ACTIONS/INTERVENTIONS | RATIONALE |
| --- | --- |

### Independent

| | |
| --- | --- |
| Determine relationship history and possibility of sexual abuse. | May contribute to current issues of self-esteem/patterns of coping. |
| Determine client's motivation for weight loss and set goals. | The individual may harbor repressed feelings of hostility, which may be expressed inward on the self. Because of a poor self-concept, the person often has difficulty with relationships. Note: When losing weight for someone else, the client is less likely to be successful/maintain weight loss. |
| Be alert to myths the client/SO may have about weight and weight loss. | Beliefs about what an ideal body looks like or unconscious motivations can sabotage efforts at weight loss. Some of these include the feminine thought of "If I become thin, men will pursue me or rape me"; the masculine counterpart of "I don't trust myself to stay in control of my feelings"; as well as issues of strength, power, or the "good cook" image. |
| Assist client to identify feelings that lead to compulsive eating. Develop strategies for doing something besides eating for dealing with these feelings, e.g., talking with a friend. | Awareness of emotions that lead to overeating can be the first step in behavior change, e.g., people often eat because of depression, anger, and guilt. |
| Graph weight on a weekly basis. | Provides ongoing visual evidence of weight changes (reality oriented). |
| Promote open communication, avoiding criticism/judgment about client's behavior. | Supports client's own responsibility for weight loss; enhances sense of control, and promotes willingness to discuss difficulties/setbacks and problem-solve. Note: Distrust and accusations of "cheating" on caloric intake are not helpful. |
| Outline/clearly state responsibilities of client and nurse. | It is helpful for each individual to understand area of own responsibility in the program so misunderstandings do not arise. |
| Be alert to binge-eating and develop strategies for dealing with these episodes, e.g., substituting other actions for eating. | The client who binges experiences guilt about it that is also counterproductive, because negative feelings may sabotage further weight loss. |
| Encourage client to use imagery to visualize self at desired weight when choosing to participate in weight loss program. | Mental rehearsal is very useful to help the client plan for and deal with anticipated change in self-image or deal with occasions that may arise (family gatherings, special dinners) where confrontations with food will occur. |
| Discuss the use of makeup, hairstyles, and ways of dressing to maximize figure assets. | Enhances positive feelings of self-esteem, promotes improved body image. |
| Encourage buying clothes as a reward for weight loss instead of food treats. | Properly fitting clothes enhance the body image as small losses are made and the individual feels more positive. Waiting until the desired weight loss is reached can become discouraging. |

408

| ACTIONS/INTERVENTIONS | RATIONALE |
|---|---|
| **Independent** | |
| Suggest client dispose of "fat clothes." | Removes the "safety valve" of having clothes availabe "in case" the weight is regained. Retaining fat clothes can convey the message that the weight loss will not occur/be maintained. |
| Help staff be aware of and deal with own feelings when caring for this client. | Judgmental attitudes, feelings of disgust, anger, and weariness can interfere with care/be transmitted to client, reinforcing negative self-esteem/image. |
| Help client identify positive self-attributes. Focus on strengths/past accomplishments (unrelated to physical appearance). | It is important that self-esteem not be tied solely to size of the body. Client needs to recognize that obesity need not interfere with positive feelings regarding self-concept and self-worth. |
| **Collaborative** | |
| Refer to support and/or therapy group. | Support groups can provide companionship, increase motivation, decrease loneliness and social ostracism, and give practical solutions to common problems. Group therapy can be helpful in dealing with underlying psychologic concerns. |

| **NURSING DIAGNOSIS:** | **SOCIAL INTERACTION, IMPAIRED** |
|---|---|
| **May Be Related To:** | Verbalized or observed discomfort in social situations. |
| | Self-concept disturbance. |
| **Possibly Evidenced By:** | Reluctance to participate in social gatherings. |
| | Verbalization of a sense of discomfort with others. |
| **Desired Outcomes/Evaluation Criteria— Client Will:** | Verbalize awareness of feelings that lead to poor social interactions. |
| | Be involved in achieving positive changes in social behaviors and interpersonal relationships. |

| ACTIONS/INTERVENTIONS | RATIONALE |
|---|---|
| **Independent** | |
| Review family patterns of relating and social behaviors. Assess weight issues among family of origin, especially mother/father. | Social interaction is primarily learned within the family of origin. When inadequate patterns are identified, actions for change can be instituted. |
| Encourage client to express feelings and perceptions of problems. | Helps to identify and clarify reasons for difficulties in interacting with others: client may feel unloved/unlovable or insecure about sexuality. |

409

| ACTIONS/INTERVENTIONS | RATIONALE |
|---|---|

### Independent

| | |
|---|---|
| Assess client's use of coping skills and defense mechanisms. | May have coping skills that will be useful in the process of weight loss. Defense mechanisms used to protect the individual may contribute to feelings of aloneness/isolation. |
| Have client list behaviors that cause discomfort. | Identifies specific concerns and suggests actions that can be taken to effect change. |
| Involve in role-playing new ways to deal with identified behaviors/situations. | Practicing these new behaviors enables the individual to become comfortable with them in a safe environment. |
| Discuss negative self-concepts and self-talk, e.g., "No one wants to be with a fat person," "Who would be interested in talking to me?" | May be impeding positive social interactions. |
| Encourage use of positive self-talk such as telling oneself "I am OK" or "I can enjoy social activities and do not need to be controlled by what others think or say." | Positive strategies enhance feelings of comfort and support efforts for change. |

### Collaborative

| | |
|---|---|
| Refer for ongoing family or individual therapy as indicated. | Client derives support and encouragement from involvement of family/SO. |

| | |
|---|---|
| **NURSING DIAGNOSIS:** | **KNOWLEDGE DEFICIT [LEARNING NEED] regarding condition, prognosis, and treatment needs** |
| **May Be Related To:** | Lack of/misinterpretation of information. |
| | Lack of interest in learning, lack of recall. |
| | Inaccurate/incomplete information presented. |
| **Possibly Evidenced By:** | Questions/request for information about obesity and nutritional requirements. |
| | Verbalization of problem with weight reduction. |
| | Inadequate follow-through with previous diet and exercise instruction. |
| **Desired Outcomes/Evaluation Criteria— Client Will:** | Assume responsibility for own learning. |
| | Begin to look for information about nutrition and ways to control weight. |
| | Verbalize understanding of need for lifestyle changes to maintain/control weight. |
| | Establish individual goal and plan for attaining goal. |

| ACTIONS/INTERVENTIONS | RATIONALE |
|---|---|

### Independent

| | |
|---|---|
| Determine level of nutritional knowledge and what client believes is most urgent need. | Necessary to know what additional information to provide. When client's views are listened to, trust is enhanced. |
| Identify individual holistic long-term goals for health, e.g., lowering blood pressure, controlling serum lipid and glucose levels. | A high relapse rate at 5 year follow-up suggests obesity cannot be reliably reversed/cured. Shifting the focus from initial weight loss/percentage of body fat to overall wellness may enhance rehabilitation. |
| Provide information about ways to maintain satisfactory food intake in settings away from home. | "Smart" eating when dining out or when traveling helps to maintain weight at desired level while still enjoying social outlets. |
| Identify other sources of information, e.g., books, tapes, community classes, groups. | Using different avenues of accessing information will further client's learning. Involvement with others who are also losing weight can provide support. |
| Stress necessity of continued follow-up care/counseling, especially when plateaus occur. | As weight is lost, changes in metabolism occur, interfering with further loss by creating a plateau as the body activates a survival mechanism, attempting to prevent "starvation." This requires new strategies and aggressive support to continue weight loss. |
| Identify alternatives to chosen activity program to accommodate weather, travel, and so on. Discuss use of mechanical devices/equipment for reducing. | Promotes continuation of program. Note: Fat loss occurs on a generalized overall basis, and there is no evidence that spot reducing or mechanical devices aid in weight loss in specific areas. However, specific types of exercise or equipment may be useful in *toning* specific body parts. |
| Discuss necessity of good skin care, especially during summer months. | Prevents skin breakdown/yeast infections in moist skinfolds. |
| Identify alternative ways to "reward" self/family for accomplishments or to provide solace. | Reduces likelihood of relying on food to deal with feelings. |
| Encourage involvement in social activities that are not centered around food, e.g., bike ride/nature hike, attending muscial event, group sporting activities. | Provides opportunity for pleasure and relaxation without "temptation." Activities/exercise may also use calories to help maintain desired weight. |

# CHAPTER 14

# ADJUSTMENT DISORDERS

## ADJUSTMENT DISORDERS: (Specify)

**DSM IV**
**ADJUSTMENT DISORDER (ACUTE/CHRONIC)**
309.24  With Anxiety
309.0   With Depressed Mood
309.3   With Disturbance of Conduct
309.4   With Mixed Disturbance of Emotions and Conduct
309.28  With Mixed Anxiety and Depressed Mood

**DSM III-R**
**ADJUSTMENT DISORDER WITH:**
309.24  Anxious Mood
309.00  Depressed Mood
309.30  Disturbance of Conduct
309.40  Mixed Disturbance of Emotions and Conduct
309.28  Mixed Emotional Features
309.82  Physical Complaints
309.83  Withdrawal
309.23  Work (or Academic) Inhibition
309.90  Adjustment Disorder NOS

The essential feature of adjustment disorder is a maladaptive reaction to an identifiable psychosocial stressor that occurs within 3 months of the onset of the stressor. The stressor does not represent bereavement (death of a loved one) and does not meet the criteria for any specific Axis I disorder or represent an exacerbation of a preexisting Axis I or Axis II disorder.

The response is considered maladaptive because there is impairment in social or occupational functioning or because the behaviors are exaggerated beyond the usual, expected response to such a stressor. Duration of the symptoms for more than 6 months indicates a chronic state. By definition, an Adjustment Disorder must resolve within 6 months of the termination of the stressor (or its consequences).

## ETIOLOGIC THEORIES

### Psychodynamics

Factors implicated in the predisposition to this disorder include unmet dependency needs, fixation in an earlier level of development, and underdeveloped ego.

The predisposition to adjustment disorder is seen as an inability to complete the grieving process in response to a painful life change. The presumed cause of this inability to adapt is believed to be psychic overload, a level of intrapsychic strain exceeding the individual's ability to cope. Normal functioning is disrupted, and psychologic or somatic symptoms occur.

### Biologic

The presence of chronic disorders is thought to limit the general adaptive capacity of an individual. The normal process of adaptation to stressful life experiences is impaired, causing increased vulnerability to adjustment disorders. A high family incidence suggests a possible hereditary influence.

The autonomic nervous system discharge that occurs in response to a frightening impulse and/or emotion is mediated by the limbic system, resulting in the peripheral effects of the autonomic nervous system seen in the presence of anxiety.

Some medical conditions have been associated with anxiety and panic disorders, such as abnormalities in the hypothalamic-pituitary-adrenal and hypothalamic-pituitary-thyroid axes; acute myocardial infarction; pheochromocytomas; substance intoxication and withdrawal; hypoglycemia; caffeine intoxication; mitral valve prolapse; and complex partial seizures.

### Family Dynamics

The individual's ability to respond to stress is influenced by the role of the primary caregiver (her or his ability to adapt to the infant's needs) and the child-rearing environment (allowing the child gradually to gain independence and control over own life). Difficulty allowing the child to become independent leads to problems with adjustment in later life.

Individuals with adjustment difficulties have experienced negative learning through inadequate role-modeling in dysfunctional family systems. These dysfunctional patterns impede the development of self-esteem and adequate coping skills, which also contribute to maladaptive adjustment reponses.

### CLIENT ASSESSMENT DATABASE

Symptoms of affective, depressive, and anxiety disorders are manifested dependent on the individual's specific response to a stressful situation.

### Activity/Rest

Fatigue.
Insomnia.

### Ego Integrity

Reports occurrence of personal stressor/loss (e.g., job, financial, relationship) within past 3 months.
May appear depressed and tearful and/or nervous and jittery.
Feelings of hopelessness.

### Neurosensory

**Mental Status:** Depressed mood, tearful, anxious, nervous, jittery.
Attention and memory span may be impaired (depends on presence of depression, level of anxiety, and/or substance use).
Communication and thought patterns may reveal negative ruminations of depressed mood or flight of ideas/loose associations of severely anxious condition.

413

### Pain/Discomfort

Various physical symptoms such as headache, backache, other aches and pains (maladaptive response to a stressful situation).

### Safety

Anger expressed inappropriately.
Involvement in high risk behaviors, e.g., fighting, reckless driving.
Suicidal ideations may be present.

### Social Interactions

Difficulties with performance in work/social setting, when no difficulties had been experienced prior to the occurrence of the stressor.
Socially withdrawn/refuses to interact with others (e.g., isolates self in own room).
Reports of vandalism, reckless driving, fighting, defaulting on legal responsibilities, violation of the rights of others or age-appropriate norms and rules.
May display manipulative behavior (e.g., testing limits, playing individuals/family members against each other).

### Teaching/Learning

Academic difficulties, failure to attend class/complete course work.
Substance use/abuse may be present.

## DIAGNOSTIC STUDIES

As indicated to rule out underlying pathophysiologic condition, e.g., a differential diagnosis with the affective, anxiety, conduct, or antisocial personality disorders must be considered.
**Drug Screen:** Determine substance use.

## NURSING PRIORITIES

1. Provide safe environment/protect client from self-harm.
2. Assist client to identify precipitating stressor.
3. Promote development of effective problem-solving techniques.
4. Provide information and support for necessary lifestyle changes.
5. Promote involvement of client/family in therapy process/planning for the future.

## DISCHARGE GOALS

1. Relief from feelings of depression and/or anxiety is noted, with suicidal ideation reduced.
2. Anger is expressed in an appropriate manner.
3. Maladaptive behaviors are recognized and rechanneled into socially accepted actions.
4. Client is involved in social situations/interacting with others.
5. Ability and willingness to manage life situations are displayed.

| **NURSING DIAGNOSIS:** | **ANXIETY [moderate to severe]** |
| --- | --- |
| **May Be Related To:** | Situational/maturational crisis. |
| | Threat to self-concept; threat (or perceived threat) to physical integrity. |

|  | Unmet needs. |
|---|---|

**Possibly Evidenced By:**

Fear of failure.

Dysfunctional family system; unsatisfactory parent/child relationship resulting in feelings of insecurity.

Fixation in earlier level of development.

Overexcitement/restlessness; increased tension; insomnia.

Feelings of inadequacy; fear of unspecified consequences.

Poor eye contact, focus on self; difficulty concentrating.

Continuous attention-seeking behaviors; selective inattention.

Sympathetic stimulation; numerous physical complaints.

**Desired Outcomes/Evaluation Criteria—Client Will:**

Verbalize awareness of feelings of/indicators of increasing anxiety.

Demonstrate/use appropriate techniques to interrupt escalation of anxiety.

Appear relaxed and report anxiety is reduced to a manageable level.

| ACTIONS/INTERVENTIONS | RATIONALE |
|---|---|
| **Independent** | |
| Establish a trusting relationship with the client. Be honest, consistent in responses, and available. Show genuine positive regard. | Honesty, availability, and unconditional acceptance promote trust, which is necessary for the development of a therapeutic relationship. |
| Provide activities geared toward reduction of tension and decreasing anxiety, e.g., walking or jogging, musical exercises, housekeeping chores, group games/activities. | Tension and anxiety can be released safely, and physical activity may provide emotional benefit to the client through release in the brain of morphine-like substances (endorphins) that promote sense of well-being. |
| Encourage client to identify true feelings and to acknowledge ownership of those feelings. | Anxious clients often deny a relationship between emotional problems and their anxiety. Use of the defense mechanisms of projection and displacement are exaggerated. |
| Maintain a calm atmosphere and approach to client. | Can help to limit transmission of anxiety to those surrounding client. |
| Assist client to recognize specific events that precede onset of elevation in anxiety. Provide information about signs and symptoms of increasing anxiety and ways to intervene before behaviors become disabling. | Recognition of precipitating stressors and a plan of action to follow should they recur provides client with feelings of security and control over similar situations in the future. This in itself may help to control anxiety response. |

415

| ACTIONS/INTERVENTIONS | RATIONALE |
|---|---|

### Independent

Offer support during times of elevated anxiety. Provide physical and psychologic safety. (Refer to ND: Violence, high risk for, directed at self/others.)

Presence of a trusted individual may provide needed security/client safety.

### Collaborative

Administer medications as necesary, e.g., benzodiazepines: alprazolam (Xanax).

Antianxiety medications induce a calming effect and work to maintain anxiety at a manageable level while providing the opportunity for client to develop other ways to manage stress.

| **NURSING DIAGNOSIS:** | **VIOLENCE, HIGH RISK FOR, DIRECTED AT SELF/OTHERS** |
|---|---|
| **Risk Factors May Include:** | Depressed mood, hopelessness, powerlessness; inability to tolerate frustration; rage reactions. |
| | Low self-esteem; unmet needs. |
| | Negative role modeling; lack of support systems. |
| | Substance use/abuse. |
| | History of previous suicide attempts. |
| **Possible Indicators:** | Increased motor activity (pacing, excitement, irritability, agitation). |
| | Muscle tension (e.g., clenched fists, tense facial expressions, rigid posture, tautness). |
| | Hostile, threatening verbalizations; provocative behavior (argumentative, dissatisfied, overreactive, hypersensitive). |
| | Suicide ideation. |
| **Desired Outcomes/Evaluation Criteria— Client Will:** | Verbalize understanding of behavior and precipitating factors. |
| | Participate in care and meet own needs in an assertive manner. |
| | Rechannel anger/hostile feelings into socially acceptable behaviors. |
| | Demonstrate self-control as evidenced by relaxed posture, absence of violent behavior, etc. |
| | Use resources/support systems in an effective manner. |

| ACTIONS/INTERVENTIONS | RATIONALE |
|---|---|

### Independent

Observe client's behavior frequently during routine activities and interactions; avoid appearing watchful and suspicious.

Close observation is required so that intervention can occur if required to ensure the safety of others. Instilling suspicion may provoke aggressive behaviors.

Ask client direct questions regarding intent, plan, and availability of the means for self-harm. Evaluate and prioritize on a scale of 1–10 according to severity of threat, availability of means.

Direct questions, if presented in a caring, concerned manner, provide the necessary information to assist the nurse in formulating an appropriate plan of care for the suicidal client.

Provide a safe environment: reduce stimuli (e.g., low lighting, few people, simple decor, low noise level).

A stimulating environment may increase agitation and provoke aggressive behavior.

Remove potentially dangerous objects, such as straps, belts, ties, sharp objects, glass items, and drugs, as indicated.

External control of environment aids in preventing impulsive actions at a time when client lacks own internal controls.

Secure contract from client that she or he will not harm self and will seek out staff member if suicidal ideations emerge.

A contract encourages the client to share in the responsibility of own safety. A degree of control is experienced, and the attitude of acceptance of the client as a worthwhile individual is conveyed.

Promote verbalizations of honest feelings. Through exploration and discussion, help client identify symbols of hope in own life.

May be difficult for client to express negative feelings. Verbalization of these feelings in a nonthreatening environment may help client come to terms with unresolved issues and identify reasons for wanting to change life/continue living.

Help client identify true source of anger/hostility and underlying feelings.

Because of weak ego development, client may be using the defense mechanism of displacement. Helping the client to recognize this in a nonthreatening environment may help reveal unresolved issues so that they may be confronted, regardless of the discomfort involved.

Convey an attitude of acceptance toward the client. Impart a message that it is not the client but the behavior that is unacceptable.

An attitude of acceptance promotes feelings of self-worth. These feelings are further enhanced as person and behavior are viewed separately, communicating unconditional positive regard.

Explore with client alternative ways of handling frustration/pent-up anger that channel hostile energy into socially acceptable behavior, e.g., brisk walks, jogging, physical exercises, volleyball, punching bag, exercise bike.

Physically demanding activities help to relieve pent-up tension.

Maintain a calm attitude toward the client if behavior escalates. Have sufficient staff available to convey a show of strength to the client if it becomes necessary.

Anxiety is contagious and can be transferred from person to person. A calm attitude provides client with a feeling of safety and security. A display of strength provides reassurance for the client that the staff is in control of the situation and will provide physical security for the client, staff, and others.

Be alert to increased potential for suicidal action as mood elevates.

Client may mobilize self for suicidal attempt as decrease in depression results in increased energy and motivation.

417

| ACTIONS/INTERVENTIONS | RATIONALE |
|---|---|

## Collaborative

| | |
|---|---|
| Administer medication as indicated, e.g.:<br>  tricyclic drugs: amitriptyline (Elavil), desipramine (Norpramin), doxepin (Sinequan), imipramine (Tofranil); | Antidepressant medication may elevate the mood, as it increases level of energy and decreases feelings of fatigue. |
|   serotonin reuptake inhibitors: fluoxetine (Prozac), sertraline (Zoloft), paroxetine (Paxil); | |
|   monoamine-oxidase inhibitors: isocarboxazid (Marplan), phenelzine (Nardil); | |
|   benzodiazepines: diazepam (Valium), chlordiazepoxide (Librium), alprazolam (Xanax); | Antianxiety medication may provide needed relief from anxious feelings, inducing a calming effect and inhibiting aggressive behavior. |

| NURSING DIAGNOSIS: | COPING, INDIVIDUAL, INEFFECTIVE |
|---|---|
| May Be Related To: | Situational/maturational crises. |
| | Dysfunctional family system; negative role modeling; inadequate support systems. |
| | Unmet dependency needs; low self-esteem; retarded ego development. |
| Possibly Evidenced By: | Inability to cope/problem-solve. |
| | Chronic worry, depressed/anxious mood. |
| | Alteration in societal participation; manipulation of others. |
| | Inability to meet role expectations; increased dependency; refusal to follow rules of the unit. |
| | Numerous physical complaints. |
| | Destructive behavior, substance abuse. |
| Desired Outcomes/Evaluation Criteria—Client Will: | Assess the current situation accurately. |
| | Identify ineffective coping behaviors and consequences. |
| | Meet psychologic needs as evidenced by appropriate expression of feelings, identification of options, and use of resources. |
| | Avoid manipulating others for own gratification. |

| ACTIONS/INTERVENTIONS | RATIONALE |
|---|---|

## Independent

| | |
|---|---|
| Explain rules of the unit and consequences of lack of cooperation. Set limits on manipulative behavior. Be consistent in enforcing the consequences when rules are broken and limits tested. | Negative reinforcement may work to decrease undesirable behaviors. Consistency among all staff members is vital if intervention is to be successful. |

| ACTIONS/INTERVENTIONS | RATIONALE |
|---|---|

### Independent

Ignore negative behaviors when possible and provide feedback when positive behaviors are noted, encouraging client to give self-acknowledgment of success.

Negative behaviors diminish when they provide no reward of attention. When client gives self positive feedback, inner rewards are enhanced.

Encourage client to discuss angry feelings. Help client identify the true object of the hostility. Provide physical outlets for healthy release of the hostile feelings, e.g., punching bags, pounding boards. Involve in outdoor recreation program, if available.

Verbalization of feelings with a trusted individual may help client work through unresolved issues. Physical excercise provides a safe and effective means of releasing pent-up tension, as well as of developing self-confidence and trust in others.

Take care not to reinforce dependent behaviors. Allow client to perform as independently as possible and provide feedback.

Independent accomplishment and positive reinforcement enhance self-esteem and encourage repetition of desirable behaviors.

Help client to recognize some aspects of life over which a measure of control is maintained/possible. (Refer to ND: Powerlessness.)

Recognition of personal control, however minimal, diminishes the feeling of powerlessness and decreases the need for manipulation of others.

Give minimal attention to the physical condition if client is coping through numerous somatic complaints and organic pathology has been ruled out. Increase attention during times when client is not focusing on physical complaints.

Organic pathology must always be considered. Failure to do so may place the client in physical jeopardy. Lack of attention to maladaptive behaviors may work to decrease their repetition. Positive reinforcement encourages desirable behaviors.

Discuss the negative aspects of substance abuse as a response to stress. Help client recognize difficult life situations that may be contributing to use of substances.

Denial of problems related to use of substances is common. Client needs to recognize relationship between use of substances and personal problems before rehabilitation can begin.

Assist client with problem-solving process. Suggest alternatives, and help to select more adaptive strategies for coping with stress.

Because of level of anxiety and delayed development, client may require assistance in determining which methods of coping are most individually appropriate. Increased anxiety interferes with the ability to solve problems.

Encourage client to learn relaxation techniques, use of imagery.

These skills can be helpful to the development of new coping methods to deal with/reduce stress.

### Collaborative

Refer client to substance rehabilitation program if problem is identified.

A greater likelihood of success can be expected if client seeks professional assistance with this problem.

---

| NURSING DIAGNOSIS: | **ADJUSTMENT, IMPAIRED [when stressor is a change in health status]** |
|---|---|
| **May Be Related To:** | Change in health status requiring modification in lifestyle (e.g., development of chronic disease/disability, changes associated with aging process). |
| | Assault to self-esteem. |
| | Inadequate support systems. |

| | |
|---|---|
| **Possibly Evidenced By:** | Verbalization of nonacceptance of health status change. |
| | Difficulty in problem-solving, decision-making, or goal setting; lack of future-oriented thinking. |
| | Lack of movement toward independence. |
| **Desired Outcomes/Evaluation Criteria— Client Will:** | Recognize reality of situation and individual needs/options. |
| | Assume personal responsibility for care, problem-solve needs. |
| | Initiate necessary lifestyle changes. |
| | Plan for future needs/changes. |

## ACTIONS/INTERVENTIONS

### Independent

Encourage client to talk about lifestyle prior to the change in health status. Discuss coping mechanisms that were used at stressful times in the past.

Help client to discuss the change or loss and particularly to express anger associated with it.

Have client express fears associated with the change/loss or the alteration in lifestyle that the change or loss has created.

Provide assistance with activities of daily living as required, but encourage independence to the limit that client's ability will allow. Give positive feedback for activities accomplished independently.

Help client with decision-making regarding incorporation of change or loss into lifestyle. Identify problems the change or loss is likely to create. Discuss alternative solutions, weighing potential benefits and consequences of each alternative. Support client's decisions.

Use role-play when stressful situations that might occur in relation to the health status change are anticipated.

Provide information regarding the physiology of the change in health status and its necessity for optimal wellness. Encourage client and family to ask questions. Provide printed material explaining the change.

## RATIONALE

It is important to identify the client's strengths so that they may be used to facilitate adaptation to the change or loss that has occurred.

Some individuals may not realize that anger is a normal stage in the grieving process. If it is not released in an appropriate manner, it may be turned inward on the self, leading to pathologic depression.

Change often creates a feeling of disequilibrium, and the individual may respond with fears that are irrational or unfounded. Client may benefit from feedback that corrects misperceptions about how life will be with the change in health status.

Independent accomplishments and positive feedback enhance self-esteem and encourage repetition of desired behaviors. Successes also provide hope that adaptive functioning is possible and decrease feelings of powerlessness.

The high degree of anxiety that usually accompanies a major lifestyle change often interferes with an individual's ability to solve problems and to make appropriate decisions. Client may need assistance with this process in an effort to progress toward successful adaptation.

Role-play decreases anxiety and provides a feeling of security by preparing the client with a plan of action to respond in an appropriate manner when a stressful situation occurs.

Helps client and family understand what has happened, clarifies information, and provides opportunity to review information at individual's leisure.

| ACTIONS/INTERVENTIONS | RATIONALE |
| --- | --- |

### Collaborative

Refer to resources within the community, e.g., self-help/support groups, public health nurse, counselor, or social worker.

Provides assistance in adapting to the change in health status.

| NURSING DIAGNOSIS: | GRIEVING, DYSFUNCTIONAL |
| --- | --- |
| **May Be Related To:** | Real or perceived loss of any concept of value to the individual; bereavement overload (cumulative grief from multiple unresolved losses, **excluding the death of a loved one**). |
| | Absence of anticipatory grieving; thwarted grieving response to loss. |
| | Feelings of guilt generated by ambivalent relationship with the lost concept/person. |
| **Possibly Evidenced By:** | Idealization of the lost concept. |
| | Difficulty in expressing loss; denial of loss. |
| | Excessive anger, expressed inappropriately; labile affect. |
| | Developmental regression. |
| | Alterations in concentration and/or pursuit of tasks. |
| **Desired Outcomes/Evaluation Criteria—Client Will:** | Express emotions appropriately. |
| | Demonstrate progress in dealing with stages of grief at own pace. |
| | Carry out activities of daily living independently. |
| | Express feeling of hope for the future. |

| ACTIONS/INTERVENTIONS | RATIONALE |
| --- | --- |

### Independent

Determine stage of grief in which client is fixed. Identify behaviors associated with this stage. (Most depressed people are fixed in the anger stage, with the anger directed inward on the self.)

Accurate baseline assessment data are necessary to choose appropriate interventions/provide effective care and evaluate progress.

Develop trusting nurse/client relationship. Show empathy and caring. Be honest and keep all promises.

Trust is the basis for a therapeutic relationship that supports client in dealing with loss/reality.

Convey an accepting attitude; encourage client to express self openly.

An accepting attitude enhances trust and communicates to the client that you believe the client is a worthwhile person, regardless of what may be expressed.

421

| ACTIONS/INTERVENTIONS | RATIONALE |
|---|---|

### Independent

Encourage client to express anger. Do not become defensive if initial expression of anger is displaced on nurse/therapist. Assist client to explore angry feelings and direct them toward the intended object/person or other loss.

Verbalization of feelings in a nonthreatening environment may help client come to terms with unresolved issues related to the loss.

Encourage participation in large motor activities.

Physical activity provides a safe and effective method for discharging pent-up tension/anger.

Provide information about the stages of grief and the behaviors associated with each stage. Help client understand that feelings, such as anger directed toward the loss, are appropriate during the grief process.

Knowledge of the acceptability of the feelings associated with normal grieving may help relieve some of the guilt that these responses generate.

Encourage client to review relationship with loss. With support and sensitivity, point out reality of the situation in areas where misrepresentations are expressed.

Client needs to give up idealized perception and accept both positive and negative aspects about the loss before resolution of grief can occur.

Assist client to determine methods for more adaptive coping with the experienced loss. Provide positive feedback for strategies identified and decisions made.

Feelings of depression may interfere with client's problem-solving ability, resulting in need for assistance. Positive feedback enhances self-esteem and encourages repetition of desirable behaviors.

### Collaborative

Determine client's perception of spiritual needs as support in the grieving process. Involve chaplain or appropriate spiritual leader as indicated.

Some individuals derive great strength from spiritual support. This strength may be used by the client in the task of grief resolution.

| NURSING DIAGNOSIS: | HOPELESSNESS |
|---|---|
| May Be Related To: | Lifestyle of helplessness (repeated failures, dependency). |
| | Incomplete grief work of losses in life. |
| | Lost belief in transcendent values/God. |
| Possibly Evidenced By: | Verbal cues/despondent content (e.g., "I can't," sighing). |
| | Apathy/passivity, decreased response to stimuli. |
| | Lack of initiative, nonparticipation in care or decision-making when opportunities are provided. |
| Desired Outcomes/Evaluation Criteria—Client Will: | Recognize and verbalize feelings. |
| | Demonstrate independent problem-solving techniques to take control over life. |
| | Verbalize acceptance of life situations over which one does not have control. |

| ACTIONS/INTERVENTIONS | RATIONALE |
|---|---|
| **Independent** | |
| Identify use of maladaptive behaviors/defense mechanisms (e.g., withdrawal, substance use, regression.) | Personal attempts to overcome feelings of hopelessness may have resulted in ineffective/harmful behaviors. Recognizing the behaviors provides opportunity for change. |
| Encourage client to explore and verbalize feelings and perceptions. | Identification of feelings underlying behaviors helps client to begin process of taking control of own life. |
| Identify individual signs of hopelessness, e.g., decreased physical activity, social withdrawal. | Helps to individualize interventions, focus attention on areas of need. |
| Express hope to client in positive, low-key manner. | Even though client feels hopeless, it is helpful to hear positive expressions from others. |
| Help client identify areas of life situation that are under own control. | Client's emotional condition may interfere with ability to problem-solve. Assistance may be required to perceive the benefits and consequences of available alternatives accurately. |
| Encourage client to assume responsibility for own self-care, e.g., setting realistic goals, scheduling activities, making independent decisions. | Providing the client with choices increases feelings of control. Note: Unrealistic goals set the client up for failure and reinforce feelings of hopelessness. |
| Help client identify areas of life situation that are not within ability to control. Discuss feelings associated with this lack of control. | Client needs to identify and resolve feelings associated with inability to control certain life situations before level of acceptance can be achieved. |

| NURSING DIAGNOSIS: | SELF-ESTEEM DISTURBANCE [specify] |
|---|---|
| **May Be Related To:** | Maturational transitions. |
| | Unmet dependency needs; retarded ego development. |
| | Repeated negative feedback, diminished self-worth. |
| | Dysfunctional family system. |
| **Possibly Evidenced By:** | Self-negating verbalization, inability to deal with events. |
| | Difficulty accepting positive feedback. |
| | Lack of eye contact; nonassertive/passive behaviors; indecision, difficulty making decisions. |
| | Hesitancy to undertake new tasks; fear of failure. |
| | Social isolation; nonparticipation in therapy. |
| | Manipulation of one staff member against another. |
| | Self-destructive ideas/behavior. |

| Desired Outcomes/Evaluation Criteria— Client Will: | Identify feelings and underlying dynamics for negative perception of self. |
|---|---|
| | Demonstrate behaviors/lifestyle changes to promote positive self-esteem. |
| | Accept recognition for personal accomplishments/abilities. |
| | Verbalize increased sense of self-esteem. |

| ACTIONS/INTERVENTIONS | RATIONALE |
|---|---|

### Independent

| | |
|---|---|
| Discuss goals, making sure they are realistic. Plan activities in which success is likely. | Achievement/success enhance self-esteem. |
| Convey unconditional positive regard for the client. Promote understanding of acceptance for client as a worthwhile human being. | Unconditional acceptance of an individual serves to counteract feelings of worthlessness by reinforcing that individual is worthy of another person's respect. |
| Spend time with client both on a 1:1 basis and in group activities. | Conveys that the nurse sees the client as someone worth spending time with. |
| Assist client in identifying positive aspects of self and in developing plans for changing the characteristics viewed as negative. | Individuals with low self-esteem often have difficulty recognizing positive attributes. They may also lack problem-solving ability and require assistance to formulate a plan for implementing the desired changes. |
| Encourage and support client in confronting the fear of failure by attending therapy activities and undertaking new tasks. Offer recognition of successful endeavors and positive reinforcement of attempts made. | Recognition and positive reinforcement enhance self-esteem and encourage repetition of desirable behaviors. |
| Assist client to avoid ruminating about past failures. Withdraw attention if client persists. | Lack of attention to these undesirable behaviors may discourage their repetition. Client needs to focus on positive attributes if self-esteem is to be enhanced. |
| Minimize negative feedback to client. Enforce limit setting in matter-of-fact manner, imposing previously established consequences for violations. | Negative feedback can be extremely threatening to a person with low self-esteem, possibly aggravating the problem. Consequences need to convey unacceptability of the behavior but not the person. |
| Encourage independence in the performance of personal responsibilities, as well as in decision-making related to own self-care. Offer recognition and praise for accomplishments. | The ability to perform self-care activities independently enhances self-esteem. Positive reinforcement encourages repetition of desirable behaviors. |
| Support client in critical examination of feelings, attitudes, and behaviors. Help client understand that it is acceptable for attitudes and behaviors to differ from those of others, as long as they do not become intrusive. | The need for judging the behavior of others diminishes as client increases self-esteem through greater self-awareness and the achievement of self-acceptance. |

| NURSING DIAGNOSIS: | SOCIAL INTERACTION, IMPAIRED |
|---|---|
| May Be Related To: | Unmet dependency needs; retarded ego development |
| | Negative role-modeling. |
| | Low self-esteem. |
| Possibly Evidenced By: | Verbalized/observed discomfort in social situations; use of unsuccessful/dysfunctional social interaction behaviors. |
| | Verbalized or observed inability to receive or communicate a satisfying sense of belonging, caring, interest. |
| | Exhibits behaviors unacceptable for age, as defined by dominant cultural group. |
| Desired Outcomes/Evaluation Criteria— Client Will: | Verbalize awareness of factors resulting in difficulty in forming satisfactory relationships with others. |
| | Identify feelings that lead to poor social interactions. |
| | Interact with staff and peers with little/no indication of discomfort. |
| | Participate in group activities appropriately and willingly. |
| | Identify/develop effective social support system. |

## ACTIONS/INTERVENTIONS

## RATIONALE

### Independent

| ACTIONS/INTERVENTIONS | RATIONALE |
|---|---|
| Establish 1:1 relationship with client, which serves as role model for testing new behaviors. | Client needs to learn to interact appropriately with nurse, so that behaviors may then be generalized to others. |
| Encourage client to engage in activities out of room. Offer to attend initial group interactions with client. Provide feedback for appropriate interactions. | Decreases opportunity for client to isolate self. Presence of a trusted individual may provide a feeling of security and decrease the anxiety generated by difficult social situation. Positive reinforcement enhances self-esteem and encourages repetition of desirable behaviors. |
| Confront client and withdraw attention when interactions with others are manipulative or exploitative. | Attention to the unacceptable behavior may reinforce it. |
| Assist client to understand how unacceptable behaviors have interfered with the ability to form satisfactory relationships in the past. | Client may not realize how others actually perceive actions. Correction of these misperceptions may assist in the improvement of ability to interact with others. |
| Act as role model for client through appropriate interactions with client, other clients, and staff members. | Because of weak ego development, client is inclined to imitate the actions of those individuals admired or trusted. |

425

## ACTIONS/INTERVENTIONS

## RATIONALE

### Independent

Establish schedule of group activities for client.

It is through these group interactions, with positive and negative feedback from peers, that client learns socially acceptable behavior.

| **NURSING DIAGNOSIS:** | **FAMILY PROCESSES, ALTERED** |
| --- | --- |
| **May Be Related To:** | Situational/maturational crisis. |
| **Possibly Evidenced By:** | Needs of family members not being met; confusion within family system regarding how needs should be met. |
| | Impaired family communication; dissonance among family members. |
| | Impairment of family decision-making process; family developmental tasks not being fulfilled. |
| | Reduced/restricted social involvement. |
| **Desired Outcomes/Evaluation Criteria—Family Will:** | Express feelings freely and appropriately. |
| | Develop effective patterns of communication, encouraging honest input from all members. |
| | Identify source(s) of dysfunction and effectively problem-solve to achieve desired resolution. |
| | Demonstrate pattern of functioning improved from premorbid state, having gained knowledge and achieved growth from crisis situation. |

## ACTIONS/INTERVENTIONS

## RATIONALE

### Independent

Assess family developmental stage, communication patterns, and extent of dysfunction.

Identifies specific needs and provides direction for care.

Meet with the total family group as often as possible.

The family as a system operates as a single unit. Each member affects, and is affected by, all other members. Therapy is most effective when directed toward the functioning of the family system.

Construct a client/family genogram.

Genograms help to identify emotional closeness among family members over several generations. Family process is clarified, and configuration and dynamics are clearly illustrated.

Assist family to identify true source of conflict. Help them recognize that "identified patient's" adjustment disorder may be a way to avoid confronting the real problem.

Conflict creates high levels of anxiety within the family system. Common defense mechanisms, such as denial, displacement, projection, and rationalization, are used by the family to decrease anxiety and avoid conflict.

| ACTIONS/INTERVENTIONS | RATIONALE |
|---|---|
| **Independent** | |
| Assist family members to set goals and identify alternatives. Support efforts directed toward positive change. Assist with necessary modifications of original plan. | Life crises interfere with family decision-making and problem-solving ability. Assistance with this process may be required to promote adaptation and growth. |
| Promote separation and individuation and clear, functional boundaries between members. | Emotional connectedness among family members (enmeshment) discourages individual growth and ability to function autonomously. |
| Assist client-family to identify actions/problem-solve for potential life crises. | Anticipatory guidance/knowing what to expect and having a plan of action for management of situations may help to avert a crisis in the future. |
| **Collaborative** | |
| Involve family in group therapy. | Interacting with others in family/multifamily groups can be helpful to identify dysfunctional patterns and assist in learning new skills and solutions for family problems. |
| Refer family to other resources, such as support groups, classes, e.g., parenting/assertiveness training. | Sharing with others who have had similar experiences can provide support and assist family members to learn new ways to deal with situation. |

# CHAPTER 15

---

# PERSONALITY DISORDERS

Note: Coded on Axis II.

## ANTISOCIAL PERSONALITY DISORDER

**DSM IV**
301.7 Antisocial Personality Disorder

**DSM III-R**
301.70 Antisocial Personality Disorder

The terms "sociopath" and "psychopath" are often used to describe the individual with antisocial personality. The disorder is extremely difficult to treat. Imprisonment has been society's major method for controlling the most dangerous behaviors.

## ETIOLOGIC THEORIES
### Psychodynamics

Psychodynamically, this individual remains fixed in an earlier level of development. Because of parental rejection or indifference, needs for satisfaction and security remain unmet, and the ego is underdeveloped. Because of a lack of ego strength, behavior is id directed and results in the need for immediate gratification. An immature superego allows this individual to pursue gratification, regardless of means and without experiencing feelings of guilt.

### Biologic

Genetic involvement has been implicated in studies that showed that individuals with antisocial personality, and their parents, showed excessive EEG abnormalities when these examinations were conducted on both groups. (Despite genetic or environmental factors, sociopaths choose their lifestyle; therefore, it is up to them to choose to change it.)

### Family Dynamics

Family functioning has been implicated as an important factor in determining whether or not an individual develops this disorder. The following circumstances may predispose to the disorder: absence of parental discipline (teaching/guidance), extreme poverty, removal from the home, growing up without parental figures of both sexes, erratic and inconsistent limit setting, being "rescued" each time the person is in trouble (never having to suffer the consequences of own behavior), and maternal deprivation.

## CLIENT ASSESSMENT DATABASE

### Circulation

**Heart Rate:** Slight increase may be demonstrated when anticipating stress (correlates with electrodermal responses indicating minimal anxiety).

### Ego Integrity

Lacks motivation for change, often not seeking therapy voluntarily (unless client can no longer tolerate the mess he or she has made of own life/is facing long-term imprisonment).

Absence of feelings of guilt/shame.

Use of aliases.

### Neurosensory

**Mental Status:** Personality appears charming, engaging, and is usually intelligent.

Demeanor is often a pretense intended to deceive others or to facilitate exploitation of others.

Manipulation is style of operating, e.g., needs and demands immediate gratification; low tolerance level results in feelings of frustration when desires are not immediately gratified.

Signs of personal distress may be evident, e.g., tension and poor tolerance for boredom.

Lacks emotional attachment to others, even parents.

Displays preference for stimulation rather than isolation.

**Mood:** Adaptive to individual's intended goal, ranging from charming and pleasant to intense anger.

**Affect:** Emotional reactions may be erratic and extreme, with lack of concern for other people's feelings.

**Thought Processes:** Preoccupied with own interests, grandiose expressions of own importance; insight/judgment poor; impulsivity or failure to plan ahead.

### Safety

Experiences low level of autonomic arousal and responds to dangerous or painful stimuli with minimal anxiety.

Reckless disregard for safety of self/others.

### Sexuality

Early, aggressive, sexual acting-out behaviors.

### Social Interactions

Occurs most frequently in lower socioeconomic populations.

Family may be dysfunctional with little positive interaction; may be history of violence in the home.

Displays chronic antisocial behavior incompatible with the value system of general society, e.g., lying, stealing, fighting, frequent conflicts with the law, conning others for personal profit or pleasure.

Repeatedly violates the rights of others without remorse, i.e., is indifferent to or rationalizes behavior (thought to be without a conscience).

Rejects authority, has contempt for morality, does not learn from the past, and does not care about the future.

History often reveals significant impairment in social, marital, and occupational functioning (generally has poor employment history, fails to honor financial obligations).

## Teaching/Learning

More prevalent in males (onset occurring in childhood) than females (with onset at puberty).

History/evidence of conduct disorder with onset before age 15 with antisocial behaviors occurring since age 15 and usually diminishing after age 30, when the individual seems to "mellow out"/get tired of the situation.

Alcohol/substance abuse.

## DIAGNOSTIC STUDIES

**EEG:** Abnormally higher amounts of slow-wave activity, reflecting a possible deficit in inhibitory mechanisms, which may lessen impact of punishment.

**Aversive Stimuli:** Tends to be slower in learning to avoid shock, associated with a lower than normal level of physiologic arousal. Heightened ability to tune out aversive stimuli.

**Psychopathy Checklist:** Recently developed rating scale identifies 2 sets of characteristics (impulsiveness and instability; callousness, egocentricity, and limitation of capacity for anxiety) that are useful in predicting client outcome and likelihood of future violent crime activity.

**Drug Screen:** Determines substance use.

## NURSING PRIORITIES

1. Limit aggressive behavior; promote socially acceptable responses.
2. Develop a trusting relationship.
3. Assist client to learn healthy ways to deal with anxiety.
4. Increase sense of self-worth.
5. Promote development of alternate, constructive methods of interacting with others.

## DISCHARGE GOALS

1. Self-control is maintained.
2. Assertive behaviors are used to gain desired responses.
3. A trusting relationship initiated.
4. Anxiety is recognized and diminished/managed.
5. Client/family are involved in ongoing therapy/support groups.

| NURSING DIAGNOSIS: | VIOLENCE, HIGH RISK FOR, DIRECTED AT OTHERS |
|---|---|
| **Risk Factors May Include:** | Contempt for authority/rights of others (antisocial character). |
| | Inability to tolerate frustration; need for immediate gratification; easy agitation. |
| | Vulnerable self-esteem; inability to verbalize feelings. |
| | Use of maladjusted coping mechanisms including substance use. |
| | Negative role modeling; suspiciousness of others. |
| **Possible Indicators:** | Body language (muscle tension, facial expression, rigid posture); increased motor activity, irritability, agitation. |

|  | Hostile, threatening verbalizations (boasting of prior abuse of others); possession of destructive means. |
|---|---|
|  | Becoming assaultive when angry; choice of aggression to meet needs; overt and aggressive acts. |
|  | Substance abuse. |
| **Desired Outcomes/Evaluation Criteria— Client Will:** | Verbalize understanding of why behavior occurs, its consequences, and how it affects outcome(s). |
|  | Develop and use assertive/nonaggressive, socially acceptable behaviors to gratify needs and interact with others. |
|  | Demonstrate self-control as evidenced by relaxed posture and manner. |

| ACTIONS/INTERVENTIONS | RATIONALE |
|---|---|

### Independent

| | |
|---|---|
| Convey accepting attitude toward client. Work on development of trust. Be honest, keep all promises, and convey message that the behavior, not the client, is unacceptable. | Feelings of rejection are undoubtedly familiar to client. An attitude of acceptance promotes feelings of self-worth. Trust is the basis of a therapeutic relationship. Note: Major obstacles in working with the sociopath lie in an inherent inability to form a trusting, open relationship with a therapist. |
| Maintain low level of stimuli in client's environment (low lighting, few people, simple decor, low noise level). | A stimulating environment may increase agitation and promote aggressive behavior. |
| Provide structured environment, set firm limits, e.g., consistent schedule, ward rules, expectations of the client for cooperating. Involve client in process and follow through with consequences. | Sociopaths often function better in a controlled setting. Structure discourages escalation of aggressive behaviors and facilitates therapeutic intervention by reducing the anxiety caused by ambiguity. |
| Encourage verbalization of feelings and provide outlet for expression. | Increases client's self-awareness of feelings and stressors. |
| Help client identify the true object of his or her hostility (e.g., "You seem to be upset with . . ."). | Because of weak ego development, client may be misusing the defense mechanism of displacement. Helping client recognize this in a nonthreatening manner may help reveal unresolved issues so that they may be confronted. |
| Note distortions of the truth, manipulation. Confront client with these behaviors in a calm but firm manner, pointing out discrepancies in statements and behaviors. | Confronting unacceptable behaviors helps to increase client's awareness of own feelings and the effect these feelings and behaviors have on others. |
| Monitor escalating behaviors, e.g., increased psychomotor activity, threats, attempts to intimidate. Isolate if observed to be losing control. | Client can become dangerous very quickly with or without provocation. Early detection provides opportunity to alter behavior before violence occurs. |

431

| ACTIONS/INTERVENTIONS | RATIONALE |
|---|---|

### Independent

Be aware of prior history of violent behavior, seriousness of homicidal tendency, gestures, threats. (Use scale of 1–10 and prioritize according to severity of threat, availability of means.)

Therapist needs to be aware of client's style of acting out behaviors to provide a safe environment and protect client and others.

Remove all dangerous objects from client's environment, as appropriate.

Decreases availability of objects that can compromise safety of client/others.

Remain calm and nonaggressive in communicating with client. Avoid responding to client's verbal hostility with anger.

Anger is released through others. Not responding to client's anger breaks cycle, providing opportunity for change.

Assist client to identify when feelings of loss of control began and to identify events that led to this situation.

Recognition of these events provides an opportunity for resolution/adaptation of more effective behaviors. (Note: Sociopaths have often been victims of child abuse and need to deal with these feelings.)

Explore with client how aggressive, destructive behaviors have affected interpersonal relationships, e.g., with children, spouse, parents, peers.

Needs to realize own role and responsibility in personal interactions.

Discuss ways to detect potentially provocative/volatile situations before becoming involved. Help client learn to anticipate situations that usually result in anger, and develop a plan to handle anger before losing control.

Sociopaths tend to tune out aversive stimuli and need to increase awareness of environment to avoid becoming involved in volatile situations. Restructuring helps to eliminate old behavioral patterns that result in acting out. A plan of action provides client with a feeling of control.

Review with client the benefits of using assertive behaviors and the consequences of aggression. Ask client to identify situations when aggression was used and discuss alternate methods for handling those situations.

Consequences serve as the best motivation for changing behavior. Client needs a rehearsed plan of action to aid in handling situations differently.

Encourage client to engage in healthy outlets for anger, e.g., telling other person in an assertive manner, use of large motor skill activities/relaxation techniques.

Developing new ways of reacting is essential to breaking the maladaptive pattern of responding.

| NURSING DIAGNOSIS: | COPING, INDIVIDUAL, INEFFECTIVE |
|---|---|
| **May Be Related To:** | Very low tolerance for external stress. |
| | Lack of experience of internal anxiety such as guilt or shame. |
| | Personal vulnerability; unmet expectations; conflict; difficulty delaying gratification. |
| | Inadequate support systems. |
| | Multiple life changes. |

| Possibly Evidenced By: | Inability to cope, problem-solve; choice of aggression and manipulation to handle problems and conflicts. |
|---|---|
| | Inappropriate use of defense mechanisms (e.g., denial, projection). |
| | Chronic worry, anxiety, depression; poor self-esteem. |
| | High rate of accidents; destructive behavior toward self (substance use/abuse) or others. |
| Desired Outcomes/Evaluation Criteria—Client Will: | Identify maladaptive coping behaviors and consequences. |
| | Verbalize awareness of own positive coping abilities. |
| | Demonstrate increased tolerance for external stress and meet needs with assertive behaviors. |
| | Verbalize feelings congruent with behavior. |

| ACTIONS/INTERVENTIONS | RATIONALE |
|---|---|
| **Independent** | |
| Provide outlet for expression of feelings/concerns. Assist client to recognize anxiety by describing feeling states. | Individual needs to get in touch with own feelings, own them, and be responsible for them before he or she can begin to change behavior. Identifying sources of fears and anxieties increases understanding and self-awareness of feelings, which facilitates appropriate actions. |
| Assist to identify/recognize early warning signs of increased anxiety. | Establishing a plan in advance helps client, on becoming aware of feelings, to apply new skills that aid in controlling/reducing anxiety and impulsive actions. |
| Explore anxiety-producing situations. Help to formulate possible rationales for feelings. | Clarifying basis of anxious feelings may help eliminate unnecessary worry. Establishing a possible cause-effect relationship provides opportunity for insight. |
| Discuss present patterns of coping with feelings and effectiveness of these mechanisms. | Client needs to become aware that present patterns are self-destructive as well as harmful to others. |
| Investigate pattern of attempting to control environment through anger and intimidation and use of denial and projection. | Increases client's awareness of inappropriate mode of interaction and the consequences. |
| Provide information about constructive, effective coping strategies, e.g., discussing feelings with staff, running or jogging, relaxation techniques. | Client has likely not learned effective coping skills and needs information to begin to replace maladaptive skills/modify stressors. |
| Confront client with manipulative and intimidating behaviors when they occur. | Helps reinforce the need to stop this pattern. |
| Explore the implications/consequences of continuing antisocial activities. | Needs to be constantly aware of the direction life is taking and the effect these behaviors have on society and self. |

433

| ACTIONS/INTERVENTIONS | RATIONALE |
|---|---|

### Independent

| | |
|---|---|
| Discuss the importance of being responsible for own actions and not blaming others for own behaviors. | Sociopaths tend to externalize blame onto others and do not accept responsibility for own actions. |
| Give positive feedback when client demonstrates use of constructive alternatives. | Enhances self-esteem and reinforces acceptable behaviors. |
| Evaluate with client effectiveness of new behaviors and discuss modifications. | If client's new methods of coping are not working, assistance will be needed to reassess and develop new strategies. |
| Discuss fears or anxieties of others' responses to client's new behaviors and feelings concerning these responses. | Gives client a sense of what might be expected from others to help alleviate fears. |
| Encourage participation in unit activities, groups, outdoor education program (e.g., hiking, wall/rock climbing, caving). | Interaction with others provides opportunities for client to begin to experience success, feel good about self, get needs met in positive ways. |
| Acknowledge difficulties of therapy and slow progress. Discuss likelihood of discouragement and ways to deal with these feelings. | Difficulty in developing therapeutic relationship, degree of impairment, and need for total life restructuring require prolonged intervention. |

| | |
|---|---|
| **NURSING DIAGNOSIS:** | **SELF-ESTEEM, CHRONIC LOW** |
| **May Be Related To:** | Lack of positive feedback; repeated negative feedback. |
| | Unmet dependency needs; retarded ego development. |
| | Dysfunctional family system. |
| **Possibly Evidenced By:** | Acting-out behaviors, such as excessive use of alcohol and other drugs, sexual promiscuity. |
| | Feelings of inadequacy/diminished self-worth; inability (difficulty) accepting positive reinforcement. |
| | Nonparticipation in therapy. |
| **Desired Outcomes/Evaluation Criteria— Client Will:** | Acknowledge self as an individual who has responsibility for own actions. |
| | Verbalize a sense of worthwhileness. |
| | Make healthy choices regarding management of/be involved in meeting own care needs. Demonstrate prosocial functioning. |
| | Recognize and incorporate change into self-concept in accurate manner without negating self-esteem. |

| ACTIONS/INTERVENTIONS | RATIONALE |
| --- | --- |

### Independent

Encourage verbalization of feelings of inadequacy, worthlessness, fear of rejection, and need for acceptance from others.

Client may relate acting-out behaviors to a poor self-concept, and acceptance of reality of own behaviors in relation to others' reactions can assist decision to change.

Assist client to identify positive aspects about self related to social skills, work abilities, education, talents, and appearance.

Helps to build on positive aspects of personality and use them to improve self-concept.

Provide clear, consistent, verbal/nonverbal communication. Be truthful and honest.

Client's perception is keen and can instantly detect insincerity.

Explore the relationship between feelings of inadequacy and aggressive behaviors, use of drugs, sexual promiscuity.

Provides opportunity for client to understand relationship between low self-esteem and ineffective measures taken to "feel" better.

Discuss how companions are chosen. Ask if these people reinforce client's own antisocial activities/values.

Aids client to see how much peers can influence thinking and thereby reinforce antisocial behavior.

Ask client to describe interpersonal relationships, their quality and depth. If relationships are superficial, discuss how this came about.

Sociopaths have great difficulty forming close relationships. Perhaps exploring early relationships with parents or siblings may provide insight into the problem.

Review ways to improve the quality of interaction with others.

Learning to recognize/respect feelings of others in relation to own helps client to develop more satisfactory relationships.

Assist client in identifying positive aspects of the self and in developing ways to change the characteristics that are socially unacceptable.

Individuals with low self-esteem often have difficulty recognizing their positive attributes. They may also lack problem-solving ability and require assistance to formulate a plan for implementing the desired changes.

Minimize negative feedback to client. Enforce limit-setting in a matter-of-fact manner, imposing previously established consequences for violations.

Negative feedback can be extremely threatening to a person with low self-esteem, possibly aggravating the problem. Consequences should convey unacceptability of the behavior but not of the person.

Encourage independence in the performance of personal responsibilities and in decision-making related to own self-care. Offer recognition and praise for accomplishments.

Positive reinforcement enhances self-esteem and encourages repetition of desirable behaviors.

Provide instruction about assertiveness techniques, especially the ability to recognize the difference between passive, assertive, and aggressive behaviors and the importance of respecting the human rights of others while protecting one's own basic human rights.

These techniques increase self-esteem while enhancing the ability to form satisfactory interpersonal relationships.

Identify individual goals for therapy and activities to enhance feelings of success and self-esteem.

Focusing on practical realities helps the client to move ahead step by step.

435

| NURSING DIAGNOSIS: | FAMILY COPING, ineffective: compromised/disabling |
|---|---|
| **May Be Related To:** | Temporary family disorganization and role changes. |
| | Client providing little support in turn for the primary person. |
| | Prolonged disability progression that exhausts the supportive capacity of significant people. |
| | Highly ambivalent family relationships. |
| **Possibly Evidenced By:** | Expressions of concern or complaint about significant other's response to client's problem. |
| | Significant person reporting preoccupation with personal reactions regarding condition. |
| | Significant person displaying protective behavior disproportionate (too little or too much) to client's abilities or need for autonomy. |
| **Desired Outcomes/Evaluation Criteria— Family Will:** | Identify/verbalize resources within individual members to deal with the situation. |
| | Interact appropriately with the client/each other, providing support and assistance as indicated. |
| | Provide opportunity for client to deal with situation in own way. |
| | Express feelings openly and honestly. |

| ACTIONS/INTERVENTIONS | RATIONALE |
|---|---|
| **Independent** | |
| Identify behaviors/interactions of family members. Note factors affecting abilities of family members to provide needed support. | Provides information about patterns within family and whether they are helpful to resolution of current problems. Personality disorder/mental illness of other family members inhibits coping abilities. |
| Listen to client/significant others' comments and expressions of concern, noting nonverbal behaviors and/or responses. | Provides clues to underlying feelings, unconscious motivations/defenses. |
| Discuss basis for client's behavior(s). | Helps family begin to understand and accept/deal with unacceptable actions. |
| Assist family and client to understand "who owns the problem" and who is responsible for resolution. | When each individual begins to assume responsibility for own actions, each one can begin to problem-solve without expectation that someone else will take care of him or her. |
| Encourage free expression of feelings, including frustration, anger, hostility, and hopelessness. | Expression of feelings can be the beginning of recognition and resolution of short-/long-term problems. |

## ACTIONS/INTERVENTIONS

### Independent

Assist family members to identify coping skills being used and how these skills are/are not helping them to deal with the situation.

### Collaborative

Refer to additional resources as needed, e.g., family therapy, financial counseling, spiritual.

## RATIONALE

Identification of what is helpful and what is not will allow for learning new ways to cope with behaviors/situation.

May need further assistance to help with resolution of current/long-term problems.

| NURSING DIAGNOSIS: | SOCIAL INTERACTION, IMPAIRED |
|---|---|
| May Be Related To: | Factors contributing to the absence of satisfying personal relationships, e.g., inadequate personal resources (shallow feelings), immature interests, underdeveloped conscience, unaccepted social values. |
| Possibly Evidenced By: | Difficulty meeting expectations of others; lack of belief that rules pertain to them. |
| | Sense of emptiness/inadequacy covered up by expressions of self-conceit, arrogance, and contempt. |
| | Behavior unaccepted by dominant cultural group. |
| Desired Outcomes/Evaluation Criteria— Client Will: | Identify causes and actions to correct isolation. |
| | Express increased sense of self-worth. |
| | Participate willingly in activities/programs without use of manipulation. |
| | Demonstrate behavior congruent with verbal expressions. |

## ACTIONS/INTERVENTIONS

### Independent

Note expressions of hopelessness/worthlessness, e.g., "I'm a loser," "It's fate."

Listen to expressions of feelings and "insight," pointing out discrepancies between what is said versus behaviors.

## RATIONALE

These may be the only genuine emotions this individual feels and may be expressed in subtle ways when failures can no longer be denied. Although these feelings may be dismissed quickly, this may be the time when the client is most accessible to change.

Client may be very good at saying what others want to hear. However, behavior is the ultimate determinant of real change. It is almost impossible for this person to understand the feelings of others.

437

### Independent

Confront expressions of powerlessness, inability to control situation/make difference in relationships/commitments.

Consistent confrontation with reality of how client's behavior affects interactions with and trust of others may force client to begin to look at own responsibility for problems in these areas. This person's refusal to accept criticism and/or projection of failure as the fault of others make it difficult to change behavior.

Encourage client to make requests/ask for what is wanted in a clear, straightforward manner and express feelings clearly to others.

As needs are met by direct action, client may begin to see the value of this approach.

Explore client's need for immediate gratification. Ask client to describe feelings when someone says "no."

Client needs to understand own feelings in order to work on resolution.

Review with client feelings regarding authority and violating rights of others.

Client often experiences pleasure through antisocial behaviors and needs to gain insight regarding personal motives.

Discuss with client thoughts and fantasies present before committing crimes. Ascertain how much planning went into the crimes. Did the client "experience" the crime "mentally" before commission?

Antisocial behavior may lead to involvement in criminal activity. Fantasizing about crime plays a large role in eventual commission. In order to restructure cognitive processes, client needs to break this pattern.

Have client discuss thoughts/feelings about family, peers, authority figures, opposite sex, violence, and victims. Give feedback on the "correctness" of thinking process.

Reinforces positive values or attitudes and exposes problem areas in thinking process. This is important for cognitive restructuring.

Help client recognize behaviors that do not get intended response and discuss possible modifications.

Sociopaths have difficulty interpreting others' feelings and need guidance in this area.

### Collaborative

Involve in group activities, e.g., occupational/vocational therapy, psychotherapy, outdoor education program, codependency meetings.

Provides opportunity for interaction with others to learn new behaviors, gain support for change.

# BORDERLINE PERSONALITY DISORDER

## DSM IV
301.83 Borderline Personality Disorder

## DSM III-R
301.83 Borderline Personality Disorder

The term "borderline" has been used to identify clients who seem to fall on the border between the standard categories of neuroses or psychoses. It has been refined to indicate a client with a pervasive pattern of instability of interpersonal relationships, self-image, affect, and control over impulses beginning in early adulthood, and includes such factors as feelings of abandonment, impulsivity, reactivity of mood, chronic feelings of emptiness, and problems with anger.

## ETIOLOGIC THEORIES
### Psychodynamics

Unconscious processes that are believed to shape personality are set in motion by drives or instincts that are then influenced by conflicts among them as well as instinctual wishes and demands of reality. Defensive maneuvers are unconsciously developed to protect against anxiety arising from this conflict. This personality is seen as a painstaking but poorly constructed defense.

It is also seen as resulting from a fixation of libido at stages of psychosexual development associated with certain body parts. Although it is difficult to agree on how personality is formed, it is believed that severe personality disorders do begin early in childhood and that milder forms are influenced by factors during later development.

### Biologic

Personality is believed to have a hereditary basis known as "temperament" and biologic dispositions that affect mood and level of activity, e.g., cranky, placid, self-contained, outgoing, impulsive, cautious. There is little agreement about how this affects the development of personality disorders.

### Family Dynamics

The social environment of the child, particularly the family, is assumed to be the main force that shapes personality. The theory of object relations provides a basis for personality development and an explanation of the dynamics that manifest the borderline characteristics. It has been suggested that the individual with borderline personality is fixed in the rapprochement phase of development (18–25 months of age). In this phase the child is experiencing increasing autonomy, while still requiring "emotional refueling" from the mothering figure. The mother feels threatened by the child's efforts at independence, so strives to keep the child dependent. Nurturing and emotional support become bargaining tools. They are withheld when the child exhibits independent behaviors and used as rewards for clinging, dependent behaviors. This engenders a deep fear of abandonment in the child that persists into adulthood as the child continues to view objects (people) as parts, either good or bad. This is called splitting, which is the primary dynamic of borderline personality.

Current studies suggest that borderline personality disorders are strongly associated with a history of physical or sexual abuse by family members, and incest may be a major reason for the disproportionate ratio (2:1) of female clients.

## CLIENT ASSESSMENT DATABASE

### Ego Integrity

Markedly disturbed/distorted sense of self.

Experiences ambivalence toward being independent; does not like to be alone (frantic attempts to avoid real or imagined abandonment).

Reports feelings of emptiness and boredom; depression, sadness.

May conform to current companions, sharing beliefs and values based on imitation.

### Food/Fluid

Binge eating may be reported (impulsivity).

### Neurosensory

**Mental Status:**

**Behavior:** May be erratic, impulsive, intense, clinging; may indulge in unpredictable/impulsive behaviors, e.g., irresponsible spending, reckless driving, gambling, substance abuse.

**Mood:** Marked reactivity of mood (e.g., intense episodes of anxiety, irritability, dysphoria).

**Emotions:** Intense emotions with rapid, unpredictable, strong mood swings; quick to anger (may be intense, inappropriate), lacks ability to control; may exhibit hostile attitude.

**Affect:** May appear genuine but not necessarily appropriate to the situation.

**Thought Processes:** Displays overall poor reality base with difficulty making decisions; engages in concrete "all or nothing"/black or white thinking; lacks insight and does not learn from past experience; unable to form long-term goals or values.

> Magical thinking, difficulty in identifying the self occur; severely impaired self-concept.
>
> Lying and fabrication habitual, almost delusional.
>
> Self-centered, often to the point of narcissism, inordinately hypersensitive, and inflexible; relationships may be transient, shallow and/or demanding, with little flexibility and unstable interpersonal behavior; may use and exploit others; lacks empathy for others.
>
> Major defense mechanism used is projection (seeing in others those attitudes one fails to see in self).
>
> May border on neuroses and psychoses, exhibiting transient psychotic symptoms when experiencing extreme stress; transient episodes of paranoid ideation or severe dissociative symptoms.
>
> May be associated with other personality disorders that have histrionic, narcissitic, schizotypal, or antisocial features.

### Safety

May reveal evidence of self-mutilative acts (nonlethal actions), e.g., cutting, burning.

History of recurrent suicidal behavior, gestures, threats.

### Sexuality

May present a profound disturbance in gender identity.

Sexual promiscuity.

Possible history of incest/sexual abuse.

### Social Interactions

Significant impairment in social, marital, and occupational functioning; interpersonal relationships unstable and intense, alternate between extremes of overidealization and devaluation; often attempts to provoke guilt in others, makes endless demands.

History of recurrent physical fights.

## Teaching/Learning

More prevalent in females.

Substance abuse (especially alcohol) may be reported.

Higher incidence found in families with history of both chronic schizophrenia and major affective disorders.

## DIAGNOSTIC STUDIES

**P-300** (a change in brain electrical activity that occurs in most people about 300 milliseconds after they perceive a tone, light, or other signal indicating that they have to perform a task): May be abnormal, smaller than average, and slightly delayed.

**CSF5-HIAA (5-Hydroxyindoleacetic Acid):** Decreased in some clients.

**Prolacting Response:** Diminished response to serotonin releaser fenfuramine.

**Drug Screen:** Identifies substance use.

## NURSING PRIORITIES

1. Limit aggressive behavior; promote socially acceptable responses.
2. Encourage assertive behaviors to attain sense of control.
3. Assist client to learn healthy ways of controlling anxiety/developing positive self-concept.
4. Promote development of effective coping skills.
5. Assist client to learn alternate, constructive methods of interacting with others.

## DISCHARGE GOALS

1. Impulsive behavior(s) recognized and controlled.
2. Establishing goals and asserting control over own life.
3. Problem-solving techniques are used constructively to resolve conflicts.
4. Interacting with others in socially appropriate manner.
5. Client/family involved in behavioral therapy/support programs.

| NURSING DIAGNOSIS: | VIOLENCE, HIGH RISK FOR, DIRECTED AT SELF/OTHERS/SELF-MUTILATION, HIGH RISK FOR |
|---|---|
| **Risk Factors May Include:** | Use of projection as a major defense mechanism. |
| | Pervasive problem with negative transference. |
| | Feelings of guilt/need to "punish" self; distorted sense of self. |
| | Inability to cope with increased psychologic/physiologic tension in a healthy manner. |
| **Possible Indicators:** | Vulnerable self-esteem. |
| | Easily agitated, angry when frustrated (may become assaultive). |
| | Provocative behavior: argumentative, dissatisfied, overreactive, hypersensitive; use of unprovoked anger, hostility toward others. |
| | Choice of maladjusted ways of getting needs met (e.g., splitting, projection, provocation, depression). |

| **Desired Outcomes/Evaluation Criteria— Client Will:** | Self-mutilative acts; substance abuse. |
| --- | --- |
| | Verbalize understanding of why behavior occurs. |
| | Recognize precipitating factors. |
| | Demonstrate self-control, using appropriate, assertive coping skills. |
| | Clarify feelings of negative transference and eliminate the use of projection. |

| ACTIONS/INTERVENTIONS | RATIONALE |
| --- | --- |

### Independent

| | |
| --- | --- |
| Establish therapeutic nurse/client relationship. Maintain a firm, consistent approach. | Building rapport and trust is imperative, although difficult, for this client. |
| Determine negative transference feelings and clarify the actual source of anger, hostility. | Heightens self-awareness of these feelings to assist with resolution. |
| Assist to identify how much anger is "elicited" by significant other(s) and how much results from own unresolved feelings. | Becoming aware of the use of projection helps to break this maladjusted pattern. Note: Feelings of anger and hostility, not depression, are more often the basis for destructive behaviors/suicidal acts. |
| Intervene immediately in a nondefensive manner when acting out occurs. Set firm, consistent limits. | Intervention is critical to prevent dangerous situation for either client or others. Therapeutic milieu helps client to manage self and develop self-control. Environmental safety provides external control until internal control is regained. |
| Make an agreement or "no harm" contract to discuss angry or hurt feelings when they begin instead of "internalizing" and displacing anger/hurt onto others and acting on the feelings. | Agreeing not to engage in violent behaviors involving self, others, or property promotes safety and enhances feelings of self-worth by having client assume control of own behavior. Helps client learn to work through feelings as they occur to prevent intensification and promote resolution. |
| Encourage client to evaluate situations in which angry feelings develop. Is the amount of anger appropriate to the actual event? | Needs to listen to recognize/assess inappropriate, unwarranted anger directed at others. |
| Explore what client expects from others, and self, in interpersonal relationships. | Assists client to learn to define roles and recognize own responsibility in the situation. |
| Define expectations and rules of the situation clearly, and state what the client can/cannot do. | Structure reduces ambiguity and anxiety, providing sense of security and minimizing escalation of violent behavior. |
| Determine prior suicidal gestures/attempts. Evaluate seriousness of suicidal expressions/ideation. Use scale of 1–10 and prioritize according to seriousness of threat, availability of means, timing of previous attempts, current age. | It is important to take suicidal threats seriously, listening carefully to underlying messages and providing a safe environment to prevent client from following through on plan, especially when scale is in upper range. Note: Risk of suicide completion is highest during first few years after initial presentation, declining as client ages. |

| ACTIONS/INTERVENTIONS | RATIONALE |
|---|---|

### Independent

| | |
|---|---|
| Provide close supervision as indicated. | Allows for early recognition of escalating behavior and timely intervention. |
| Note substance use/withdrawal. (Refer to Ch. 6, specific plan of care as appropriate.) | Substance use, especially alcohol, increases likelihood of suicide 6-fold. |
| Provide care for client's wounds, if self-mutilation occurs, in a matter-of-fact manner. Do not offer sympathy or provide additional attention. | Additional attention and sympathy can provide positive reinforcement for the maladaptive behavior and may encourage its repetition. A matter-of-fact attitude can convey empathy/concern. |

### Collaborative

| | |
|---|---|
| Have client participate in group therapy sessions with feedback given by peers. | Group setting aids in promoting diffusion of anger; provides insight as to how negative, aggressive behaviors affect others, making feedback easier to digest. |
| Support substance withdrawal. Refer to support group, e.g., Alcohol/Narcotics Anonymous, etc. | Provides assistance to enable client to maintain abstinence. |
| Administer medication as indicated, e.g., carbamazepine (Tegretol), tranylcypromine (Parnate). | May reduce frequency of impulsive/self-destructive acts while other therapeutic interventions are initiated. |

| | |
|---|---|
| **NURSING DIAGNOSIS:** | **ANXIETY [severe to panic]** |
| **May Be Related To:** | Unconscious conflicts (experience of extreme stress). |
| | Perceived threat to self-concept; unmet needs. |
| **Possibly Evidenced By:** | Easy frustration and feelings of hurt. |
| | Abuse of alcohol/other drugs. |
| | Transient psychotic symptoms (disorganized thinking; misinterpretation of environment, interference with ability to think clearly and logically). |
| | Performing self-mutilating acts. |
| **Desired Outcomes/Evaluation Criteria— Client Will:** | Verbalize awareness of feelings of anxiety and healthy ways to deal with them. |
| | Recognize warning signs of increasing anxiety and validate perceptions before drawing conclusions. |
| | Develop and implement effective methods for decreasing anxiety. |
| | Report anxiety reduced to manageable level. |
| | Use resources effectively. |

| ACTIONS/INTERVENTIONS | RATIONALE |
|---|---|

### Independent

| | |
|---|---|
| Maintain open communication and provide consistency of care. | Provides for accurate information and reduces anxiety. |
| Assess escalating anxiety and observe client contact with reality, e.g., presence/development of psychotic symptoms, delusions/hallucinations, disorganized thinking, confusion, altered communication patterns. (Refer to CP: Delusional Disorder.) | Underlying feelings of worthlessness, inadequacy, powerlessness can lead to increasing anxiety with resultant inability to think clearly. |
| Note rapid changes in behavior, e.g., from cooperative to angry, demanding, argumentative. | Need for immediate gratification can lead to frustration and changes in behavior, which may indicate loss of touch with reality. |
| Monitor for substance use; note physical symptoms of abuse, e.g., slurred speech, mood swings, dilated/constricted pupils, abnormal vital signs, needle marks. | May cloud symptomatology, potentiate erratic behavior, and interfere with progress, requiring therapeutic intervention. |
| Provide information in brief, clear, calm manner. | Specific instructions and expectations about what is happening help client maintain contact with reality. |
| Maintain calm, quiet, nonstimulating environment. | Auditory and visual stimulation may increase labile affect and potential for acting out. |
| Correct misinterpretations of environment as expressed by the client. | Confronting misinterpretations honestly, with a caring and accepting attitude, provides a therapeutic orientation to reality and preserves client's feelings of dignity and self-worth. |
| Encourage client to identify events that precipitate stress/anxious feelings; e.g., real or anticipated anxiety about relationships with others. | Helps to establish a cause-effect relationship, enhancing awareness and promoting change. |
| Explore how client has dealt with these feelings, including times when substances were taken to relieve tension, anxiety. | Provides an understanding of the relationship between anxiety and drug use. |
| Have client keep an "anger journal" describing when anger occurs, how it is handled, and outcome of situation. | When reviewed periodically with primary nurse/therapist, can provide insight into development of feelings, effectiveness of response and create opportunity to develop new coping strategies. |
| Assist in learning to identify early warning signs that anxiety is escalating and request intervention before it becomes overwhelming. | Promotes development of internal control. |
| Ask client to describe events/feelings preceding cutting or hurting self. Explore ways to relieve anxiety without self-damaging acts. (Refer to ND: Violence, high risk for, directed at self/others/Self-Mutilation, high risk for.) | Provides knowledge for adapting new effective coping skills and breaking the pattern of self-destructive acts. |
| Identify constructive ways of releasing tension, e.g., jogging, talking with nurse/therapist, use of relaxation/imagery techniques, involvement in outdoor education programs, e.g., hiking, wall/rock climbing, caving. | Client needs to learn constructive methods of coping to replace the maladjusted behaviors that have been used. |

| ACTIONS/INTERVENTIONS | RATIONALE |
|---|---|

### Independent

Discuss fears involving interactions with parents, spouse, children, or significant other(s).

Knowledge of specific fear may provide insight into problem areas.

Encourage client to develop a relationship with more than 1 person.

Helps client to achieve object constancy. Client may feel abandoned when therapist leaves and have a feeling that the person ceases to exist. Dependency can be avoided, and client can begin to develop independent activities in this atmosphere.

### Collaborative

Administer medications as indicated:
   antipsychotics, e.g., haloperidol (Haldol), thio-thixine (Navene), thioridazine (Mellaril);

May help reduce anxiety, hostility, ideas of reference, illusions, increasing receptiveness to other therapeutic approaches.

   antidepressants.

A number of agents have been used with varying success to help alleviate symptoms of severe depression.

| NURSING DIAGNOSIS: | SELF-ESTEEM DISTURBANCE/PERSONAL IDENTITY DISTURBANCE |
|---|---|
| **May Be Related To:** | Lack of positive feedback; unmet dependency needs. |
| | Retarded ego development/fixation at an earlier level of development. |
| **Possibly Evidenced By:** | Difficulty identifying self or defining self-boundaries; feelings of depersonalization, derealization. |
| | Extreme mood changes; lack of tolerance of rejection or being alone. |
| | Unhappiness with self, striking out at others. |
| | Peformance of ritualistic, self-damaging acts, such as "cutting veins and watching the blood flow to cleanse the soul"; belief that punishing self is necessary. |
| **Desired Outcomes/Evaluation Criteria— Client Will:** | Verbalize a sense of worthwhileness. |
| | Demonstrate increased self-worth/respect with reduction in punishing/mutilative behaviors. |
| | Use 1 self-image to promote good interpersonal relationships. |

465

| ACTIONS/INTERVENTIONS | RATIONALE |
|---|---|
| **Independent** | |
| Encourage client to describe and verbalize feelings about self. | Aids in assessing in which areas negative feelings are most intense. |
| Provide safe, supportive environment to discuss issues of abuse/incest and ownership of behaviors. (Refer to CP: Problems Related to Abuse or Neglect.) | Studies suggest a high percentage of these clients may be victims of physical/sexual abuse, which is a significant factor in the development of the disorder. Failure to address these issues potentiates continued problems with relationships and self-destructive acts. |
| Explore need to punish self. When did this begin, and what events precipitated these acts? | May help to establish a cause-effect relationship. |
| Discuss what stressors usually bring on anger/depression. Explore ways to deal with feelings before they become overwhelming. | Information can be used to learn and implement effective methods to prevent onset of depression, destructive acts. |
| Note attitude of superiority, arrogant behaviors, exaggerated sense of self, resentment, and anger. | Indicative of attempt to compensate for feelings of worthlessness, inadequacy, and powerlessness. |
| Note personality traits such as extreme shyness, chaotic impulsiveness, chronic irascibility, antisocial tendencies, refusal of treatment for substance abuse. | Research suggests these traits are associated with poor outcomes. Recognition of this provides opportunity to deal with these issues, possibly influencing therapeutic efforts in a positive manner to improve individual response. |
| Encourage client to verbalize feelings of insecurity and need for constant reassurance from others. | Provides insight into sources of insecurities. |
| Discuss feelings of worthlessness and how these feelings relate to need for acceptance by others. | Gives client the message that life cannot be spent trying to meet others' expectations. |
| Identify situations in which client pushed others away. Help client to look at reality of behavior in context of this situation. | Pattern of relationships has often been one of approach-avoidance conflicts characterized by intense feelings, crises, and stormy episodes. Fearing engulfment, client pushes others away, then, fearing abandonment, tries to draw them back in. Awareness of this pattern of behavior and underlying dynamics provides opportunity for change. |
| Identify positive, realistic behaviors the client possesses. | Helps client begin to look at possibility of making desired changes to meet needs in a more satisfying way. |
| Give feedback regarding nonverbal behaviors. | Increases awareness of the possibility of double messages that client may be giving. |
| Encourage increased sense of responsibility for own behaviors. | Use of projection has enabled client to blame others for own problems/consequences of behavior. |
| Define sexual identity and what areas create confusion, fears. | Helps to assess possible knowledge deficit or which direction to take in alleviating anxiety. |
| Assess knowledge of human sexuality and supply needed information. | Provides information appropriate to learning needs. |

| NURSING DIAGNOSIS: | POWERLESSNESS |
|---|---|
| May Be Related To: | Lifestyle of helplessness; need for control (history of abuse/incest as a child). |
| Possibly Evidenced By: | Becoming enraged and hurt. |
| | Manipulative behavior; self-centered and hyper-sensitive attitude. |
| | Provoking guilt in others; making endless demands; using and exploiting others. |
| | Ambivalence toward being independent; alternating clinging and distancing behaviors. |
| Desired Outcomes/Evaluation Criteria— Client Will: | Express sense of control over present situation and future outcome. |
| | Develop a sense of being in charge of own life. |
| | Interact with others without abusing or violating their rights. |
| | Make choices related to and be involved in care. |

## ACTIONS/INTERVENTIONS

### Independent

Develop alliance with the client and assist to overcome fear of closeness and intimacy.

Identify behaviors used to gain control of others, e.g., manipulation, attempts to influence, intimidate.

Explore areas of life in which client is feeling inadequate or having no control.

Encourage verbalization of how feelings of anger, hurt, and loss of control relate to desire to strike out at others.

Confront inconsistencies in statements; discuss what needs these statements serve.

Recognize client manipulations and respond differently.

Provide opportunities to learn how to get needs met in an acceptable, truthful way.

Ask to discuss feelings about someone in life who seems self-centered. Compare behaviors.

## RATIONALE

This individual is generally frightened by close relationships; an alliance demonstrates that it is possible to trust. Note: Evidence indicates incest/physical abuse in childhood are strongly associated with a poor outcome and high rates of suicide/violent crime.

Increases awareness of modes of interaction that are used to get own way and feel in control of the situation.

Provides insight into feelings that are necessary for learning adaptive behaviors.

Enhances understanding of how the use of projection has become a pervasive pattern.

Reinforces that lying and manipulation are maladaptive and lead to feelings of low self-esteem.

Redirection stops the manipulation, allowing for straight, congruent communication.

Promotes inner strength and adaptive functioning.

By comparing behaviors, client may understand how others perceive self-centeredness and the feelings about these behaviors.

| ACTIONS/INTERVENTIONS | RATIONALE |
|---|---|

### Independent

| | |
|---|---|
| Assist client to learn to listen to others and consider their feelings by putting self in their place. | Promotes feelings of empathy for others. |
| Encourage client to participate in developing treatment plan. | Aids in promoting a sense of control over life and helps client assume greater responsibility for own life. |
| Role-play behaviors, e.g., appropriate anger, admitting mistakes, shared humor. | Avoiding angry confrontations, maintaining sense of humor help client learn new ways of control. |

| NURSING DIAGNOSIS: | COPING, INDIVIDUAL, INEFFECTIVE |
|---|---|
| **May Be Related To:** | Use of maladjusted defense mechanisms (e.g., projection, denial, externalizing). |
| | Chronic feelings of emptiness, boredom. |
| | Repetitive use of ineffective coping strategies. |
| **Possibly Evidenced By:** | Inability to cope, problem-solve, or ask for assistance. |
| | Not learning from previous experiences. |
| | Inappropriate use of defense mechanisms (e.g., projection, manipulation). |
| | Relief of anxiety through destructive acts (sexual promiscuity, impulsive spending, gambling, substance abuse). |
| **Desired Outcomes/Evaluation Criteria— Client Will:** | Identify ineffective coping behaviors and consequences. |
| | Verbalize awareness of own coping abilities. |
| | Meet psychologic needs as evidenced by appropriate expression of feelings, identification of options, and effective use of resources. |
| | Verbalize feelings congruent with behavior. |

| ACTIONS/INTERVENTIONS | RATIONALE |
|---|---|

### Independent

| | |
|---|---|
| Ask client to describe present coping patterns and their consequences. | Identifies which defenses are maladjusted, ineffective, and destructive in order to effect change. |
| Have client identify problems and perceptions of their cause. | Exposes problem areas in thinking process and possible cognitive distortions. |
| Promote development of effective ways to deal with stress, anger, frustration. | Client will need help in learning new behaviors, e.g., acceptable expression of anger, "I-messages." |

| ACTIONS/INTERVENTIONS | RATIONALE |
|---|---|

## Independent

Develop with/have client sign a behavioral contract to include minimum standards of acceptable behaviors, management of anger.

Fosters collaborative relationship between client and nurse that can be generalized to others as progress is made. Encourages client to assume control of own behavior and, as specified outcomes are achieved, enhances sense of self-worth and encourages repetition of successful behaviors.

Discuss ways of dismissing feelings of boredom and assist client to understand that these feelings can be controlled.

Client needs to get in touch with own feelings and own/be responsible for them before they can be resolved.

Be aware of attempts to split staff. Avoid manipulative games and be consistent in dealing with the client.

Staff splitting can be a major problem. Client may behave in one way (quiet/cooperative) with some staff and in another way (angry/demanding) with others.

Confront manipulative and other maladaptive behaviors.

Consistent confrontation removes the reward and reinforces need for the client to adopt new behavior and to stop directing anger at others. Consistency in approach provides a stable environment and reinforces sense of trust.

Give feedback on how effectively client is handling situations and discuss suggestions for improvement.

May need assistance and guidance in modifying behaviors that are not working.

Give positive feedback when client demonstrates use of appropriate, constructive behaviors.

Reinforces use of positive techniques, enhances self-esteem.

Evaluate antisocial behaviors and resulting problems. (Refer to CP: Antisocial Personality.)

Destructive behaviors may lead to legal involvements and other problems in which client needs to learn new behaviors.

Encourage client to discuss issues related to family. Involve family in therapeutic process when possible.

High incidence of incest/physical abuse is associated with the diagnosis of borderline personality disorder. Additionally, clients whose families accept and support them demonstrate more positive outcomes.

## Collaborative

Involve entire team in planning and evaluating care.

When team is committed to a single approach and information is shared by all, issues of splitting and countertransference can be minimized.

| NURSING DIAGNOSIS: | SOCIAL ISOLATION |
|---|---|
| May Be Related To: | Immature interests; unaccepted social behavior. |
| | Inadequate personal resources. |
| | Inability to engage in satisfying personal relationships. |
| Possibly Evidenced By: | Alternating clinging and distancing behaviors. |
| | Difficulty meeting expectations of others. |

449

| **Desired Outcomes/Evaluation Criteria— Client Will:** | Experiencing feelings of difference from others. |
| | Expressed interests inappropriate to developmental age. |
| | Exhibiting behavior unaccepted by dominant cultural group (including sexual promiscuity). |
| | Identify causes and actions to correct isolation. |
| | Verbalize willingness to be involved with others. |
| | Participate in activities at level of desire. |
| | Express increased sense of self-worth. |

| ACTIONS/INTERVENTIONS | RATIONALE |
|---|---|
| **Independent** | |
| Determine presence of factors contributing to sense/choice of isolation. | Identification of individual factors allows for developing appropriate plan of care/interventions. |
| Differentiate isolation from solitude and aloneness. | The latter are acceptable or by choice, and this differentiation helps client to identify which is applicable to self so steps to deal with problem can be taken. |
| Let client know the nurse will not abandon the client. | Client is often fearful that the therapist will become angry or discouraged and give up. |
| Ask client to identify significant other(s) with whom client can talk. If there is no one, ascertain how this came about. | Aids in seeing a pattern of interaction that is ineffectual. |
| Examine guilt feelings involving significant other(s). Discuss how these feelings occurred. | May have unrealistic guilt feelings that need resolution before work on the relationship can begin. |
| Discuss/define fears about being alone. Develop a schedule to "practice" being alone a few minutes each day, gradually increasing the time. | Provides knowledge for developing adaptive coping skills and desensitizes person to feelings of anxiety. |
| Identify how fears, anxieties have affected quality and depth of interpersonal relationships. | Reinforces a sense that projection does indeed cripple relationships. |
| Develop a plan of action with client, e.g., look at available resources, support risk-taking behaviors. | Structure of a plan with support of a trusted person helps client to try out new behaviors. |
| Discuss ways to identify and confront inappropriate behaviors. Talk about how others may respond to these behaviors and suggest ways in which client can deal with them. Use role-play to practice new skills. | When plan is agreed on, client is involved and willing to look at behaviors that create problems in relationships. Provides a beginning to develop more appropriate ways to interact with others. |
| Encourage client to identify positive, realistic behaviors currently being used. | As client recognizes that there are already some positive behaviors to build on, self-confidence will be enhanced, and client may be willing to take more risks. |
| **Collaborative** | |
| Encourage involvement in classes/group therapy, e.g., assertiveness, vocational, sex education; psychotherapy. | Provides opportunity to learn social skills, enhance sense of self-esteem, and promote appropriate social involvement. |

450

# PERSONALITY DISORDER NOS: Passive-Aggressive Personality Disorder

## DSM IV
301.9 Personality Disorder NOS

## DSM III-R
301.84 Passive-Aggressive Personality Disorder

A pervasive pattern of passive resistance, expressed indirectly rather than directly to demands for adequate social/occupational performance.

## ETIOLOGIC THEORIES

### Psychodynamics

These clients are unaware that ongoing difficulties are the result of own behaviors. They experience conscious hostility toward authority figures but do not connect own passive-resistant behaviors with hostility or resentment. They do not trust others, are not assertive, are intentionally inefficient, and try to get back at others through aggravation. Anger and hostility are released through others, who become angry and may suffer because of the inefficiencies. This disorder can lead to more serious psychologic dysfunctions such as major depression, dysthymic disorder, and alcohol and other drug abuse/dependence.

These behaviors are not disturbing to the client but are to those in the environment who interact with the client. Therapy is not usually sought, but client is generally referred by family members.

### Biologic

Personality disturbance is attributed to constitutional abnormalities. It is suggested that there is a biologic base to behavioral and emotional deviations, and researchers hope to demonstrate a correlation between chromosomal and neuronal abnormalities and a person's behavior.

### Family Dynamics

Theories of development implicate environmental factors occurring in the very early years of the child's life. Feelings of rejection or inadequate nurturing by the primary caregiver result in anger that is then turned inward on the self. Depression is common.

## CLIENT ASSESSMENT DATABASE

### Neurosensory

Covert aggressive behaviors are chosen over self-assertive behaviors.

Passively resists demands (to increase or maintain certain level of performance) through behaviors such as dawdling, stubbornness, procrastination, and "forgetfulness."

**Mental Status:**

**Behavior:** May not appear uncomfortable in social situations but is cold and indifferent, reflecting stiff perfectionism.

**Mood and Affect:** Displays a seriousness with difficulty expressing warm feelings, may sulk and pout, passively acquiesce/conform, resentment is unspoken.

**Emotion:** Display/report anxiety, depression; expresses low self-esteem, lack of self-confidence; may be dependent and passive.

**Thought Processes:** Views world in a negativistic manner but fails to connect behavior to others' reactions, feels resentful, and believes others are being unfair; sees the world as a hostile and unfair environment.

451

## Social Interactions

Habitually "forgets" commitments, arrives late for appointments.

Demands for adequate performance are met with resistance expressed indirectly, resulting in pervasive social or occupational ineffectiveness, which interferes with job performance and leads to difficulty adjusting to close relationships.

Strained interpersonal relationships.

## DIAGNOSTIC STUDIES

**Drug Screen:** Identifies substance use.

## NURSING PRIORITIES

1. Assist client to learn methods to control anxiety and express anger appropriately.
2. Promote effective, satisfying coping strategies.
3. Promote development of positive self-concept.
4. Encourage client/family to become involved in therapy/support programs.

## DISCHARGE GOALS

1. Resolving feelings of anger, hostility.
2. Assertive techniques learned and used.
3. Self-esteem increased.
4. Client/family involved in therapy programs.

| NURSING DIAGNOSIS: | ANXIETY [moderate to severe] |
|---|---|
| **May Be Related To:** | Unconscious conflict; unmet needs; threat to self-concept. |
| | Difficulty in asserting self directly; feelings of resentment toward authority figures. |
| **Possibly Evidenced By:** | Difficulty resolving feelings/trusting others. |
| | Passive resistance to demands made by others. |
| | Extraneous movements: foot-shuffling, hand/arm movements. |
| | Irritability, argumentativeness. |
| **Desired Outcomes/Evaluation Criteria— Client Will:** | Define and use effective methods for decreasing anxiety. |
| | Demonstrate problem-solving skills. |
| | Report anxiety is reduced to a manageable level. |
| | Use resources effectively. |

| ACTIONS/INTERVENTIONS | RATIONALE |
|---|---|
| **Independent** | |
| Encourage direct expression of feelings. Help client to recognize when open, honest feelings are not being expressed. | Client has established a pattern of expressing feelings indirectly through covert aggression. Needs to learn to express feelings directly as they occur. |

| ACTIONS/INTERVENTIONS | RATIONALE |
|---|---|

### Independent

Explore situations that lead to feelings of anger, hostility. Discuss possible causes.

Client needs to gain insight into areas that cause resentment and anger in order to plan resolution.

Examine feelings toward authority figures. Discuss how these feelings come about.

Authority figures are a common target for client's aggression. May have started in early childhood, leaving multiple unresolved conflicts.

Assist client to be in tune to own feelings and increasing internal anxiety.

Client is often unaware that responses are consequences of anxiety.

Discuss fears concerning intimate relationships. Does client feel betrayed by significant other(s)?

Inability to trust is a significant problem for this client. Examining situations in past provides opportunity for insight.

Review how the inability to express feelings has resulted in covert acting-out behaviors.

Important for establishing the correlation between hostility and covert maneuvers.

Aid client in establishing a possible cause-and-effect relationship of "forgetfulness," dawdling, procrastination, etc., to internal resentment toward the person making demands.

Important for heightened awareness of own feelings and behaviors manifested.

Encourage client to recognize need to act out with covert aggression to "get back" at others. Together develop effective methods to alter response.

Client is not always aware of own feelings/needs, and assistance in redirecting aggression can help client to change behaviors.

Support verbalization of feelings in an assertive manner instead of using flight response.

Client needs to learn to face issues directly, using assertive techniques.

Discuss client's fears regarding new assertive behaviors. Help define ways to alleviate these fears.

Self-assertion is a new experience for this client. Discussing fears helps diminish them.

Explore with client how often anger is displaced onto others because client believes the target of the anger cannot be approached.

Reinforces need for client to deal directly with target of feelings.

Explain "pressure cooker" effect of "stuffing" feelings.

This individual usually has established a lifelong pattern of internalizing feelings, and this eventually leads to exploding inappropriately. Education is necessary to understand relationship between thoughts, feelings, and behavior.

Define methods of expression that effectively control anxiety, e.g., relaxation, use of "I-messages."

This is a new approach for the client, who therefore needs guidance in learning effective anxiety control.

Give positive feedback for new behaviors. Discuss any needed modifications.

Provides reassurance and encourages repetition of newly learned skills. Client may have difficulty trusting own judgment.

Involve family/SO(s) in treatment plan and practice sessions.

Longstanding patterns of interaction need to be changed to enable client and SO(s) to develop new style of communication/behavior.

| NURSING DIAGNOSIS: | COPING, INDIVIDUAL, INEFFECTIVE |
|---|---|
| **May Be Related To:** | Inability to cope, problem-solve; inadequate coping method (does not use self-assertive behaviors). |

| | |
|---|---|
| **Possibly Evidenced By:** | Personal vulnerability. |
| | Unrealistic perceptions; unmet expectations. |
| | Lack of recognition of relationship between passive-aggressive behaviors and internal anxiety. |
| | Use of maladaptive, temporary relief behaviors that do not last or really satisfy; lack of assertive behaviors. |
| | Real issues remaining unaddressed and unresolved. |
| | Maneuvers such as dawdling, procrastination, stubbornness, forgetfulness, habitual tardiness. |
| | Difficulty meeting basic needs. |
| | Alteration in societal participation. |
| **Desired Outcomes/Evaluation Criteria—Client Will:** | Identify ineffective coping behaviors and consequences. |
| | Develop and implement repertoire of coping strategies that are based on problem-solving techniques and that provide effective relief of conflicts. |

| ACTIONS/INTERVENTIONS | RATIONALE |
|---|---|
| **Independent** | |
| Discuss present patterns of coping and evaluate their effectiveness. | Client needs to recognize pattern and see that current methods do not bring positive results. |
| Assist client to identify how passive-resistant behaviors are maladaptive relief behaviors. | Needs to associate behaviors with an attempt to gain relief from anxiety and hostility. |
| Confront client with what needs the behaviors are really serving when forgetfulness and procrastination are used. | Confrontation heightens awareness of problem, providing stimulus for change to get needs met in more constructive ways. |
| Review what unmet needs are and why present coping patterns do not afford lasting relief. | Brings to light that client's needs are really not being satisfied. |
| Discourage client from justifying current automatic relief behaviors. Point out the inadequacies of these behaviors. | Client will have difficulty changing old behaviors and has already spent a lifetime justifying them to self. |
| Encourage client to identify examples of situations when the client felt imposed upon or angered but did not speak up. Discuss alternate ways to handle those situations. | Promotes understanding that avoidance of dealing directly with anger often leads to a negative outcome. Realization is crucial to learning new coping skills. |
| Suggest client ask family members/SO(s) to let him or her know when they feel imposed on or angered by client's behavior. | Helps develop new awareness and opportunity to change old ineffective ways of responding. |
| Ask client to discuss how it feels when others are habitually forgetful and do not keep commitments. Discuss importance of following through with what is promised. | Developing empathy may help break this pattern. |

454

| ACTIONS/INTERVENTIONS | RATIONALE |
|---|---|

### Independent

| | |
|---|---|
| Give feedback on how passive-resistant behaviors affect others. | Client needs to realize how destructive the behaviors can be and how difficult it is to maintain intimate relationships with family/SO(s). |
| Provide information about problem-solving techniques to provide base for effective, satisfying coping behaviors. | Aids client in learning to think through problems and arriving at well-thought-out solutions that are successful. |
| Give positive feedback when client demonstrates use of adaptive skills and makes suggestions for improvement. | Aids in reinforcing positive behaviors. |

| NURSING DIAGNOSIS: | SELF-ESTEEM, CHRONIC LOW |
|---|---|
| **May Be Related To:** | Retarded ego development. |
| | Unmet dependency needs; early rejection by significant other(s). |
| | Lack of positive feedback. |
| **Possibly Evidenced By:** | Lack of self-confidence; feelings of inadequacy, fear of asserting self. |
| | Dependency on others. |
| | Directing frustrations toward others by using covert aggressive tactics. |
| | Not accepting own responsibility for what happens as a result of maladaptive behaviors. |
| | Not verbalizing negative feelings and working through them. |
| **Desired Outcomes/Evaluation Criteria— Client Will:** | Verbalize a sense of worthwhileness. |
| | Use assertive, effective behaviors to interact with others. |
| | Actively participate in program(s) to develop positive self-esteem. |

| ACTIONS/INTERVENTIONS | RATIONALE |
|---|---|

### Independent

| | |
|---|---|
| Encourage client to describe self and perceived inadequacies and how these relate to others. Note whether client compares self to others and in what terms. | Negative self-image often comes from comparing oneself unfavorably to others. |
| Assess client's self-concept. Determine if client is realistic about strengths and limitations. | May not have accurate perceptions of own strengths and shortcomings. |
| Encourage client to make adjustments in thinking if expectations of self and others are unrealistic. | Cannot improve self-esteem if expectations are not realistic/achievable. |

455

| ACTIONS/INTERVENTIONS | RATIONALE |
|---|---|

### Independent

| | |
|---|---|
| Discuss how evaluations by others might have negatively affected the client. | Often people are hypersensitive to others' comments and allow them to stick as a "label." |
| Explore past relationships. Determine if client feels let down or hurt by significant other(s). | Client may be hanging onto old pain that needs to be worked through or let go. |
| Assist client to learn how to express feelings assertively, e.g., "I feel hurt, angry, rejected, discounted, etc." This mode of interaction promotes more comfortable relationships. | Expressing feelings assertively is self-enhancing. |
| Explain that being willing to take some risks by allowing others to get close is necessary, even though getting hurt is a possible outcome. | Taking risks and experiencing success can do much to enhance self-esteem. Likewise, knowledge that one can survive failure can enhance confidence in ability to handle difficult situations as they arise. |
| Discuss specific objectives for self-improvement and enhancing relationships. | Client needs to take action on newly gained knowledge in order to achieve success. |
| Encourage client to learn more about others to gain a clearer perspective of their motives and feelings. | Client uses defense mechanism of projection of own feelings on others. Anger and hostility can be diffused by gaining more information about others and their situations. |
| Ask client to describe what is defined as success in others and perceptions of what made them successful, and compare with own life successes. | May already have qualities for success but has overshadowed them with negative feelings. |
| Explore how the desired attributes can be adopted and put into practice. | Helps client to apply goals to daily life situations. |
| Encourage client to accept self with strengths and liabilities and learn to like self. | Self-acceptance is necessary to build self-esteem and improve relationships with others. |

| | |
|---|---|
| **NURSING DIAGNOSIS:** | **POWERLESSNESS** |
| **May Be Related To:** | Interpersonal interaction. |
| | Lifestyle of helplessness; dependency feelings. |
| | Difficulty connecting own passive-resistant behaviors with hostility or resentment. |
| **Possibly Evidenced By:** | Experiencing conscious hostility toward authority figures. |
| | Releasing anger and hostility through others, who may become angry or suffer because of client's inefficiencies. |
| | Getting back at others through aggravation. |
| **Desired Outcomes/Evaluation Criteria— Client Will:** | Express sense of control over present/future outcomes. |
| | Verbalize resolution of hostile feelings |

Use assertive (instead of aggressive) behaviors to deal with feelings, anxiety-producing situations, and interactions with others.

| ACTIONS/INTERVENTIONS | RATIONALE |
|---|---|
| **Independent** | |
| Examine hostile feelings toward authority figures. Determine when this began and what painful experiences have come about because of those in authority. | A major dynamic for this personality disorder is resentment of authority and the resulting sense of powerlessness. It helps the nurse to know what experiences client has had that led to this situation, especially relationship with primary caregiver during early years, when client may have felt particularly helpless. |
| Explore areas of life in which feeling inadequate or having a sense of no control occurs. | Provides insight into feelings necessary for learning adaptive behaviors. |
| Identify covert aggressive behaviors used to gain control of others. | Increases awareness of mode of interaction used and attempts to maintain sense of own control. |
| Encourage verbalization of how feelings of anger, hurt, and loss of control relate to desire to strike out at others. | Enhances understanding of how use of covert aggression has become a pervasive pattern. |
| Provide opportunity to learn how to get needs met in an acceptable, assertive manner. | Promotes inner strength and adaptive functioning, enhancing sense of control. |
| Assist client to learn to listen to others and consider their feelings by putting self in their place. | Promotes empathy for others and sense of own self-worth. |
| Have client assist in developing treatment plan. | Aids in promoting a sense of control and involvement in own care/future. This sense of participation enhances cooperation. |

# CHAPTER 16

# OTHER CONDITIONS THAT MAY BE A FOCUS OF CLINICAL ATTENTION

## PSYCHOLOGICAL FACTORS AFFECTING MEDICAL CONDITION

### DSM IV
316 (Psychological Factors) Affecting Medical Condition

Choose name based on nature of/most prominent factor:

Mental Disorder Affecting Medical Condition
Psychological Symptoms Affecting Medical Condition
Personality Traits or Coping Style Affecting Medical Condition
Maladaptive Health Behaviors Affecting Medical Condition
Stress-Related Physiological Response Affecting Medical Condition
Unspecified Psychological Factors Affecting Medical Condition

(Refer to DSM IV list for specific definitions.)

### DSM III-R
316.00 Psychological Factors Affecting Physical Condition (Specify physical condition on Axis III.)

These disorders represent a group of ailments in which emotional stress is a contributing factor to physical problems (coded on Axis III) involving an organ system under involuntary control. Any organ system may be affected and is dependent on the individual's susceptibility. The result is the development or exacerbation of, interference with therapy for, and/or delayed recovery from a medical condition.

Lists of related medical conditions are subject to change as research progresses, although to date a clear psychologic-biologic connection has been inferred but not yet scientifically proved.

### ETIOLOGIC THEORIES

Although the etiology of psychosomatic disorders is unknown, it is believed that an individual's emotional state and life circumstances significantly affect the onset, form, and

458

course of psychosomatic illness. The interaction of psychologic, social, and biologic factors becomes evident as physical symptoms appear and diminish in direct relationship to the amount of stress the person is experiencing. Psychophysiologic disorders do occur without known psychologic components, but generally these disorders have some genetic predisposition in order to respond to stress pathologically.

## Psychodynamics

Thought to center around issues of unresolved dependency conflicts, undischarged aggressive feelings, repressed anger, hostility, resentment, and anxiety, these conflicts are expressed somatically. Physiologic responses correspond to unconscious emotional conflict instead of directly through verbalization, indicating inadequate or maladaptive defense mechanisms.

Interpersonal theory proposes that individuals with specific personality traits are predisposed to develop or precipitate certain disease processes, e.g., those who are dependent may develop asthma; depression has been linked to cancer and aggressiveness to chest pain or dysrhythmia.

## Biologic

A new field of psychoneuroimmunology is developing around research of the biologic factors that underlie these illnesses. It has been demonstrated that the immune response can be affected by behavior modification. Skills are being taught to assist people to modify responses that are thought to lead to illness.

In extensive stress studies, it was found that specific physiologic responses under direct control of the pituitary/adrenal axis occurred in response to stress. When these stress responses are prolonged, psychosomatic disorders can develop. It is postulated that the specific organ system involved and type of psychosomatic disorder the individual develops may be genetically determined.

The Selye stress theory proposes three levels of response—the alarm reaction, the stage of resistance, and the stage of exhaustion—called the general adaptation syndrome, which have an effect on physical functioning. The belief of the individual regarding the degree of stress is related to the effect of the stressor on the physiologic condition.

## Family Dynamics

Children who grow up observing the attention, increased dependency, or other secondary gain an individual receives because of illness see these behaviors as a desirable response and subsequently imitate them. The dysfunctional family system uses these psychophysiologic problems to cover up interpersonal conflicts. Anxiety is thus shifted from the conflict to the ailing member. As anxiety decreases, conflict is avoided, and positive reinforcement is given for the symptoms of the sick person.

## CLIENT ASSESSMENT DATABASE
## General

These clients do not present a calm, relaxed demeanor but rather a pattern of anxiety and problems of coping with stress that occurs in their lives. Data obtained are dependent on organ system involved, e.g.:

### CORONARY ARTERY DISEASE
Activity/Rest

May exhibit an abrupt, fast-talking presentation, and are constantly moving, e.g., jiggling knees or tapping fingers.

Usually are "too busy" to notice quiet, beautiful surroundings; work overload, do not take vacations.

459

### Circulation
Elevated blood pressure, tachycardia, palpitations, angina.

### Ego Integrity
Measures success by material goods/personal accomplishments.

### Neurosensory
**Mental Status:** Psychologic factors linking stress and personality traits include life stressors, ongoing emotional turmoil/anger, and overexertion. There is an intense need to compete and win, even if competing with a child. May be overdutiful to job; hostile, angry, and aggressive toward others; feel a need to do everything in a hurry and become impatient if asked to wait; may not tolerate waiting in lines. Driving, idealistic, dominant, compulsive individual, with passive-aggressive tendencies, strict superego, feelings of insecurity, and difficulty managing anger.

### Teaching/Learning
Males have higher incidence.
Risk factors most frequently reported: cigarette smoking, hypertension, elevated serum cholesterol and triglyceride levels, left ventricular hypertrophy, diabetes, and age.

## PEPTIC ULCER
### Ego Integrity
May express an intense need for perfection and feelings of not having enough control over stressors and environment.

### Food/Fluid
History of multiple stomach complaints, e.g., gastritis/ulcers, hyperacidity; heartburn, reflux; food intolerances.

### Neurosensory
**Mental Status:** Longstanding feelings of anxiety, repressed anger, hostility, resentment, and a sense of helplessness, with difficulty in coping; highly developed superego, conscientious/dutiful; may be insecure/nervous.

### Teaching/Learning
Family history may reveal other affected members.

## ESSENTIAL HYPERTENSION
### Activity/Rest
Fatigue, sleep disturbances.

### Circulation
Chronic high blood pressure with no known organic origin.
Dizziness, nervousness, palpitations.

### Ego Integrity
May report emotional trauma, presence of stressful situations in daily life; controlled emotionality.
Increased incidence in urban areas rather than in rural or tropical areas (may reflect a more relaxed lifestyle).

### Food/Fluid
Obesity, sensitivity to salt.

*Neurosensory*

**Mental Status:** Conflicted over expression of hostile and aggressive feelings, struggle with dependency vs. achievement needs; tends to hold anger in and to feel guilty if anger is expressed, inhibits aggressive wishes; may show greater reactivity to stressful stimuli, even in normal situations.

*Pain/Discomfort*

Headaches.

*Social Interactions*

Social isolation.

*Teaching/Learning*

More prevalent in black population; onset usually in early adult life (mean age in early 30s).

## BRONCHIAL ASTHMA

*Neurosensory*

**Mental Status:** Dependent, meek, sensitive, nervous, compulsive, and perfectionistic. Feelings of insecurity and oppression, insufficient superego, compulsive, overdutiful attitudes, tendency to be passive-aggressive. May be shy, irritable, impatient, stubborn, and tyrannical at times. Anxiety, anger, depression, tension, frustration, and anticipation of a pleasurable event can contribute to exacerbation of symptoms.

*Respiratory*

Wheezing, shortness of breath, restlessness, cyanosis; hyperventilation, sighing, hiccups. Smoking in the home.

*Social Interactions*

Strong correlation between asthma attacks and tension in the home/estranged relationships with parents.

*Teaching/Learning*

Can occur at any age (1/3 are children; 2/3 of these are boys).
Respiratory infections/induced emotionality may trigger/exacerbate attacks.

## ULCERATIVE COLITIS

*Activity/Rest*

Fatigue.

*Ego Integrity*

Precipitating stressors center around real or feared threats to significant interpersonal relationships or deaths.

*Elimination*

Diarrhea (with/without blood).

*Food/Fluid*

Weight loss, pallor, anemia.

*Neurosensory*

**Mental Status:** Compulsive, especially regarding punctuality and neatness; difficulty expressing anger/hostility directly, timidity, obstinacy, hyperintellectualism, lack of humor. May perceive even the slightest criticism as rejection and feel a loss of self-esteem and may respond by using avoidance or by becoming suspicious.

Social Interactions

Difficulty in interpersonal relationships/dependency on others.

Ambivalence/hypersensitivity toward significant others who have been a source of hurt or perceived rejection.

Feels hurt or humiliated and unable to/not inclined to meet the demands of those on whom they feel dependent.

Teaching/Learning

Can occur at any age.

### MIGRAINE HEADACHE

Activity/Rest

Fatigue.

Food/Fluid

Nausea, vomiting

Neurosensory

**Mental Status:** Compulsive/perfectionistic, conscientious, intelligent, neat, inflexible, rigid, resentful, experiences guilt feelings.

Sensitivity to light/noise; visual disturbances; sensory/motor disturbances (e.g., tingling of face, hands; staggering gait).

Pain/Discomfort

Head pain, unilateral or bilateral; aching, throbbing.

### OTHER SYMPTOMS/CONDITIONS THAT MAY BE NOTED

**Genitourinary:** Menstrual and urinary disturbances; dyspareunia, impotence.

**Musculoskeletal:** Joint stiffness/pain, backache, muscle cramps, tension headaches.

**Skin:** Pruritus, cutaneous inflammation (neurodermatitis), excessive sweating (hyperhidrosis).

**Others:** Autoimmune diseases, manifested as rheumatoid arthritis, systemic lupus erythematosus, myasthenia gravis, and pernicious anemia, etc.

## DIAGNOSTIC STUDIES

Dependent on specific presenting condition/symptoms.

## NURSING PRIORITIES

1. Encourage verbalization of feelings and stressors.
2. Assist client to develop coping skills and assertiveness techniques to reduce/manage anxiety.
3. Promote development of positive self-esteem.
4. Help client to accomplish a sense of autonomy and independence.

## DISCHARGE GOALS

1. Assertive techniques used as a more productive, effective means of expression.
2. Stress management methods used to reduce anxiety.
3. Positive self-esteem that satisfies client's needs without compromising self/others is displayed.
4. Client/family involved in group therapy/community support programs.

Note: This plan of care deals with the psychiatric component of these conditions. Ongoing evaluation of physical condition is required to ensure timely intervention and client well-being. The user is referred to a medical-surgical resource (such as *Nursing Care Plans: Guidelines for Planning and Documenting Patient Care*, by Doenges, Moorhouse, Geissler, 1993) for physiologic considerations.

| NURSING DIAGNOSIS: | ANXIETY [moderate to severe] |
|---|---|
| May Be Related To: | Internalized feelings of inadequacy, resentment, frustration, anger; negative self-talk. |
| | Inability to obtain relief from stress; unmet needs. |
| | Perceived threat to self-concept. |
| Possibly Evidenced By: | Stimulation of the fight-or-flight reaction; sympathetic stimulation, increase in blood pressure/somatic complaints. |
| | Focus on self. |
| | Denial of relationship between physical symptoms and emotional problems. |
| Desired Outcomes/Evaluation Criteria— Client Will: | Verbalize understanding of relationship between feelings of anxiety and physical symptoms. |
| | Develop effective methods for decreasing anxiety. |
| | Report anxiety reduced to manageable level. |
| | Experience marked decrease in somatic complaints. |

| ACTIONS/INTERVENTIONS | RATIONALE |
|---|---|
| **Independent** | |
| Explore situations that lead to feelings of anger, resentment. Discuss possible causes and explore stressors or events that trigger illness. Discuss ways to stop the escalation of anxiety. | Helps client define problem areas and begin to establish goals to work through them. Client reacts to stress psychologically and needs to learn to control/deal effectively with emotional responses. |
| Assist client to learn to be in tune with feelings and recognize situations that cause increase in anxiety. | Client may be out of touch with body and not aware of feelings, therefore does not experience "signal anxiety," which helps to recognize beginning development of anxiety so steps can be taken for control. |
| Encourage direct expression of feelings. Help client to recognize times when the feelings are internalized. | The client who internalizes feelings is not always aware of doing that and may have trouble even identifying feelings. |
| Identify the amount of anxiety experienced if not perceiving self as "perfect" in job performance and interpersonal relationships. | May put pressure on self to be "perfect," while at the same time not recognizing/accepting feelings and resultant anxiety, which is then expressed in physical illness. |
| Examine possible cause-effect relationship between "internalizing" feelings and somatic symptoms. | Client needs to see the relationship between physical discomfort and turning feelings inward, so steps can be taken to intervene/deal more appropriately with the stress. |

463

| ACTIONS/INTERVENTIONS | RATIONALE |
|---|---|

### Independent

Assist client to relate pattern of resurgence of symptoms and stressful life situations. Have client keep a diary of appearance, duration, and intensity of physical symptoms. Compare with a separate record of stressful situations.

Reinforces the fact that client does transfer stress to body (GI upset, tension headache, chest pain, respiratory distress, etc.) and needs to learn how to stop this unhealthy reaction. Comparison of these records may provide objective data from which to observe the relationship between physical symptoms and stress.

Help client recognize difference between assertive and aggressive behaviors. Instruct in assertiveness techniques. Discuss importance of respecting rights of others while protecting one's own basic rights.

Assertiveness training is of utmost importance for the client who does not know how to directly express self, in order to defuse inner tension and relieve resulting physiologic effects of anxiety. Also promotes self-esteem and may improve ability to form satisfactory interpersonal relationships.

Demonstrate/encourage use of relaxation, visualization, imagery techniques, e.g., progressive relaxation, meditation.

Studies show that these techniques decrease anxiety and work to moderate the stimulation of the sympathetic nervous system.

Use gentle, supportive therapeutic approach to develop a positive rapport.

Skill of the therapist is crucial. Care needs to be taken to avoid alienating the client.

Be cautious in using confrontative techniques or making demands for achievement.

Client has low tolerance for stress. It is most critical not to exacerbate onset of symptoms.

Explore possible recreational activities to alleviate and rechannel stress productively (e.g., brisk walks/jogging, volleyball, bowling, swimming).

Physical activity is very effective for relieving stress, and it provides opportunity to develop new skills to dissipate anxiety.

| NURSING DIAGNOSIS: | COPING, INDIVIDUAL, INEFFECTIVE |
|---|---|
| May Be Related To: | Personal vulnerability. |
| | Inadequate repertoire of coping mechanisms. |
| | Compelling, intense desire to compete and win, excessive need to achieve success. |
| | Feeling pressured to hurry, preoccupation with the urgency of passing time; work overload, too many deadlines; no vacations. |
| | Unrealistic perceptions; unmet expectations. |
| Possibly Evidenced By: | Inability to cope/problem-solve or to ask for help. |
| | Internalizing stress/build-up of frustration; failure to obtain relief from and/or not resolving negative feelings; inadequate discharge of aggressive feelings/desires. |
| | Use of maladaptive coping methods; use of passive-aggressive maneuvers. |
| | Somatic complaints, rise in blood pressure. |

| Desired Outcomes/Evaluation Criteria— Client Will: | Develop and implement repertoire of coping strategies based on problem-solving techniques. |
| --- | --- |
| | Use assertive techniques in place of passive-aggressive, maladaptive behaviors. |
| | Demonstrate a more moderate lifestyle. |
| | Verbalize understanding of health risks. |

| ACTIONS/INTERVENTIONS | RATIONALE |
| --- | --- |
| **Independent** | |
| Assist client to identify present coping patterns and the consequences and to evaluate their effectiveness. | A realistic picture of how effective current mechanisms are provides insight and enables client to acknowledge ineffectiveness of these methods and begin to look at healthy alternatives. |
| Help client identify/understand unmet needs and how present coping patterns relate to relief of anxiety. | Developing a keen sense of self-awareness and how these factors are interrelated provides opportunity for change. |
| Demonstrate/practice problem-solving techniques. Encourge client to think through problems, identify goals for own care. | Learning to arrive at thought-out solutions provides base for effective, satisfying coping behaviors. Personal involvement in own care provides a feeling of control, increases chances for positive outcome, and enhances self-esteem. |
| Ask client to give examples of situations when resentment and anger were felt but were not expressed. Discuss/role-play alternate ways to handle those situations. | Behavior rehearsal helps client to learn how to handle troublesome situations much more effectively. |
| Examine how needs are expressed, passively or aggressively. | Client may not be aware of use of passive or aggressive approach. Awareness offers choice to change behavior. |
| Have client identify and discuss personal dynamics. Determine if they are used to prevent guilt or win approval. | Many interactions may be based on trying to relieve guilt or to please others while ignoring own wishes. |
| Confront with behaviors that are used to prevent rejection or disapproval by others. | Increases self-awareness of maladaptive pattern(s). |
| Encourage client to assume control over own reactions to stressful events, even though the circumstances cannot always be controlled. | The client can learn to control how much a stressful event affects feelings, behavior, and becoming upset by changing the way these events are viewed. |
| Identify competitive behaviors and explore reasons for feeling a compulsion to achieve/win. | Realization that the compulsive drive for achievement can be strong enough to endanger health may provide stimulus for change. |
| Evaluate the effect these compulsive feelings have had on physical and emotional health. | Heightens awareness of the possible toll on health, longevity. |
| Explore how these behaviors have affected interpersonal relationships. | Client may be intolerant of others and aggressive in relationships, resulting in problems interacting with others. |

465

| ACTIONS/INTERVENTIONS | RATIONALE |
|---|---|

### Independent

| | |
|---|---|
| Assist client to identify what needs are really being met by competitive behaviors. | Recognition of own self-esteem needs provides opportunity to meet these needs in a more direct/successful manner. |
| Discuss consequences of "driving" oneself and how to moderate lifestyle to reduce stress. | Reinforces the negative effects of continuing an intense lifestyle. |
| Discuss importance of leisure time and how to develop and use it. Explain how pacing oneself can be a more productive and efficient use of time. | Client has not been used to taking time out to relax, and learning how to relax and enjoy recreation can relieve anxiety and promote effective coping. |

| | |
|---|---|
| **NURSING DIAGNOSIS:** | **POWERLESSNESS** |
| **May Be Related To:** | Unresolved dependency conflicts; sacrificing own wishes for others. |
| | Feelings of insecurity, resentment; repression of anger and aggressive feelings. |
| **Possibly Evidenced By:** | Lack of a sense of control in stressful situations. |
| | Difficulty expressing self directly and assertively. |
| | Passive/docile or aggressive behavior. |
| | Internalizing of stress/increased anxiety expressed through somatic complaints, elevated blood pressure. |
| **Desired Outcomes/Evaluation Criteria— Client Will:** | Recognize and work through feelings of insecurity, resentment. |
| | Use assertive behaviors to deal with feelings, anxiety-producing situations, and interactions with others. |
| | Verbalize awareness of own control over self and how stress is handled in situations over which client does not have control. |
| | Demonstrate less frequent episodes of illness with fewer physical complaints. |

| ACTIONS/INTERVENTIONS | RATIONALE |
|---|---|

### Independent

| | |
|---|---|
| Have client describe events that lead to feeling inadequate or having no control. | Helpful in identifying sources of frustration and defining problem areas so action can be taken. |
| Examine together how client feels when not "perfectly" competent or adequate in performance. | Client may be self-deprecating and believe she or he has failed unless self is perceived as "perfect." |

| ACTIONS/INTERVENTIONS | RATIONALE |
|---|---|

### Independent

Assess client's attitude toward making mistakes, e.g., able to admit and accept or feels inadequate and worthless.

When client indulges in self-punishment, client needs to learn a rational way of "thinking" regarding mistakes. Failure is seldom a catastrophe and often leads to learning important lessons when the client is open to the opportunity.

Discuss how worry and anxiety prevent dealing with problems efficiently and cause more feelings of incompetency.

Worry and anxiety can prevent objective evaluation of a situation and lead to poor judgment.

Encourage client to do the feared activity. Provide support for these efforts.

Avoiding dreaded events increases unnecessary fears and causes further loss of self-confidence. Confronting the situation provides opportunity for client to test reality, consequences, and ability to cope with whatever happens, thus increasing self-confidence.

Discuss behaviors that are self-defeating and explore new, productive behaviors, e.g., looking at problem as a challenge instead of a threat, developing a sense of commitment to something, and gaining a sense of control over own life.

Past solutions to problems may not be relevant at this time, and previous failed experiences are not sufficient reason to discount their reevaluation.

Ask client to describe significant others' behaviors that are perceived as intimidating and how fear of these behaviors can be overcome.

Identifying successful actions to use can improve self-esteem. As self-confidence is gained, the client will be less easily intimidated.

Explain how a lack of self-confidence in one's own judgment and abilities can result in feeling powerless in stressful situations.

Loss of self-confidence serves only to "immobilize"/prevent using effective mechanisms in dealing with problems.

Use role-playing techniques to demonstrate how to assert feelings and help client learn direct self-expression when faced with frustration or aggression.

Behavior rehearsal is an effective way to practice self-expression/learn to deal with troublesome situations, get the desired need met, and enhance sense of control.

Have client describe people seen as dynamic or powerful individuals and how they achieved personal power. Explore how client can achieve these desired attributes.

Helps client to clearly define goals and values and look at how these relate to own self.

Examine sources of resentment. Identify what has been done to resolve these feelings and whether an effort has been made to get information to justify resentment.

More information can diffuse an angry or resentful response. Situations are not always as they appear, and an individual's perceptions may be distorted. Checking out reality can help the client decide on appropriate follow-up.

Encourage client to be open and direct in verbal expression. Confront when guarding of feelings is noted.

Learning new ways of expression is difficult. Reinforcing open/direct expression promotes continuation of activity.

Assess client's pattern of response to aggression or frustration, and together evaluate the effectiveness of these reponses.

Client first needs to recognize own pattern of maladaptive defense mechanisms in order to learn new adaptive responses.

Examine situations that produce anger or guilt in client and discuss what triggers these feelings.

Unresolved guilt and anger lead to feelings of frustration or powerlessness.

| ACTIONS/INTERVENTIONS | RATIONALE |
|---|---|
| **Independent** | |
| Discuss causes of difficulty in making own needs known to others and fears surrounding these issues. | The client does not assert own needs and either passively accepts things as they are or ineffectively tries to assert control, increasing feelings of powerlessness. Discussion and awareness provide opportunity for change. |
| Explore guilt feelings when expressing anger and ways to work through this problem. | Client needs to learn that it is acceptable to feel and express anger appropriately. |
| Examine causes of hostility and how these feelings can be adequately discharged, e.g., pounding pillows, yelling appropriately; expressing feelings assertively, not aggressively, to the other person. | Client may be harboring undischarged hostility that needs resolution or release instead of allowing these feelings to affect body negatively (e.g., increased blood pressure, tension headache). |
| Ask client to verbalize how and why feelings of helplessness and dependency began. Discuss ways to put these feelings into perspective. | Being aware of emotional dependency and how these dynamics originate provides opportunity to change behavior/outcomes. |
| Explore with client fears of loss/rejection and evaluate together how realistic these concerns are. | May tend to exaggerate slight criticism into unrealistic fears. |
| Assist client to think through these concerns and identify ways to deal with them. | Client needs to learn to accept the positive and negative aspects of relationships without becoming dysfunctional. |
| Have client identify what will happen if client functions independently. Assist to learn how to use own capabilities. | Functioning autonomously and capitalizing on own strengths promote client's sense of control over own life/outcomes. |

| NURSING DIAGNOSIS: | SELF-ESTEEM DISTURBANCE [specify] |
|---|---|
| **May Be Related To:** | Lack of positive feedback, repeated negative feedback resulting in diminished self-worth. |
| | Dysfunctional family system; unmet dependency needs. |
| | Retarded ego development. |
| | Unrealistic expectations of self and/or others. |
| **Possibly Evidenced By:** | Belief that individual should be "perfect." |
| | Not expressing needs directly, lacking self-confidence, being dependent, not verbalizing/not working through negative feelings. |
| | Feelings of worthlessness. |
| **Desired Outcomes/Evaluation Criteria— Client Will:** | Verbalize view of self as a worthwhile, important person who functions well both interpersonally and occupationally. |
| | Demonstrate self-confidence by setting realistic goals and actively participating in life situations. |
| | Experience a decrease in somatic complaints. |

| ACTIONS/INTERVENTIONS | RATIONALE |
|---|---|
| **Independent** | |
| Assess client's strengths and limitations and compare with client's own assessment of self. | An accurate picture of the client's sense of self-worth is important in developing the plan of care. |
| Assist client to learn to accept disapproval from others without feeling a sense of failure. | Helps to develop confidence in own abilities and judgment despite what others think. |
| Discuss client's goals. Are they what the client really wants or are they what the client thinks they "should" or "ought" to be? | Typically tends to ignore own wishes and do what client thinks others expect. |
| Explain why it is necessary to take risks in order to build self-esteem. | Self-confidence is built on taking risks and learning from success and/or failure. |
| Ask client to discuss feelings about criticism from others. Discuss ways to cope with these feelings. | May have unrealistic feelings when criticized and needs to learn how to apply constructive criticism for personal growth rather than becoming devastated. |
| Identify what needs are being met by preoccupation with neatness and orderliness. Relate these needs to self-esteem needs. | Client more than likely experiences a sense of failure if unable to keep environment perfect. |
| Discuss possible feelings of ambivalence toward significant other(s) who have been a source of disappointment, rejection, or loss. | Often experiences ambivalent feelings toward significant others due to inability to deal with negative feelings directly and having a fear of rejection if negative feelings are expressed. |
| Explore expectations family and/or significant others hold for client. | Client may be trying to meet unrealistic expectations, further increasing sense of failure and anxiety. |
| Assist to identify realistic needs for change in relation to self, family/significant other(s). | Without guidance, may misinterpret/block needs, setting self up for failure. |
| Reinforce client's ability to assume responsibility and rely on own abilities. | Needs emotional support and encouragement to become self-reliant. |

| | |
|---|---|
| **NURSING DIAGNOSIS:** | **ROLE PERFORMANCE, ALTERED** |
| **May Be Related To:** | Chronic illness. |
| | Situational crisis, conflicts. |
| | Developmental crisis regarding values/beliefs. |
| **Possibly Evidenced By:** | Changes in usual patterns of responsibility; inability (perceived/actual) to resume role. |
| | Change in self/others' perception of role. |
| | Assumption of dependent role. |
| **Desired Outcomes/Evaluation Criteria— Client Will:** | Verbalize realistic perception of role expectations/obligations. |
| | Assume role-related responsibility. |
| **Client and Family Will:** | Verbalize plan for attempt at conflict resolution. |

| ACTIONS/INTERVENTIONS | RATIONALE |
|---|---|

### Independent

Determine client's usual role within the family system. Identify roles of other family members.

Accurate database is required to formulate appropriate plan of care for client.

Assess specific disabilities related to role expectations. Note relationship of disability to actual physical condition.

It is necessary to determine the validity of the client's/family's role expectations in light of client's physical ability to make realistic plans to modify role and encourage adaptation.

Encourage client to discuss conflicts evident within the family system. Identify how client and other family members have responded to this conflict.

Identifies specific stressors, as well as adaptive and maladaptive responses within the system, so that individualized assistance can be provided in an effort to create change.

Help client identify feelings associated with family conflict, the subsequent exacerbation of physical symptoms, and the accompanying disabilities.

Client may be unaware of the relationship between physical symptoms and emotional problems. An awareness of the correlation is the first step toward creating change.

Help client identify changes he or she would like to occur within the family system.

Involving client helps to focus thinking on positive ways to adapt to problems in the family.

Encourage family participation in the development of plans to effect positive change, and work to resolve the conflict for which the client's sick role provides relief.

Input from the individual who will be directly involved in the change will increase the likelihood of a positive outcome.

Promote all family members having input into the plan for change as well as knowledge of benefits and consequences for each alternative, selection of appropriate alternatives, methods for implementation of alternatives, alternate plan in the event initial change is unsuccessful.

Family may require assistance with this problem-solving process. When all members are involved, chances for success are enhanced.

Ensure that client has accurate perception of role expectations within family system. Use role-play to practice areas associated with role that client perceives as painful.

Repetition through practice may help to desensitize client to the anticipated distress.

Discuss more adaptive coping strategies that may be used to prevent interference with performance of role during times of stress.

As client is able to understand the relationship between exacerbation of physical symptoms and existing conflict, more effective skills can be used.

---

| NURSING DIAGNOSIS: | **FAMILY COPING, ineffective: compromised/disabling** |
|---|---|
| **May Be Related To:** | Inadequate or incorrect information or understanding by a primary person. |
| | Prolonged disease progression that exhausts supportive capacity of significant other(s). |

| Possibly Evidenced By: | Significant person with chronically unexpressed feelings of guilt, anxiety, hostility, despair. |
|---|---|
| | Client providing little support for primary person. |
| | Client expresses despair regarding family reactions/lack of involvement. |
| | Intolerance/abandonment; psychosomatic tendency. |
| | Taking on illness signs of client. |
| | Distortion of reality regarding the client's health problem. |
| | Significant other(s) display protective behavior disproportionate (too little or too much) to client's abilities or need for autonomy. |
| **Desired Outcomes/Evaluation Criteria— Family Will:** | Identify/verbalize resources within themselves to deal with situation. |
| | Interact appropriately with the client and each other, providing support and assistance as indicated. |
| | Verbalize knowledge and understanding of illness. |
| | Participate actively in treatment program. |

## ACTIONS/INTERVENTIONS

### Independent

Explore past relationships and feelings about successes and failures.

Discuss precipitating stresses regarding real or feared threats to significant personal relationships.

Determine extent of "enabling" behaviors evidenced by family members; explore with family/client.

Assist to develop communication skills that enable needs to be met by using assertive expressions, e.g., "I-messages."

Explore possible negative feelings or fears caused by feeling compelled to meet demands of others.

Discuss ways of handling troublesome situations by using newly learned coping skills.

## RATIONALE

May help identify a pattern of interacting that may be counterproductive and lead to failure.

Unrealistic fears may be dictating relationships.

"Enabling" is doing for the client what he or she needs to do for own self. People want to be helpful and do not want to feel powerless to help their family member to be well. When the family members' "roles" are to "help" the client stay ill, they need to learn new ways of interacting to attain/maintain health for each individual.

Using assertive, direct communication can make significant differences in communicating needs and having these needs met in more effective ways.

May frustrate own wishes to please others due to fear of rejection or loss of the relationship.

Having a plan for handling situations before they arise helps increase successful interactions.

471

| ACTIONS/INTERVENTIONS | RATIONALE |
|---|---|
| **Independent** | |
| Give positive feedback for efforts toward using constructive new behaviors. | Client may lack self-confidence and require emotional support and assurance of capability. |
| **Collaborative** | |
| Refer to support groups, family therapy, if indicated. | May need additional assistance to promote healthy ways of interacting and assist client to deal effectively with illness/improve quality of life. |

# PROBLEMS RELATED TO ABUSE OR NEGLECT

## DSM IV

V61.21  Physical Abuse of Child
V61.21  Sexual Abuse of Child
V61.21  Neglect of Child
V61.1   Phsyical Abuse of Adult
V61.1   Sexual Abuse of Adult

Abuse affects all populations and is not restricted to specific socioeconomic or ethnic/cultural groups. While violence is defined as the use of force or physical compulsion to abuse or damage, the term "abuse" is much broader and includes physical or mental maltreatment and neglect that result in emotional, physical, or sexual injury. In the case of children, the disabled, or elderly, abuse can be the result of direct actions or omissions on the part of those responsible for the care of the individual. Additionally, one's perception of abuse is impacted by cultural and religious practices, values, and biologic predispositions. The problem can be generational, with victimizers often being victims of abuse themselves as children.

Violence is not a new problem; in fact, it is probably as old as humankind. However, in the United States, medicine has focused on these issues only since 1946. Therefore, the parameters of abuse are being identified and redefined on what may be perceived as an almost daily basis. For example, until recently women and children were considered to be the personal property of men and did not own property or have rights of their own. Women viewed themselves as sexual objects and were expected to subjugate themselves/defer to the will of men. Harsh treatment of children was justified by the belief that corporal and/or excessive punishment was necessary to maintain discipline and instill values. Changes in societal beliefs and the enactment of new laws have done little to curb abuse. Today, battering is the single most common cause of injury to women, and there has been an increase in the incidence of child abuse and neglect-related fatalities reported to child protection service agencies in the United States. Whether these statistics represent an increase in incidents or are the result of changing attitudes and/or better reporting is much debated.

This plan of care addresses the problems of abuse and neglect in both adults and children.

## ETIOLOGIC THEORIES

### Psychodynamics

Psychoanalytic theory suggests that unmet needs for satisfaction and security result in an underdeveloped ego and a poor self-concept. Aggression and violence supply this individual with a sense of power and prestige that boosts the self-image and provides a significance or purpose to the individual's life that is lacking. Some theorists have supported the hypothesis that aggression and violence are the overt expressions of powerlessness and low self-esteem.

### Biologic

Various components of the neurologic system have been implicated in both the facilitation and inhibition of aggressive impulses. The limbic system in particular appears to be involved. In addition, higher brain centers play an important role by constantly interacting with the aggression centers. It is also believed that various neurotransmitters, such as epinephrine, norepinephrine, dopamine, acetylcholine, and serotonin, may play a role in the facilitation and inhibition of aggressive impulses. This theory is consistent with the "fight-or-flight" arousal in response to stress.

Some studies suggest the possibility of a direct genetic link; however, the evidence has not been firmly established. Organic brain syndromes associated with various cerebral disorders have been linked to violent behavior. Particularly, areas of the limbic system and

473

temporal lobes, trauma to the brain, and diseases such as encephalitis and epilepsy have been implicated in aggressive behavior.

## Family Dynamics

Child abuse is often the consequence of the interactions of parental vulnerabilities (e.g., mental illness, substance abuse); child vulnerabilities (e.g., low birth weight, difficult temperament); a particular developmental stage, such as adolescence, toddler; and social stressors (e.g., lack of social supports, young parental age, single parenthood, poverty, minority ethnicity, lack of acculturation, exposure to family violence).

Learning theory states that children learn to behave by imitating their role models, usually parents, although as they mature they are influenced by teachers, friends, and others. Individuals who were abused as children or whose parents disciplined with physical punishment are more likely to behave in a violent manner as adults. Television and movies are believed to have an influence on developing both adaptive and maladaptive behavior. Some theorists believe that individuals who have a biologic influence toward aggressive behavior are more likely to be affected by external models than those without this predisposition.

The influence of culture and social structure cannot be discounted. Difficulty in negotiating interpersonal conflict has led to a general acceptance of violence as a means of solving problems. When individuals/groups of people discover they cannot meet their needs through conventional methods, they are more likely to resort to delinquent behaviors. This may contribute to a subculture of violence within society.

## CLIENT ASSESSMENT DATABASE

### Activity/Rest

Sleep problems, e.g., sleeplessness or oversleeping, nightmares, sleepwalking, sleeping in strange places (avoiding perpetrator).
Fatgiue.

### Ego Integrity

Negative appraisal of self, accepts self-blame/makes excuses for the actions of others.
Feelings of guilt, anger, fear and shame, helplessness, and/or powerlessness.
Minimization or denial of significance of behaviors (most prominent defense mechanism).
Avoidance or fear of certain people, places, objects; submissive, fearful manner (particularly in presence of abuser).
Report of stress factors (e.g., family unemployment; financial, lifestyle changes; marital discord).
Hostility toward/mistrust of others.

### Elimination

Enuresis, encopresis.
Recurrent urinary infections.

### Food/Fluid

Frequent vomiting; changes in appetite (anorexia, overeating).
Changes in weight; failure to gain weight appropriately/signs of malnutrition, repeated pica (neglect).

### Hygiene

Wearing clothing that covers body in a manner that is inappropriate for weather conditions or clothing that is inadequate to provide protection (neglect).
Excessive/anxiety about bathing; dirty/unkempt appearance (neglect).

## Neurosensory

Behavioral extremes (very aggressive/demanding conduct); extreme rage or passivity and withdrawal; age-inappropriate behavior.

**Memory:** Blackouts, periods of amnesia; reports of flashbacks.

Disorganized thinking; difficulty concentrating/making decisions.

Inappropriate affect; may be hypervigilant, anxious, depressed.

Poor impulse control.

Rocking, thumb sucking, or other habitual problems; restlessness.

Psychiatric manifestations, e.g.: dissociative phenomena including multiple personalities (sexual abuse); borderline personality disorder (adult incest survivors).

Presence of neurologic deficits/CNS damage without external injuries evident may indicate shaken baby syndrome.

## Pain/Discomfort

Dependent on specific injuries/form of abuse.

Multiple somatic complaints (e.g., stomach pain, chronic pelvic pain, spastic colon, headache).

## Safety

Bruises, bite marks, skin welts, burns (e.g., scalding, cigarette), bald spots, fractures, lacerations, unusual bleeding, internal injuries, brain damage; rashes/itching in the genital area; anal fissures, skin tags, hemorrhoids, scar tissue, changes in tone of sphincter.

Recurrent injuries; history of multiple accidents.

Description of incident incongruent with injury, delay in seeking treatment.

Lack of age-appropriate supervision, inattention to avoidable hazards in the home (neglect).

Intense episodes of rage directed at self or others.

Self-injurious/suicidal behavior; involvement in high-risk activities.

History of suicidal behavior of family members.

## Sexuality

Changes in sexual awarenese or activity: compulsive masturbation, precocious sex play, tendency to repeat or reenact incest/abuse experience; excessive curiosity about sex; sexually abusing another child; promiscuity; overly anxious/inhibited about sexual anatomy or behavior.

May display feminine sex-role stereotypes; confusion about sexuality (male survivors).

Reports of decreased sexual desire (as adult), erectile dysfunction, premature ejaculation, and/or anorgasmia; dyspareunia, vaginismus; flashbacks during intercourse; inability to engage in sex without anxiety.

Episodes of marital rape or forced intercourse.

Vaginal bleeding; linear laceration of hymen, vaginal mucosa.

Presence of STD, vaginitis, genital warts, or pregnancy (especially child).

## Social Interactions

Multiple family/relationship stressors reported.

Household members may include steprelatives or a paramour.

History of frequent moves/relocation.

Few/no support systems.

Inability to form satisfactory peer relationships; withdrawal in social settings; inappropriate attachment to imaginary companion.

Lack of assertive communication skills; difficulty negotiating interpersonal conflicts.

Cheating, lying; low achievement or drop in school performance.

Running away from home/relationship.

Memories of childhood may contain blank periods, excessive fantasizing/daydreaming; report of violence/neglect in family of origin.

Family interaction pattern—less verbally responsive, increased use of direct commands and critical statements, decreased verbal praise or acknowledgment, belittling, denigrating, scapegoating, ignoring; significant imbalance of power/use of hitting as control measure, patterns of enmeshment, closed family system.

### Teaching/Learning

May be any age, race, religion/culture, or educational level; from all socioeconomic groups (usual child profile is under age 3 or perceived as different due to temperamental traits, congenital abnormalities, chronic illness).

Learning disabilities include attention-deficit disorders, conduct disorders.

Delay in achieving developmental tasks, declines on cognitive testing; habitual truancy/absence from school for nonlegitimate reasons (neglect).

Substance abuse by client or family member(s) (most often cocaine, crack, amphetamines, alcohol).

Use of multiple health-care providers/resources (limits awareness of repeated nature of problem); lack of age-appropriate health screening/immunization, dental care, absence of necessary prostheses, such as eyeglasses, hearing aid (neglect).

## DIAGNOSTIC STUDIES

Dependent on individual situation/needs.

Screening tests, e.g., Child Behavior Checklist: Elevated scores on the internalization scale reveal behaviors described as fearful, inhibited, depressed, overcontrolled or undercontrolled, aggressive, antisocial.

## NURSING PRIORITIES

1. Provide physical/emotional safety.
2. Develop a trusting therapeutic relationship.
3. Enhance sense of self-esteem.
4. Improve problem-solving ability.
5. Involve family/partner in therapeutic program.

## DISCHARGE GOALS

1. Physical/emotional safety maintained.
2. Trusting relationship with one person established.
3. Self-growth and positive approaches to problems evident.
4. Client/SOs participating in ongoing therapy.

| NURSING DIAGNOSIS: | TRAUMA, HIGH RISK FOR |
| --- | --- |
| Risk Factors May Include: | Dependent position in relationship(s). |
| | History of previous abuse/neglect. |
| | Lack of, or nonuse of, support systems/resources. |
| Possibly Evidenced By: | [Not applicable; presence of signs and symptoms establishes an **actual** diagnosis.] |
| Desired Outcomes/Evaluation Criteria—Client Will: | Be free of injury/signs of neglect. |
| Client/Family Will: | Recognize need for/seek assistance to prevent abuse. |
| | Identify and access resouces to assist in promoting a safe environment. |

| ACTIONS/INTERVENTIONS | RATIONALE |
|---|---|

### Independent

Note age/developmental level of client, mentation agility, physical abilities/limitations.

Children under 3, those perceived as having different temperament, or those with congenital problems/chronic illness are at increased risk of being abused/neglected. Additionally, elderly people who are dependent on others because of age or infirmities or individuals with significant disabilities are also at risk. Individuals who are incapable of meeting their own needs/directing their personal affairs may require alternate placement/court-ordered advocate.

Review physical complaints/injuries including those that suggest possibility of sexual abuse (e.g., bladder infection, bruises in the genital area, reports of aggression or inappropriate sexual behavior). Note affect and demeanor.

The visible evidence of physical abuse/neglect makes it more easily recognized. While these individuals display signs of emotional involvement, inappropriate affect, and behaviors such as withdrawal, acting out, or suicidal gestures in the absence of physical evidence of abuse/neglect, suggests presence of emotional abuse. Child sexual abuse is particularly difficult to diagnose. While the signs noted here are not definitive, they suggest need for further investigation.

Identify individual concerns of client.

Concerns of client will vary dependent on circumstances and affect choice of interventions, possible options.

Interview perpetrator(s)/family in a nonjudgmental manner, displaying tact and professional concern for individual(s).

Can provide insight into risks to client and potential for repetition of behavior. The need for power over or control of client, excessive jealousy/over-possessiveness, frequency of verbal arguments that can escalate to violence, substance abuse, severity of past injuries inflicted, history of forced or threatened sexual acts, and/or threats to kill client (especially when perpetrator indicates a belief he or she cannot live without partner) greatly increases the level of concern for client's safety and choice of interventions.

Maintain objectivity and avoid blame or accusations during interview process.

Individuals will be defensive and may react with hostility and anger, or may withdraw, making it difficult to obtain accurate information. Initially, perpetrator may not be known, and even if family is not involved in situation, members will feel guilt that they did not protect the victim. Avoiding blame promotes open communication and therapeutic interactions and may enhance the investigation process.

Use open-ended questions with gentle, caring manner. Speak at individual's level (e.g., child vs. adult, or developmentally disabled individual). Provide privacy as indicated by age, circumstances of the situation.

Client and parent will respond more positively to caring approach and be more available for help to correct underlying problems when dealt with in this way. Note: Care must be taken to avoid leading the client or suggesting answers to questions. As these individuals are vulnerable, they are suggestible and may provide answers to "please" the therapist, resulting in questionable information.

477

| ACTIONS/INTERVENTIONS | RATIONALE |
|---|---|

### Independent

Use techniques of play therapy to obtain information from children. Videotape session(s) as appropriate.

The child may be afraid to tell/be unable to adequately verbalize what has happened. Play therapy is a nonthreatening method of observation/Active-listening that allows for free expression of the child's feelings and perceptions without undue influence from adults. Videotaping allows various parties (legal and counseling) to view the same data, reducing risk of misinterpretation and negating need for child to submit to repeated questioning, which may color data over time. In addition, this can provide safeguards for both therapist and client.

Note sequence of events as related by parent(s)/ caregivers and partner, paying particular attention to inconsistencies and contradictory reports.

May reveal reality of what happened. Perpetrator(s)/ family members are upset and afraid about what has happened/the potential consequences and may try to cover up circumstances of injury.

Evaluate family and home environment. Note particularly areas of stress related to abusive occurrence.

Provides clues to need for change to prevent further problems. Families who move frequently and are socially isolated and stepfamilies are at greater risk. Children who have been separated from parents because of prematurity or neonatal illness also may be more at risk owing in part to problems with bonding.

Identify individual risk factors for recidivism of abuse/neglect.

Perpetrator's resistance to ongoing therapy, substance abuse, immaturity, and narcissistic personality traits increase risk that violent behavior will recur.

Help adult client develop a safety plan incorporating available personal and community resources.

Typically, these individuals have few/are separated from support systems and require assistance to identify options and initiate a plan. Additionally, availability of resources such as women's shelters, counseling services, or ombudsman for the elderly/disabled varies according to locality.

Discuss importance of involved adults participating in therapeutic program. Identify consequences of abusive behaviors.

Without outside intervention, the behavior is likely to continue. Loss of family (divorce, separation, restraining order, alternate placement), loss of property/income, possible loss of job, as well as potential for incarceration can occur. Studies indicate skilled specialized counseling has a success rate of 50%–75% in eliminating violent behavior.

### Collaborative

Follow correct procedures and be familiar with reporting protocols of institution/community.

Legal obligations vary from state to state but most have mandatory reporting of suspected child abuse. Sensitive handling of this procedure can provide protection for the client and direct families to the help they need to promote improved functioning.

| ACTIONS/INTERVENTIONS | RATIONALE |
|---|---|
| **Collaborative** | |
| Arrange for home-based interventions (e.g., visiting nurse) as indicated. | Home visitation provides opportunity for teaching/modeling of effective child rearing behaviors, ongoing monitoring of home situation, and early identification of/intervention for developing problems to help maintain the family unit. |
| Refer to individual/family therapy. | As in the case of violent behavior, involved individuals need to distinguish between validity of emotions and the inappropriateness of the behavior. Violence is the choice of the perpetrator, is under his or her control, and is his or her sole responsibility although the dynamics of relationship(s) may be a factor. |
| Refer client/SOs to substance abuse program as appropriate. | Substance abuse negatively impacts the therapeutic process and increases likelihood that behavior will recur/continue. |

| **NURSING DIAGNOSIS:** | **SELF-ESTEEM, CHRONIC LOW** |
|---|---|
| **May Be Related To:** | Personal vulnerability, feelings of abandonment, circular process of self-negation. |
| | Life choices perpetuating failure/abuse. |
| **Possibly Evidenced By:** | Self-negating verbalization, expressions of shame/guilt. |
| | Evaluating self as unable to deal with events. |
| | Rationalizing away/rejecting positive feedback and exaggerating negative feedback about self. |
| | Hesitancy to try new things/situations; nonassertive/passive, indecisive, or overly conforming behaviors. |
| **Desired Outcomes/Evaluation Criteria—Client Will:** | Verbalize understanding of negative evaluation of self and reasons for this problem. |
| | Participate in treatment program to promote change in self-evaluation. |
| | Demonstrate behaviors/lifestyle changes to promote positive self-esteem. |
| | Verbalize increased sense of self-esteem in relation to current situation. |

| ACTIONS/INTERVENTIONS | RATIONALE |
|---|---|

### Independent

| | |
|---|---|
| Develop therapeutic relationship. Be attentive, validate client's communication, provide encouragement for efforts, maintain open communication, use skills of Active-listening and "I-messages." | Promotes self-esteem by validating the individual as a worthwhile person who has important things to say and has value in situation. This relationship may be slow to develop as client's feelings of betrayal will impact client's ability to trust others as well as him- or herself. Note: Males who have been sexually abused may have difficulty with self-disclosure to male therapists, while young children may fear being seduced by male therapist and also be concerned that female therapist will not act in a protective manner. |
| Note body language and hypervigilant attitude. | After period of testing reliability of caregiver/therapist, client may begin to relax vigilance, indicating initiation of trust relationship and openness to progress in therapy. |
| Assess content of negative self-talk. | "Damaged goods" syndrome and self-blame for what has occurred are common. Additionally, this may be reinforced by negative responses by individuals/peers, hostility from family members, and inner feelings of shame/guilt. Depending on severity, this will likely be the initial focus of therapy once client safety is assured. |
| Discuss client perceptions of self related to what is happening. Confront misconceptions. | Client frequently believes he or she is "lacking" or in some way causing the behavior in the other person. Gently confronting these misperceptions can help the client accept the reality that he or she is not responsible for the other's behavior. |
| Emphasize need for client to avoid comparing self to others. | Pattern has been established to make unfavorable comparisons, and stopping this thought process is a step toward increasing self-esteem. |
| Be aware that people are not programmed to be rational, rather it is a learned behavior/skill. | In order to develop positive self-esteem, individual needs to seek information/facts, choose to learn, choose to think rather than merely accepting/reacting to what is happening, to respect self and value honesty. |
| Confront client's tendency to minimize situation. Discuss impact of abuse/neglect on individual. | Gentle confrontation can help the client begin to accept the reality of what has happened. Giving up the "fantasy" of "things as you wish they were" provides a stronger base for client to build on, enhancing likelihood of successful outcome. |
| Proceed with caution when helping client recall/investigate areas of life that are forgotten. | While the concept of repression has long been accepted in psychology, the phenomenon of "false memories" has raised questions regarding the validity of what is remembered. The suggestion of questioning and the client's own misperceptions and fantasies can lead to inaccurate conclusions and accusations that may be damaging to the client and family. |

480

| ACTIONS/INTERVENTIONS | RATIONALE |
|---|---|
| **Independent** | |
| Identify what behavior does for client (positive intention, i.e., maintains dependent position). Ask what options are available to the client/SO. | Promotes awareness of why things are the way they are and provides a starting point for making changes. |
| Set limits on aggressive or problem behaviors, such as acting out, suicide preoccupation, or rumination. (Refer to ND: Violence, high risk for, directed at self/others). | These behaviors diminish self-esteem, and continuation of them interferes with recovery. Rumination locks client into a circular path rather than allowing him or her to move forward and "get on" with life. |
| Discuss inaccuracies in self-perception with client/significant other(s). Help client to recognize view of self as "the victim." | Client may not see positive aspects of self that others see, and bringing it to awareness may help change perception. Dwelling on/sense of being "the victim" can interfere with sense of worth and impede recovery. |
| Have client list current/past successes and strengths. Provide feedback using positive "I-messages" rather than praise. | Helps client to develop internal sense of self-worth, new coping behaviors. |
| Discuss past choices, helping client identify future options. Avoid blaming client, assuring client that his or her decision was the best he or she could make at the time. | Negative view of self and perceived lack of options can interfere with client taking control of own life and developing new behaviors to prevent future abusive situations. Note: Appropriately attributing responsibility for the abuse to other(s) is an important part of healing, allowing client to stop criticizing self and to begin self-nurturing and protection. |
| Assist client to identify goals that are personally achievable and supportive of self. | Provides direction for client to work toward. Note: Clients not only need to feel differently about themselves but also need to *treat* themselves differently. |
| Allow client to progress at own rate. | Adaptation to a change in self-concept depends on its significance to individual, disruption of lifestyle, and length of illness/debilitation. Note: Emotional abuse (e.g., rejecting, terrorizing, ignoring, isolating, or corrupting) may have continued for a prolonged period of time before being diagnosed and therefore may be more pervasive and more difficult to overcome than physical abuse. |
| Involve in activities/exercise program. | Provides opportunities to practice new skills and promotes socialization. |
| Encourage development of social/vocational skills. | Participation in classes/activities/hobbies that client enjoys or would like to experience promotes successful accomplishments, enhancing self-esteem. Also provides options for increased independence and future options. |
| Give positive reinforcement for progress noted. | Helps client to accept self as a worthwhile person. Positive words of encouragement support development of coping behaviors. |
| Evaluate educational placement. | Special program may be needed to help client overcome educational deficiencies and catch up to appropriate grade level. |

481

| ACTIONS/INTERVENTIONS | RATIONALE |
| --- | --- |

### Independent

Identify family dynamics past and present.

Family interactions contribute to development of self-esteem in family members and provide clues to problems contributing to abuse.

Provide age-/situation-appropriate bibliotherapy.

Reading information supplements and supports other therapeutic intervention.

### Collaborative

Provide therapy in a team setting and seek peer consultation as appropriate.

Opportunity for open discussion increases therapist's awareness of personal feelings regarding abuse behavior/victimization of client, overidentifying with client, or need to "rescue" client, which could lead to countertransference problems and interfere with the progress of therapy. Note: This concern may be of greater significance when client is a child who has been sexually abused and the therapist has discomfort regarding own sexuality and unconscious childhood fantasies.

Involve in classes such as assertiveness training, positive self-image, communication skills.

Assists with learning skills to promote self-esteem.

Provide information about available community programs and opportunities for involvement.

Influencing one's community through volunteer or paid service (e.g., abuse prevention programs or as a victim advocate) allows client to be proactive and view self as a contributing member of society, aiding in client's own recovery process.

Refer to clinical nurse specialist, psychologist/psychiatrist, group therapy as indicated.

Type, severity, frequency, duration, and age of client at time of abuse affect recovery. Client may require long-term and/or specialized therapy, such as hypnosis. Additionally, group therapy provides an opportunity for client to share his or her healing with other survivors and learn new skills to enhance sense of self-worth.

| NURSING DIAGNOSIS: | POWERLESSNESS |
| --- | --- |
| **May Be Related To:** | Legitimate dependency on other(s) (child, elderly, disabled individual), personal vulnerability. Interpersonal interaction (e.g., misuse of power, force, abusive relationships). |
| | Lifestyle of helplessness (e.g., repeated failures, dependency). |
| **Possibly Evidenced By:** | Verbal expressions of having no control. |
| | Reluctance to express true feelings, fearing alienation from caregiver(s). |
| | Apathy (withdrawal, resignation, crying), passivity; anger. |

| **Desired Outcomes/Evaluation Criteria— Client Will:** | Express sense of control over future. |
| | Identify areas over which individual has control. |
| | Engage in problem-solving activities. |

| ACTIONS/INTERVENTIONS | RATIONALE |
|---|---|
| **Independent** | |
| Identify circumstances of individual situation contributing to client's sense of powerlessness. | Promotes understanding of factors involved and enables client to begin to develop sense of control over self and future. |
| Determine client locus of control. | Client who believes problems are caused by others (external) will need to begin to accept own responsibility for being in charge of self. Making a decision to take control of own life is crucial to making changes needed to support growth. |
| Help client to identify factors that are under own control. | Provides a starting point for client to begin to assume control over own life. |
| Identify use of manipulative behavior and reactions of client, SO(s), and health-care providers. | Manipulation is used for management of powerlessness because of distrust of others, fear of intimacy, and search for approval. This can interfere with personal and therapeutic relationships. |
| Discuss needs openly with client. Set agreed-on routines for meeting identified needs. | Promotes meeting needs directly and decreases the need for client to use manipulation. |
| Identify when flashbacks are problem for client and how they may be minimized. | May occur with fatigue or stress and generally intensify feelings of loss of control. Avoidance of individual "triggers" may reduce occurrence. |
| **Collaborative** | |
| Refer to assertiveness program. | As client learns these skills and becomes more active/assertive in relationships, she or he is more likely to set limits on the behaviors of others, express feelings more openly/directly, and take control of own life. |

| **NURSING DIAGNOSIS:** | **COPING, INDIVIDUAL, INEFFECTIVE** |
|---|---|
| **May Be Related To:** | Situational/maturational crises. |
| | Overwhelming threat to self, personal vulnerability. |
| | Inadequate support systems. |
| **Possibly Evidenced By:** | Verbalization of inability to cope/ask for help. |
| | Chronic worry, anxiety, depression, poor self-esteem. |
| | Inability to problem-solve, lack of assertive behaviors. |

483

| | |
|---|---|
| | Inappropriate use of defense mechanisms (e.g., denial, withdrawal). |
| | High illness rate, destructive behavior toward self/others. |
| **Desired Outcomes/Evaluation Criteria—Client Will:** | Assess the current situation accurately (related to age, individual condition). |
| | Identify ineffective coping behaviors and consequences. |
| | Verbalize feelings congruent with behavior. |

| ACTIONS/INTERVENTIONS | RATIONALE |
|---|---|
| **Independent** | |
| Help client separate issues of vulnerability from blame. | Client blames self/others for situation without looking at own responsibility for victim stance. Although this does not excuse abuse, client needs to change victim behaviors to gain control of self. |
| Active-listen and identify client perceptions/understanding of current situation. Evaluate decision-making ability. | Client often enters the health-care system in response to a crisis. This is an opportunity to help the client look at reality of abuse and begin to make changes. |
| Identify previous methods of dealing with life problems. Note use of denial. | Provides clues to coping skills that can be used for personal growth. Denial is the most prominent defense mechanism used by client/family members to protect against shame/guilt and to preserve intactness of the family, and it must be dealt with before progress can be made. |
| Encourage verbalization of fears and anxieties and expression of feelings of denial, depression, and anger. Let client know that these are normal reactions. | Expressing feelings helps client to become aware of the feelings, recognize and deal with what is happening. |
| Encourage and support client in evaluating lifestyle. Assess stressors and make plan for necessary change. | Identifying areas of life that promote abusive reactions/interactions helps client make changes in coping methods to prevent recurrences. |
| **Collaborative** | |
| Refer to appropriate resources as indicated by individual situation. | May need additional therapy/group involvement to learn new coping skills. |

| | |
|---|---|
| **NURSING DIAGNOSIS:** | **VIOLENCE, HIGH RISK FOR, DIRECTED AT SELF/OTHERS** |
| **Risk Factors May Include:** | Negative role modeling; developmental crises. |
| | History of abuse. |
| | Rage reactions; suicidal behavior. |
| | Organic brain syndrome; temporal lobe epilepsy. |

| **Possible Indicators:** | Anger, rage, fear of others. |
|---|---|
| | Increasing anxiety level, motor activity. |
| | Hostile threatening verbalizations; body language indicating effort to control behavior. |
| | Overt and aggressive acts. |
| | Expressed intent/desire to harm self/others; self-destructive behaviors, substance abuse. |
| **Desired Outcomes/Evaluation Criteria— Client Will:** | Acknowledge realities of the situation. |
| | Verbalize understanding of why behavior occurs. |
| | Identify precipitating factors/responses. |
| | Demonstrate new skills/methods for dealing with own responses. |

| ACTIONS/INTERVENTIONS | RATIONALE |
|---|---|
| **Independent** | |
| Determine underlying dynamics of individual situation, e.g., pattern of abuse, contributing factors to violent behavior, relationship of involved persons (parent/child, spouse or lover), family pattern of communication. | Necessary to determine needs/safety concerns. |
| Note signs of suicidal/homicidal intent, e.g., statements of intent/threats, development of a plan, giving away belongings, possession of means. | Allows for initiation of safety measures to protect client/others. Note: Association between suicidal behavior and physical abuse may be related to modeling of aggressive behavior within family/exposure to suicidal behavior of family member(s) as well as biologic risk in family for disorders associated with suicide, e.g., substance abuse and affective or impulsive conduct disorders. |
| Determine client's perception of self, impact of abuse on life, and future expectations. | May see self as useless, damaged goods without hope for positive change/productive future, which may result in feelings of hopelessness and the perception of lacking options. Depth of rage and extent of feelings of powerlessness may predict potential for violent behavior. |
| Explore death fantasies when expressed (e.g., "They'll be sorry"). | Discussion of fantasies helps client to look at reality of ideas and begin to deal with them. |
| Note coping behaviors being used currently by the client, e.g., denial, helplessness, rage reaction. | Provides information about mechanisms client uses to maintain the status quo, which may also increase risk for violent behavior. |
| Acknowledge reality of suicide/homicide as an option. Discuss consequences of actions if they were to follow through on intent. Ask how it will help client resolve problems. | Acknowledging feelings helps the client begin to look at what might happen if actions were acted on and own ability to control self and make choices regarding recovery. |
| Encourage appropriate expression of feelings. Acknowledge reality and normalcy of these feelings. Set limits on acting-out behaviors. | Promotes awareness of feelings and ability to deal with them in acceptable ways. |

485

| ACTIONS/INTERVENTIONS | RATIONALE |
|---|---|

### Independent

| | |
|---|---|
| Accept client's anger without reacting on an emotional basis. | Client's anger is directed at situation and those involved, not at health-care provider, so remaining separate from the client allows therapist to be helpful to the resolution of the anger. |
| Contract with client for safety. | Provides parameters to help client deal with destructive thoughts/actions and helps to keep client safe. |
| Assist client to learn new coping skills, e.g., assertive rather than nonassertive/aggressive behavior, effective parenting techniques. | Promotes sense of self-worth and ability to control own actions/situation. |

### Collaborative

| | |
|---|---|
| Administer antidepressants as indicated. | Helps client to deal with feelings of sadness and hopelessness and move forward in therapy. Age of client as well as nature of abusive situation affects depth of depression client may experience. |
| Refer to inpatient program as appropriate. | May require more intensive therapy to deal with covert forms of self-destructive behavior, e.g., substance abuse, heavy risk-taking/runaway behavior. |
| Refer to community resources. | Helps to attain/maintain recovery program. |

| NURSING DIAGNOSIS: | FAMILY PROCESSES, ALTERED [dysfunctional]/PARENTING, ALTERED |
|---|---|
| May Be Related To: | Situational crises (e.g., economic, illness, change in roles), developmental transitions (loss/gain of family member[s], blending of families). |
| | Poor role model, lack of support systems; unrealistic expectation for self, infant, partner; physical/pyschosocial abuse of nurturing figure. |
| Possibly Evidenced By: | Family system does not meet physical, emotional, spiritual, or security needs of its members. |
| | Inability of family members to relate to each other for mutual growth and maturation. |
| | Rigidity in functions, rules, roles; verbalization of inability to control child, resentment toward child, unresolved disappointment in gender or physical characteristics of child. |
| | Inattention to child needs, inappropriate caretaking behaviors, history of child/abuse or abandonment, incidence of physical/psychologic trauma. |

| Desired Outcomes/Evaluation Criteria—Client Will: | Express feelings freely and appropriately. |
|---|---|
| | Demonstrate individual involvement in problem-solving process. |
| | Demonstrate appropriate parenting behaviors. |

| ACTIONS/INTERVENTIONS | RATIONALE |
|---|---|
| **Independent** | |
| Identify composition of family, developmental stage, presence/involvement of extended family, use of social supports. | Knowing this information helps to create plan to change abusive situation. Lack of/ineffective use of support systems increases risk of recidivism. |
| Review type, severity, duration of problem and contribution of, as well as impact on, individual family members. | Affects choice of interventions. Abuse is an act of commission, while neglect is considered an act of omission. These behaviors indicate the presence of problems with relationships and/or parenting skills and individual problems such as inability to deal with stressors, substance abuse, mental illness, cognitive limitations, or criminality. Even if the behavior is the result of a single individual, all family members may be involved in the denial/coverup or even passive condoning of the behavior. Additionally, *all* family members *will be* impacted by the disclosure of the behavior. |
| Assess boundaries of family members. Do members share family identity and have little sense of individuality? Do they seem emotionally distant, not connected with one another? | These factors are critical to understanding individual family dynamics and developing strategies for change. Family that pressures client to heal quickly/forgive offender, blames client for causing pain by disclosing situation, fails to acknowledge significance of abuse, or minimizes/negates need for counseling is nonsupportive and will likely impede recovery process. |
| Discuss parenting techniques and parents' expectations. Review developmental levels of children. | Ineffective parenting and unrealistic expectations contribute to abuse. Understanding normal responses, progression of developmental milestones may help parents cope with changes. (Refer to ND: Growth and Development, altered.) |
| Note cultural and religious factors. | Beliefs about family roles, parenting style may contribute to practices that are abusive. |
| Discuss negative mode of individual interactions. Stress importance of continuous, open dialogue between family members using therapeutic communication skills. | Promotes successful interactions to break cycle of abuse. Keeping family secrets is destructive. |
| Determine current "family rules." Identify areas of needed change. | Rules may be imposed by adults rather than through a democratic process involving all family members, leading to conflict and angry confrontations. Setting positive family rules with all family members participating can promote functional family. |

487

| ACTIONS/INTERVENTIONS | RATIONALE |
|---|---|

### Independent

Identify and encourage use of previous successful coping behaviors.

Everyone has positive ways of dealing with life stressors, and when these are identified and enhanced they can help to change abusive situation.

Discuss concept of forgiveness for covert acts as well as acts of omission.

Forgiving others and oneself frees individuals from the past, allowing them to move forward with life. While forgiving does not condone the actions, it may help heal relationships.

Acknowledge realities of situation and inability to change others.

Family may not change, or relationship may be permanently destroyed. Individual needs to go forward with own life and healing process.

### Collaborative

Encourage family participation in multidisciplinary team conference/group therapy as appropriate.

Participation in family and group therapy for 13–18 months increases likelihood of success as interactional issues (e.g., marital conflict, scapegoating of the abused child) can be addressed/dealt with. Involvement with others can help family members to experience new ways of interacting and gain insight into their behavior, providing opportunity for change.

Refer to classes (e.g., Parent Effectiveness), specific disease/disability support groups (including substance abuse resources), clergy as indicated.

Can assist family to effect positive change/enhance conflict resolution. Parents may require positive role modeling to learn nonpunitive child-rearing techniques. Presence of substance abuse problems requires all family members to seek support/assistance in dealing with situation to promote a healthy outcome.

Refer family to community programs/resources.

When the individual is willing to accept responsibility for past behavior, self-help organizations help families overcome stigma of situation and achieve greater self-esteem while providing professionally supervised treatment. Note: High dropout rates have been reported when abusive parents are referred to traditional community mental health clinics. Parents often view authority figures with suspicion and mistrust and require more personal approaches, e.g., 24-hour availability of counselors, evening/after-hours appointments.

---

| **NURSING DIAGNOSIS:** | **GROWTH AND DEVELOPMENT, ALTERED** |
|---|---|
| **May Be Related To:** | Inadequate caretaking (physical/emotional neglect or abuse). |
| | Indifference, inconsistent responsiveness, multiple caretakers. |
| | Environmental and stimulation deficiencies. |

| | |
|---|---|
| **Possibly Evidenced By:** | Delay or difficulty in performing skills typical of age group. |
| | Altered physical growth. |
| | Inability to perform self-care or self-control activities appropriate for age. |
| | Loss of previously acquired skills, precocious or accelerated skill attainment. |
| | Flat affect, listlessness, decreased responses. |
| **Desired Outcomes/Evaluation Criteria— Client Will:** | Perform motor, social, and/or expressive skills typical of age group, within scope of individual capabilities. |
| | Perform self-care and self-control activities appropriate for age/developmental level. |
| **Parents/Caregivers Will:** | Verbalize understanding of developmental delay/deviation and plan(s) for intervention. |

| ACTIONS/INTERVENTIONS | RATIONALE |
|---|---|
| **Independent** | |
| Determine existing condition(s) that contribute to developmental deviation. Note severity/pervasiveness of situation. | May be long-term physical/emotional abuse, situational disruption, or inadequate assistance during period of crisis or transition. Identifying individual situation of abuse/neglect guides choice of interventions. |
| Ascertain nature of parenting/caretaking activities and parents' expectations of the child (e.g., inadequate, inconsistent, unrealistic/insufficient expectations; lack of stimulation, inappropriate limit-setting and responsiveness). | Provides information about needs of family/child. Parents' unrealistic expectations of the abilities/ independence needs of the child may lead to demands for behavior that the child is unable to accomplish or may interfere with the developmental process. Note: Conflict may especially arise during the preschool and teen years, when separation issues are paramount. |
| Identify developmental age/stage of child, expected skills/activities using authoritative texts (e.g., Gesell) or assessment tools (e.g., Draw-a-Person, Denver Developmental Screening Test). | Baseline information notes areas of deviation, skills affected, whether pervasive or one area of difficulty. |
| Provide information regarding normal growth and developmental process and appropriate expectations for individual child. | Helps parents/caregivers to have realistic expectations about child's abilities. |
| Note significant stressful events that have occurred recently in the family. | Losses and separation such as the death of a parent, divorce, or unemployment may tax the supportive abilities of the parents/caregivers. |
| Avoid blame when discussing contributing factors. | Parents usually feel inadequate and blame themselves for being "a poor parent." Note: Adding blame will not be helpful for changing behavior. |
| Support parents'/caretakers' attempts to maintain or return to optimal level of self-control or self-care activities. | Providing assistance enables parents to progress in learning new skills and helping child develop to fullest potential. |

489

| ACTIONS/INTERVENTIONS | RATIONALE |
|---|---|

### Independent

| | |
|---|---|
| Involve parents/caregivers in role-play, group activities. | Provides opportunities to practice new behaviors. |
| Provide pertinent reference materials. | Bibliotherapy provides information to encourage questions and additional learning. |

### Collaborative

| | |
|---|---|
| Consult appropriate professional resources, e.g., occupational/rehabilitation/speech therapists, special education teacher, job counselor. | Necessary to coordinate an individual plan of care to optimize child's growth and development. |
| Encourage attendance at appropriate educational programs, e.g., Parent Effectiveness classes, infant stimulation sessions, nurturing programs. | Participation in these activities will provide parent with new skills to enable avoidance of abusive/neglectful behaviors. |

| NURSING DIAGNOSIS: | SEXUAL DYSFUNCTION/SEXUALITY PATTERNS, ALTERED |
|---|---|
| **May Be Related To:** | Ineffectual or absent role models; impaired relationship with a significant other. |
| | Vulnerability. |
| | Physical/psychosocial abuse (e.g., harmful relationships). |
| | Misinformation or lack of knowledge. |
| **Possibly Evidenced By:** | Verbalization of a problem; reported difficulties, limitations, or changes in sexual behaviors or activities. |
| | Inability to achieve desired satisfaction. |
| | Conflicts involving values. |
| | Seeking of confirmation of desirability. |
| **Desired Outcomes/Evaluation Criteria— Client Will:** | Verbalize understanding of sexual anatomy/function. |
| | Identify individual reasons/stressors contributing to situation. |
| | Discuss satisfying/acceptable sexual practices. |
| | Demonstrate improved communication and relationship skills. |

| ACTIONS/INTERVENTIONS | RATIONALE |
|---|---|

### Independent

| | |
|---|---|
| Discuss client's perceptions of sexuality as learned in family/relationships. Ask client about past sexual abuse during history taking. | Gives permission to the client to talk about sex and abuse in a safe environment. Many abused individuals feel guilty about sharing family secrets, fear reaction of others, and are concerned that they will not be believed. |

| ACTIONS/INTERVENTIONS | RATIONALE |
|---|---|

### Independent

Determine usual pattern of functioning and level of desire as well as vocabulary used by the client.

Provides information about how client views sexual activity and areas of lack of knowledge/misinformation.

Identify sexual problems present for the client, e.g., avoiding/afraid of sex; promiscuous behavior; seeing sex as an obligation; fear, anger, or disgust with touching (particularly sexual touching); feeling emotionally distant during sexual activity; painful intercourse; or orgasmic difficulty.

Sexual abuse is demonstrated in many different ways depending on the extent, duration, and presence of threat/fear of violence. Survivors require long-term therapy to change attitudes about sex, sense of self as a person/sexual being, and general feelings related to the abuse.

Identify cultural, religious, and/or value factors and conflicts present.

Beliefs/values of client will affect view of what has happened and feelings about situation, influencing therapeutic treatment program.

Note substance use/abuse.

May affect sexual function/satisfaction, requiring therapeutic intervention.

Avoid making value judgments and be aware of own feelings and response to client expressions, revelations, and/or concerns.

Judgments and negative responses do not help client to cope with situation and may result in client withdrawing and not talking further.

Provide information about anatomy and physiology and individual situation according to client needs.

Lack of accurate knowledge may contribute to problems client is experiencing.

Note coping style exhibited.

Client may use repetition and reenactment of the molestation/abuse incident(s) or may avoid sexual stimuli.

Encourage use of higher-level defenses (e.g., repression, sublimation, and intellectualization) by limit-setting, education, interpretation, and desensitization.

Successful intervention focuses on having the client become gradually aware of the painful memories and verbalize them instead of acting them out or avoiding them.

Set limits on seductive behavior when displayed. Help client distinguish the difference between acceptable and unacceptable behaviors.

The difference between acceptable physically affectionate behavior and behavior with sexual intent, as well as respect for own and others bodily privacy, needs to be learned. The sexually abused child may have difficulty differentiating affectionate from sexual relationships and may be aroused by routine physical or psychologic closeness.

Help client learn to say "No" to sex.

It is difficult for survivors to learn to say "Yes" to sex until they can learn to say "No" at any time.

Encourage careful selection of future sexual partner and delaying sexual activity until a friendship is established.

Helps incest/abuse survivors develop a positive sexual experience. Individuals heal best in relationships high in emotional intimacy and support and low in expectations of sexual interaction.

Encourage client to share thoughts/concerns with partner.

Appropriate self-disclosure in current/future relationships will help couple develop positive relationship.

| ACTIONS/INTERVENTIONS | RATIONALE |
|---|---|
| **Independent** | |
| Identify sights, sounds, smells, and types of touch that are associated with the event/trigger flashbacks for the client. Discuss ways to minimize flashbacks/deal with triggers. | Triggers can cause the feelings and fears to recur. Avoiding or learning to deal with triggers helps client to remain in the safety of the present. For example, a specific sexual position may trigger anxious feelings/flashbacks. Sexual partner "allowing" client to take control, choose alternate position can lessen these feelings, promoting trust and enhancing emotional growth. Reexperiencing the event in a flashback is a traumatic occurrence and affects current relationship/intimacy. |
| Tell the client that recovery is possible. | Client may believe that problems will last forever, and it can be reassuring to hear that therapy can help the client gain a positive, healthy perspective on sex and engage in positive relationships. |
| **Collaborative** | |
| Refer to clinical nurse specialist, professional sex therapist, family counseling as appropriate. | Problems may be deep-seated and require specialized/prolonged therapy. |

# PREMENSTRUAL DYSPHORIC DISORDER:
## (Premenstrual Syndrome)

### DSM IV
Premenstrual Dysphoric Disorder (provided for further study)

### DSM III-R
Late Luteal Dysphoric Disorder

Recommended for further systematic clinical study and research, Premenstrual Dysphoric Disorder (popularly called PMS) is characterized by multiple symptom clusters occurring during the menstrual cycle, becoming progressively disabling. Some research suggests these symptoms may be a delayed effect of hormonal changes earlier in the menstrual cycle, or the result of an independent cyclical mood disorder that is synchronized with the menstrual cycle. Although the physical symptoms produce discomfort, the mood change or premenstrual negative affect symptoms are often more distressing, interfering with familial, social, and work-related activities. The condition usually improves after the onset of menses; however, for some women, symptoms persist through and after menses. The symptoms cannot be the sole result of cyclic or environmental stress, but may be enhanced by these stressors. This diagnosis is not used when the person is experiencing a late luteal phase exacerbation of another disorder, such as major depression, panic disorder, or dysthymia.

## ETIOLOGIC THEORIES
### Psychodynamics

Although etiology is not understood, symptoms are believed to be related to the interaction of psychologic, social, and biological factors. Underlying personality and psychiatric conditions contribute to how any particular individual deals with these physical problems. It has been suggested that an individual's past and present negative attitudes toward menstruation likely influence the symptomatology of Premenstrual Dysphoric Disorder. Emotion is the result of complex interactions between hormonal changes and cognitive variables. Hormonal changes during the menstrual cycle are likely to increase the female's susceptibility to negative psychologic experiences rather than to cause such experiences.

### Biologic

Although not completely understood, it may be related to the alterations (fluctuations) in estrogen and progesterone and the fluid-retaining action of estrogen during the menstrual cycle. Estrogen excess/deficiency, progesterone deficiency, vitamin deficiency, hypoglycemia, and fluid retention have all been proposed to contribute to Premenstrual Dysphoric Disorder. In addition, levels of androgen, adrenal hormones, and prolactin have been hypothesized to be important in the etiology of this syndrome. Finally, an increase in prostaglandins secreted by the uterine musculature has been implicated in accounting for the pain associated with this disorder.

### Family Dynamics

It is possible that the behaviors associated with this disorder are learned through modeling during the socialization process. Children may observe and identify with this behavior in significant adults and incorporate it into their own responses as they grow up. Positive reinforcement in the form of primary or secondary gains for these behaviors may serve to perpetuate the learned patterns of disability.

# CLIENT ASSESSMENT DATABASE

## Activity/Rest

Decreased interest in usual activities; lack of regular exercise.
Sleep disorders (insomnia).
Fatigue, lethargy; restlessness.

## Circulation

Heart pounding/palpitations.
Increased sweating/diaphoresis.

## Ego Integrity

History of personality changes not unlike Jekyll and Hyde (e.g., feeling happy or serene during the follicular phase of the menstrual cycle and tense, irritable, and depressed beginning any time in the luteal phase but primarily during the last week), occurring during a majority of menstrual cycles and ceasing at the onset of the menstrual period.
Changes in body image; feeling fat, ugly, etc.
Anxiety, feelings of being unable to cope, sense of loss of control/powerlessness.

## Elimination

Urinary retention, oliguria; recurrent cystitis.
Constipation; diarrhea.

## Food/Fluid

Nausea, vomiting.
Poor nutritional habits; increased appetite/overeating; sugar and other specific food cravings.
Difficulty maintaining a stable weight/transient weight gain.
Abdominal bloating.
Swelling of extremities.

## Neurosensory

Headaches (classic migraine); dizziness or fainting, vertigo, syncope.
Aggravation of seizure activity.
Paresthesias of extremities.
Visual disturbances.
**Mental Status:** Decreased concentration, forgetfulness, confusion.
Sense of depersonalization may be reported.
Affective changes of dysphoria or depressed mood, irritability, nervous tension, sudden mood swings, impatience, crying spells.
Depression, anger, and anxiety; hostility, aggressiveness, nagging.
Irrational thought processes involving suicide.

## Pain/Discomfort

Abdominal cramping.
Breast tenderness, joint pain/swelling, backache.

## Respiration

Nasal congestion.
Hoarseness.
Aggravation of asthmatic episodes.

## Safety

Skin changes: acne, neurodermatitis; easy bruising.
Conjunctivitis.
Suicidal ideation/attempts.

## Sexuality

Intolerance or multiple side effects to birth control pills (however, a small percentage of women report improvement in condition).
Breast swelling.
Changes in sexual drive.
History of pregnancy-induced hypertension.

## Social Interactions

Reports interference with the quality of life (home, social, and work).

## Teaching/Learning

Age of onset may be any time after menarche but may not be noticeable until the 20s (may not seek treatment until 30s or 40s, when the symptoms worsen).
May have close female relative(s) with similar problems.
Alcohol intolerance.

## DIAGNOSTIC STUDIES

As indicated by individual situation, dependent on age, medication, therapy, family history, and symptomatology.
In nonmenstruating females who have had a hysterectomy, the timing of luteal and follicular phases may require measurement of circulating reproductive hormones and/or daily self-ratings.

**Serum Progesterone and Estradiol 17 (Midluteal Phase):** Assesses inadequate luteal phase.

**Serum Prolactin and TSH:** Rules out pituitary/thyroid abnormalities in client with galactorrhea.

**Adrenal Suppresssion Test:** Locates source of androgen excess and serves as a guide for therapy for clients with hirsutism.

**Abraham Menstrual System Questionnaire (MSQ), the Dalton Diagnostic Checklist (or similar premenstrual symptom worksheet), and calendar of premenstrual symptoms (minimum 2 months):** Self-reporting tools to determine cycles of symptoms and degree of impairment.

**Psychologic Assessment:** Minnesota Multiphasic Personality Inventory (MMPI) twice, once during the follicular phase of the menstrual cycle and again during the luteal phase (preferably the client's most critical day) of the menstrual cycle to identify psychologic components and degree of disability.

## NURSING PRIORITIES

1. Provide emotional support and relief of symptoms.
2. Present information about condition/health-care needs/resources.
3. Encourage adoption of a lifestyle promoting health and diminishing premenstrual symptoms.

## DISCHARGE GOALS

1. Assertive behavior/stress-management techniques used to manage problems.
2. Condition understood and sources for assistance identified.
3. Lifestyle changes to promote health/diminish symptoms implemented.
4. Family/SO participating in treatment process.

495

| NURSING DIAGNOSIS: | ANXIETY [moderate to panic] |
|---|---|
| **May Be Related To:** | Cyclic changes in female hormones affecting other systems. |
| **Possibly Evidenced By:** | Increased tension; apprehension, jitteriness. |
| | Impaired functioning, feelings of inability to cope/loss of control; depersonalization. |
| | Somatic complaints. |
| **Desired Outcomes/Evaluation Criteria—Client Will:** | Verbalize awareness of feelings of anxiety. |
| | Identify healthy ways to deal with feelings. |
| | Appear relaxed and report anxiety is reduced to a manageable level. |
| | Use resources/support systems effectively. |

| ACTIONS/INTERVENTIONS | RATIONALE |
|---|---|
| **Independent** | |
| Assess level of anxiety and degree of interference with daily activities/interpersonal relationships. | Degree to which this disorder is affecting life will indicate need for/type of intervention. |
| Review history and have client maintain a premenstrual symptom calendar, noting occurrence of nervous tension, mood swings, irritability, and feelings of anxiety. | Identifies established patterns of symptoms, allowing for proactive intervention to break cycle of increasing irritability, muscle tension, and escalating anxiety. |
| Review with client the premenstrual worksheet, confidential personal data sheets, and Life Events Stress Scale. | Joint evaluation of all the data, noting the interaction between life stress and premenstrual symptoms, is essential to making a correct diagnosis and developing an appropriate treatment program. |
| Encourage client to acknowledge and express feelings, accepting client's perception of the situation. | Listening to the client promotes feelings of worthwhileness and normalcy, thereby reducing anxiety. |
| Have client keep a diary of feelings and precipitating factors. | Helps client become more in tune with own body/responses, enhancing ability to intervene/control situation. |
| Demonstrate/encourage use of stress reduction techniques, relaxation and visualization skills. | Enhances ability to relax and flow with the discomfort/pain, provides sense of control, and helps to reduce anxiety. |
| Recommend involvement in regular aerobic exercise program such as fast walking, jogging, dancing. | Provides outlet for tension, promotes release of endorphins, increases sense of general well-being. |
| Assist the client to use anxiety to promote understanding and deal with situation. | A moderate degree of anxiety can be helpful to heighten awareness, and when client learns to use this, problem-solving can be enhanced. |
| Identify helpful resources/people, e.g., physicians, nurse practitioners/clinicians, psychiatrist/psychologist, lay support groups. | Professionals who specialize in this disorder can assist the client to accept self-feelings as reality-based and begin to identify necessary lifestyle changes. |

## ACTIONS/INTERVENTIONS

## RATIONALE

### Collaborative

Administer medications, as indicated:
    antianxiety, e.g., alprazolam (Xanax), diazepam (Valium);

May be used for short-term control of anxiety. Dose may be increased as necessary to prevent panic attacks during the luteal phase.

    B complex vitamins, especially B$_6$.

Helpful in reducing feelings of anxiety, depression.

Refer client who does not respond to treatment regimen within 3 months for further evaluation of premature menopause, hypoglycemia, diabetes, hypothyroidism, polycystic ovaries, and ovarian failure.

Although 1/3 of clients seeking treatment respond to an initial multifaceted, nonhormonal treatment, it is important to rule out hormonal abnormalities, as the client will respond best to treatment for specific need.

| NURSING DIAGNOSIS: | PAIN, CHRONIC |
| --- | --- |
| May Be Related To: | Changes in estrogen/progesterone levels; increased secretion of prostaglandins. |
| | Vitamin deficiency; hypoglycemia. |
| | Fluid retention. |
| Possibly Evidenced By: | Reports of headache, breast tenderness; lower abdominal pain, backache. |
| | Nervousness and irritability; changes in sleep patterns. |
| | Physical and social withdrawal. |
| Desired Outcomes/Evaluation Criteria—Client Will: | Initiate individually appropriate lifestyle changes. |
| | Verbalize relief from pain/discomforts associated with condition. |
| | Actively engage in routine ADLs and social activities. |

## ACTIONS/INTERVENTIONS

## RATIONALE

### Independent

Note and record type, duration, and intensity of pain.

Background assessment data are necessary to formulate an accurate plan of care for the client.

Provide/recommend comfort measures with a matter-of-fact approach that does not provide added attention to the pain behavior (e.g., back rub, warm bath, heating pad).

May serve to provide some temporary relief of pain. Secondary gains from solicitous response may provide nontherapeutic reinforcement to the behavior.

Encourage client to get adequate rest and sleep and avoid stressful activity during the premenstrual period.

Fatigue exaggerates associated symptoms. Stress elicits heightened symptoms of anxiety during this period, affecting perception of pain.

497

| ACTIONS/INTERVENTIONS | RATIONALE |
|---|---|

### Independent

| | |
|---|---|
| Assist client with activities that distract from focus on self and pain. Demonstrate techniques, such as visual or auditory distractions, guided imagery, breathing exercises, massage, application of heat or cold, and relaxation techniques that may provide symptomatic relief. | Use of techniques described may help to reduce muscle tension, refocus attention, and provide a sense of control, preventing the discomfort from becoming disabling. |
| Provide positive reinforcement for times when client is not focusing on self and personal discomfort and is functioning independently. | May encourage repetition of desired independent behaviors while eliminating the secondary gain of dependency for the client. |
| Support use of biofeedback techniques. | May be useful in relieving tension and reducing severity of headaches. |

### Collaborative

| | |
|---|---|
| Administer medication as indicated: | When other measures are insufficient to bring about relief, symptomatic drug therapy may be necessary/useful. |
| diuretics, e.g., hydrochlorothiazide (Esidrix, HydroDIURIL), furosemide (Lasix); | Provides relief from discomfort of bloating and edema when fluid retention is extreme and does not respond to other measures, e.g., diet and sodium restriction. |
| nonsteroidal antiinflammatory agents, e.g., ibuprofen (Motrin), naproxen (Naprosyn); | May be effective for relief of pain due to increased prostaglandin secretion. |
| propranolol (Inderal); | May be used for prophylactic treatment of migraine. |
| muscle relaxants, diazepam (Valium); | Useful in relieving severe muscular tension. |
| bromocriptine (Parlodel); | Although studies do not show clear benefit, some women report control of pain of mastodynia and other premenstrual symptoms that may be caused by elevated prolactin, although side effects (especially nausea) may preclude use in some clients. |
| vitamin E supplement; | May reduce breast tenderness. |
| sumatriptin (Imitrex). | Highly effective in the treatment of acute migraine attack. |

| | |
|---|---|
| **NURSING DIAGNOSIS:** | **COPING, INDIVIDUAL, INEFFECTIVE** |
| **May Be Related To:** | Personal vulnerability; threat to self-concept. |
| | Multiple stressors (premenstrual symptoms) repeated over period of time. |
| | Poor nutrition. |
| | Work overload, lack of leisure activities. |

| | |
|---|---|
| **Possibly Evidenced By:** | Verbalization of difficulty coping/problem-solving or inability to ask for help. |
| | Emotional/muscular tension. |
| | Chronic fatigue, insomnia, lack of appetite or overeating. |
| | High illness rate. |
| | Inability to meet role expectations; alteration in societal participation. |
| **Desired Outcomes/Evaluation Criteria—Client Will:** | Identify ineffective coping behaviors and consequences. |
| | Meet psychologic needs as evidenced by appropriate expression of feelings, identification of options, and use of resources. |
| | Participate in ongoing treatment program. |

| ACTIONS/INTERVENTIONS | RATIONALE |
|---|---|
| **Independent** | |
| Assess current functional level/coping ability, noting substance use, smoking habits, eating patterns. | Identifies needs and appropriate interventions for individual situation. |
| Note understanding of current situation and previous methods of dealing with life problems. | Provides information about how the client views what is happening and provides opportunity for her to look at previous methods of coping that may be helpful now. |
| Determine effect(s) of problem on client's relationships/family. Include partner/SOs in process, as appropriate. | Destructive impact of symptoms can seriously undermine family systems, resulting in alienation , divorce. Including family promotes open communication and provides opportunity for increased understanding and problem-solving. |
| Identify extent of feelings and situations when loss of control occurs. Discuss/problem-solve behaviors to protect self/others, e.g., call support person, remove self from situation. | Recognition of potential for harm to self/others and development of plan enables client to take effective actions to meet safety needs. |
| Discuss importance of learning new coping strategies and developing more supportive relationships (based on information from psychologic testing). | Realization that past behaviors have contributed to current situation/lack of support may provide impetus for change. |
| Encourage client to reduce or shift workload and social activities during the premenstrual period as part of a total stress-management program. | By coping realistically with life stresses, the decreased responsibility should relieve stress and therefore help relieve symptoms. |
| Have client identify most troublesome symptoms, which may persist after initial therapy trials. | If other measures are inadequate/unsuccessful, pharmacologic treatment may be needed to enhance coping abilities. |

499

| ACTIONS/INTERVENTIONS | RATIONALE |
|---|---|
| **Collaborative** | |
| Review psychologic assessments, e.g., Minnesota Multiphasic Personality Inventory (MMPI) and clinical interview. (The first MMPI should be taken during the follicular phase, and a second MMPI should be taken during the most critical day of the luteal phase.) | Evaluation of these tests can determine the difference in emotional overlay and psychologic functioning. MMPI results can show very different patterns of emotional and personality functioning between these two phases. Consideration of these results is essential to an accurate picture of an individual's dynamics, coping skills, and stresses, which play such a significant role in this problem. |
| Provide for counseling at each appointment, reviewing past month's charting and evaluating symptoms and effects of therapy, as well as client relationship(s). | This opportunity for assessing ongoing problems and making needed changes helps both client and nurse to know whether program is successful. |
| Administer medications as indicated, e.g.: | |
|     hormonal manipulation: oral contraceptive, progesterone vaginal suppositories or injections; | May be useful for some clients to relieve premenstrual symptoms when nonpharmacologic measures have not been effective. |
|     tricyclic antidepressants: amitriptyline (Elavil); | Used for depression that does not respond as other symptoms are resolved. |
|     antiprostaglandins; | Relieves dysmenorrhea. |
|     lithium carbonate (Eskalith). | May be used in the presence of affective lability when other treatments have not been successful. |
| Encourage participation in support group, psychotherapy, marital counseling on a regular basis. | May help client/family members learn effective coping strategies and support indicated lifestyle changes. |

| | |
|---|---|
| **NURSING DIAGNOSIS:** | **KNOWLEDGE DEFICIT [LEARNING NEED] regarding condition, treatment, and prognosis** |
| **May Be Related To:** | Lack of exposure to/misinterpretation of/unfamiliarity with resources. |
| | Inaccurate/incomplete information presented. |
| **Possibly Evidenced By:** | Verbalization of the problem; request for information; statement of misconception. |
| | Inappropriate or exaggerated behaviors, e.g., hysteria, hostility, agitation. |
| | Exacerbation of symptoms. |
| **Desired Outcomes/Evaluation Criteria— Client Will:** | Identify relationship of signs/symptoms to the disease process and correlate symptoms with causative factors. |

| | |
|---|---|
| | Assume responsibility for own learning, begin to look for information and ask questions. |
| | Initiate necessary lifestyle changes. |
| | Participate in ongoing treatment regimen. |

| ACTIONS/INTERVENTIONS | RATIONALE |
|---|---|
| **Independent** | |
| Determine client's knowledge of and misconceptions about condition. | May have incomplete information and misunderstandings about problem. |
| Provide information about condition in written/verbal form. | Provides different methods for accessing/reinforcing information and enhances opportunity for learning/understanding. |
| Have client do a nutritional survey/record entire food and liquid intake for 1 month. | Assists in interpretation of whether the client's diet is a contributing/aggravating factor. (Commercial computer analysis may be available for interpretation of the survey.) |
| Encourage client to limit/stop smoking. | Smoking decreases the absorption of vitamins. |
| Suggest participation in regular exercise program. | Exercise increases the release of certain neurotransmitters in the brain (endorphins), which are important in determining mood and anxiety and can reduce premenstrual symptoms. |
| Demonstrate procedure/encourage client to do self-exam of breasts regularly. | While an important practice for all women, statistics have suggested that some clients have a higher incidence of breast cancer. |
| Review medication regimen, importance of follow-up visits to health-care provider. | Understanding enhances cooperation and promotes ongoing evaluation/adjustment of treatment program. |
| Suggest client keep diary recording symptoms and interventions used. | Useful in determining effectiveness of therapy/need for change. |
| Discuss recommended diet plan, e.g.: | Beginning an early self-help program may relieve clinical symptoms and encourage the client emotionally. |
|     limit red meat to 3 ounces/day, reduce intake of fats, especially saturated fats; | Decreases arachidonic acid, which helps balance $PGE_1$ ("good") with $PGE_2$ ("bad") prostaglandin, improving many premenstrual symptoms. |
|     limit intake of dairy products to 2 servings a day; | Excessive dairy products block the absorption of magnesium. |
|     increase intake of complex carbohydrates (vegetables, legumes, cereals, and whole grains) and cislinoleic acid-containing foods, e.g., safflower oil; | Stimulates insulin release in a less abrupt and more sustained manner. Although the value of cislinoleic acid has not been proved, some women have found it to be helpful for the relief of premenstrual symptoms. |

501

| ACTIONS/INTERVENTIONS | RATIONALE |
|---|---|

**Independent**

decrease intake of refined and simple sugars;

Reduces possibility of rapid release of insulin, which could lower the blood sugar and initiate the craving for sweets, thus creating a vicious cycle. Additionally, excess sugar is thought to cause nervous tension, palpitations, headache, dizziness, drowsiness, and excretion of magnesium in the urine, thus preventing the body from breaking down sugar for energy.

decrease salt intake to 3 g/day, but not less than 0.5 g/day;

Insulin prevents the kidneys from excreting salt; however, too little salt stimulates norepinephrine and causes sleep disturbances. Salt restriction also prevents edema.

limit intake of methylxanthines (coffee and chocolate) and alcohol (1 or 2 drinks a week).

Increase breast tenderness and pain, may negate the therapeutic effect of vitamins. Alcohol can cause reactive hypoglycemia and fluid retention, and it may be the biggest reason for treatment failure.

Review need for complete vitamin therapy program, such as Optivite.

Women with this disorder tend to eat more junk food and to be too busy to eat a well-balanced diet. Therefore, the client may be short of vitamins and minerals, which act as cofactors in a number of chemical reactions in the body that are involved in making, using, and excreting hormones. Abnormal levels of hormones are thought to be a cause of premenstrual symptoms.

Refer to available support groups/research centers.

Provides additional resources to understand and deal with condition.

# Appendix 1: Bibliography

## General References

### Books

Berkow, R (ed): The Merck Manual, ed 16. Merck Research Laboratories, Rahway, NJ, 1992.

Capers, CF: Culture and Nursing Practice: An Applied View, Holistic Nursing Practice, 6(3). Aspen Pub, Frederick, MD, April, 1992.

Deglin, J and Vallerand, AH: Davis's Drug Guide for Nurses, ed 3. FA Davis, Philadelphia, 1993.

Doenges, M and Moorhouse, MF: Nurse's Pocket Guide: Nursing Diagnoses with Interventions, ed 4. FA Davis, Philadelphia, 1993.

Doenges, M, Moorhouse, MF, and Geissler, A: Nursing Care Plans, Guidelines for Planning and Documenting Patient Care, ed 3. FA Davis, Philadelphia, 1993.

DSM IV. American Psychiatric Association, Washington, DC, 1994.

DSM III-R. American Psychiatric Association, Washington, DC, 1987.

Giger, J and Davidhizar, R: Transcultural Nursing. Mosby, St. Lous, 1991.

Hyman, SE and Tesar, GE: Manual of Psychiatric Emergencies, ed 3. Little, Brown and Company, Boston, 1994.

McFarland, GK, Wasli, EL, and Gerety, EK: Nursing Diagnoses & Process in Psychiatric Mental Health Nursing, ed 2. JB Lippincott, Philadelphia, 1992.

Moir, A and Jessel, D: Brain Sex. Dell Pub, NY, 1991.

Nicholi, A, Jr: The New Harvard Guide to Psychiatry. Harvard University Press, Cambridge, 1988.

Restak, R: The Brain Has a Mind of Its Own. Harmony Books, NY, 1991.

Shader, RI (ed): Manual of Psychiatric Therapeutics, ed 2. Little, Brown and Co, Boston, 1994.

Stuart, G and Sundeen, S: Principles and Practice of Psychiatric Nursing, ed 4. Mosby Year Book, St Louis, 1991.

Thomas, CL (ed): Taber's Cyclopedic Medical Dictionary, ed 17. FA Davis, Philadelphia, 1993.

Townsend, MC: Drug Guide for Psychiatric Nursing, ed 2. FA Davis, Philadelpha, 1994.

Towsend, MC: Nursing Diagnosis in Psychiatric Nursing: A Pocket Guide for Care Plan Construction, ed 3. FA Davis, Philadelphia, 1994.

Townsend, MC: Psychiatric Mental Health Nursing: Concepts of Care. FA Davis, Philadelphia, 1993.

Wilson, HS and Kneisl, CR: Psychiatric Nursing, ed 4. Addison-Wesley, Redwood City, CA, 1992.

### Articles

Dumas, RG: Psychiatric nursing in an era of change. J Psychosoc Nurs 32(1):11–14, January 1994.

Dunn, JK: Medical skills and knowledge: How necessary are they for psychiatric nurses? 31(12):25–28, December 1993.

Goldstein, SV: You are what you read: The use of bibliotherapy to facilate psychotherapy. J Psychosoc Nurs 28(9):6, September 1990.

Outlaw, FH and Lowery, B: Seclusion: The nursing challenge. J Psychosoc Nurs 30(4):13, April 1992.

Sebastian, L: Promoting object constancy: Writing as a nursing intervention. J Psychosoc Nurs 29(1):21–23, January 1991.

Stevenson, S: Heading off violence with verbal de-escalation. J Psychosoc Nurs 29(9):6–10, September 1991.

Stilling, L: The pros and cons of physical restraints and behavior controls. J Psychosoc Nurs 30(3):18, March 1992.

Turnbull, J, Black, L, and Patterson, B: Turn it around: Short-term management for aggression and anger. J Psychosoc Nurs 28(6):7, June 1990.

White, K and Vincent, M: Patient violence toward a nurse. J Psychosoc Nurs 32(2):30–32, February 1994.

## Chapter 1

### Books

Boaz, JT: Delivering Mental Health Care, A Guide for HMOs. Pluribus Press, Chicago, 1988.

Restak, R: The Brain Has a Mind of Its Own. Harmony Books, NY, 1991.

### Articles

Beeber, LS, et al: Challenge of diversity. J Psychosoc Nurs 31(8):23–29. August 1993.

Brooks, AMT, et al: Continuing journey: Health care reform and mental health—To the Rose Garden, the White House, and more. J Psychosoc Nurs (Editorial) 31(8):5–7, August 1993.

Brooks, AMT, et al: New partnerships: Creating the future. J Psychosoc Nurs 31(8):37–40, August 1993.

Campbell-Heider, NC and Hanna, ND: Nursing's new

political era, in chronic illness. Holistic Nursing Practice 8(1):78–87, Aspen Pub, Frederick, MD, October 1993.

Carter, R: Don't forget the mentally ill. The Denver Post, Sunday, August 22, 1993, Section E, 1–5.

Caverly, S: Coordinating psychosocial nursing care across treatment settings. J Psychosoc Nurs 29(1): 26–29, August 1991.

Connolly, PM: Professionally speaking: Case management. 30(3):35–39, March 1992.

Connors, N: Employers seek alternative treatments for adolescent mental health care. Business and Health, 27–29, July 1992.

Cravener, P: Establishing therapeutic alliance across cultural barriers. J Psychosoc Nurs 30(12):10–14, December 1992.

Cronin, CT and Maklebust, T: Case-management care: Capitalizing on the CNS. Nursing Management 20(3): 38–47, March 1989.

Dibner, LA and Mursphy, JS: Nurse entrepreneurs. J Psychosoc Nurs 29(5):30–34, May 1991.

Fox, JC: The role of nursing in public policy reform. J Psychosoc Nurs 3(8):9, 1993.

Kanter, J: Clinical case management: Definition, principles, components. Hospital and Community Psychiatry 40(4):361–368, April 1989.

Kelly, J and Beaven, J: Establishing therapeutic programs in the public sector psychiatric hospital: Rethinking the possibilities and priorities. J Psychosoc Nurs 29(8): 19–25, August 1991.

Kunes, R: Mental health mega-trends. Managing Employee Health Benefits 52–57, Fall 1993.

Managed care: Where will your hospital fit in? Hospitals, April 5, 1993, pp 18–24.

Merrill, JC: Defining case management. Business and Health, July/August 1985, pp 5–9.

Mound, B, et al: The expanded role of nurse case managers. J Psychosoc Nurs 29(6):18–22, 1991.

Osborne, OH and Thomas, MD: On public sector psychosocial nursing: A conceptual framework. J Psychosoc Nurs 28(8):13–18, August 1991.

Paterson, DY: Managed care: An approach to rational psychiatric treatment. Hospital and Community Psychiatry 41(10):1092–1095, October 1990.

Pittman, DC: Nursing case management, holistic care for the deinstitutionalized and chronically mentally ill. J Psychosoc Nurs 27(11):23–27, 1989.

Rosenzweig, L: Psychiatric triage: A cost-effective approach to quality management in mental health. J Psychosoc Nurs 30(6):5–8, June 1992.

Smith, GB: Hospital case management for psychiatric diagnoses: Focusing on quality and cost outcomes. J Psychosoc Nurs 32(2):3–4, February 1994.

Tischler, GL: Utilization management of health services for private third parties. Am J Psychiatry 147(8): 967–973, August 1990.

Van Dongen, CJ and Jambunathan, J: Pilot study results: The psychiatric RN case manager. J Psychosoc Nurs 30(11):11–14, November 1992.

## Chapter 2

American Nurses Association: Nursing: A Social Policy Statement. Pub code NP-63 3SM, 12/80, Kansas City, 1980.

American Nurses Association: Standards of Nursing Practice. Pub code NO-41, 10M 1:77, Kansas City, 1991.

Statement on Psychiatric-Mental Health Clinical Nursing Practice and Standards of Psychiatric-Mental Health Clinical Nursing Practice, American Nurses Publishing, Washington, DC, 1994.

### Books

Alfaro-LeFevre, RA: Application of Nursing Process: A Step-by-Step Guide to Care Planning, ed 3. JB Lippincott, Philadelphia, 1994.

Brooks, KL: Critical Thinking in Clinical Practice, Holistic Nursing Practice, 7(3). Aspen Pub, Frederick, MD, April 1993.

Cox, HC, et al: Clinical Applications of Nursing Diagnosis, ed 2. FA Davis, Philadelphia, 1993.

Doenges, ME and Moorhouse, MF: Application of Nursing Process and Nursing Diagnosis: An Interactive Text. FA Davis, Philadelphia, 1992.

Lampe, SS: Focus Charting®: Creative Nursing Management, ed 4. Minneapolis, 1986.

### Articles

Dolan, M: Why nurses and doctors should be partners in diagnosis. Nursing 90, 20(11):42, 1990.

Mosher, C, et al: Upgrading practice with critical pathways. AJN 22(2):41, 1992.

Radwin, LE: Research on diagnostic reasoning in nursing. Nursing Diagnosis 1(2):70–77, 1990.

Rasmussen, N and Gengler, T: Clinical pathways of care: The route to better communication. Nursing 94, 24(2): 47–49, February 1994.

## Chapter 3
### Books

Bates, B: A Guide to Physical Examination, ed 5. JB Lippincott Co, Philadelphia, 1991.

DeGowin, EL and DeGowin, RL: Bedside Diagnostic Examination, ed 4. Macmillan, NY, 1981.

### Articles

Wheeland, RM: Focus Charting® in a psychiatric facility. J Psychosoc Nurs 31(12):15–20, December 1993.

## Chapter 4
### Books

Aichhorn, A: Wayward Youth. Viking Press, NY, 1965.

Barbee, MA: The disruptive child: Conduct disorder, discharge planning. In Babich, K and Brown, L (eds): A Manual for Psychiatric Nurses. Slack, Inc, Thorofare, NJ, 1991.

Family Guide: Child Behavior. Cleo Wallace Center, Westminster, CO, 1993.

Family Guide: Adolescent Behavior. Cleo Wallace Center, Westminster, CO, 1993.

Gordon, T: Teaching Children Self-Discipline at Home and at School. Random House, NY, 1989.

Lewis, M (ed): Child and Adolescent Psychiatry, A Comprehensive Textbook. Williams & Wilkins, New Haven, CT, 1991.

Lauer, JW: Attention Deficit Disorder (ADD), ed 2. Cleo Wallace Center, Westminster Campus, CO, 1992.

Popper, C and Famularo, R: Child and adolescent psychopharmacology. In Levine, MD (ed): Developmental-Behavioral Pediatrics. WB Saunders, Philadelphia, 1983.

Safer, D and Allen, R: Hyperactive Children. University Park Press, Baltimore, 1976.

Wender, PH: The Hyperactive Child, Adolescent and Adult: Attention Deficit Disorder through the Life Span. Oxford University Press, NY, 1987.

## Articles

Becker-Fritz, FT and Barbee, MA: What are the warning signs for suicidal adolescents? J Psychosoc Nurs 31(2):37–41, February 1993.

Bernstein, G, et al: Comparative studies of pharmacotherapy for school refusal. J Am Acad Child Adolesc Psychiatry 29(5):773–781, September 1990.

Biederman, T and Jellinek, M: Current concepts of psychopharmacology in children. N Engl J Med 310(15): 968–972, April 1984.

Biederman, J, et al: Diagnosis of attention-deficit hyperactivity disorder from parent reports predict diagnosis based on teacher reports. J Am Acad Child Adolesc Psychiatry 32(2):315–317, March 1993.

Boyle, MH and Offord, DR: Primary prevention of conduct disorder, issues and prospects. J Am Acad Child Adolesc Psychiatry 29(2):227–233, March 1990.

Carrey, NJ and Adams, L: How to deal with sexual acting-out on the child psychiatric inpatient ward. J Psychosoc Nurs 30(5):19–23, May 1992.

Childhood psychoses. The Harvard Mental Health Letter 6(11):1–4, May 1990.

Children's conduct disorders—Part I. The Harvard Mental Health Letter 5(9):1–3, March 1989.

Conners, C: A teacher rating scale for use in drug studies with children. Am J Psychiatry, 126:84–88, 1969.

Delaney, KR: Nursing in child psychiatric milieus, Part I. JCPN 5(1):10–14, 1992.

Delaney, KR: Nursing in child psychiatric milieus, Part II. JCPN 5(1):15–18, 1992.

Dulcan, MK: The psychopharmacologic treatment of children and adolescents with attention deficit disorder. Psychiatr Annals 15(2):69–86, February 1985.

DuPaul, G and Rapport, M: Does methylphenidate normalize the classroom performance of children with ADD? J Am Acad Child Adolesc Psychiatry 32(1): 190–197, January 1993.

Fischer, M, et al: The adolescent outcome of hyperactive children: Predictors of psychiatric, academic, social and emotional adjustment. J Am Acad Child Adolesc Psychiatry 32(2):322–324, March 1993.

Haswell, KL, Hock, E, and Wenai, C: Techniques for dealing with oppositional behavior in preschool children. Young Children pp 13–18, March 1992.

Hawkins, JD, et al: Reducing early childhood aggression, results of a primary prevention program. J Am Acad Child Adolesc Psychiatry 30(2):208–214, March 1991.

Hill, P: Assessing faecal soiling in children. Nursing Times 87(14):61–64, April 1991.

Hirshfeld, DR, et al: Stable behavioral inhibition and its association with anxiety disorders. J Am Acad Child Adolesc Psychiatry 31(1):103–110, January 1992.

Jones, RN, O'Brien, P, and McMahon, WM: Contracting to lower precaution status for child psychiatric inpatients. J Psychosoc Nurs 31(1):6–10, January 1993.

Kaplan, S, et al: A comparison of three nocturnal enuresis treatment methods. J Am Acad Child Adolesc Psychiatry 28(2):282–286, March 1989.

Kaplan, S, et al: Helping a child overcome enuresis. Med Aspects Human Sexuality 25(2):36–38, February 1991.

Lahey, B, et al: Are attention deficit disorders with and without hyperactivity similar or dissimilar disorders? J Am Acad Child Psychiatry 23(3):302–309, May 1984.

Levine, M: The unhappy wanderers: Children with attention deficits. Pediatr Clin North Am 29(1), February 1982.

Loeber, R: Oppositional defiant disorder and conduct disorder. Hosp Community Psychiatry 42(11):1099–1102, November 1991.

Loranger, N: Play intervention strategies for Hispanic toddler with separation anxiety. Psychiatr Nursing 18(6):571–575, November–December 1992.

Lovaas, I: Autism: A new behavioral treatment. The Harvard Mental Health Letter 5(12):4–6, June 1989.

Newcomb, P: Tricyclic antidepressants and children. Nurse-Practitioner 16(5):26–29, May 1991.

NIMH Research conference: Research recommendations for anxiety disorders and ADHD. J Am Acad Child Adolesc Psychiatry 32(5):1099, September 1993.

Pine, DS: Child-adult anxiety disorders, letter to editor. J Am Acad Child Adolesc Psychiatry 33(2):280–281, February 1994.

Raymer, G: Cognitive restructuring for antisocial adolescents. Unpublished article, February 1991.

Sadler, C: Enuresis getting dry. Community Outlook, pp 33–35, September 1990.

Scahill, L: Nursing diagnosis vs goal-oriented treatment planning in inpatient child psychiatry. Image: J Nursing Scholarship 23(2):95–98, Summer 1991.

Silverman, WK and Eisen, AR: Age differences in reliability of parent and child reports of child anxiety symptomatology using a structured interview. J Am Acad Child Adolesc Psychiatry 31(1):117–123, January 1992.

Steinhouse, HC, et al: Enuresis in child psychiatric clinic patients. J Child Adolesc Psychiatry 28(2):279–281, March 1989.

Teets, JM: Enuresis: Nursing diagnosis and treatment. J Community Health Nursing 9(2):95–101, 1992.

Tosches, R: Neglected, abused, deadly, a special report. Colorado Springs Gazette Telegraph, January 23, 1994, pp. A1, A4-A5.

Venn, ES and Derdyn, AP: Working with a difficult adolescent. J Psychosoc Nurs 26(6):28–31, June 1988.

Wagner, WG: The behavioral treatment of childhood nocturnal enuresis. J Counseling Dev 165(1):262–264, January 1987.

Wender, PH: Hyperactivity in children and adults. The Harvard Mental Health Letter 7(5):4–7, November 1990.

Wilens, T, et al: Nortriptyline in the treatment of ADHD: A chart review of 58 cases. J Am Acad Child Adolesc Psychiatry 32(2):343–349, March, 1993.

## Chapter 5

### Books

Flaskerud, JH and Ungvarski, P: HIV/AIDS, ed 2. WB Saunders, Philadelphia, 1992.

505

## Articles

AIDS and mental health—Part I. The Harvard Mental Health Letter 10(7):1–4, January 1994.

AIDS and mental health—Part II. The Harvard Mental Health Letter 10(8):1–4, February 1994.

Alzheimer's disease—Part I. The Harvard Mental Health Letter 9(2):1–4, August 1992.

Alzheimer's disease—Part II. The Harvard Mental Health Letter 9(3):1–4, September 1992.

Bower, B: HIV-linked mental loss takes job toll. Science News 145(9):132, February 26, 1994.

Cowles, KV and Rodgers, BL: When a loved one has AIDS: Care for the significant other. J Psychosoc Nurs 29(4):6–12, April 1991.

Davies, HD and Zeiss, A: 'Til death do us part: Intimacy and sexuality in the marriages of Alzheimer's patients. J Psychosoc Nurs 30(11):5–10, November 1992.

Elder, G and Sever, J: AIDS & neurological disorders: An overview. Ann Neurol 23(suppl):54–56, 1988.

Grabbe, L and Brown, L: Identifying neurologic complications of AIDS. Nursing 89, 19(5):66, May 1989.

Grant, I, et al: Evidence of early central nervous system involvement in the acquired immunodeficiency syndrome (AIDS) and other human immunodeficiency virus (HIV) infections. Ann Intern Med 6(107):828–836, December 1987.

Hanks, N: The effects of Alzheimer's disease on the sexual attitudes and behavhiors of married caregivers and their spouses. Sexuality and Disability 10(3):137–152, Fall 1992.

Hilton, G and Sisson, R: The Neurobehavioral Rating Scale: An interrater reliability study in the HIV seropositive population. Presentation at the Association of Nurses in AIDS Care Conference, November 1989.

Jones, PS and Martinson, IM: The experience of bereavement in caregivers of family members with Alzheimer's disease. Image: J Nursing Scholarship 224(3):172, March 1992.

Liken, MA and Collins, CE: Grieving: Facilitating the process for dementia caregivers. J Psychosoc Nurs 31(1):21–26, January 1993.

Manuel, CO: Rifabutin. J Assoc Nurses in AIDS Care 5(1):45–50, January–February 1994.

McArthur, J: AIDS dementia: Your assessment can make all the difference. RN 53(3):36, March 1990.

Pillard, RC: Does homosexuality have a biological basis? The Harvard Mental Health Letter 8(12):5–6, June 1992.

Regan-Kubinski, MJ and Sharts-Engel, N: The HIV-infected woman. J Psychosoc Nurs 30(2):11–15, February 1992.

Swanson, B, et al: Dementia and depression in persons with AIDS: Causes and care. J Psychosoc Nurs 28(10):33–39, October 1990.

Yarchoan, R, et al: Long-term administration of 3[1]-azido-2[1], 3[1]-dedeoxythymedine to patients with AIDS-related neurologic disease. Ann Neurol 23(suppl):582–587, 1988.

## Chapter 6

## Articles

Addiction—Part I. The Harvard Mental Health Letter 9(4):1–4, October 1992.

Addiction—Part II. The Harvard Mental Health Letter 9(5):1–4, November 1992.

Amphetamines. The Harvard Mental Health Letter 6(10):1–4, April 1990.

Drug abuse and dependence—Part I. The Harvard Mental Health Letter 6(4):1–4, October 1989.

Dual diagnosis: Part I. The Harvard Mental Health Letter 8(2):1–4, August 1991.

Dual diagnosis: Part II. The Harvard Mental Health Letter 8(3):1–4, September 1991.

Espeland, K: Inhalant abuse: Assessment guidelines. J Psychosoc Nurs 31(3):11–14, March 1993.

Malloy, GB and Berkery, AC: Codependency: A feminist perspective. J Psychosoc Nurs 31(4):15–19, April 1993.

McLellan, AT, et al: Which services for addicts. The Harvard Mental Health Letter 10(11):6–7, May 1994.

Naltrexone against alcohol. The Harvard Mental Health Letter 9(11):6, May 1993.

Psychedelic drugs. The Harvard Mental Health Letter 6(8):1–4, February 1990.

Self-help groups—Part I. The Harvard Mental Health Letter 9(9):1–4, March 1993.

Self-help groups—Part II. The Harvard Mental Health Letter 9(10):1–4, April 1993.

Update on cocaine—Part I. The Harvard Mental Health Letter 10(2):1–4, August 1993.

Update on cocaine—Part II. The Harvard Mental Health Letter 10(3):1–4, September 1993.

## Chapter 7

## Articles

Davidson, J: New type of medications for schizophrenia. The Menninger Letter 2(2):7, February 1994.

Dzurec, LC: How do they see themselves? Self-perceptions and functioning for people with chronic schizophrenia. J Psychosoc Nurs 28(8):10–14, August 1990.

Families in the treatment of schizophrenia—Part I. The Harvard Mental Health Letter 5(12):1–4, June 1989.

Families in the treatment of schizophrenia—Part II. The Harvard Mental Health Letter 6(1):1–4, July 1989.

Malone JA: Schizophrenia research update: Implications for nursing. J Psychosoc Nurs 28(8):4–9, August 1990.

Meltzer, H: Clozapine: A major advance in the treatment of schizophrenia. The Harvard Mental Health Letter 10(2):4–6, August 1993.

Moller, M and Wer, J: Interview. J Psychosoc Nurs 28(8):22–24, August 1990.

Ricci, MS: The new after-care clinic: Treating individuals rather than masses. J Psychosoc Nurs 28(8):18–21, August 1990.

Schiller, L: Waking from the nightmare of schizophrenia (my side). J Psychosoc Nurs 30(5):48, May 1992.

Schizophrenia: The present state of understanding, Part II. The Harvard Mental Health Letter 8(12):1–5, June 1992.

## Chapter 8

## Articles

Anderson, DB: Never too late: Resolving the grief of suicide. J Psychosoc Nurs 29(3):29–31, March 1991.

Atypical depression. The Harvard Mental Health Letter 6(12):1–3, June 1990.

Bailey, K and Glod, CA: Update on psychopharmacology: Seasonal affective disorder: A new light? J Psychosoc Nurs 29(3):38–39, March 1991.

Becker-Fritz, T and Barbee, MA: Professionally speaking: What are the warning signs for suicidal adolescents? J Psychosoc Nurs 31(2):37–41, February 1993.

Conrad, N: Where do they turn? Social support systems of suicidal high school adolescents. J Psychosoc Nurs 29(3):14–20, March 1991.

Cugino, A, et al: Searching for a pattern: Repeat suicide attempts. J Psychosoc Nurs 29(2):26, February 1991.

Depression in primary care: Detection, diagnosis, and treatment. US Department of Health and Human Services, Public Health Service, Agency for Health Care Policy and Research 31(6):19–28, June 1993.

Dunham, KL: Seasonal affective disorder: Light makes right. AJN 92(12):44–46, December 1992.

Dysthymia and other mood disorders. The Harvard Mental Health Letter 7(11):1–3, May 1991.

Fink, M: Can ECT be an effective treatment for adolescents? The Harvard Mental Health Letter 10(11):8, May 1994.

Glod, CA and Mathieu, J: Expanding uses of anticonvulsants in the treatment of bipolar disorder (update on psychopharmacology). J Psychosoc Nurs 31(11):15–20, November 1993.

Loving, RT and Kripke, DF: Daily light exposure among psychiatric impatients. J Psychosoc Nurs 30(11):15–19, November 1992.

Richards, R: Mood swings and everyday creativity. The Harvard Mental Health Newsletter 8(10):4–6, April 1992.

Seasonal affective disorder. The Harvard Mental Health Letter 9(8):1–4, February 1993.

Zerhusen, JD, Boyle, K, and Wilson, W: Out of the darkness: Group cognitive therapy for depressed elderly. J Psychosoc Nurs 29(9):16–21, September 1991.

## Chapter 9
## Articles

Bailey, K and Glod, CA: Update on psychopharmacology: Posttraumatic stress disorder. J Psychosoc Nurs 29(9):42–43, September 1991.

Bille, DA: Road to recovery: Post-traumatic stress disorder—The hidden victim. J Psychosoc Nurs 31(9):19–28, September 1993.

Blair, DT, and Hildreth, NA: PTSD and the Vietnam veteran: The battle for treatment. J Psychosoc Nurs 29(1):15–20, October 1991.

Butler, K: The enigma of EMDR: too good to be true? The Family Therapy Networker 17(6):18–31, November/December 1993.

Childs-Clarke, A and Sharpe, J: Keeping the faith: Religion in the healing of phobic anxiety. J Psychosoc Nurs 29(2):22–24, February 1991.

Cohen, MV: Sexual abuse and post-traumatic stress disorder. Sexuality and Disability. 11(4):255–258, Winter 1993.

Cumbie, B: Action stat! Treating a P.T.S.D. flashback. Nursing 94, 24(2):33, February 1994.

Gerlock, AA: Vietnam: Returning to the scene of the trauma. J Psychosoc Nurs 29(2):4–8, February 1991.

Ledray, LE and Arndt, S: Examining the sexual assault victim: A new model for nursing care. J Psychosoc Nurs 31(2):7–12, February 1994.

Ture, W, et al: Hereditary and environment in posttraumatic stress reactions. The Harvard Mental Health Letter 10(7):7, January 1994.

Whitley, GG: Ritualistic behavior: Breaking the cycle. J Psychosoc Nurs 29(1):31–35, January 1991.

## Chapter 10
## Books

Barsky, AJ: Somatoform disorders. In Kaplan, HI and Sadock, BJ (eds): Comprehensive Textbook of Psychiatry/V, ed 3. Williams & Wilkins, Baltimore, 1989.

## Articles

Barsky, AJ and Klerman, GL: Overview: Hypochrondriasis, bodily complaints, and somatic styles. Am J Psychiatry 140:273–283, 1983.

Corbin, LJ, et al: Somatoform disorders: How to reduce over utilization of health care services. J Psychosoc Nurs 26(9):31, September 1988.

Goldberg, D, Gask L, and O'Dowd, T: The treatment of somatization: Teaching techniques of reattribution. J Psychosom Res 33:689–695, 1989.

Mabe, PA, Jones, LF, and Riley, WT: Managing somatization phenomena in primary care. In Hall RCW (ed): Psychiatry Med 8(4):117–127, 1990.

Mechanic, D: Social psychologic factors affecting the presentation of bodily complaints. N Engl J Med 286:1132–1139, 1972.

Wise, TN: The somatizing patient. Ann Clin Psychiatry 4:9–17, 1992.

## Chapter 11
## Articles

Curtin, SL: Recognizing multiple personality disorder. J Psychosoc Nurs 31(2):29–33, February 1993.

Dissociation and dissociative disorders: Part I. The Harvard Mental Health Letter 8(9):1–4, March 1992.

Dissociation and dissociative disorders: Part II. The Harvard Mental Health Letter 8(10):1–4, April 1992.

Stafford, LL: Dissociation and multiple personality disorder: A challenge for psychosocial nurses. J Psychosoc Nurs 31(1):15–20, January 1993.

## Chapter 12
## Books

Hyde, J: Understanding Human Sexuality, ed 4. McGraw-Hill, NY, 1990.

## Articles

Bailey, M, and Pillard, R: The innateness of homosexuality. The Harvard Mental Health Letter 10(7):4–6, January 1994.

Bradford, JM: Can pedophilia be treated? The Harvard Mental Health Letter 10(9):8, March 1994.

Byne, W and Parsons, B: Biology and human sexual orientation. The Harvard Mental Health Letter 10(8):5–7, February 1994.

Deevy, S: Lesbian self-disclosure: Strategies for success. J Psychosoc Nurs 31(4):21–26, April 1993.

LeVay, S: Is homosexuality all in the brain? The Harvard Mental Health Letter 8(9):7, March 1992.

McGown, A: How to help your lesbian teenager (my side). J Psychosoc Nurs 31(8):48, August 1993.

Perilstein, RD, et al: Antidepressants for sexual disorders? The Harvard Mental Health Letter 8(5):7, November 1991.

Sexual disorders—Part I. The Harvard Mental Health Letter 6(6):1–4, December 1989.

Sexual disorders—Part II. The Harvard Mental Health Letter 6(7):1–4, January 1990.

Smith, GB: Nursing Care Challenges: Homosexual psychiatric patients. J Psychosoc Nurs 30(12):15–21, December 1992.

## Chapter 13

### Articles

Bennett, WI: Obesity is not an eating disorder. The Harvard Mental Health Letter 8(4):4–6, October 1991.

Brentin, L and Sick, A: Caring for the morbidly obese. AJN 91(8):40, 1991.

Eating disorders—Part I. The Harvard Mental Health Letter 9(6):1–4, December 1992.

Eating disorders—Part II. The Harvard Mental Health Letter 9(7):1–4, January 1993.

Fairburn, CC, et al: Comparing treatments for bulimia. The Harvard Mental Health Letter 10(11):7, May 1994.

Hofland, SL and Dardis, PO: Bulimia nervosa: Associated physical problems. J Psychosoc Nurs 30(2):23–27, February 1992.

Hofland, SL and O'Brian, DP: Bulimia nervosa: Associated problems. J Psychosoc Nurs 30(2):46, February 1992.

O'Connell, KA: Compulsive exercise and the eating disorders: Toward an integrated theory of activity (book review). J Psychosoc Nurs 31(6):35–36, June 1993.

Staples, NR and Schwartz, M: Anorexia nervosa support group: Providing transitional support. J Psychosoc Nurs 28(2):6, February 1990.

## Chapter 14

### Books

Sappington, A: Adjustment: Theory, Research, and Personal Applications. Brooks/Cole Pub Co., Pacific Grove, CA, 1989.

### Articles

Esper, J: Reactions to violence: Normal adjustment is not psychopathology. Issues in Radical Therapy 12(1): 52–54, January 1986.

Strain, J, et al: Considering changes in adjustment disorder. Hosp Community Psychiatry 44(1):13–15, January 1993.

Svanborg, P, Carlsson, A, and Herlofson, J: Crisis reactions: As problems in differential diagnosis at a community mental health center. Is the DSM-III-R useful in the diagnostic procedure? Nordic J Psychiatry 47(2): 133–139, February 1993.

Wise, MG and Rieck, SO: Diagnostic considerations and treatment approaches to underlying anxiety in the medically ill. J Clin Psychiatry 54(suppl):22–26, May 1993.

## Chapter 15

### Articles

Borderline personality. The Harvard Mental Health Letter 10(11):1–3, May 1994.

Hare, RD, et al: New test for psychopathy. The Harvard Mental Health Letter 8(7):7, January 1992.

Peccinino, S: The Nursing care challenge: Borderline patients. J Psychosoc Nurs 28(4):22–41, April 1990.

Stone, MH: The fate of borderline patients. The Harvard Mental Health Letter 8(9):4–6, March 1992.

## Chapter 16

### Books

Green, AH: Child sexual abuse and incest. In Lewis, M (ed): Child and Adolescent Psychiatry. Williams & Wilkins, New Haven, CT, 1991.

Kaplan, S: Physical abuse and neglect. In Lewis, M (ed): Child and Adolescent Psychiatry. Williams & Wilkins, New Haven, CT, 1991.

Olds, S, London, M, and Ladewig, P: Maternal Newborn Nursing, ed 4. Addison-Wesley Nursing, Redwood City, CA, 1992.

### Articles

Baladerian, NJ: Sexual abuse of people with developmental disabilities. Sexuality and Disability 9(4): 323–336, Winter 1991.

Burgess, AW, et al: Assessing child abuse: The TRIADS checklist. J Psychosoc Nurs 28(4):7–14, April 1990.

Carparulo, F: Identifying the developmentally disabled sex offenders. Sexuality and Disability 9(4):311–322, Winter 1991.

Child abuse—Part I. The Harvard Mental Health Letter 9(11):1–3, May 1993.

Child abuse—Part II. The Harvard Mental Health Letter 9(12):1–4, June 1993.

Child abuse—Part III. The Harvard Mental Health Letter 10(1):1–5, July 1993.

Chuong, CJ, and Gibbons, WE: Premenstrual syndrome: Update on therapy. Med Aspects of Human Sexuality 24(5):58–65, May 1990.

Corwin, DL: How to recognize and prevent child sexual abuse. Med Aspects of Human Sexuality 23(12):40–49, December 1989.

Devlin, BK and Reynolds, E: Child abuse: How to recognize it, how to intervene. AJN 94(3):26–32, March 1994.

Draucker, CB: The healing process of female adult incest survivors: Constructing a personal residence. Image: J Nursing Scholarship 24(1):4–8, Spring 1992.

Elliott, DM and Briere, J: The sexually abused boy: Problems in manhood. Med Aspects of Human Sexuality 26(2):68–71, February 1992.

Garlock, AA: Vietnam: Returning to the scene of the trauma. J Psychosoc Nurs 29(2):5, February 1991.

Gise, LH: Premenstrual syndrome—Which treatments help? Med Aspects of Human Sexuality 25(2):62–68, February 1991.

Greenfield, M: Disclosing incest: The relationships that make it possible. J Psychosoc Nurs 28(5):20, May 1990.

Hamberger, LK, et al: Detecting the wife batterer. Med Aspects of Human Sexuality 24(9):32–38, September 1990.

Kreidler, MC and Carlson, RE: Breaking the incest cycle: The group as a surrogate family. J Psychosoc Nurs 29(4):28–32, April 1991.

Maltz, W: Adult survivors of incest—How to help them overcome the trauma. Med Aspects of Human Sexuality 24(12):42–47, December 1990.

Miller, EA and Hergenroeder, AC: Taking a teenager's sexual history. Med Aspects of Human Sexuality 24(12):32–36, December 1990.

Moss, VA: Battered women and the myth of masochism. J Psychosoc Nurs 29(7):18–23, July 1991.

Muram, D and Gale, CL: Clinical assessment of the sexually abused girl. Med Aspects of Human Sexuality 24(9):43–50, September 1990.

Rew, L and Shirejian, P: Seuxally abused adolescent: Conceptualization of sexual trauma and nursing interventions. J Psychosoc Nurs 31(12):29–33, December 1993.

Ridley, PJ: Kaufman's theory of shame and identity in treating childhood sexual abuse in adults. J Psychosoc Nurs 31(6):13–17, June 1993.

Ruckman, L: Rape: How to begin the healing. AJN 92(9): 48–51, September 1992.

Salzinger, S, et al: Abused children and their friends. The Harvard Mental Health Letter 10(9):5–6, March 1994.

Schmidt, PJ, et al: PMS after menstruation. The Harvard Mental Health Letter 8(7):5, January 1992.

Taylor, DL: Evaluating therapeutic change in symptom severity at the level of the individual woman experiencing severe PMS. Image: J Nursing Scholarship 26(1):25–34, Spring 1994.

The mind, the body, and the immune system: Part I. The Harvard Mental Health Letter 8(7):1–5, January 1992.

The mind, the body, and the immune system: Part II. The Harvard Mental Health Letter 8(8):1–5, February 1992.

Weingourt, R: Wife rape in a sample of psychiatric patients. Image: J Nursing Scholarship 22(3):144–147, Fall 1990.

What is late luteal phase dysphoric disorder and why is there a controversy surrounding it? The Harvard Mental Health Letter 6(8):8, February 1990.

Zavodnick, JM: Clinical assessment of the sexually abused boy. Med Aspects of Human Sexuality 24(7): 47–49, July 1990.

# Appendix 2: Taxonomy 1R

The underlined entries are the nursing diagnoses approved by NANDA for clinical use and testing, which have been organized into categories reflecting the 9 human response patterns. Additional listings indicate "holes" in the taxonomic tree requiring further study and development of the progressive levels of specificity inherent in a taxonomic structure.

TAXONOMY 1 Revised (1992)

1. **EXCHANGING:** A human response pattern involving mutual giving and receiving. (To give, relinquish, or lose something while receiving something in return; the substitution of one element for another; the reciprocal act of giving and receiving.)
  1.1 Alterations in Nutrition
      1.1.2.1 More Than Body Requirements
      1.1.2.2 Less Than Body Requirements
      1.1.2.3 High Risk for More Than Body Requirements
  1.2 (Alterations in Physical Regulation)
      1.2.1.1 High risk for Infection
    1.2.2 (Alteration in Body Temperature)
      1.2.2.1 High risk
      1.2.2.2 Hypothermia
      1.2.2.3 Hyperthermia
      1.2.2.4 Ineffective Thermoregulation
    1.2.3 ( * )
      1.2.3.1 Dysreflexia
  1.3 (Alterations in Elimination)
      1.3.1.1 Constipation
        1.3.1.1.1 Perceived
        1.3.1.1.2 Colonic
      1.3.1.2 Diarrhea
      1.3.1.3 Bowel Incontinence
    1.3.2 Altered Urinary Elimination
      1.3.2.1 (Incontinence)
      1.3.2.1.1 Stress
      1.3.2.1.2 Reflex
      1.3.2.1.3 Urge
      1.3.2.1.4 Functional
      1.3.2.1.5 Total
      1.3.2.2 Retention
  1.4 (Alterations in Circulation)
    1.4.1 (Vascular)
      1.4.1.1 Tissue Perfusion
        [1.4.1.1.1] Renal
        [1.4.1.1.2] Cerebral
        [1.4.1.1.3] Cardiopulmonary
        [1.4.1.1.4] Gastrointestinal
        [1.4.1.1.5] Peripheral
      1.4.1.2 Fluid Volume
      1.4.1.2.1 Excess
      1.4.1.2.2.1 Deficit
      1.4.1.2.2.2 High risk
    1.4.2 (Cardiac)
      1.4.2.1 Decreased Cardiac Output
  1.5 (Alterations in Oxygenation)
    1.5.1 (Respiration)
      1.5.1.1 Impaired Gas Exchange
      1.5.1.2 Ineffective Airway Clearance
      1.5.1.3 Ineffective Breathing Pattern
        1.5.1.3.1 Inability to Sustain Spontaneous Ventilation
        1.5.1.3.2 Dysfunctional Ventilatory Weaning Response
  1.6 (Alterations in Physical Integrity)
    1.6.1 High risk for Injury
      1.6.1.1 High risk for Suffocating
      1.6.1.2 High risk for Poisoning
      1.6.1.3 High risk for Trauma
      1.6.1.4 High risk for Aspiration
      1.6.1.5 High risk for Disuse Syndrome
    1.6.2 Altered Protection
      1.6.2.1 Impaired Tissue Integrity
        1.6.2.1.1 Altered Oral Mucous Membrane
        1.6.2.1.2.1 Impaired Skin Integrity
        1.6.2.1.2.2 High risk

2. **COMMUNICATING:** A human response pat-

tern involving sending messages (To converse; to impart, confer, or transmit thoughts, feelings, or information, internally or externally, verbally or nonverbally.)
2.1 (Alterations in Communication)
    2.1.1 (Verbal)
        2.1.1.1 Impaired
3. **RELATING:** A human response pattern involving establishing bonds. (To connect, to establish a link between, to stand in some association to another thing, person, or place; to be borne or thrust in between things.)
3.1 (Alterations in Socialization)
    3.1.1 Impaired Social Interaction
    3.1.2 Social Isolation
3.2 (Alterations in Role)
    3.2.1 Altered Role Performance
        3.2.1.1.1 Altered Parenting
        3.2.1.1.2 High risk
      3.2.1.2 (Sexual)
        3.2.1.2.1 Dysfunction
    3.2.2 Altered Family Processes
      3.2.2.1 Caregiver Role Strain
      3.2.2.2 Caregiver Role Strain, high risk for
      3.2.3.1 Parental Role Conflict
3.3 Altered Sexuality Patterns
4. **VALUING:** A human response pattern involving the assigning of relative worth. (To be concerned about, to care; the worth or worthiness; the relative status of a thing, or the estimate in which it is held, according to its real or supposed worth, usefulness, or importance; one's opinion or like for a person or thing; to equate in importance.)
4.1 (Alterations in Spiritual State)
    4.1.1 Spiritual Distress
5. **CHOOSING:** A human response pattern involving the selection of alternatives. (To select between alternatives, the action of selecting or exercising preference in regard to a matter in which one is a free agent; to determine in favor of a course; to decide in accordance with inclinations.)
5.1 (Alterations in Coping)
    5.1.1 (Individual)
      5.1.1.1 Ineffective
        5.1.1.1.1 Impaired Adjustment
        5.1.1.1.2 Defensive Coping
        5.1.1.1.3 Ineffective Denial
    5.1.2 (Family)
      5.1.2.1 (Ineffective)
        5.1.2.1.1 Disabling
        5.1.2.1.2 Compromised
      5.1.2.2 Potential for Growth
5.2 (Alterations in Participation)
    5.2.1 (Individual)

5.2.1 Therapeutic Regimen, ineffective management of
    5.2.1.1 Noncompliance (specify)
5.2.2 (Family)
5.2.3 (Community)
    5.3.1.1 Decisional Conflict (specify)
5.4 Health Seeking Behaviors (specify)
6. **MOVING:** A human response pattern involving activity. (To change the place or position of a body or any member of the body, to put and/or keep in motion; to provoke an excretion or discharge; the urge to action or to do something, leave in; to take action.)
6.1 (Alterations in Activity)
    6.1.1 (Physical Mobility)
      6.1.1.1 (Impaired)
        6.1.1.1.1 Peripheral Neurovascular Dysfunction, high risk for
      6.1.1.2 Activity Intolerance
        6.1.1.2.1 Fatigue
      6.1.1.3 High Risk for Activity Intolerance
6.2 (Alterations in Rest)
    6.2.1 Sleep Pattern Disturbance
6.3 (Alterations in Recreation)
    6.3.1 (Diversional Activity)
      6.3.1.1 Deficit
6.4 (Alterations in Activities of Daily Living)
    6.4.1 (Home Maintenance Management)
      6.4.1.1 Impaired
    6.4.2 Altered Health Maintenance
6.5 (Alterations in Self-Care)
    6.5.1 Feeding
      6.5.1.1 Impaired Swallowing
      6.5.1.2 Ineffective Breastfeeding
        6.5.1.2.1 Interrupted Breastfeeding
      6.5.1.3 Effective Breastfeeding
      6.5.1.4 Ineffective Infant Feeding Pattern
    6.5.2 Bathing/Hygiene
    6.5.3 Dressing/Grooming
    6.5.4 Toileting
6.6 Altered Growth and Development
6.7 Relocation Stress Syndrome
7. **PERCEIVING:** A human response pattern involving the reception of information. (To apprehend with the mind; to become aware of by the senses; to apprehend what is not open or present to observation; to take in fully or adequately.)
7.1 (Alterations in Self-Concept)
    7.1.1 Body Image Disturbance
    7.1.2 Self-Esteem Disturbance
      7.1.2.1 Chronic Low Self-Esteem
      7.1.2.2 Situational Low Self-Esteem
    7.1.3 Personal Identity Disturbance
7.2 Sensory/Perceptual Alteration
    [7.2.1] Visual

7.2.1.1 Unilateral Neglect
[7.2.2] Auditory
[7.2.3] Kinesthetic
[7.2.4] Gustatory
[7.2.5] Tactile
[7.2.6] Olfactory
7.3 (Alterations In Meaningfulness)
  7.3.1 Hopelessness
  7.3.2 Powerlessness
8. **KNOWING:** A human response pattern involving the meaning associated with information. (To recognize or acknowledge a thing or a person; to be familiar with by experience or through information or report; to be cognizant of something through observation, inquiry, or information; to be conversant with a body of facts, principles, or methods of action; to understand.)
8.1 (Alterations in Knowledge)
  8.1.1 Deficit (specify)
8.2 (Alterations in Learning)
8.3 Altered Thought Processes
9. **FEELING:** A human response pattern involving the subjective awareness of information. (To ex-

perience a consciousness, sensation, apprehension, or sense; to be consciously or emotionally affected by a fact, event, or state.)
9.1 (Alterations in Comfort)
  9.1.1 Pain
    9.1.1.1 Chronic
    [9.1.1.2 Acute]
  9.1.2 (Discomfort)
9.2 (Alterations in Emotional Integrity)
  9.2.1 (Grieving)
    9.2.1.1 Dysfunctional
    9.2.1.2 Anticipatory
  9.2.2 High Risk for Violence: Self-Directed/Directed at Others
    9.2.2.1 Self-Mutilation, high risk for
  9.2.3 Post Trauma Response
    9.2.3.1 Rape Trauma Syndrome
      9.2.3.1.1 Compound Reaction
      9.2.3.1.2 Silent Reaction
  9.3.1 Anxiety
  9.3.2 Fear
[Brackets indicate author additions provided for further clarity.]

# Appendix 3: Gordon's Functional Health Patterns

## (CLASSIFICATION OF NANDA NURSING DIAGNOSES BY GORDON'S FUNCTIONAL HEALTH PATTERNS—M. Gordon, 6th ed, 1993)

1. **HEALTH PERCEPTION–HEALTH MANAGEMENT PATTERN**
   Altered health maintenance
   Ineffective management of therapeutic regimen (Individuals)
   Noncompliance (specify)
   Health-seeking behaviors (specify)
   High risk for infection
   High risk for injury (trauma)
   High risk for poisoning
   High risk for suffocation

2. **NUTRITIONAL-METABOLIC PATTERN**
   Altered nutrition: high risk for more than body requirements
   Altered nutrition: more than body requirements
   Altered nutrition: less than body requirements
   Ineffective breastfeeding
   Effective breastfeeding
   Interrupted breastfeeding
   Ineffective infant feeding pattern
   High risk for aspiration
   Impaired swallowing
   Altered oral mucous membrane
   High risk for fluid volume deficit
   Fluid volume deficit
   Fluid volume excess
   High risk for impaired skin integrity
   Impaired skin integrity
   Impaired tissue integrity (specify type)
   High risk for altered body temperature
   Ineffective thermoregulation
   Hyperthermia
   Hypothermia

3. **ELIMINATION PATTERN**
   Constipation
   Colonic constipation
   Perceived constipation
   Diarrhea
   Bowel incontinence
   Altered urinary elimination patterns
   Functional incontinence
   Reflex incontinence
   Stress incontinence
   Urge incontinence
   Total incontinence
   Urinary retention

4. **ACTIVITY-EXERCISE PATTERN**
   High risk for activity intolerance
   Activity intolerance (specify level)
   Fatigue
   Impaired physical mobility
   High risk for disuse syndrome
   Bathing/hygiene self-care deficit
   Dressing/grooming self-care deficit
   Feeding self-care deficit
   Toileting self-care deficit
   Diversional activity deficit
   Impaired home maintenance management
   Dysfunctional Ventilatory Weaning Response (DVWR)
   Inability to sustain spontaneous ventilation
   Ineffective airway clearance
   Ineffective breathing pattern
   Impaired gas exchange
   Decreased cardiac output
   Altered tissue perfusion (specify)
   Dysreflexia

High risk for peripheral neurovascular dysfunction
Altered growth and development

## 5. SLEEP-REST PATTERN
Sleep pattern disturbance

## 6. COGNITIVE-PERCEPTUAL PATTERN
Pain
Chronic pain
Sensory perceptual alteration (specify)
Unilateral neglect
Knowledge deficit (specify)
Altered thought process
Decisional conflict (specify)

## 7. SELF-PERCEPTION–SELF-CONCEPT PATTERN
Fear
Anxiety
Hopelessness
Powerlessness
Self-esteem disturbance
Chronic low self-esteem
Situational low self-esteem
Body image disturbance
High risk for self-mutilation
Personal identify disturbance

## 8. ROLE-RELATIONSHIP PATTERN
Anticipatory grieving
Dysfunctional grieving
Altered role performance
Social isolation
Impaired social interaction
Relocation stress syndrome
Altered family processes
High risk for altered parenting
Altered parenting
Parental role conflict
Caregiver role strain
High risk for caregiver role strain
Impaired verbal communication
High risk for violence: self-directed or directed at others

## 9. SEXUALITY-REPRODUCTIVE PATTERN
Sexual dysfunction
Altered sexuality patterns
Rape-trauma syndrome
Rape-trauma syndrome: compound reaction
Rape-trauma syndrome: silent reaction

## 10. COPING-STRESS TOLERANCE PATTERN
Ineffective individual coping
Defensive coping
Ineffective denial
Impaired adjustment
Post-trauma response
Family coping: potential for growth
Ineffective family coping: compromised
Ineffective family coping: disabling

## 11. VALUE-BELIEF PATTERN
Spiritual distress (distress of the human spirit)

# INDEX OF NURSING DIAGNOSES